Ten Cate's

Oral Histology

Development, Structure, and Function

Ten Cate's
Oral Histology
Development, Structure, and Function

Antonio Nanci, PhD

Professor and Director
Laboratory for the Study of Calcified Tissues
and Biomaterials
Director, Department of Stomatology
Faculty of Dentistry
University of Montreal
Montreal, Quebec
Canada

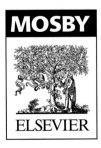

MOSBY

ELSEVIER

11830 Westline Industrial Drive
St. Louis, Missouri 63146

TEN CATE'S ORAL HISTOLOGY: DEVELOPMENT,
STRUCTURE, AND FUNCTION

ISBN: 978-0-323-04557-5

Library of Congress Control Number 2007930316

ISBN: 978-0-323-04557-5

Publishing Director: Linda Duncan
Senior Editor: John J. Dolan
Managing Editor: Jaime Pendill
Publishing Services Manager: Patricia Tannian
Senior Project Manager: Anne Altepeter
Cover Design Direction: Paula Catalano
Interior Design Direction: Paula Catalano

Printed in China

Last digit is the print number: 9 8 7 6 5 4 3 2

Contributors

ANDERS BENNICK, DDS, PhD, MScD
Professor Emeritus
Department of Biochemistry
University of Toronto
Toronto, Ontario, Canada
Chapter 11: Topics for Consideration: Xerostomia

ERMANNO BONUCCI, MD, PhD
Department of Experimental Medicine and Pathology
University La Sapienza
Rome, Italy
Chapter 1: Topics for Consideration: Matrix Vesicles
Chapter 6: Topics for Consideration: Organic-Inorganic Relationships During the Early Phases of the Calcification Process

SAMANTHA A. BRUGMANN, PhD
Postdoctoral Fellow
Children's Surgical Research Laboratory
School of Medicine
Stanford University
Stanford, California
Chapter 3: Topics for Consideration: What's in a Face?

JENNIFER F. CRANE, MS
Stowers Institute for Medical Research
Kansas City, Missouri
Chapter 2: Topics for Consideration: Neural Crest Cells and Their Potential for Tissue-Specific Repair

RENA N. D'SOUZA, DDS, MS, PhD
Department of Biomedical Sciences
Baylor College of Dentistry
Texas A&M Health Science Center
Dallas, Texas
Chapter 5: Topics for Consideration: Tooth Agenesis
Chapter 10: Topics for Consideration: Physiologic Tooth Movement: Eruption and Shedding

WILLIAM V. GIANNOBILE, DDS, DMSc
Najjar Professor of Dentistry
Director, Michigan Center for Oral Health Research
University of Michigan Clinical Research Center
Ann Arbor, Michigan
Chapter 14: Topics for Consideration: Future Prospects for Gene Therapy in Periodontology

ARTHUR R. HAND, DDS
Professor
Department of Pediatric Dentistry
School of Dental Medicine
University of Connecticut
Farmington, Connecticut
Chapter 4: Cytoskeleton, Junctions, Fibroblasts, and Extracellular Matrix
Chapter 11: Salivary Glands
Chapter 4: Topics for Consideration: Intercellular Communication
Chapter 9: Topics for Consideration: Fibroblast Contractility
Chapter 11: Topics for Consideration: Xerostomia

JILL A. HELMS, DDS, PhD
Associate Professor
Department of Surgery
School of Medicine
Stanford University
Stanford, California
Chapter 3: Topics for Consideration: What's in a Face?

JAN C-C HU, DDS, PhD
Department of Orthodontics and Pediatric Dentistry
University of Michigan Dental Research Laboratory
Ann Arbor, Michigan
Chapter 7: Topics for Consideration: Genetic Basis of Inherited Tooth Defects

ADEL KAUZMAN, DMD, MSC, FRCD(C)
Specialist in Oral Pathology and Oral Medicine
Associate Professor
Department of Stomatology
Faculty of Dentistry
University of Montreal
Montreal, Quebec
Canada
Chapter 12: Topics for Consideration: Oral Epithelium, Premalignant and Malignant Lesions

JOSÉ LUIS MILLÁN, PhD
Professor
Burnham Institute for Medical Research
La Jolla, California
Chapter 6: Topics for Consideration: Alkaline Phosphatase: Its Role in Skeletal Mineralization

PAUL T. SHARPE, PhD

Professor
Department of Craniofacial Development
Dental Institute
Kings College London
London, England
Chapter 5: Topics for Consideration: Biologic Tooth Replacement
Chapter 5: Topics for Consideration: Human and Mouse Tooth Genetics

JAMES P. SIMMER, DDS, PhD

Department of Biologic and Materials Sciences
University of Michigan Dental Research Laboratory
Ann Arbor, Michigan
Chapter 7: Topics for Consideration: Genetic Basis of Inherited Tooth Defects
Chapter 8: Topics for Consideration: Dentin and Dentin Sialophosphoprotein

ANTHONY (TONY) J. SMITH, PhD

Unit of Oral Biology
School of Dentistry
University of Birmingham
Birmingham, England
Chapter 8: Topics for Consideration: Dentin-Pulp: A Biologic Basis to Restorative Dentistry

CHARLES E. SMITH, DDS, PhD

Senior Scientist
Faculty of Dentistry
University of Montreal
Montreal, Quebec
Canada
Chapter 7: Topics for Consideration: The Organic Matrix of Enamel: Why Is There So Much Complexity and Protein Diversity in an Environment That Is Essentially Destructive?

NAOTO SUDA, DDS, PhD

Lecturer, Maxillofacial Orthognathics
Graduate School
Tokyo Medical and Dental University
Tokyo, Japan
Chapter 13: Topics for Consideration: Characteristic Origin and Differentiation of Condylar Cartilage

IRMA THESLEFF, DDS, PhD

Professor, Research Director
Institute of Biotechnology
University of Helsinki
Helsinki, Finland
Chapter 5: Topics for Consideration: Dental Placodes: Roles in Tooth Formation and in Ectodermal Dysplasia Syndromes

PAUL A. TRAINOR, PhD

Stowers Institute for Medical Research
Kansas City, Missouri
Chapter 2: Topics for Consideration: Neural Crest Cells and Their Potential for Tissue-Specific Repair

YASUO YAMAKOSHI, PhD

University of Michigan Dental Research Laboratory
Ann Arbor, Michigan
Chapter 8: Topics for Consideration: Dentin and Dentin Sialophosphoprotein

To my parents, Giuseppe and Angelina, whose personal sacrifices have allowed me to pursue my dreams

Preface

As for any new edition, one major objective is to update information either by integrating new information or by covering more comprehensively and clarifying well-established literature. Since the last edition of *Ten Cate's Oral Histology: Development, Structure, and Function,* new information on the biology of oral tissues has dealt largely with molecular events. Although the scope of this textbook is histology, molecular information has been extended because it is essential for understanding embryogenesis and development, cell function, and tissue formation. Particular attention has been given to clarifying and simplifying the text where possible, and adding tables and schematic illustrations. That the textbook now includes many micrographs and illustrations also facilitates visualization of structures. The bibliography has been replaced by a list of "Recommended Readings" that complement the content of each chapter. Finally, again we are fortunate to have contributions in the form of "Topics for Consideration" from key protagonists in various areas of oral biology.

As in the previous edition, a CD-ROM is included with the textbook; its content has been expanded by the addition of multiple-choice questions and interactive labeling exercises.

The textbook is intended to serve as a learning guide for students in a variety of disciplines. The first chapter provides an overview of the subject matter covered in the textbook and sets the stage for a subsequent detailed treatise by topics. Although coverage is exhaustive, the text has been structured such that individual chapters and even selected sections can be used independently. Also, focus is on learning and understanding concepts rather than on memorization of detail. Thus dental hygienists, medical students, and undergraduate and graduate dental students can all find a degree of coverage suited for their respective needs.

Finally, as for the previous edition, a major objective is to sensitize students to the concept that, in addition to helping understand certain clinical conditions, better understanding of the development and biology of oral tissues is expected to engender novel therapeutic approaches based on biologics. Such information is necessary for obtaining predictive clinical outcomes and applying tissue engineering approaches and gene therapy to heal and rebuild oral tissues, a prospect likely to be realized in the foreseeable future.

ACKNOWLEDGMENTS

The present edition integrates material from the six previous editions. I am most grateful to all previous contributors for their input over the years. Particular recognition goes to Dr. A. Richard Ten Cate for having created almost 30 years ago a didactic style that is still fully relevant today and that has helped to train several classes of oral health practitioners. His many years of teaching and profound belief in research are an inspiration and are reflected in this seventh edition.

It must be noted that many of the chapters in the current edition have evolved from the participation of previous authors. In particular, I recognize the inputs of P. Mark Bartold, Paolo Bianco, Michael W. Finkelstein, Stéphane Roy, Paul T. Sharp, Martha J. Somerman, Christopher A. Squier, S. William Whitson, and A. Richard Ten Cate himself in the previous edition. A particular appreciation goes to my friend and colleague Arthur R. Hand for maintaining co-authorship of Chapter 4 and for his excellent coverage of salivary glands (see Chapter 11) in this edition. I also thank all contributors to "Topics for Consideration."

For the illustrations not provided by previous contributors, I have attempted to make accurate attribution based on the information available to me. Although there may be solace in knowing that your work will be seen by successive generations of students, I would like to eventually recognize the input of each individual who has contributed images to the textbook. If you recognize some of your figures, please let me know and I will make the necessary adjustments in the next edition.

Finally, I thank Jaime Pendill, Anne Altepeter, and John Dolan at Elsevier for their editorial help and patience; the personnel in my laboratory—Annie Bélanger, Micheline Fortin, and, in particular, Sylvia Francis Zalzal—whose expert and dedicated assistance over the years has been instrumental in obtaining both light and electron illustrations; Rima M. Wazen for her invaluable help with imaging and preparing multiple-choice questions; and the various individuals at Precision Graphics for their creative input with several of the color illustrations.

Antonio Nanci

Contents

Features of the Companion CD-ROM

The companion CD-ROM is an exciting teaching tool for classroom and individual student use. System requirements are included on the card that is packaged with the CD in the envelope bound into the textbook. Valuable electronic resources include:

IMAGE COLLECTIONS

The complete electronic image collection from the textbook is included for instructors and students. A bonus color image collection is also included as a separate menu item.

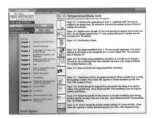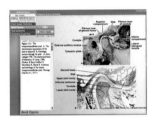

Click on a thumbnail image to enlarge any figure.

TEST QUESTIONS

Students can self-test their knowledge with more than 400 multiple-choice questions divided by topic.

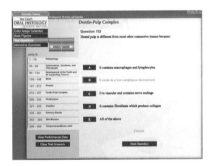

The program gives immediate feedback for correct or incorrect answer choices, and keeps track of performance data.

INTERACTIVE EXERCISES

More than 100 labeling exercises help students to assess their comprehension of content and prepare for examinations.

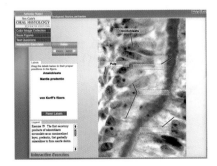

Labels must be placed correctly to complete the exercises.

Structure of the Oral Tissues

This chapter presents a brief description of the histology of the tooth and its supporting tissues (Figure 1-1). The salivary glands, the bones of the jaw, and the articulations between the jaws (temporomandibular joints) also are discussed. The intention is to provide an overview of the subject matter in this book, setting the stage for more detailed consideration.

THE TOOTH

Teeth constitute approximately 20% of the surface area of the mouth, the upper teeth significantly more than the lower teeth. Teeth serve several functions. Mastication is the function most commonly associated with the human dentition, but teeth also are essential for proper speech and, in modern times, for esthetics. In the animal kingdom, teeth have important roles as weapons of attack and defense. Teeth must be hard and firmly attached to the bones of the jaws to fulfill most of these functions. In most submammalian vertebrates the teeth are fused directly to the jawbone. Although this construction provides a firm attachment, it is a brittle arrangement, and such teeth frequently are broken and lost during normal function. In these cases, many successional teeth form to compensate for tooth loss and ensure continued function of the dentition.

The tooth proper consists of a hard, inert, acellular *enamel* formed by epithelial cells supported by the less mineralized, more resilient, and vital hard connective tissue *dentin*, which is formed from and supported by the dental *pulp*, a soft connective tissue (Figure 1-2; see also Figure 1-1). In mammals, teeth are attached to the bones of the jaw by tooth-supporting connective tissues consisting of the *cementum, periodontal ligament* (PDL), and *alveolar bone*, which provide an attachment with enough flexibility to withstand the forces of mastication. In human beings and most mammals, a limited succession of teeth still occurs, not to compensate for continual loss of teeth but to accommodate the growth of the face and jaws. The face and jaws of a human child are small and consequently can carry only a few teeth of small size. These small teeth constitute the *deciduous* or *primary* dentition. A large increase in the size of the jaws occurs with growth, necessitating not only more teeth but also larger ones. Because the size of teeth cannot increase after they are formed, the deciduous dentition becomes inadequate and must be replaced by a *permanent* or *secondary* dentition consisting of more and larger teeth.

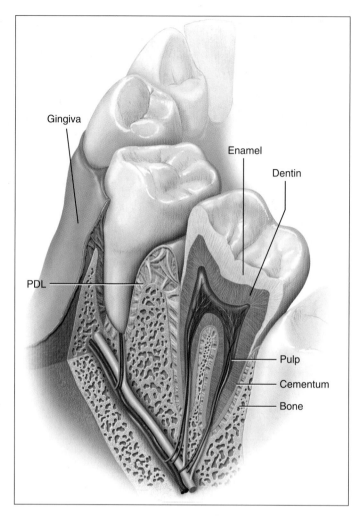

Figure 1-1 The tooth and its supporting structure. *PDL,* Periodontal ligament.

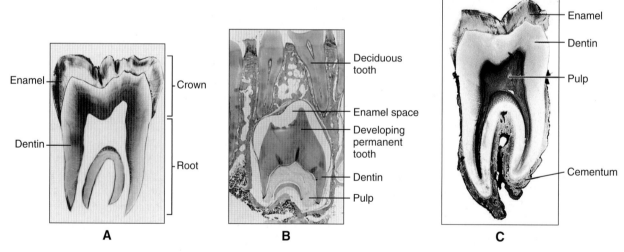

Figure 1-2 Various ways of preparing the tooth for histologic observation with the light microscope. **A,** Ground section whereby a diamond disk is used initially to prepare a tooth slice, which is progressively thinned using an abrasive paste. Only hard tissue is retained. **B,** Demineralized section whereby mineral is first removed to permit sectioning. In such sections the highly mineralized enamel is entirely lost. The section shows deciduous teeth and underneath, a developing permanent tooth. **C,** Specially prepared thick (100 μm) section in which both the hard and soft tissues have been retained.

Anatomically the tooth consists of a *crown* and a *root* (see Figure 1-2, *A*); the junction between the two is the *cervical margin*. The term *clinical crown* denotes that part of the tooth visible in the oral cavity. Although teeth vary considerably in shape and size (e.g., an incisor compared with a molar), histologically they are similar.

ENAMEL

Enamel has evolved as an epithelially derived protective covering for the anatomic crown of the teeth (see Figures 1-1 and 1-2). The enamel is the most highly mineralized tissue in the body, consisting of more than 96% inorganic material in the form of *apatite* crystals and traces of organic material. The cells responsible for the formation of enamel, the *ameloblasts*, cover the entire surface of the layer as it forms but are lost as the tooth emerges into the oral cavity. The loss of these cells renders enamel a nonvital and insensitive tissue that, when destroyed by any means (usually wear or caries), cannot be replaced or regenerated. To compensate for this inherent limitation, enamel has acquired a high degree of mineralization and a complex organization. These structural and compositional features allow enamel to withstand large masticatory forces and continual assaults by acids from food and bacterial sources. The apatite crystals within enamel pack together differentially to create a structure of enamel *rods* separated by an *interrod substance* (Figure 1-3). Although enamel is a dead tissue in a strict biologic sense, it is permeable; ionic exchange can occur between the enamel and the environment of the oral cavity, in particular the saliva.

DENTIN

Because of its exceptionally high mineral content, enamel is a brittle tissue, so brittle that it cannot withstand the forces of mastication without fracture unless it has the support of a more resilient tissue, such as dentin. Dentin forms the bulk of the tooth, supports the enamel, and compensates for its brittleness.

Dentin is a mineralized, elastic, yellow-white, avascular tissue enclosing the central pulp chamber (Figure 1-4; see also Figures 1-1 and 1-2). The mineral is also apatite, and the organic component is mainly the fibrillar protein collagen. A characteristic feature of dentin is its permeation by closely packed tubules traversing its entire thickness and containing the cytoplasmic extensions of the cells that once formed it and later maintain it (see Figure 1-4, *B*). These cells are called *odontoblasts*; their cell bodies are aligned along the inner edge of the dentin, where they form the peripheral boundary of the dental pulp. The very existence of odontoblasts makes dentin a vastly different tissue from enamel. Dentin is a sensitive tissue, and more importantly, it is capable of repair, because odontoblasts or cells in the pulp can be stimulated to deposit more dentin as the occasion demands.

PULP

The central pulp chamber, enclosed by dentin, is filled with a soft connective tissue called pulp (see Figure 1-4, *B*). Anatomically, it is the practice to distinguish between dentin and pulp. Dentin is a hard tissue; the pulp is soft (and is lost in dried teeth, leaving a clearly recognizable empty chamber; see Figure 1-2, *A*). Embryologically and

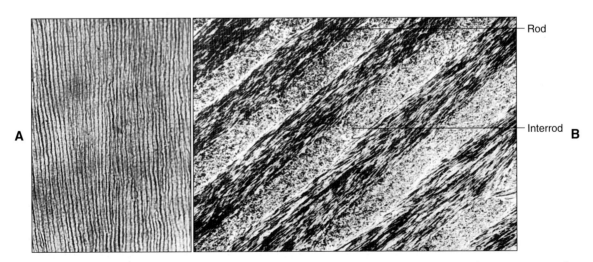

Figure 1-3 Enamel. **A,** Its rod structure as seen in ground sections with the light microscope. **B,** Electron micrography shows that enamel consists of crystallites organized into rod and interrod enamel.

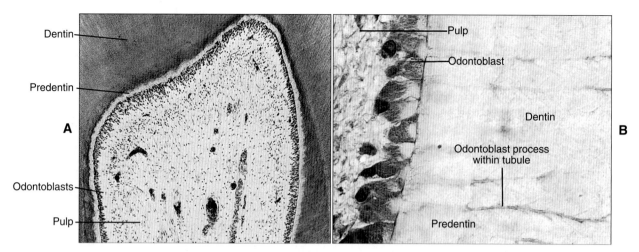

Figure 1-4 Dentin and pulp. **A,** The odontoblasts (cells that form dentin) line the pulp. **B,** These cells at higher magnification show processes extending into dentin.

functionally, however, dentin and pulp are the same and should be considered together. This unity is exemplified by the classic functions of the pulp: it is (1) formative, in that it produces the dentin that surrounds it; (2) nutritive, in that it nourishes the avascular dentin; (3) protective, in that it carries nerves that give dentin its sensitivity; and (4) reparative, in that it is capable of producing new dentin when required.

In summary, the tooth proper consists of two hard tissues: the acellular enamel and the supporting dentin. The latter is a specialized connective tissue the formative cells of which are in the pulp. These tissues bestow on teeth the properties of hardness and resilience. Their indestructibility also gives teeth special importance in paleontology and forensic science, for example, as a means of identification.

SUPPORTING TISSUES OF THE TOOTH

The tooth is attached to the jaw by a specialized supporting apparatus that consists of the *alveolar bone*, the PDL, and the cementum, all of which are protected by the *gingiva* (see Figure 1-1).

PERIODONTAL LIGAMENT

The PDL is a highly specialized connective tissue situated between the tooth and the alveolar bone (Figure 1-5). The principal function of the PDL is to connect the tooth to the jaw, which it must do in such a way that the tooth will withstand the considerable forces of mastication. This requirement is met by the masses of collagen fiber bundles that span the distance between the bone

and the tooth and by ground substance between them. At one extremity the fibers of the PDL are embedded in bone; at the other extremity the collagen fiber bundles are embedded in cementum. Each collagen fiber bundle is much like a spliced rope in which individual strands can be remodeled continually without the overall fiber losing its architecture and function. In this way the collagen fiber bundles can adapt to the stresses placed on them. The PDL has another important function, a sensory one. Tooth enamel is an inert tissue and therefore insensitive, yet the moment teeth come into contact with each other, we know it. Part of this sense of discrimination is provided by sensory receptors within the PDL.

CEMENTUM

Cementum covers the roots of the teeth and is interlocked firmly with the dentin of the root (see Figures 1-1 and 1-2, C). Cementum is a mineralized connective tissue similar to bone except that it is avascular; the mineral is also apatite, and the organic matrix is largely collagen. The cells that form cementum are called *cementoblasts*.

The two main types of cementum are *cellular* and *acellular*. The cementum attached to the root dentin and covering the upper (cervical) portion of the root is acellular and thus is called acellular, or *primary*, cementum. The lower (apical) portion of the root is covered by cellular, or *secondary*, cementum. In this case, cementoblasts become trapped in lacunae within their own matrix, very much as the osteocytes occupy lacunae in bone; these entrapped cells are now called *cementocytes*. Acellular cementum anchors the PDL fiber bundles to the tooth; cellular cementum has an adaptive role. Bone, the PDL, and cementum together form a functional unit

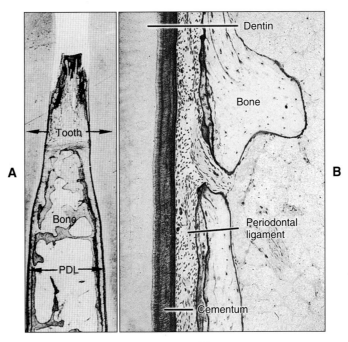

Figure 1-5 Light microscopic histologic sections of the periodontal ligament *(PDL)*. **A,** Supporting apparatus of the tooth in longitudinal section. **B,** At higher magnification, note the fibrocellular nature of the periodontal ligament.

of special importance when orthodontic tooth movement is undertaken.

ORAL MUCOSA

The oral cavity is lined by a mucous membrane that consists of two layers: an epithelium and connective tissue (the *lamina propria;* Figure 1-6). Although its major functions are lining and protecting, the mucosa also is modified to serve as an exceptionally mobile tissue that permits free movement of the lip and cheek muscles. In other locations it serves as the organ of taste.

Histologically, the oral mucosa can be classified in three types: (1) *masticatory,* (2) *lining,* and (3) *specialized.* The masticatory mucosa covers the gingiva and hard palate. The masticatory mucosa is bound down tightly by the lamina propria to the underlying bone (see Figure 1-6, B), and the covering epithelium is keratinized to withstand the constant pounding of the food bolus during mastication. The lining mucosa, by contrast, must be as flexible as possible to perform its function of protection. The epithelium is not keratinized; the lamina propria is structured for mobility and is not tightly bound to underlying structures (see Figure 1-6, C). The dorsal surface of the tongue is covered by a specialized mucosa consisting of a highly extensible masticatory mucosa containing papillae and taste buds.

A unique feature of the oral mucosa is that the teeth perforate it. This anatomic feature has profound implications in the initiation of periodontal disease. The teeth are the only structures that perforate epithelium anywhere in the body. Nails and hair are epithelial appendages around which epithelial continuity is always maintained. This perforation by teeth means that a junction must be established between the gum and the tooth.

The mucosa immediately surrounding an erupted tooth is known as the *gingiva.* In functional terms the gingiva consists of two parts: the part facing the oral cavity, which is masticatory mucosa, and the part facing the tooth, which is involved in attaching the gingiva to the tooth and also forms part of the periodontium. The junction of the oral mucosa and the tooth is permeable, and thus antigens can pass easily through it and initiate inflammation in gum tissue (marginal gingivitis).

SALIVARY GLANDS

Saliva is a complex fluid that in health almost continually bathes the parts of the tooth exposed within the oral cavity. Consequently, saliva represents the immediate environment of the tooth. Saliva is produced by three paired sets of major salivary glands—the *parotid, submandibular,* and *sublingual* glands—and by the many minor salivary glands scattered throughout the oral cavity. A precise account of the composition of saliva is difficult because not only are the secretions of each of the major and minor salivary glands different, but also

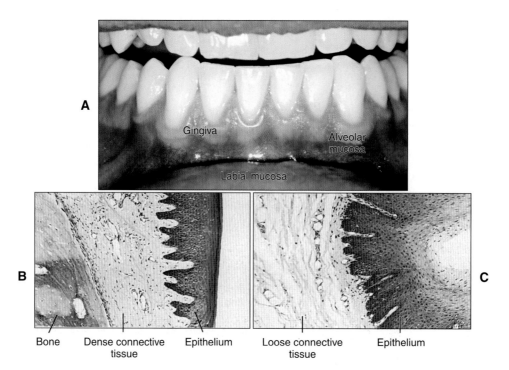

Figure 1-6 Oral mucosa. **A,** Note the difference between tightly bound mucosa of the gingiva (gum) and mobile of the labial sulcus (alveolar mucosa). **B** and **C,** In histologic sections, the gingival epithelium is seen to be tightly bound to bone by a dense fibrous connective tissue, whereas the epithelium of the sulcus is supported by a much looser connective tissue.

their volume may vary at any given time. In recognition of this variability, the term *mixed saliva* is used to describe the fluid of the oral cavity. Regardless of its precise composition, saliva has several functions. Saliva moistens the mouth, facilitates speech, lubricates food, and helps with taste by acting as a solvent for food molecules. Saliva also contains a digestive enzyme (amylase). Saliva not only dilutes noxious material mistakenly taken into the mouth but also cleanses the mouth. Furthermore, it contains antibodies and antimicrobial substances and by virtue of its buffering capacity plays an important role in maintaining the pH of the oral cavity.

The basic histologic structure of the major salivary glands is similar. A salivary gland may be likened to a bunch of grapes. Each "grape" is the *acinus* or *terminal secretory unit*, a mass of secretory cells surrounding a central space. The spaces of the acini open into ducts running through the gland that are called successively the *intercalated, striated,* and *excretory* ducts (Figure 1-7), analogous to the stalks and stems of a bunch of grapes. These ducts are more than passive conduits, however; their lining cells have a function in determining the final composition of saliva.

The ducts and acini constitute the *parenchyma* of the gland, the whole of which is invested by a connective tissue stroma carrying blood vessels and nerves. This connective tissue supports each individual acinus and divides the gland into a series of lobes or lobules, finally encapsulating it (Figure 1-8).

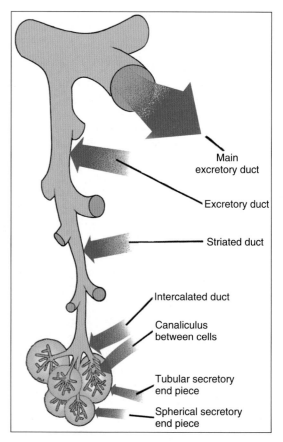

Figure 1-7 Diagrammatic illustration of the ductal system of a salivary gland.

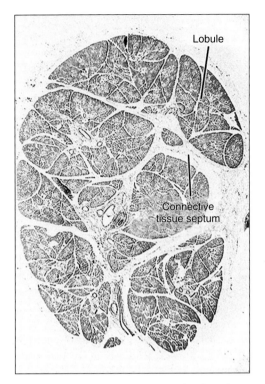

Figure 1-8 Low-power photomicrograph of a salivary gland showing its lobular organization.

fossa of the temporal bone. This articulation, the *temporomandibular joint* (TMJ), is a synovial joint with special features that permit the complex movements associated with mastication. The specialization of the TMJ is reflected in its histologic appearance (Figure 1-9). The TMJ cavity is formed by a fibrous capsule lined with a synovial membrane and is separated into two compartments by an extension of the capsule to form a specialized movable disk. The articular surfaces of the bone are covered not by hyaline cartilage but by a fibrous layer that is a continuation of the periosteum covering the individual bones. A simplified way to understand the function of a TMJ is to consider it as a joint with the articular disk being a movable articular surface.

HARD TISSUE FORMATION

The hard tissues of the body—bone, cementum, dentin, and enamel—are associated with the functioning tooth. Because the practice of dentistry involves manipulation of these tissues, a detailed knowledge of them is obligatory (and each is discussed separately in later chapters). The purposes of this section are (1) to explain that a number of common features are associated with hard tissue formation, even though the final products are

BONES OF THE JAW

As stated before, teeth are attached to bone by the PDL. This bone, the *alveolar bone*, constitutes the *alveolar process*, which is in continuity with the basal bone of the jaws. The alveolar process forms in relation to the teeth. When teeth are lost, the alveolar process is gradually lost as well, creating the characteristic facial profile of the edentulous person whose chin and nose approximate because of a reduction in facial height. Although the histologic structure of the alveolar process is essentially the same as that of the basal bone, practically it is necessary to distinguish between the two. The position of teeth and supporting tissues, which include the alveolar process, can be modified easily by orthodontic therapy. However, modification of the position of the basal bone is usually much more difficult; this can be achieved only by influencing its growth. The way these bones grow is thus important in determining the position of the jaws and teeth.

TEMPOROMANDIBULAR JOINT

The relationship between the bones of the upper and lower jaws is maintained by the articulation of the condylar process of the mandible with the glenoid

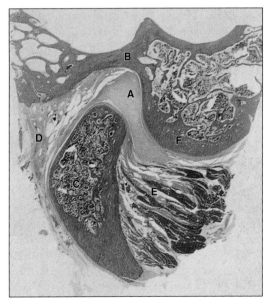

Figure 1-9 Sagittal section through the temporomandibular joint. The disk (dividing the joint cavity into upper and lower compartments) is apparent. *A,* Intra-articular disc; *B,* mandibular (glenoid fossa); *C,* condyle of mandible; *D,* capsule; *E,* lateral pterygoid muscle; *F,* articular eminence. (*From Berkovitz BKB, Holland GR, Moxham BJ: Oral anatomy, histology, and embryology, ed 3, London, 2002, Mosby, courtesy S. Kariyawasam.*)

structurally distinct; (2) to indicate that the functional role of a number of these features is still not understood; and (3) to describe the common mechanism of hard tissue breakdown.

Three of the four hard tissues in the body (i.e., bone, cementum, and dentin) have many similarities in their composition and formation. They are specialized connective tissues, and collagen (principally type I) plays a large role in determining their structure. Although enamel is not a connective tissue and no collagen is involved in its makeup, its formation still follows many of the principles involved in the formation of hard connective tissue. Hard tissue formation may be summarized as the production by cells of an organic matrix capable of accepting mineral. This rather simple concept, however, embraces a number of complex events, many of which are still not fully understood. For example, how is mineralization initiated in the organic matrix? Or, for that matter, how are mineral ions brought to the mineralization site?

THE ORGANIC MATRIX IN HARD TISSUES

A hallmark of calcified tissues is the various matrix proteins that attract and organize calcium and phosphate ions into a structured mineral phase based on carbonated apatite. The formative "blast" cells of calcified tissues produce the organic matrix constituents that interact with the mineral phase. These cells specialize in protein synthesis and secretion, and they exhibit a polarized organization for the vectorial secretion and appositional deposition of matrix proteins.

Of great interest is the fact that the proteins involved, with one exception (enamel), are similar, composing a predominant supporting meshwork of type I collagen with various added noncollagenous proteins functioning primarily as inducers, inhibitors, or both, of mineralization. Table 1-1 provides a comparative analysis of the characteristics of the various calcified tissues. This basic similarity of constituents is consistent with the general role of collagen-based hard tissues in providing rigid structural support and protection of soft tissues in vertebrates. Enamel, however, serves no "scaffolding" role; instead it has evolved to function specifically as an abrasion-resistant, protective coating that relies on its uniquely large mineral crystals for its function. However, enamel is not the only calcified tissue without collagen. Mineralization of cementum situated along the cervical margin of the tooth occurs within a matrix composed largely of noncollagenous matrix proteins also found in bone. In invertebrates, the shell of mollusks consists of laminae of calcium carbonate separated by a thin layer of organic material, acidic macromolecules among others.

MINERAL

The inorganic component of mineralized tissues consists of biologic apatite, which is essentially a calcium phosphate salt approximating in composition to *calcium hydroxyapatite*, represented as $Ca_{10}(PO_4)_6(OH)_2$ and which has undergone a number of substitutions with other ions. This formula indicates only the atomic content of a conceptual entity known as the *unit cell*, which is the least number of calcium, phosphate, and hydroxyl ions able to establish ionic relationships. The unit cell of biologic apatite is hexagonal; when stacked together, these cells form the lattice of a crystal. The number of repetitions of this arrangement produces crystals of various sizes. Generally the crystals are described as needlelike or platelike and, in the case of enamel, as long, thin ribbons. Some believe that the formation of crystals is preceded by an unstable amorphous calcium phase.

A layer of water, called the *hydration shell*, exists around each crystal. Each apatite crystal has three compartments: the crystal interior, the crystal surface, and the hydration shell, all of which are available for the exchange of ions. Thus magnesium and sodium can substitute in the calcium position, fluoride and chloride in the hydroxyl position, and carbonate in the hydroxyl and phosphate positions. Fluoride substitution decreases the solubility of the crystals, whereas carbonate increases it. Magnesium inhibits crystal growth. Furthermore, ions may be adsorbed to the crystal surface by electrostatic attraction or bound in the hydration layer. The apatite crystal can retain its structural configuration while accommodating these substitutions.

In summary, biologic apatite is built on a definite ionic lattice pattern that permits considerable variation in its composition through substitution, exchange, and adsorption of ions. This pattern of ionic variability reflects the immediate environment of the crystal and is used clinically to modify the structure of crystals by exposing them to a fluoride-rich environment.

MINERALIZATION

Over the past few years, there has been a shift in the perception of biologic mineralization, from a physiologic process highly dependent on sustained active promotion to one relying more on rate-limiting activities. Essentially, once calcium phosphate deposition is initiated, the crux is then to control spontaneous precipitation from tissue fluids supersaturated in calcium and phosphate ions and limit it to well-defined sites. Formative cells achieve this by creating microenvironments that facilitate mineral ion handling and by secreting proteins that stabilize calcium and phosphate ions in body fluids and/or control their deposition onto a

TABLE 1-1   Comparative Relationship Between Vertebrate Hard Tissues

	ENAMEL	DENTIN	FIBRILLAR CEMENTUM	BONE
Matrix Support proteins	Amelogenin (several isoforms) Globular with supramolecular aggregates	Collagen (type I) (+ type III, traces of V, VI) Random fibrils	Collagen (type I) (+ type III, XII, traces of V, VI, XIV) Fibrils • Bundles (AEFC) • Sheets (CIFC)	Collagen (type I) (+ type III, traces of V, XII, XIV) Fibrils as random • Random (woven) • Sheets (lamellar)

Other matrix proteins
Types
	Nonamelogenins
	1. Ameloblastin
		Noncollagenous
		1. Dentin sialophosphoprotein as transcript
		  • Dentin glycoprotein
		  • Dentin phosphoprotein
		  • Dentin sialoprotein
			Noncollagenous
			1. Bone sialoprotein
				Noncollagenous
				1. Bone sialoprotein

	2. Enamelin 3. Sulfated protein	2. Dentin matrix protein 1 3. Bone sialoprotein 4. Osteopontin 5. Osteocalcin 6. Osteonectin 7. Matrix extracellular phosphoglycoprotein	2. Osteopontin 3. Osteocalcin 4. Osteonectin 5. Dentin matrix protein 1 6. Dentin sialoprotein	2. Osteopontin 3. Osteocalcin 4. Osteonectin 5. Bone acidic glycoprotein-75 6. Dentin matrix protein 1 7. Dentin sialophosphoprotein as transcript 8. Matrix extracellular phosphoglycoprotein
Status	Degraded along with amelogenins	Remain in matrix; also present in peritubular dentin	Remain in matrix, but some may be degraded; also present in resting lines	Remain in matrix, but some may be degraded; also present in resting and reversal lines
Proteoglycans Matrix proteinases	Controversial 1. MMP-20 (enamelysin) 2. KLK-4	SLRP Collagen-processing enzymes and others needed to degrade matrix	SLRP Collagen-processing enzymes and others needed to degrade matrix	SLRP Collagen-processing enzymes and others needed to degrade matrix
Mineral	Hydroxyapatite >90% ribbons (R) expand (mature rod crystallites can be millimeters in length)	Hydroxyapatite 67% Uniform small plates	Hydroxyapatite 45% to 50% Uniform small plates	Hydroxyapatite 50% to 60% Uniform small plates
Location Nucleated from	Between amelogenin nanospheres Controversial—Amelogenins? Nonamelogenins? Dentin?	Inside or at periphery of type I collagen fibril Matrix vesicles then moving mineralization front, although additional mechanisms are most likely involved	Inside or at periphery of type I collagen fibril Matrix vesicles then moving mineralization front, although additional mechanisms are most likely involved	Inside or at periphery of type I collagen fibril Matrix vesicles then moving mineralization front, although additional mechanisms are most likely involved
Prematrix	None present; crystallites abut plasma membrane of ameloblasts	Always present; usually thick	Always present; usually very thin	Present only during formative phase; usually thin
Growth type	Appositional	Appositional	Appositional	Appositional
Cells Formative	Ameloblasts very tall and thin; multiple morphologies	Odontoblasts tall with long cytoplasmic processes	Cementoblasts short	Osteoblasts short

Continued

TABLE 1-1 Comparative Relationship Between Vertebrate Hard Tissues—cont'd

	ENAMEL	DENTIN	FIBRILLAR CEMENTUM	BONE
Microenvironment	Putatively sealed by secretory and ruffle-ended ameloblasts; leaky relative to smooth ended-ameloblasts	Controversial; moderately leaky junctions	Cells widely spaced	No junctions at the level of the cell body
Life span	Limited to time until crown erupts	For life of tooth with gradual loss as pulp chamber occludes	Unclear; probably for life of tooth	Limited; associated with appositional growth phase
Maintenance	None	Odontoblast process	Cementocytes	Osteocytes
Life span	NA	For life of tooth with gradual loss as pulp chamber occludes	Limited by overall thickness of the layer	Long until area of bone undergoes turnover
Degradative	None per se; cells secrete proteinases	Odontoclasts	Odontoclasts/cementoclasts	Osteoclasts (limited life span)

Updated from Nanci A, Smith CE. In Goldberg M, Boskey A, Robinson C, editors: *Chemistry and biology of mineralized tissues*, Rosemont, Ill, 1999, American Academy of Orthopaedic Surgeons.

Dentin, fibrillar cementum, and bone are collagen-based tissues. Enamel is outside rather than inside the body. Enamel, dentin, and cementum are not vascularized, and they do not turnover. Enamel, dentin, and primary cementum are acellular, but dentin contains the large, arborizing processes of odontoblasts embedded in the matrix. *AEFC*, Acellular extrinsic fiber cementum; *CIFC*, cellular intrinsic fiber cementum; *SLRP*, small leucine-rich proteoglycans (biglycan, decorin); *MMP*, metalloproteinase; *KLK-4*, kallikrein-4; *NA*, not available.

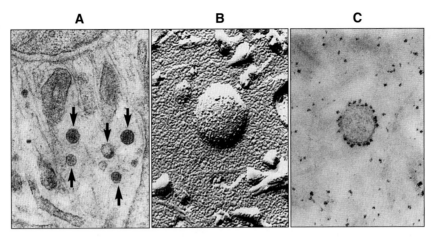

Figure 1-10 A, Matrix vesicles *(arrows)* as seen with the electron microscope. **B,** Freeze fracture of the vesicle, showing many intramembranous particles thought to represent enzymes. **C,** Histochemical demonstration of calcium-adenosinetriphosphatase activity on the surface of the vesicle. *(From Sasaki T, Garant PR: Anat Rec 245:235, 1996.)*

receptive extracellular matrix. Genome sequencing and gene mapping have shown that several of these proteins are located on the same chromosome and that there is synteny across several species. It has been proposed that all of these proteins derive from the duplication and diversification of an ancestral gene during evolution. Collectively, these proteins are referred to as the *"secretory calcium-binding phosphoprotein gene cluster"* that comprises (1) salivary proteins, (2) enamel matrix proteins, and (3) bone/cementum/dentin matrix proteins.

Spontaneous precipitation of a calcium phosphate product does not occur for the following reasons. First, tissue fluid contains macromolecules, which inhibit crystal formation, and second, the initial cluster of ions needed to form a lattice structure is unstable; although a few may form, not enough clusters remain for the critical number of crystals to develop. Furthermore, the formation of a cluster of ions requires the expenditure of energy, and an energy barrier must be overcome for crystallization to happen. Inhibitors of mineralization increase the amount of energy required.

Two mechanisms have been proposed for initiating mineralization of hard connective tissue. The first involves a structure called the *matrix vesicle* (Figure 1-10), and the second is *heterogeneous nucleation.*

In the first mechanism the vesicle exists only in relation to initial mineralization. The matrix vesicle is a small, membrane-bound structure that buds off from the cell to form an independent unit within the first-formed organic matrix of hard tissues. The first morphologic evidence of a crystallite is seen within this vesicle. The matrix vesicle provides a microenvironment in which proposed mechanisms for initial mineralization exist. Thus it contains alkaline phosphatase, calcium-adenosinetriphosphatase, metalloproteinases, proteoglycans, and anionic phospholipids, which can bind calcium and inorganic phosphate and thereby forms calcium–inorganic phosphate phospholipid complexes. These complexes are unique to mineralizing situations, and when they are selectively removed, the matrix vesicle can no longer initiate mineralization. Matrix vesicles have had an interesting history since their discovery. Initially it was questioned whether they were real structures or artifacts of tissue preparation, and questions remain regarding whether matrix vesicles are implicated only in initiation of mineralization or could still play a role in the ensuing appositional mineralization.

TOPICS FOR CONSIDERATION   Matrix Vesicles

Matrix vesicles (MVs) are organelles of cellular origin that can be observed by electron microscopy in the matrix of cartilage, bone, and other hard tissues. Originally described as "dense bodies" in normal cartilage and as "cytoplasmic fragments" in cartilage induced by the injection of cultured, human amniotic cells into the muscles of cortisone-conditioned mice, they now generally are referred to by the term *matrix*

vesicle in recognition of their often spherical shape and, above all, their location in the matrix, where they may be in contact with collagen fibrils.

Ultrastructurally, MVs consist of an amorphous, osmiophilic substance surrounded by a typical bilaminar plasma membrane. They are usually roundish, with a diameter between 100 and 200 nm, but elongated and irregular shapes sometimes

Continued

are found. Their ultrastructure prompted the hypothesis that they might be no more than cross sections of the many cellular processes that penetrate the matrix from chondrocytes and osteoblasts, but serial sectioning demonstrated that they are independent, individual structures with no direct connection with cells. Probably because of the difficulties connected with the ultrastructural study of hard tissues, doubts were once expressed about the existence of MVs. By now, they have been demonstrated in fixed or unfixed, freeze-dried and cryosectioned material by transmission and scanning electron microscopy; and, above all, they have been isolated by enzymatic and nonenzymatic methods. Moreover, they have been found not only in the longitudinal septa of hypertrophic cartilage but also in bone (chiefly woven bone and medullary bone of birds), mantle dentin, deer antlers, fish scales, turkey tendons, and in several pathologic calcifying tissues such as the arteriosclerotic wall of the arteries. However, MVs are not detectable in all calcifying tissues. They have never been reported in enamel and circumpulpal dentin, and in bone their numbers decrease as the compactness of its matrix increases so that there are few in osteonic bone.

The biologic interest attached to MVs is due to their being the initial, although not exclusive, loci of calcification, as shown by the presence within them of hydroxyapatite crystals when the intercellular matrix is still uncalcified. This finding has been questioned on the grounds that no intravesicle crystals should be visible in cartilage and bone sections prepared by anhydrous techniques. However, reports of crystals within MVs are so numerous (even when cryosections are used) that their existence is unquestionable. Moreover, MVs contain more calcium ions than the chondrocyte cytoplasm, and electron-probe analysis and K-pyroantimonate histochemistry show that their intravesicle concentration increases as the cartilage calcifying hypertrophic zone is approached. This agrees with the observation that MVs can concentrate $^{45}Ca^{2+}$ and La^{3+}.

Crystals contained in MVs are initially single or collected in small clusters; they gradually fill MVs completely and then spread through the surrounding matrix, giving rise to calcification nodules. The coalescence of nodules leads to complete matrix calcification. The mechanism by which the membrane of MVs is broken and crystals find their way into the matrix is not known.

Doubts persist about the mechanism of MV calcification. Histochemical and biochemical studies have shown that MVs contain most of the substances that are believed to play a role in the calcification process, especially alkaline phosphatase and related enzymes. The inhibition of these enzymes, or the removal of their substrate, forestalls MV calcification. It has been proposed that alkaline phosphatase might induce the hydrolysis of phosphate esters, thus producing phosphate ions, which might react with calcium ions linked to phospholipids. Lipids such as fatty acids, cholesterol, sphingomyelin, glycolipids, lysophospholipids, and phosphatidylserine are present in MVs in proportions similar to those of the plasma membrane. The role of alkaline phosphatase has in some ways been questioned by findings reported on isolated chick cartilage MVs. These may be separated into quickly and slowly calcifying MVs. The calcifying properties of the former appear to depend on the presence of unstable internal mineral (nucleational core complex) that does not require organic phosphate esters, as the latter do, so that the removal of alkaline phosphatase would have only a minor effect. These findings suggest that MVs have some degree of structural and functional heterogeneity.

There can be no doubt that MVs have a cellular origin and that, at least in the rat cartilage, their production continues through the entire life span of chondrocytes. Electron microscope studies suggest that MV biogenesis occurs through two main mechanisms, both primarily observed in calcifying cartilage: budding from cells and cellular processes, and cell disintegration. Swelling of the tip of the long chondrocyte processes, which penetrate the matrix, followed by detachment of the swollen, vesicle-like part, has been described several times. Direct release of MVs from the chondrocyte membrane also has been reported. The long known disintegration of chondrocytes, probably an apoptotic process, has been documented as a source of MVs. This mechanism could be particularly relevant in pathologic calcification and above all in the calcification of atherosclerotic arteries.

The fact that early crystals are found in MVs does not mean that initial calcification cannot occur in relationship with other structures. This is the case of collagen fibrils, the calcification of which can occur together with that of MVs, or independently of them, as often shown in compact bone, circumpulpal dentin, and other normal or pathologic hard tissues. Whether different structures calcify through the same or different processes is still unknown.

Ermanno Bonucci
*Department of Experimental Medicine and
    Pathology
University "La Sapienza"
Rome, Italy*

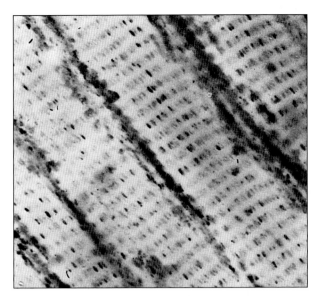

Figure 1-11 Electron micrograph showing the disposition of crystals in collagen fiber bundles. The gaps in the collagen fibrils are where mineral has been deposited. *(From Nylen MV et al: Calcification in biological systems, Pub No. 64, Washington, 1960, American Association for the Advancement of Science.)*

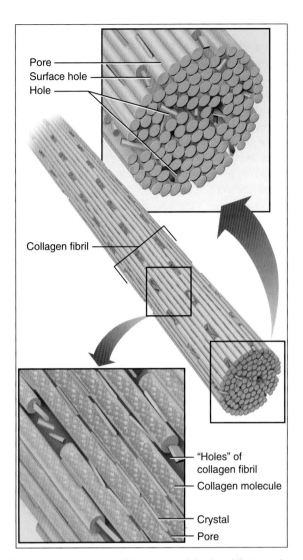

Figure 1-12 Schematic illustration of the localization of mineral within the collagen fibril. *(Redrawn from Glimcher ML. In Veis A, editor: The chemistry and biology of mineralized connective tissues, New York, 1981, Elsevier-North Holland.)*

In the second mechanism, during the formation of collagen-based calcified tissues, deposition of apatite crystals is catalyzed by specific atomic groups associated with the surface, holes, and pores of collagen fibrils (Figures 1-11 and 1-12). Although a direct role by collagen has not been excluded, regulation of this process is believed to be achieved by noncollagenous proteins; but the precise function of these proteins and manner by which they achieve their effect are still not fully understood (see Table 1-1). One item of particular interest is how these molecules interact with type I collagen. In bone, 70% to 80% of mineral is located within the collagen fibril; the rest is located in the spaces between fibrils. Mineral nucleation also can occur at these sites in relation to noncollagenous matrix proteins.

Neither of these mechanisms is involved in the mineralization of enamel; matrix vesicles are absent, and enamel contains no collagen. Initiation of enamel mineralization is believed to be achieved by crystal growth from the already mineralized dentin, by matrix proteins secreted by the ameloblasts, or by both processes.

CRYSTAL GROWTH

Once an apatite crystal has been initiated, its initial growth is rapid. Later, slower growth results in crystals that exceed their initial size by 10 to 20 times. Such growth plays an important part in mineralization, especially in enamel formation.

Several factors influence crystal growth and composition, but especially important is the immediate environment of the growing crystal. For example, noncollagenous proteins can bind selectively to different surfaces of the crystal, preventing further growth and thereby determining the final size of the crystal. Pyrophosphate accumulation on the crystal surface also blocks further growth.

ALKALINE PHOSPHATASE

Alkaline phosphatase activity is always associated with the production of a mineralized tissue. In all cases, alkaline phosphatase exhibits a similar pattern of distribution and is involved with the blood vessels and cell membrane of hard tissue–forming cells. In hard connective tissues, alkaline phosphatase also is found in the organic matrix, associated with matrix vesicles (when present) and occurring free within the matrix.

Although the enzyme alkaline phosphatase has a clear-cut function (i.e., is hydrolyzing phosphate ions from organic radicals at an alkaline pH), its role in mineralization is not yet fully defined. A precise description of this role is complicated by at least two factors. First, the term *alkaline phosphatase* is nonspecific, describing a group of enzymes that have the capacity to cleave phosphate ions from organic substrates at an alkaline pH. Second, the enzyme may have more than one distinct function in mineralization.

When associated with cell membranes, alkaline phosphatase has been thought for many years to play some role in ion handling. It now has been shown, however, that inhibitors of alkaline phosphatase activity do not interfere with calcium transport, and therefore attention has shifted again to the possibility that the enzyme is associated with providing phosphate ions at mineralization sites—the original role proposed for it some 75 years ago.

The extracellular activity of alkaline phosphatase at mineralization sites occurs where continuing crystal growth is taking place. At these sites the enzyme is believed to have the function of cleaving pyrophosphate (inorganic phosphate). Hydroxyapatite crystals in contact with serum or tissue fluids are prevented from growing larger because pyrophosphate ions are deposited on their surfaces, inhibiting further growth. Alkaline phosphatase activity breaks down pyrophosphate, thereby permitting crystal growth to proceed.

TRANSPORT OF MINERAL IONS TO MINERALIZATION SITES

Although the subject has been studied extensively, the mechanism(s) whereby large amounts of phosphate and calcium are delivered to calcification sites is still the subject of debate. Mineral ions can reach a mineralization front by movement through or between cells. Tissue fluid is supersaturated in these ions, and it is possible that fluid simply needs to percolate between cells to reach the organic matrix, where local factors then would permit mineralization. A priori, this mechanism is more likely to occur between cells such as osteoblasts and odontoblasts that have no complete tight junctions and where serum proteins such as albumin can be found in the osteoid and predentin matrix they produce. This also applies to cementoblasts that frequently are separated from each other by PDL fibers entering cementum. A number of facts, however, complicate such a simple explanation. For example,

hormones influence the movement of calcium in and out of bone. Thus it has been proposed that osteoblasts and odontoblasts form a sort of "limiting membrane" that would regulate ion influx into their respectable tissues. The situation would seem more straightforward for enamel where tight junctions between secretory stage ameloblasts restrict the passage of calcium. It has been concluded that during the secretory phase of enamel formation some calcium likely passes between cells but that the majority of calcium entry into enamel would occur through a transcellular route. The situation is different during the maturation stage.

The possibility of transcellular transport is dictated by a particular circumstance: the cytosolic free calcium ion concentration cannot exceed 10^{-6} mol/L because a greater concentration would cause calcium to inhibit critical cellular functions, leading to cell death. Two mechanisms have been proposed that permit transcellular transport of calcium without exceeding this critical threshold concentration. The first suggests that as calcium enters the cell through specific calcium channels, it is sequestered by a calcium-binding protein that in turn is transported through the cell to the site of release. The second suggests that a continuous and constant flow of calcium ions occurs across the cell without the concentration of free calcium ions ever exceeding 10^{-6} mol/L. (Water in a hose pipe is a good analogy; regardless of the rate of flow, the amount of water in the pipe is always constant.) Finally, intracellular compartments (e.g., endoplasmic reticulum, Golgi complex, and mitochondria) also play a role in calcium handling. Calcium has been localized to these structures not only in hard tissue–forming cells but also in most other cells, and it is believed that the sequestration of calcium to these organelles is a safety device to control the calcium concentration of the cytosol.

HARD TISSUE DEGRADATION

Bone is remodeling constantly by an orchestrated interplay between removal of old bone and its replacement by new bone. The remaining hard tissues (cementum, dentin, enamel) do not remodel but are degraded and removed during the normal physiologic processes involved in the shedding of deciduous teeth. Enamel is an eccentric hard tissue in part due to its origin from epithelial cells and to the chemically distinct nature of the various noncollagenous matrix proteins expressed by ameloblasts. Like bone, enamel undergoes major changes as it ages. However, in the case of bone, formative and destructive phases result from the activity of cells derived from two separate lineages. The *osteoblasts*, originating from mesenchyme in the case of long bones, are responsible for bone formation, whereas *osteoclasts*, originating

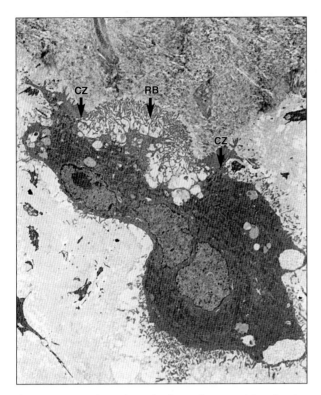

Figure 1-13 Multinucleated odontoclast resorbing dentin. Note the clear attachment zones *(CZ)* surrounding the ruffled border *(RB)*. *(From Sahara N, Okafuji N, Toyoka A et al:* Arch Histol Cytol *55:273, 1992.)*

SUMMARY

Hard tissue formation involves cells situated close to a good blood supply, producing an organic matrix capable of accepting mineral (apatite). These cells thus have the cytologic features of cells that actively synthesize and secrete protein.

Mineralization in the connective hard tissues entails an initial nucleation mechanism involving a cell-derived matrix vesicle and the control of spontaneous mineral precipitation from supersaturated tissue fluids. After initial nucleation, further mineralization is achieved in relation to the collagen fiber and spread of mineral within and between fibers. In enamel, mineralization initiates either in relation to preexisting apatite crystals of dentin or enamel matrix proteins. Alkaline phosphatase is associated with mineralization, but its role is still not fully understood. The breakdown of hard tissue involves the macrophage system, which produces a characteristic multinucleated giant cell, the osteoclast. To break down hard tissue, this cell attaches to mineralized tissue and creates a sealed environment that is first acidified to demineralize the hard tissue. After exposure to the acidic environment, the organic matrix is broken down by proteolytic enzymes. In enamel, the challenge is to maintain a relatively neutral pH environment that will prevent mineral dissolution and allow optimal activity of the enzymes that breakdown the organic matrix components.

RECOMMENDED READING

Bonnucci E: *Biological classification*, Berlin, 2007, Springer-Verlag.

Bonucci E, editor: *Calcification in biological systems*, Boca Raton, Fla, 1992, CRC Press.

Boskey AL: Biomineralization: an overview, *Connect Tissue Res* 44(suppl 1):5, 2003.

Huq NL, Cross KJ, Ung M, Reynolds EC: A review of protein structure and gene organisation for proteins associated with mineralised tissue and calcium phosphate stabilisation encoded on human chromosome 4, *Arch Oral Biol* 50:599, 2005.

Qin C, Baba O, Butler WT: Post-translational modifications of sibling proteins and their roles in osteogenesis and dentinogenesis, *Crit Rev Oral Biol Med* 15:126, 2004.

from the blood (monocyte/macrophage lineage), destroy focal areas of bone as part of normal maintenance. Enamel under ameloblasts undergoes removal of matrix proteins in a process (i.e., extracellular enzymatic processing) similar to that in the resorption lacuna under osteoclasts. The exact extent of the degradation of organic matrix constituents and the exact manner by which their fragments leave the site of resorption are still not fully defined for bone and enamel. Tissues such as cementum and dentin do not normally undergo turnover, but all hard tissues of the tooth can be resorbed under certain normal eruptive conditions (e.g., deciduous teeth) and under certain pathologic conditions, including excessive physical forces and inflammation. The cells involved in their resorption have similar characteristics as osteoclasts but generally are referred to as *odontoclasts* (Figure 1-13).

General Embryology

This chapter provides adequate information on general embryology to explain the development of the head, particularly the structures in and around the mouth. The chapter supplies a background for understanding the origins of the tissues associated with facial and dental development and clarifies the cause of many congenital defects manifest in these tissues.

GERM CELL FORMATION AND FERTILIZATION

The human somatic (body) cell contains 46 chromosomes, 46 being the *diploid* number for the cell. Two of these are *sex chromosomes*; the remainder are *autosomes*. Each chromosome is paired so that every cell has 22 homologous sets of paired autosomes, with one chromosome derived from the mother and one from the father. The sex chromosomes, designated X and Y, are paired XX in the female and XY in the male.

Fertilization is the fusion of male and female germ cells (the spermatozoa and ova, collectively called *gametes*) to form a *zygote*, which commences the formation of a new individual. The fusion of two cells with 46 chromosomes each is not possible; if it were, a cell with 92 chromosomes would result. Thus germ cells are required to have half as many chromosomes (the *haploid* number), so that on fertilization the original complement of 46 chromosomes will be reestablished in the new somatic cell. The process that produces germ cells with half the number of chromosomes of the somatic cell is called *meiosis*. *Mitosis* describes the division of somatic cells.

Before mitotic cell division begins, DNA is first replicated during the S (synthetic) phase of the cell cycle so that the amount of DNA is doubled to a value known as *tetraploid* (which is 4 times the amount of DNA found in the germ cell). During mitosis the chromosomes containing this tetraploid amount of DNA are split and distributed equally between the two resulting cells; thus both cells have a diploid DNA quantity and chromosome number, which duplicates the parent cell exactly.

Meiosis, by contrast, involves two sets of cell divisions occurring in quick succession. Before the first division, DNA is replicated to the tetraploid value (as in mitosis). In the first division the number of chromosomes is halved, and each daughter cell contains a diploid amount of DNA distributed in a haploid number of chromosomes. The second division involves the splitting and separation of the chromosomes; thus the final composition of each cell is haploid with respect to its DNA value and its chromosome number.

Meiosis is discussed in this textbook because the process occasionally malfunctions, producing zygotes with an abnormal number of chromosomes and individuals with congenital defects that sometimes affect the mouth and teeth. For example, an abnormal number of chromosomes can result from the failure of a homologous chromosome pair to separate during meiosis, so that the daughter cells contain 24 or 22 chromosomes. If, on fertilization, a gamete containing 24 chromosomes fuses with a normal gamete (containing 23), the resulting zygote will possess 47 chromosomes; one homologous pair has a third component. Thus the cells are *trisomic* for a given pair of chromosomes. If one member of the homologous chromosome pair is missing, a rare condition known as *monosomy* prevails. The best known example of trisomy is *Down syndrome*, or trisomy 21. Among features of Down syndrome are facial clefts, a shortened palate, a protruding and fissured tongue, and delayed eruption of teeth. Other types of trisomy usually result in early death of the infant a few months after birth and are beyond the scope of this book. Trisomies of other autosomes probably also occur but are likely lethal to the embryo, resulting in miscarriage. Trisomy and monosomy also can occur in relation to the sex chromosomes, but in such cases they rarely manifest themselves as dental defects.

Approximately 10% of all human malformations are caused by an alteration in a single gene. Such alterations are transmitted in several ways, of which two are of special importance. First, if the malformation results from autosomal dominant inheritance, the affected gene generally is inherited from only one parent. The trait usually appears in every generation and can be transmitted by the affected parent to statistically half of the children. Examples of autosomal dominant conditions include achondroplasia, cleidocranial dysostosis, osteogenesis imperfecta, and some forms of amelogenesis imperfecta; the latter two conditions result in abnormal formation of the dental hard tissues (Figure 2-1). Second, when the malformation is due to autosomal recessive inheritance, the abnormal gene can express itself only when it is received from both parents. Examples include chondroectodermal dysplasia, some cases of microcephaly, and cystic fibrosis. Many other congenital malformations with a genetic basis exist but are beyond the scope of this book.

All of these conditions are examples of abnormalities in the genetic makeup or *genotype* of the individual and are classified as *genetic defects*. The expression of the genotype is affected by the environment in which the embryo develops, and the final outcome of development is termed the *phenotype*. Adverse factors in the environment can result in excessive deviation from a functional and accepted norm; the outcome is described as a *congenital defect*. *Teratology* is the study of such developmental defects.

PRENATAL DEVELOPMENT

Prenatal development is divided into three successive phases. The first two, when combined, constitute the *embryonic* stage, and the third is the *fetal* stage. The forming individual is described as an embryo or fetus depending on its developmental stage.

The first phase begins at fertilization and spans the first 4 weeks or so of development. This phase involves largely cellular proliferation and migration, with some differentiation of cell populations. Few congenital defects result from this period of development because, if the perturbation is severe, the embryo is lost.

The second phase spans the next 4 weeks of development and is characterized largely by the differentiation of all major external and internal structures (*morphogenesis*). The second phase is a particularly vulnerable period for the embryo because it involves many intricate embryologic processes; during this period, many recognized congenital defects develop.

From the end of the second phase to term, further development is largely a matter of growth and maturation, and the embryo now is called a fetus (Figure 2-2).

INDUCTION, COMPETENCE, AND DIFFERENTIATION

Patterning is key in development from the initial axial (head-to-tail) specification of the embryo through its segmentation and ultimately to the development of the dentition. *Patterning* is a spatial and temporal event as exemplified by regional development of incisors, canines, premolars, and molars, which occurs at different times and involves the classical processes of *induction*, *competence*, and *differentiation*.

All the cells of an individual stem from the zygote. Clearly, they have differentiated somehow into populations that have assumed particular functions, shapes, and rates of turnover. Such a population of cells is said to be *compartmentalized*; successive generations of cells in a given compartment may remain constant or differentiate; that is, they change their characteristics and establish a new population of cells. The process that initiates differentiation is *induction*; an inducer is the agent that "persuades" cells to be induced. Furthermore, each compartment of cells must be competent to respond to the induction process. Evidence suggests that over time, populations of embryonic cells vary their competence, from no response to maximum response and then back to

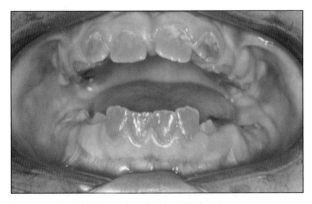

Figure 2-1 Dentition of a child with dentinogenesis imperfecta, an autosomal dominant genetic defect. *(From Ibsen O, Phelan J:* Oral pathology for the dental hygienist, *ed 4, St Louis, 2004, Saunders.)*

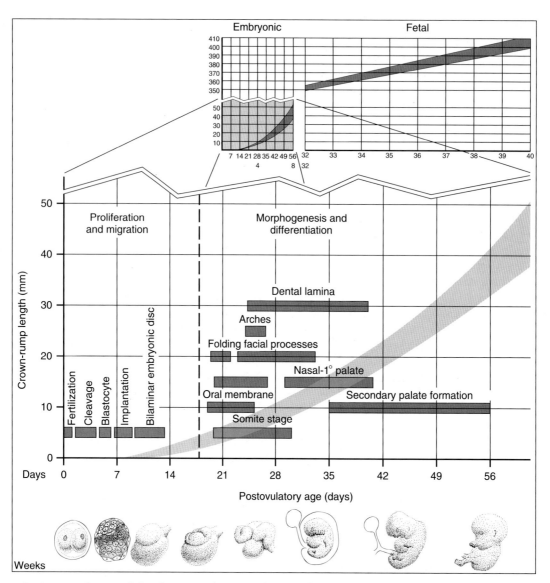

Figure 2-2 Sequences of prenatal development. The upper diagram shows the distinction between embryonic and fetal stages. The *shaded area* is expanded in the lower diagram, which distinguishes the stages of proliferation and migration and morphogenesis and differentiation. The timing of key events also is indicated. *(Redrawn and modified from Waterman RE, Meller SM. In Shaw JH et al, editors:* Textbook of oral biology, *Philadelphia, 1978, WB Saunders.)*

no response. In other words, windows of competence of varying duration exist for different populations of cells. The concepts of induction, competence, and differentiation apply in the development of the tooth and its supporting tissues and are referred to in later chapters.

Molecular biology and immunocytochemistry have helped to explain the processes of patterning, induction, and competence. Using probes composed of specific nucleic acid sequences, recombinant DNA technology can identify not only specific genes but also whether genes are transcriptionally active. By using specific antibodies for specific proteins, immunocytochemistry provides precise identification and localization of molecules within a cell. These two technologies have led to the recognition of *homeobox genes* and *growth factors*, both of which play crucial roles in development.

All homeobox genes contain a similar region of 180 nucleotide base pairs (the homeobox) and function by producing proteins (transcription factors) that bind to the DNA of other downstream genes, thereby regulating their expression. By knocking out such genes or by switching them on, it has been shown that they play a fundamental role in patterning. Furthermore, combinations of differing homeobox gene provide "codes" or sets of assembly rules to regulate development; one such code is involved in dental development (see Chapter 5).

Homeobox genes act in concert with other groups of regulatory molecules, namely, *growth factors* and

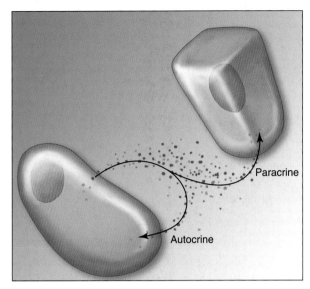

Figure 2-3 Autocrine and paracrine regulation. On the left the cell captures its own cytokine (autocrine); on the right the cytokine is captured by a nearby target cell (paracrine).

retinoic acids. Growth factors are polypeptides that belong to a number of families. For them to have an effect, cells must express *cell-surface receptors* to capture them. Once captured by the receptors, there is transfer of information across the plasma membrane and activation of cytoplasmic signaling pathways to cause alteration in the gene expression. Thus a growth factor is an inductive agent, and the appropriate expression of cell-surface receptors bestows competency on a cell. A growth factor produced by one cell and acting on another is described as *paracrine* regulation, whereas the process of a cell that recaptures its own product is known as *autocrine* regulation (Figure 2-3). The extensive and diverse effects of a relatively few growth factors during embryogenesis can be achieved by cells expressing combinations of cell-surface receptors requiring simultaneous capture of different growth factors to respond in a given way (Figure 2-4). Such combinations represent a further example of a developmental code. By contrast, the retinoic acid family freely enters a cell to form a complex with intracellular receptors, which eventually affect gene expression. Growth factors and retinoids regulate the expression of homeobox genes, which in turn regulate the expression of growth factors, an example of the role of regulatory loops in development.

FORMATION OF THE THREE-LAYERED EMBRYO

After fertilization, mammalian development involves a phase of rapid proliferation and migration of cells, with little or no differentiation. This proliferative phase lasts until three germ layers have formed. In summary, the fertilized egg initially undergoes a series of rapid divisions that lead to the formation of a ball of cells called

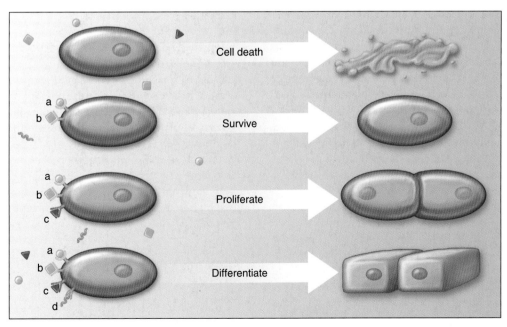

Figure 2-4 The effect of expression of cell-surface receptors to capture different combinations of growth factors on cell behavior. If no receptors are expressed, cell death ensues.

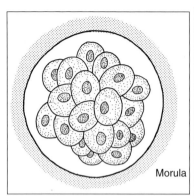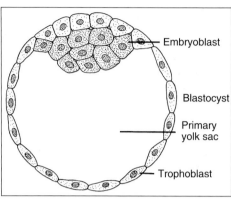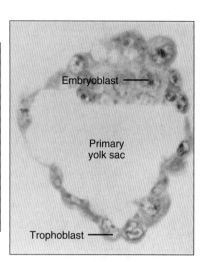

Figure 2-5 Differentiation of the morula into a blastocyst. At this time cells differentiate into the embryoblast (involved in development of the embryo) and the trophoblast (involved in maintenance). *(From Hertig AT et al:* Contrib Embryol *35:199, 1954.)*

the *morula*. Fluid seeps into the morula, and its cells realign themselves to form a fluid-filled hollow ball, the *blastocyst*. Two cell populations now can be distinguished within the blastocyst: those lining the cavity (the primary yolk sac), called *trophoblast* cells, and a small cluster within the cavity, called the inner cell mass or *embryoblast* (Figure 2-5). The embryoblast cells form the embryo proper, whereas the trophoblast cells are associated with implantation of the embryo and formation of the placenta; they are not described further here.

At about day 8 of gestation, the cells of the embryoblast differentiate into a two-layered disk, called the *bilaminar germ disk*. The cells situated dorsally, or *ectodermal layer*, are columnar and reorganize to form the *amniotic cavity*. Those on the ventral aspect, the *endodermal layer*, are cuboidal and form the roof of a second cavity (the *secondary yolk* sac), which develops from the migration of peripheral cells of the extraembryonic endodermal layer. This configuration is completed after 2 weeks of development (Figure 2-6). During that time the axis of the embryo is established and is represented by a slight enlargement of the ectodermal and endodermal cells at the head (or rostral) end of the embryo in a region known as the *prochordal plate*. Firm union exists between the ectodermal and endodermal cells at the prochordal plate.

During the third week of development the bilaminar embryonic disk is converted to a trilaminar disk. As previously described, the floor of the amniotic cavity is formed by ectoderm, and within it a structure called the *primitive streak* develops along the midline (Figure 2-7, A). This structure is a narrow groove with slightly bulging areas on each side. The rostral end of the streak finishes in a small depression called the *primitive node*, or *pit*. Cells of

the ectodermal layer divide at the node and migrate between the ectoderm and endoderm to form a solid column that pushes forward in the midline as far as the prochordal plate. Through canalization of this cord of cells, the *notochord* is formed to support the primitive embryo (Figure 2-7, A and C).

Elsewhere alongside the primitive streak, cells of the ectodermal layer divide and migrate toward the streak, where they invaginate and spread laterally between the ectoderm and endoderm. These cells, sometimes called the *mesoblast*, infiltrate and push away the extraembryonic endodermal cells of the hypoblast, except for the prochordal plate, to form the true *embryonic endoderm*. They also pack the space between the newly formed embryonic endoderm and the ectoderm to form a third layer of cells, the *mesoderm* (Figure 2-7, A and D). In addition to spreading laterally, cells spread progressively forward, passing on each side of the notochord and prochordal plate. The cells that accumulate anterior to the prochordal plate as a result of this migration give rise to the *cardiac plate*, the structure in which the heart forms. As a result of these cell migrations, the notochord and mesoderm now completely separate the ectoderm from the endoderm (Figure 2-7, C), except in the region of the prochordal plate and in a similar area of fusion at the tail (caudal) end of the embryo, the *cecal plate*.

FORMATION OF THE NEURAL TUBE AND FATE OF THE GERM LAYERS

The series of events leading to the formation of the three-layered, or *triploblastic*, embryo during the first

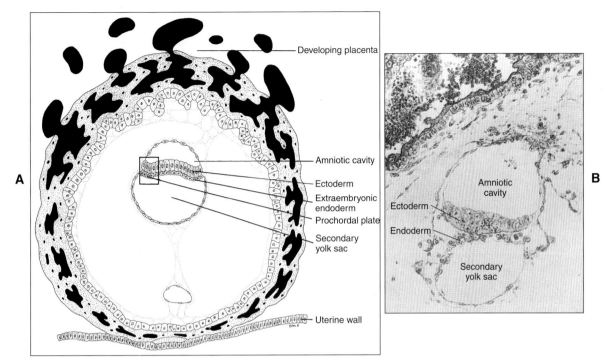

Figure 2-6 A, Schematic representation and **B,** histologic section of a human blastocyst at 13 days. An amniotic cavity has formed within the ectodermal layer. Proliferation of endodermal cells forms a secondary yolk sac. The bilaminar embryo is well established. *(****B*** *From Brewer JI:* Contrib Embryol *27:85, 1938.)*

3 weeks of development now has been sketched. These initial events involve cell proliferation and migration. During the next 3 to 4 weeks of development, major tissues and organs differentiate from the triploblastic embryo; these include the head and face and the tissues contributing to development of the teeth. Key events are the differentiation of the nervous system and neural crest tissues from the ectoderm, the differentiation of mesoderm, and the folding of the embryo in two planes along the rostrocaudal (head-tail) and lateral axes.

The nervous system develops as a thickening within the ectodermal layer at the rostral end of the embryo. This thickening constitutes the *neural plate,* which rapidly forms raised margins (the *neural folds*). These folds in turn encompass and delineate a deepening midline depression, the *neural groove* (Figure 2-8). The neural folds eventually fuse so that a *neural tube* separates from the ectoderm to form the floor of the amniotic cavity, with mesoderm intervening.

As the neural tube forms, changes occur in the mesoderm adjacent to the tube and the notochord. The mesoderm first thickens on each side of the midline to form *paraxial* mesoderm. Along the trunk of the embryo this paraxial mesoderm breaks up into segmented blocks called *somites.* Each somite has three components: the *sclerotome,* which eventually contributes to two adjacent vertebrae and their disks; the *myotome,* which

gives origin to a segmented mass of muscle; and the *dermatome,* which gives rise to the connective tissue of the skin overlying the somite. In the head region the mesoderm only partially segments to form a series of numbered *somatomeres,* which contribute in part to the head musculature. At the periphery of the paraxial mesoderm, the mesoderm remains as a thin layer, the *intermediate* mesoderm, which becomes the urogenital system. Further laterally the mesoderm thickens again to form the *lateral plate* mesoderm, which gives rise to the connective tissue associated with muscle and viscera; the serous membranes of the pleura, pericardium, and peritoneum; the blood and lymphatic cells; the cardiovascular and lymphatic systems; and the spleen and adrenal cortex.

A different series of events takes place in the head region. First, the neural tube undergoes massive expansion to form the forebrain, midbrain, and hindbrain. The hindbrain exhibits segmentation by forming a series of eight bulges known as *rhombomeres,* which play an important role in the development of the head.

FOLDING OF THE EMBRYO

A crucial developmental event is the folding of the embryo in two planes, along the rostrocaudal axis and along the lateral axis (Figure 2-9). The head fold is

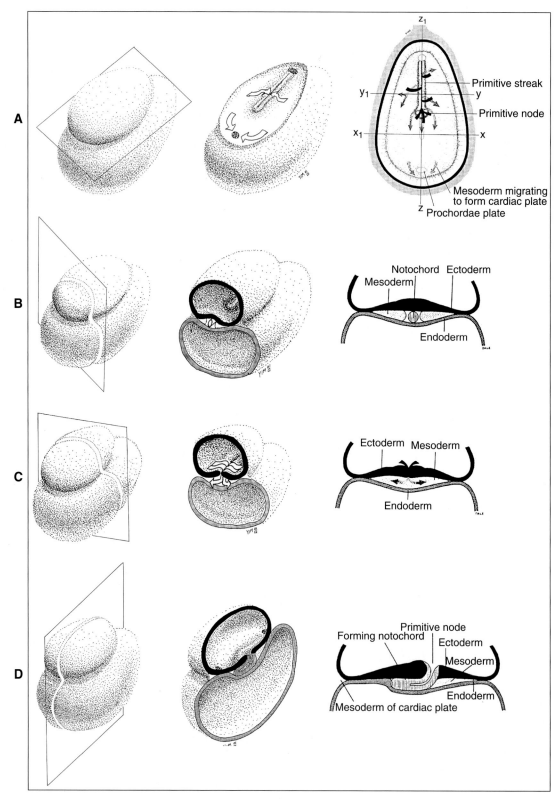

Figure 2-7 **A,** Conversion of the bilaminar embryo into a trilaminar embryo. The left column illustrates the plane of section for the middle and right columns. The middle column provides a three-dimensional view, and the right column provides a two-dimensional representation. **A** depicts the floor of the amniotic cavity, formed by the ectodermal layer of the bilaminar embryo. The primitive streak is a narrow groove *(solid line along the z-z₁ axis)* terminating in a circular depression called the primitive node. Surface ectodermal cells migrate to the streak *(shaded lines)* between the ectodermal and endodermal layers. A notochord process extends forward from the primitive node. **B,** A transverse section through x-x₁, showing the notochord flanked by mesoderm. **C,** A section through y-y₁. **D,** A section through z-z₁.

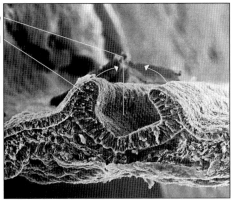

Neural groove
Neural fold

Figure 2-8 Scanning electron micrograph of neural fold elevation. *(From Tosney KW: Dev Biol 89:13, 1982.)*

critical to the formation of a primitive *stomatodeum* or oral cavity; through this fold ectoderm comes to line the stomatodeum, with the stomatodeum separated from the gut by the *buccopharyngeal membrane* (Figure 2-10).

Figure 2-11 illustrates how the lateral folding of the embryo determines this disposition of mesoderm. As another result, the ectoderm of the floor of the amniotic

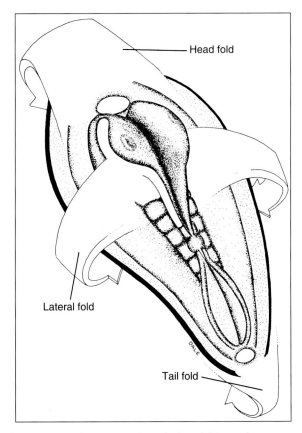

Head fold

Lateral fold

Tail fold

Figure 2-9 Embryo at 21 days, before folding. The arrows indicate where folding occurs.

cavity encapsulates the embryo and forms the surface epithelium. The paraxial mesoderm remains adjacent to the neural tube and notochord. The lateral plate mesoderm cavitates to form a space (coelom), and the mesoderm bounding the cavity lines the body wall and gut. Intermediate mesoderm is relocated to a position on the dorsal wall of the coelom. The endoderm forms the gut. The final disposition of the mesoderm and the derivatives of the ectoderm, endoderm, and neural crest are indicated in Figure 2-12.

THE NEURAL CREST

As the neural tube forms, a group of cells separate from the neuroectoderm. These cells have the capacity to migrate and differentiate extensively within the developing embryo (Figure 2-13), and they are the basis for structures such as the spinal sensory ganglia, sympathetic neurons, Schwann cells, pigment cells, and meninges. In the avian embryo these cells can be distinguished differentiating and separating at the crest of the neural folds, hence the name *neural crest cells* (Figure 2-14). In the mammalian embryo these cells separate from the lateral aspect of the neural plate (Figure 2-15) rather than from its crest; even so, the term *neural crest* is retained. During their induction, neural crest cells undergo an epithelial-mesenchymal transformation, a process whereby their cell adhesive properties and cytoskeletal organization change, allowing them to delaminate and migrate away from the neural tube. At the molecular level, neural crest cell competence is indicated by the expression of members of the Snail (*Snail* and *Slug*) zinc-finger transcription factor family that repress the expression of the cell adhesion molecule E-cadherin. Although there are still a number of unresolved issues, it is believed that bone morphogenetic proteins, Wnt (wingless homologue in vertebrates), and fibroblast growth factor signaling pathways are critical for inducing the neural crest cascade.

Neural crest cells in the head region have an important role. In addition to assisting in the formation of the cranial sensory ganglia, they also differentiate to form most of the connective tissue of the head. Embryonic connective tissue elsewhere is derived from mesoderm and is known as *mesenchyme*, whereas in the head it is known as *ectomesenchyme*, reflecting its origin from neuroectoderm. In a dental context the proper migration of neural crest cells is essential for the development of the face and the teeth. In Treacher Collins syndrome (Figure 2-16), for example, full facial development does not occur because the neural crest cells fail to migrate properly to the facial region. All the tissues of the tooth (except enamel and perhaps some cementum) and its supporting apparatus are derived directly from neural crest cells, and their depletion prevents proper dental development.

Text continued on p. 28

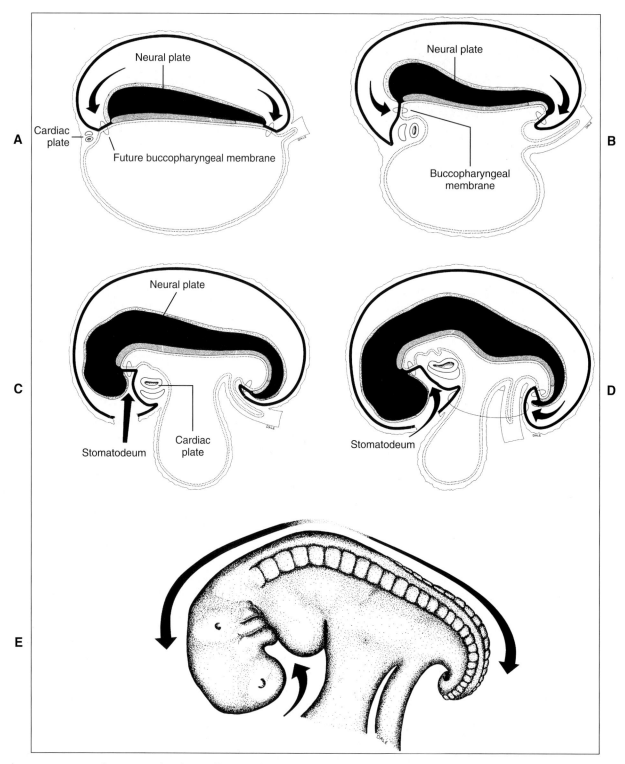

Figure 2-10 Sagittal sections of embryos illustrate the effects of the caudocephalic foldings. **A** indicates where folding begins, and **B** the onset of folding at 24 days. **C** and **D,** at 26 and 28 days, respectively, show how the head fold establishes the primitive stomatodeum, or oral cavity (*arrow*), bounded by the neural plate and the developing cardiac plate. It is separated from the foregut by the buccopharyngeal membrane. **E,** The embryo at the completion of folding.

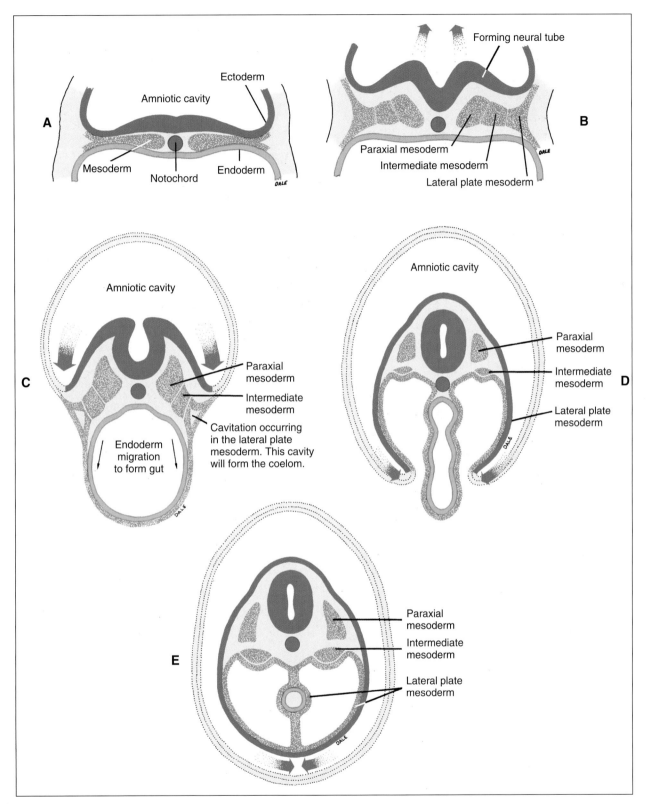

Figure 2-11 Cross-sectional profiles; **A,** The mesoderm, situated between the ectoderm and endoderm in the trilaminar disk. **B,** Differentiation of the mesoderm into three masses: the paraxial, intermediate, and lateral plate mesoderm. **C** to **E,** With lateral folding of the embryo, the amniotic cavity encompasses the embryo, and the ectoderm constituting its floor forms the surface epithelium. Paraxial mesoderm remains adjacent to the neural tube. Intermediate mesoderm is relocated and forms urogenital tissue. Lateral plate mesoderm cavitates, the cavity forming the coelom and its lining the serous membranes of the gut and abdominal cavity.

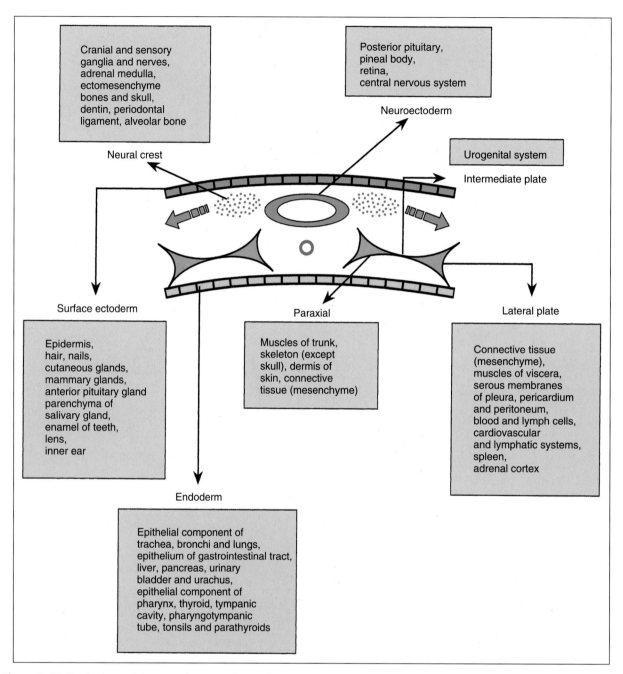

Cranial and sensory
ganglia and nerves,
adrenal medulla,
ectomesenchyme
bones and skull,
dentin, periodontal
ligament, alveolar bone

Neural crest

Posterior pituitary,
pineal body,
retina,
central nervous system

Neuroectoderm

Urogenital system

Intermediate plate

Surface ectoderm

Epidermis,
hair, nails,
cutaneous glands,
mammary glands,
anterior pituitary gland
parenchyma of
salivary gland,
enamel of teeth,
lens,
inner ear

Paraxial

Muscles of trunk,
skeleton (except
skull), dermis of
skin, connective
tissue (mesenchyme)

Lateral plate

Connective tissue
(mesenchyme),
muscles of viscera,
serous membranes
of pleura, pericardium
and peritoneum,
blood and lymph cells,
cardiovascular
and lymphatic systems,
spleen,
adrenal cortex

Endoderm

Epithelial component of
trachea, bronchi and lungs,
epithelium of gastrointestinal tract,
liver, pancreas, urinary
bladder and urachus,
epithelial component of
pharynx, thyroid, tympanic
cavity, pharyngotympanic
tube, tonsils and parathyroids

Figure 2-12 Derivatives of the germ layers and neural crest.

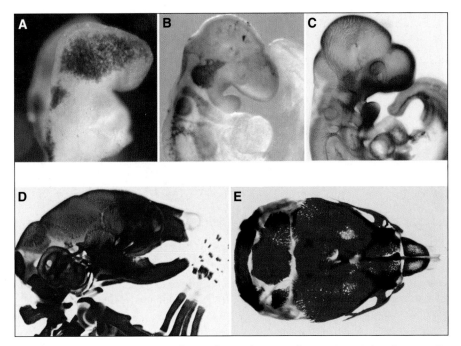

Figure 2-13 **A** to **E,** Migration and differentiation of cranial neural crest cells (nccs). **A,** Migrating ncc. **B** and **C,** Neuronal differentiation of ncc. **D,** Skeletal differentiation of ncc. **E,** Neurocranium. *(From Trainor P:* Semin Cell Dev Biol *16[6]: 683-693, 2005.)*

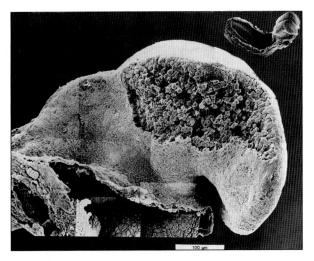

Figure 2-14 Photomicrograph illustrating the origin and development of neural crest cells in the embryo. *(From Noden DM, editor:* Receptors and recognition: specificity of embryological interactions, *London, 1978, Chapman & Hall.)*

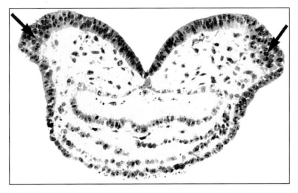

Figure 2-15 Mouse embryo. Differentiation of neural crest cells *(arrows)* from the lateral aspect of the neural plate. *(Courtesy A.G. Lumsden.)*

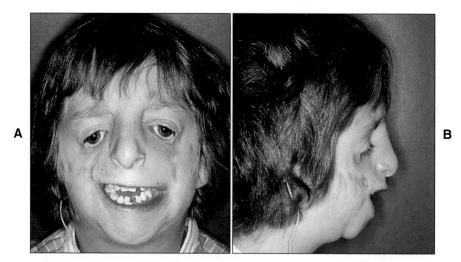

Figure 2-16 **A** and **B,** Child with mandibulofacial dysostosis (Treacher Collins syndrome). The underdevelopment results from a failure of the neural crest cells to migrate to the facial region. *(From Kaban LB, Troulis MJ:* Pediatric oral and maxillofacial surgery, *St Louis, 2004, Saunders.)*

RECOMMENDED READING

Langman J, editor: *Langman's medical embryology: human development—normal and abnormal,* ed 6, Baltimore, 1990, Williams & Wilkins.

Moore KL, Persaud TVN, editors: *The developing human: clinically orientated embryology,* ed 7, Philadelphia, 2003, WB Saunders.

Trainor PA, Melton KR, Manzanares M: Origins and plasticity of neural crest cells and their roles in jaw and craniofacial evolution, *Int J Dev Biol* 47:541, 2003.

TOPICS FOR CONSIDERATION   Neural Crest Cells and Their Potential for Tissue-Specific Repair

Stem cell transplantations have been touted as a therapeutic strategy in the treatment of numerous degenerative diseases and congenital birth defects. Although embryonic stem cells are considered the most attractive for this purpose because of their extraordinary pluripotency, their derivation remains ethically and politically controversial. In contrast, adult stem cells are abundantly available from numerous tissue sources and can be isolated free of political and ethical baggage; however, their potential may not be as great as embryonic stem cells. At this point, we consider neural crest cells, which although starting out as an embryonic population, persist in many tissues through to adulthood and may offer a unique compromise.

The neural crest is synonymous with vertebrate evolution and consists of a population of migratory, multipotential mesenchymal cells. Generated transiently in the neural plate along the entire vertebrate axis during embryonic development, the neural crest can be classified into four broad distinct axial populations—cranial, cardiac, vagal, and trunk—each of which migrates along unique pathways. Hardly a tissue or organ throughout the vertebrate body does not receive a contribution from the neural crest. In fact, neural crest cells generate an astonishingly diverse array of cell and tissue derivatives that are distinct at each axial level.

Cranial neural crest cells exhibit a unique ability to differentiate into cartilage and bone, underpinning their fundamental importance to vertebrate craniofacial evolution.[1] In addition, cranial neural crest cells also generate the odontoblasts of the teeth. Cardiac neural crest cells populate the aorticopulmonary septum and conotruncal cushions and give rise to aortic arch smooth muscle[2,3] and parasympathetic cardiac ganglia. Vagal neural crest cells generate the entire enteric nervous system (neurons and glia) that is essential for gastrointestinal function.[4] Trunk neural crest cells differentiate primarily into neurons and glia of the peripheral nervous system and pigment cells of the skin.

For a neural crest cell to be considered a stem cell, it must fulfill two important criteria. Firstly, a neural crest cell must be multipotential. In vivo single cell labeling and in vitro clonal cell culture experiments have demonstrated the presence of multipotential, bipotential, and unipotential neural crest cells.[5-8] Secondly, neural crest cells must be capable of continual self-renewal. Neural crest cells, however, are generated only transiently during a narrow window of embryonic development and at best only display a limited capacity for producing identical daughter cells.[9] Therefore the majority of neural crest cells are more akin to progenitor cells, and relatively few (1% to 3%) neural crest cells are true pluripotent stem cells.[10]

It had been assumed that any neural crest stem cells (NCSCs) that existed at the commencement of neural crest cell migration transitioned or differentiated into less potent progenitor cells fairly quickly. Surprisingly, however, the existence of NCSCs in the sciatic nerve of late-gestation rat embryos was discovered recently.[11] Furthermore, these NCSCs could be isolated by flow cytometry based on being positive for p75 (low-affinity neurotrophin receptor) and negative for P_0 (peripheral myelin protein). Subsequently, these NCSCs generate neurons and glia upon transplantation into host avian embryos. This suggested that NCSCs also might persist in other embryonic tissues and postnatally in adult tissues. Indeed, numerous reports have identified NCSCs or progenitor cells in the gut,[12] heart,[13] and epidermis.[14,15] The striking observation that these stem and progenitor cells persist throughout embryonic development and into adulthood makes their isolation and transplantation a promising avenue for tissue injury repair and regenerative medicine. Indeed, NCSCs derived from the epidermis of the skin appear to hold the greatest promise for future use in clinical treatments primarily because of their accessibility for isolation.

The hair follicle contains a mixed population of stem cells: epidermal NCSCs,[14,15] keratinocyte stem cells,[16] and melanogenic stem cells,[17] all of which represent promising candidates for diverse cell therapies because of their high degree of plasticity and accessibility. Within the hair follicle is a multilayered region of the outer root sheath called the bulge; the bulge is where new hair growth occurs and, interestingly, the inner layers of which are derived from neural crest cells.[18] Neural crest derived cells, harvested from the bulge region, have been demonstrated to undergo self-renewal, indicating that these cells are stem cells. Under differentiation conditions, the neural crest derived cells produced colonies of neurons, smooth muscle cells, rare Schwann cells, and melanocytes, highlighting their pluripotency.[14,15,19] Additionally, targeted differentiation resulted in the formation of chondrocytes,[15] a characteristic derivative of cranial neural crest cells. These neural crest derived stem cells have thus been called epidermal NCSCs, and the bulge in which they are found represents their niche.[20]

Recently, stem cells isolated from hair follicles have been shown to repair sciatic nerve function in vivo. Isolated stem cells from the hair follicle were used in transplants to treat two different injured nerves, the sciatic or tibial nerve. After transplantation, the follicle stem cells became incorporated into the nerve and resulted in the mice recovering proper nerve function. Functional studies of the gastrocnemius revealed consistent contractions upon stimulation; in contrast, control mice with a severed sciatic nerve but without transplantation displayed no muscle contraction upon stimulation. Additionally, tibial nerve function was recovered in mice that received the follicle stem cell transplant, as demonstrated by normal walking ability. Taken together, these results demonstrate that transplantation of follicle stem cells promotes regenerative axonal growth, resulting in the recovery of peripheral nerve function.[19] These experiments elegantly demonstrate the potential of follicle stem cells (of which epidermal NCSCs are a component) as a potential source of cells to be used in stem cell therapies.

Conclusions

Although the neural crest is a discrete population being generated only transiently in the embryo, numerous populations of neural crest derived stem and progenitor cells have been isolated from embryonic and adult tissues. Neural crest-derived stem cells harvested from the follicular bulge of the skin appear to be an extremely promising avenue for use in stem cell therapy. First, these cells are easily accessible and relatively easy to maintain in culture. Second, harvesting cells from the skin provides an autologous source of tissue in replacement therapies, bypassing immunorejection by the host tissue. Lastly, using neural crest derived stem cells in adult skin bypasses the ethical and political concerns surrounding the isolation and use of embryonic stem cells as a treatment for human disease.

Jennifer Crane and Paul A. Trainor
Stowers Institute for Medical Research
Kansas City, Missouri

Continued

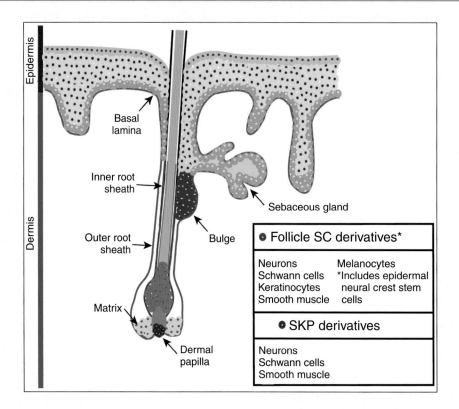

Follicle SC derivatives*

Neurons	Melanocytes
Schwann cells	*Includes epidermal
Keratinocytes	neural crest stem
Smooth muscle	cells

SKP derivatives

Neurons
Schwann cells
Smooth muscle

REFERENCES

1. Le Douarin N, Kalcheim C: *The neural crest*, ed 2, Developmental and Cell Biology Series, Cambridge, UK, 1999, Cambridge University Press.
2. Kirby ML, Gale TF, Stewart DE: Neural crest cells contribute to normal aorticopulmonary septation, *Science* 220:1059-1061, 1983.
3. Kirby ML, Stewart DE: Neural crest origin of cardiac ganglion cells in the chick embryo: identification and extirpation, *Dev Biol* 97:433-443, 1983.
4. Yntema CL, Hammond WS: The origin of intrinsic ganglia of trunk viscera from vagal neural crest in the chick embryo, *J Comp Neurol* 101:515-541, 1954.
5. Bronner-Fraser M, Fraser S: Developmental potential of avian trunk neural crest cells in situ, *Neuron* 3:755-766, 1989.
6. Sieber-Blum M, Cohen AM: Clonal analysis of quail neural crest cells: they are pluripotent and differentiate in vitro in the absence of noncrest cells, *Dev Biol* 80: 96-106, 1980.
7. Bronner-Fraser M, Fraser S: Cell lineage analysis reveals multipotency of some avian neural crest cells, *Nature* 335:161-164, 1988.
8. Stemple DL, Anderson DJ: Isolation of a stem cell for neurons and glia from the mammalian neural crest, *Cell* 71:973-985, 1992.

9. Trentin A, Glavieux-Pardanaud C, Le Douarin NM, Dupin E: Self-renewal capacity is a widespread property of various types of neural crest precursor cells, *Proc Natl Acad Sci U S A* 101:4495-4500, 2004.
10. Crane JF, Trainor PA: Neural crest stem and progenitor cells, *Annu Rev Cell Dev Biol* 22:267-286, 2006.
11. Morrison SJ, White PM, Zock C, Anderson DJ: Prospective identification, isolation by flow cytometry, and in vivo self-renewal of multipotent mammalian neural crest stem cells, *Cell* 96:737-749, 1999.
12. Kruger GM, Mosher JT, Bixby S et al: Neural crest stem cells persist in the adult gut but undergo changes in self-renewal, neuronal subtype potential, and factor responsiveness, *Neuron* 35:657-669, 2002.
13. Tomita Y, Matsumura K, Wakamatsu Y et al: Cardiac neural crest cells contribute to the dormant multipotent stem cell in the mammalian heart, *J Cell Biol* 170:1135-1146, 2005.
14. Sieber-Blum M, Grim M: The adult hair follicle: cradle for pluripotent neural crest stem cells, *Birth Defects Res C Embryo Today* 72:162-172, 2004.
15. Sieber-Blum M, Grim M, Hu YF, Szeder V: Pluripotent neural crest stem cells in the adult hair follicle, *Dev Dyn* 231:258-269, 2004.
16. Kobayashi K, Rochat A, Barrandon Y: Segregation of keratinocyte colony-forming cells in the bulge of the rat vibrissa, *Proc Natl Acad Sci U S A* 90:7391-7395, 1993.

TOPICS FOR CONSIDERATION   Neural Crest Cells and Their Potential for
Tissue-Specific Repair—cont'd

17. Nishimura EK, Jordan SA, Oshima H et al: Dominant role of the niche in melanocyte stem-cell fate determination, *Nature* 416:854-860, 2002.
18. Szeder V, Grim M, Halata Z, Sieber-Blum M: Neural crest origin of mammalian Merkel cells, *Dev Biol* 253: 258-263, 2003.
19. Amoh Y, Li L, Campillo R et al: Implanted hair follicle stem cells form Schwann cells that support repair of severed peripheral nerves, *Proc Natl Acad Sci U S A* 102:17734-17738, 2005.
20. Tumbar T, Guasch G, Greco V et al: Defining the epithelial stem cell niche in skin, *Science* 303:359-363, 2004.
21. Fernandes KJ, McKenzie IA, Mill P et al: A dermal niche for multipotent adult skin-derived precursor cells, *Nat Cell Biol* 6:1082-1093, 2004.
22. McKenzie IA, Biernaskie J, Toma JG et al: Skin-derived precursors generate myelinating Schwann cells for the injured and dysmyelinated nervous system, *J Neurosci* 26:6651-6660, 2006.
23. Toma JG, McKenzie IA, Bagli D, Miller FD: Isolation and characterization of multipotent skin-derived precursors from human skin, *Stem Cells* 23:727-737, 2005.

Embryology of the Head, Face, and Oral Cavity

CHAPTER OUTLINE

Knowledge of the evolutionary development of the skull, face, and jaws is helpful in understanding the complex events involved in cephalogenesis (formation of the head). Early chordates (creatures with a notochord) have a fairly simple anatomic plan with a notochord for support, a simple nervous system and sense organs, segmented muscle blocks, and at the beginning of the pharynx in its lateral wall, a series of branchial clefts supported by cartilage to permit gaseous exchange. The first vertebrates (possessing segmented vertebrae) evolved from this simple plan and were jawless (*agnathia*). Cartilaginous blocks (*occipital* and *parachordal*) evolved to support the notochord in the head region, along with cartilaginous *capsules* (*nasal*, *optic*, and *otic*) to protect the

sense organs. These cartilages and another cartilage derived from the branchial system (the *trabecular cartilage*) collectively form the *neurocranium*. The branchial arches, as mentioned, are supported by a series of jointed cartilaginous rods originally numbered 0, 1, 2, and so on and that constitute the *viscerocranium*. The first cartilage (cartilage 0) migrated to the neurocranium to provide additional support as the trabecular cartilage. Because of this, the actual second arch cartilage became the first arch cartilage (Figure 3-1, A and B). The neurocranium and viscerocranium together form the *chondrocranium*.

From this simple model, vertebrates came to possess jaws (*gnathostomata*) through modification of the jointed first arch cartilage, with the upper element, the *palatopterygo quadrate* bar, becoming the upper jaw and

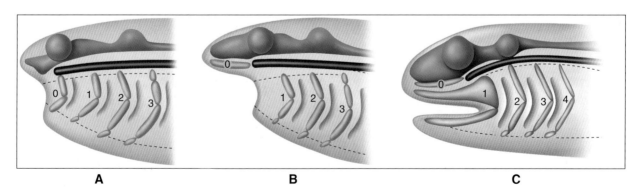

A   **B**   **C**

Figure 3-1 **A** and **B,** The viscerocranium and the movement of arch 0 to the neurocranium. **C,** The jaws developed from the first branchial arch cartilage of the viscerocranium. *(Redrawn from Osborn JW, editor:* Dental anatomy and embryology, *vol 2, Oxford, UK, 1981, Blackwell Scientific.)*

the lower elements, *Meckel's cartilage*, becoming the lower jaw (Figure 3-1, C). The fibrous connection between the two formed the jaw joint. In addition to jaws, vertebrate evolution also brought about massive expansion of the head region and associated larger neural and sensory elements. For protection, additional bony skeletal elements developed (the dermal bones) to form the vault of the skull and the facial skeleton, which included bony jaws and teeth. This cephalic expansion demanded a new source of connective tissue, and as explained in Chapter 2, this source is the neuroectoderm, from which neural crest cells migrate and differentiate

into ectomesenchyme. Comparison between the cranial components of the primitive vertebrate skull and the cranial skeleton of a human fetus is shown in Figure 3-2.

HEAD FORMATION

The folding of the three-layered embryo has been described, and the rostral or head fold is important at this point. The neural tube is produced by the formation and fusion of the neural folds, which sink beneath surface ectoderm. The anterior portion of this neural

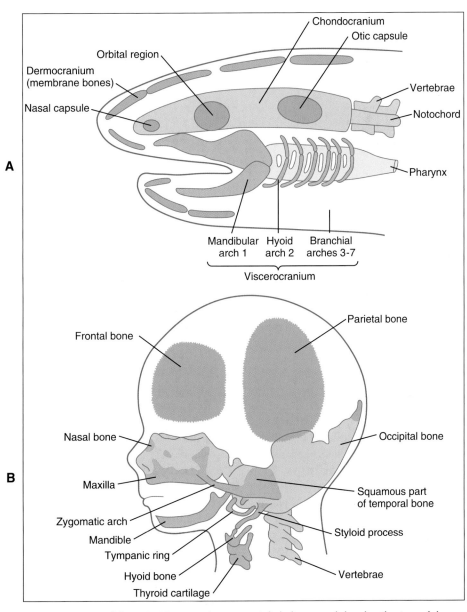

Figure 3-2 The major components of the primitive vertebrate cranial skeleton and the distribution of these same components in a human fetal head. *(From Carlson BM:* Human embryology and developmental biology, *Philadelphia, 2004, Mosby.)*

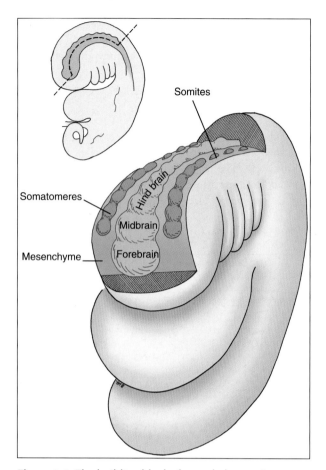

Figure 3-3 The building blocks for cephalogenesis.

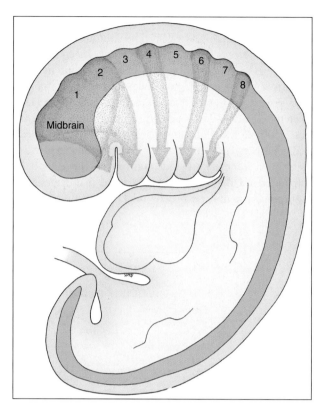

Figure 3-4 The source and pattern of neural crest migration to the developing face and branchial arch system. The midbrain and rhombomeres 1 and 2 contribute to the face and first branchial arch.

tube expands greatly as the forebrain, midbrain, and hindbrain form, but a small amount of mesenchyme (embryonic connective tissue) always remains between the developing brain and the surface epithelium except where the olfactory, orbital, and otic placodes form. At that point the neuroectoderm fuses directly with the surface epithelium. The part of the neural tube that forms the hindbrain develops a series of eight bulges, the rhombomeres (Figure 3-3). Lateral to the neural tube is paraxial mesoderm, which partially segments rostrally to form seven somatomeres and fully segments caudally to form somites, the first in the series being the occipital somites.

Migration of neural crest cells provides the embryonic connective tissue needed for craniofacial development (Figure 3-4). These neural crest cells arise from the midbrain and the first two rhombomeres as two streams. The first stream migrates forward and intermingles and reinforces the mesenchyme situated beneath the expanding forebrain. This stream provides much of the connective tissue associated with the face. The second stream is directed toward the first branchial arch.

These migrating streams of neural crest cells continue to express the homeobox genes that were expressed in the rhombomeres from which they are derived. In the case of the branchial arches, except for the first, various combinations of the *Hox* family of homeobox genes are expressed, and the details are outside the scope of this text. The stream of neural crest cells directed to the first arch is derived from the neuroectoderm of the midbrain and the first two rhombomeres. *Hox* genes are not expressed anterior to rhombomere 3 (Figure 3-5), and a different set of coded patterning homeobox genes is required to bring about the development of cephalic structures. This new set of homeobox genes (reflecting the later development of the head in evolutionary terms) includes the *Msx* gene family (*Ms* because of a relationship to the muscle homeobox in *Drosophila*), the *Dlx* family (related to *Drosophila* limb development), and the *Barx* family (related to the *Drosophila* bar locus). Some neural crest cell populations require instructions from their local microenvironment. The resulting crosstalk involves common signaling pathways such as sonic hedgehog (Shh), fibroblast growth factor (Fgf), and bone morphogenetic proteins. The molecular dialogs affect neural crest cell proliferation, differentiation, and survival. Homeobox genes also are implicated

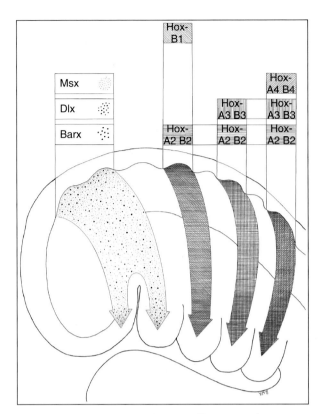

Figure 3-5 Migrating neural crest cells express the same homeobox *(Hox)* genes as their precursors in the rhombomeres from which they derive. Note that *Hox* genes are not expressed anterior to rhombomere 3. A new set of patterning genes *(Msx, Dlx, Barx)* has evolved to bring about development of cephalic structures so that a "Hox code" also is transferred to the branchial arches and developing face.

in dental development, and their effects are discussed in Chapter 5.

BRANCHIAL (PHARYNGEAL) ARCHES AND THE PRIMITIVE MOUTH

When the stomatodeum first forms, it is delimited rostrally by the *frontal prominence* and caudally by the developing cardiac bulge (Figures 3-6 and 3-7). The buccopharyngeal membrane, a bilaminar structure consisting of apposed ectoderm and endoderm, separates the stomatodeum from the foregut (see Figure 3-7), but this soon breaks down so that the stomatodeum communicates directly with the foregut. Laterally the stomatodeum becomes limited by the first pair of *pharyngeal* or *branchial arches* (Figure 3-8). The branchial arches form in the pharyngeal wall (which first consists of a sheet of lateral plate mesoderm sandwiched between ectoderm externally and endoderm internally) as a result of proliferating

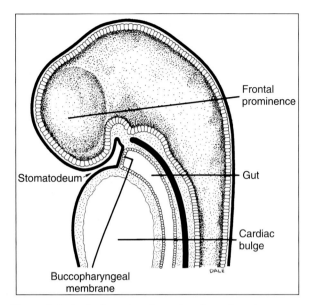

Figure 3-6 Sagittal section through a 4-week embryo showing the stomatodeum delimited by the frontal prominence above and the developing cardiac bulge below. The buccopharyngeal membrane separates the stomatodeum from the foregut.

lateral plate mesoderm and subsequent reinforcement by migrating neural crest cells. Six cylindrical thickenings thus form (the fifth and sixth are transient structures in human beings that are not visible on the surface of the embryo) that expand from the lateral wall of the pharynx, pass beneath the floor of the pharynx, and approach their anatomic counterparts expanding from the opposite side. In doing so, the arches progressively separate the primitive stomatodeum from the developing heart. The arches are seen clearly as bulges on the lateral aspect of the embryo and are separated externally by small clefts called *branchial grooves*. On the inner aspect of the pharyngeal wall are corresponding small depressions called *pharyngeal pouches* that separate each of the branchial arches internally. The derivatives of the branchial (pharyngeal) arch system are summarized in Table 3-1. In aquatic vertebrates the pharyngeal pouches and branchial grooves fuse and eventually break down to form the gill clefts. In human beings the grooves and pouches have other functions (Figure 3-9).

FATE OF GROOVES AND POUCHES

The first groove and pouch are involved in the formation of the *external auditory meatus, tympanic membrane, tympanic antrum, mastoid antrum,* and *pharyngotympanic* or *eustachian tube.* The second, third, and fourth grooves normally are obliterated by overgrowth of the second arch forming a cervical sinus that sometimes persists and opens into the side of the neck (branchial fistula) or on

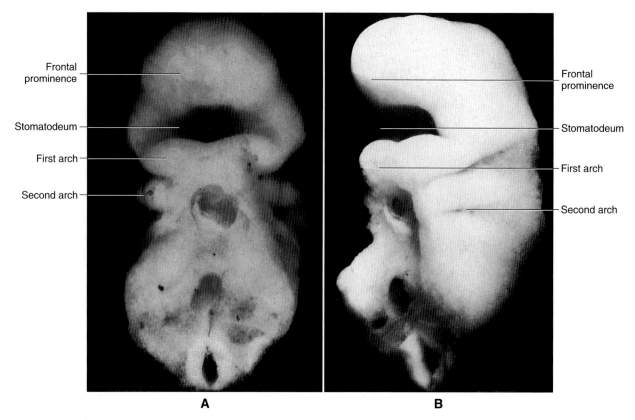

Figure 3-7 A 26-day embryo. **A,** Front view. **B,** Side view. The structures limiting the stomatodeum are clearly recognizable. *(Courtesy H. Nishimura.)*

the neck and inside the pharynx (pharyngocutaneous fistula). The second pouch also largely is obliterated by the development of the *palatine tonsil*; a part persists as the tonsillar fossa. The third pouch expands dorsally and ventrally into two compartments, and its connection

with the pharynx is obliterated. The dorsal component gives origin to the *inferior parathyroid gland,* whereas the ventral component, with its anatomic counterpart from the opposite side, forms the *thymus* gland. The fourth pouch also expands into dorsal and ventral components.

TABLE 3-1	Derivatives of the Branchial (Pharyngeal) Arch System		
	ARCH	GROOVE	POUCH

First	1. Mandible and maxilla
	2. Meckel's cartilage:
	  a. Incus and malleus of inner ear
	  b. Sphenomalleolar ligament
	  c. Sphenomandibular ligament
		1. External auditory meatus	2. Tympanic membrane
			3. Tympanic cavity
			4. Mastoid antrum
			5. Eustachian tube

Second	1. Reichert's cartilage:
	  a. Styloid process of temporal bone
	  b. Stylohyoid ligament
	  c. Lesser horns of the hyoid bone
	  d. Upper part of the body of the hyoid bone
		Obliterated by the down-growth of the second arch	1. Largely obliterated
			2. Contributes to tonsil

Third	1. Lower part of the body of the hyoid bone 2. Greater horns of the hyoid bone		Inferior parathyroid gland Thymus
Fourth	1. Cartilages of the larynx		Superior parathyroid gland Ultimobranchial body
Fifth Sixth	Rudimentary		Rudimentary

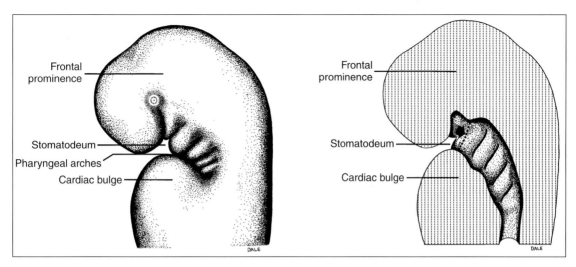

Figure 3-8 A, Development of pharyngeal arches and the clefts between them in a 35-day embryo. **B,** Midline section showing reflection of the arches on the pharyngeal wall and the pharyngeal pouches separating them. The dotted line *(arrow)* represents the site where the buccopharyngeal membrane was attached.

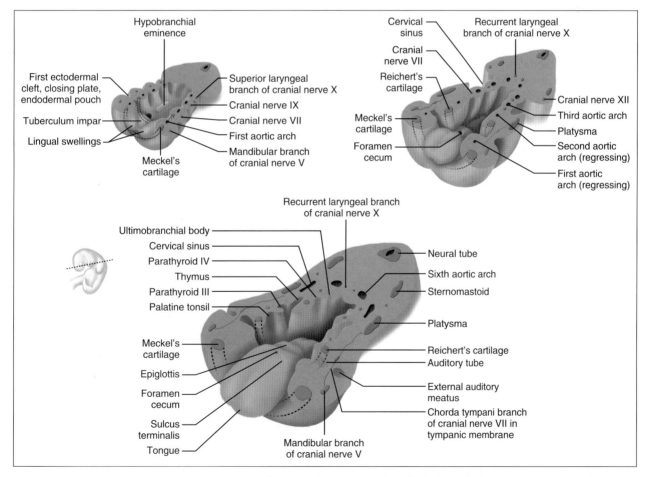

Figure 3-9 Progressive stages in development of pharyngeal arches and their derivatives during the second month in utero. *(Redrawn from Shaw JH, Sweeney EA, Cappuccino CC et al:* Textbook of oral biology, *Philadelphia, 1978, WB Saunders.)*

The dorsal component gives origin to the *superior parathyroid gland,* and the ventral portion gives rise to the *ultimobranchial body,* which in turn gives rise to the *parafollicular cells* of the thyroid gland. The fifth pouch in human beings is rudimentary and thus disappears or becomes incorporated into the fourth pouch.

ANATOMY OF AN ARCH

Every branchial arch has the same basic plan. The inner aspect is covered by endoderm (ectoderm in the case of the first arch because it forms in front of the buccopharyngeal membrane, which delineates the junction of the stomatodeum [lined by ectoderm] from the foregut [lined by endoderm]) and the outer surface by ectoderm. The central core consists of mesenchyme derived from lateral plate mesoderm, which is invaded by mesenchyme derived from the neural crest. The neural crest mesenchyme (called *ectomesenchyme*) condenses to form a bar of cartilage, the arch cartilage (see Figure 3-9). The cartilage of the first arch is called *Meckel's cartilage,* and that of the second *Reichert's,* after the anatomists who first described them. The other arch cartilages are not named. The contributions of Meckel's and Reichert's cartilages are discussed subsequently. The cartilage of the third arch gives rise to the body and greater horns of the hyoid bone and that of the fourth arch to the cartilages of the larynx.

Some of the mesenchyme surrounding this cartilaginous bar develops into striated muscle. The first arch musculature gives origin to the muscles of mastication, and the second arch musculature to the muscles of facial expression. Each arch also contains an artery and a nerve (Table 3-2). The nerve consists of two components, one motor (supplying the muscle of the arch) and one sensory. The sensory nerve divides into two branches: a *posttrematic* branch, supplying the epithelium that covers the anterior half of the arch, and a *pretrematic* branch, passing forward to supply the epithelium that covers the posterior

half of the preceding arch. The nerve of the first arch is the fifth cranial (or *trigeminal*) nerve, that of the second is the seventh cranial (or *facial*) nerve, and that of the third is the ninth cranial (or *glossopharyngeal*) nerve. Structures derived from any arch carry with them the nerve supply of that arch. Thus the muscles of mastication are innervated by the trigeminal nerve, and the muscles of facial expression, by the facial nerve.

FUSION OF PROCESSES

The first, second, and third branchial arches play an important role in the development of the face, mouth, and tongue. Classically, the formation of the face is described in terms of the formation and fusion of several processes or prominences (Figure 3-10). This terminology may be confusing, however. In some instances these processes are swellings of mesenchyme that cause furrows between apparent processes, so that the ostensible fusion of processes actually involves the elimination of a furrow.

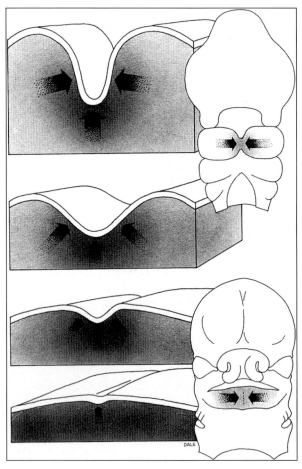

Figure 3-10 Apparent fusion of facial processes by the elimination of a furrow between them. The arrows indicate the general direction of the fusion events. Compare with Figure 3-11.

TABLE 3-2 Innervation and Vascularization of Pharyngeal Arches		
ARCH	BLOOD VESSEL	NERVE
First	First aortic arch	Mandibular (and maxillary) division of the trigeminal nerve (cranial nerve V)
Second	Second aortic arch	Facial (VII)
Third	Third aortic arch	Glossopharyngeal (IX)
Fourth	Fourth aortic arch	Vagus (X)

Only in certain instances, such as the union of the palatal processes, does actual fusion occur (Figure 3-11). With this distinction understood, the conventional term *process* rather than the more accurate terms *swelling* or *prominence* is used to describe the further development of the face and oral cavity.

To recapitulate, the primitive stomatodeum is at first bounded above (rostrally) by the frontal prominence, below (caudally) by the developing heart, and laterally by the first branchial arch. With spread of the arches midventrally, the cardiac plate is eliminated from the stomatodeum, and the floor of the mouth is formed by the epithelium covering the mesenchyme of the first, second, and third branchial arches.

At about 24 days the first branchial arch establishes another process, the *maxillary process,* so that the stomatodeum is limited cranially by the frontal prominence covering the rapidly expanding forebrain, laterally by the newly formed maxillary process, and ventrally by the first arch (now called the *mandibular process;* Figure 3-12).

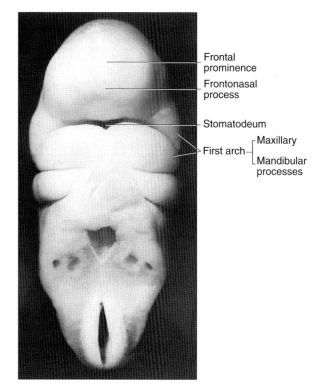

Figure 3-12 A 27-day embryo viewed from the front. The beginning elements for facial development and the boundaries of the stomatodeum are apparent. The first arch gives rise to maxillary and mandibular processes *(Courtesy H. Nishimura).*

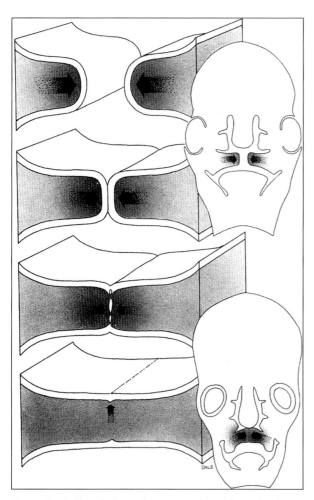

Figure 3-11 True fusion of processes (e.g., the palatal process). Such fusion involves the breakdown of surface epithelium.

FORMATION OF THE FACE

Early development of the face is dominated by the proliferation and migration of ectomesenchyme involved in the formation of the primitive nasal cavities. At about 28 days, localized thickenings develop within the ectoderm of the frontal prominence, just rostral to the opening of the stomatodeum. These thickenings are the *olfactory placodes.* Rapid proliferation of the underlying mesenchyme around the placodes bulges the frontal eminence forward and also produces a horseshoe-shaped ridge that converts the olfactory placode into the nasal pit (Figure 3-13). The lateral arm of the horseshoe is called the *lateral nasal process,* and the medial arm the *medial nasal process.* The region of the frontal prominence where these changes take place and the nose will develop also is referred to as the *frontonasal process (region).* The medial nasal processes of both sides, together with the frontonasal process, give rise to the middle portion of the nose, middle portion of the upper lip, anterior portion of the maxilla, and the *primary palate.*

The maxillary process grows medially and approaches the lateral and medial nasal processes but remains separated from them by distinct grooves (the naso-optic

TOPICS FOR CONSIDERATION   What's in a Face?

*Someone told me it's all happening at the zoo
I do believe it, I do believe it's true.*

(Paul Simon)

A quick perusal of the residents of any zoo—as well as the visitors—surely will illustrate the enormous facial variations that exist throughout the animal kingdom. An inquisitive craniofacial biologist might wonder how such diversity is created, especially because embryos—whether they are avian, mammalian, or simian—begin development looking remarkably alike. How does such variation come about, not only between animal classes but within even a single species, such as dogs? It seems as if the molecular machinery, employed so handily by Mother Nature, can be tweaked subtly to generate this multiplicity in facial forms, and we are just now getting some startling insights into how this is made possible.

Some clues have come from the study of craniofacial malformations in human beings and in other animals. Great strides have been made in recent years in pinpointing the gene mutations responsible for a wide range of craniofacial syndromes (see Online Mendelian Inheritance in Man, OMIM). These studies have brought us one step closer to understanding the genetic basis for craniofacial malformations, but they leave unanswered the question of how perturbations in a particular gene affect development of the craniofacial complex. For insights into this question, painstaking molecular and cellular analyses have to be carried out to understand how a given gene functions within the context of craniofacial development. For example, in recent years investigators have identified by in situ hybridization the temporal and spatial patterns of gene expression in the developing face. Genes with expression patterns that suggest an involvement in facial development then can be "knocked out" through homologous recombination (in mice) or through experimental manipulations (in chicks), and the consequences of this inactivation can be studied. These approaches can work exceedingly well, depending upon how well we understand a particular molecular pathway. The crucial aspect of these analyses is almost always the same: namely, we have to understand the basic cell and tissue interactions that govern craniofacial morphogenesis in order to interpret how a particular gene disrupts these interactions.

Another strategy that is now being used to understand the molecular basis for craniofacial variation is to interrogate entire genomes to find chromosomal regions that control differences in facial form. These approaches are based largely on the identification of polymorphic microsatellite markers and single nucleotide polymorphisms with a single species that shows a large dynamic range of craniofacial morphology. Think of pigeons—not those pesky feral birds that one sees decorating statues in parks but rather the spectacular show pigeons that have been selectively bred for more than 3000 years. These remarkably varied birds caught the attention of Charles Darwin, for they epitomized his theory of natural selection. We and others are using all kinds of mapping approaches in order to identify regions of the genome that control facial variations. This approach is not just for the birds, either: imagine identifying loci that distinguish the face of a borzoi from that of a bulldog, or isolating the genes responsible for the variation in fish faces. When this is accomplished, we will have gained critical clues into how craniofacial variation is controlled.

In the end, all of these approaches seek to understand the molecular basis for facial variation, but they address a more global question as well. In a larger sense, these investigations intend to provide a window into the mechanisms of evolutionary and developmental variation. Whether we focus on the face or other traits, our ultimate objective is to understand how diversification has come about. Maybe then we will have answers to the question: How did we come to look so different, when we all start off looking so alike?

Jill A. Helms, DDS, PhD
Associate Professor
Department of Surgery
School of Medicine
Stanford University
Stanford, California

Samantha A. Brugmann, PhD
Postdoctoral Fellow
Children's Surgical Research Lab
School of Medicine
Stanford University
Stanford, California

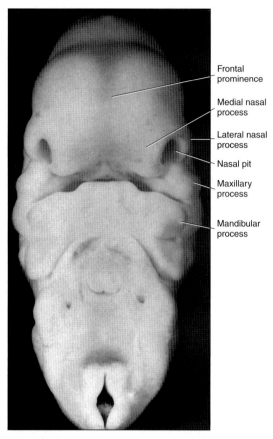

Figure 3-13 A 34-day embryo viewed from the front. The nasal pits have formed, thereby delineating the lateral and medial nasal processes. *(Courtesy H. Nishimura.)*

Labels on Figure 3-13:
- Frontal prominence
- Medial nasal process
- Lateral nasal process
- Nasal pit
- Maxillary process
- Mandibular process

groove and the bucconasal groove (Figure 3-14). The medial growth of the maxillary process pushes the medial nasal process toward the midline, where it merges with its anatomic counterpart from the opposite side. In this way the upper lip is formed from the maxillary processes of each side and the medial nasal process, with fusion occurring between the forward extent of the maxillary process and the lateral face of the medial nasal process. The lower lip is formed, of course, by merging of the two streams of ectomesenchyme of the mandibular processes. The merging of the two medial nasal processes results in the formation of that part of the maxilla carrying the incisor teeth and the primary palate and part of the lip. These steps in facial development are shown in Figure 3-15.

An unusual type of fusion occurs between the maxillary process and the lateral nasal process. As with most other processes associated with facial development, the maxillary and lateral nasal processes initially are separated by a deep furrow (see Figure 3-14). The epithelium in the floor of the groove between them forms a solid core that separates from the surface and eventually canalizes to form the nasolacrimal duct. Once the duct has separated, the two processes merge by infilling of the mesenchyme.

The face develops between the twenty-fourth and thirty-eighth days of gestation. By this time some of the epithelium covering the facial processes already can be distinguished as odontogenic, or tooth forming (see Figure 3-15). On the inferior border of the maxillary process and the superior border of the mandibular arch, where the lateral margin of the stomatodeum is formed, the epithelium begins to proliferate and thicken.

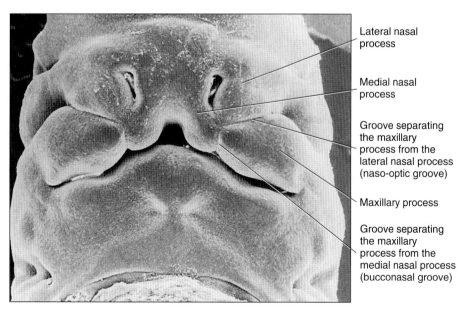

Figure 3-14 Scanning electron micrograph of a human embryo at around 6 weeks. *(Courtesy K.K. Sulik.)*

Labels on Figure 3-14:
- Lateral nasal process
- Medial nasal process
- Groove separating the maxillary process from the lateral nasal process (naso-optic groove)
- Maxillary process
- Groove separating the maxillary process from the medial nasal process (bucconasal groove)

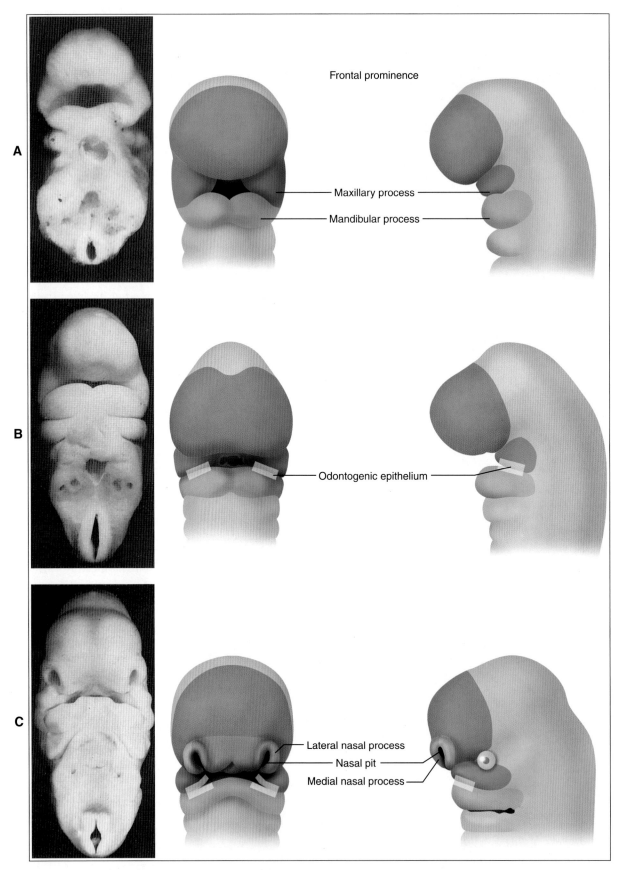

Figure 3-15 Summary of human facial development from about the fourth through the sixth week. Left-column photographs show actual embryos; the middle and right columns are diagrams of frontal and lateral views. **A,** Boundaries of the stomatodeum in a 26-day embryo. **B,** A 27-day embryo. The nasal placode is about to develop, and the odontogenic epithelium *(white bars)* can be identified. **C,** A 34-day embryo. The nasal pit, surrounded by lateral and medial nasal processes, is easily recognizable.

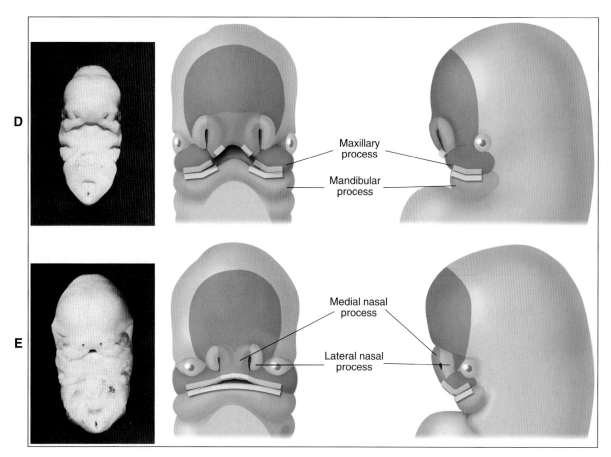

Figure 3-15—cont'd **D,** A 36-day embryo shows the fusion of various facial processes that are completed by 38 days **(E).** *(Photos courtesy H. Nishimura. Drawings adapted from Nery EB, Kraus BS, Croup M:* Arch Oral Biol *15:1315, 1970.)*

This thickened area is the odontogenic epithelium. Odontogenic epithelium also develops on the lateral aspect of the medial nasal process (see Figure 3-15, *D* and *E*), but not until the thirty-seventh day of development, when the processes fuse, can a single plate of thickened epithelium, the *primary epithelial band,* be observed. Thus the primary epithelial band is an arch-shaped continuous plate of odontogenic epithelium that forms in the upper jaw from four separate zones of epithelial proliferation; laterally one zone associated with each maxillary process and in middle one with each medial nasal process. Two zones, one in each mandibular process, form the primary epithelial band of the lower jaw.

FORMATION OF THE SECONDARY PALATE

Initially, a common oronasal cavity is bounded anteriorly by the primary palate and is occupied mainly by the developing tongue. Only after the development of the *secondary palate* is distinction between the oral and nasal cavities possible. The palate proper develops from primary and secondary components.

The formation of the primary palate from the frontonasal and medial nasal processes has been described already. The formation of the secondary palate commences between 7 and 8 weeks and completes around the third month of gestation. Three outgrowths appear in the oral cavity; the *nasal septum* grows downward from the frontonasal process along the midline, and two *palatine shelves* or processes, one from each side, extend from the maxillary processes toward the midline. The shelves are directed first downward on each side of the tongue. After the seventh week of development, the tongue is withdrawn from between the shelves, which now elevate and fuse with each other above the tongue and with the primary palate (Figures 3-16 to 3-18). The septum and the two shelves converge and fuse along the midline, thus separating the primitive oral cavity into nasal and oral cavities. The closure of the secondary palate proceeds gradually from the primary palate in a posterior direction, and involves an intrinsic force in the palatine shelves the nature of which has not been determined yet. A factor contributing to closure of the secondary palate is displacement of the tongue from between the palatine shelves by the growth pattern of the head.

Between 7 and 8 weeks the tongue and mandible in the embryo are small relative to the upper facial

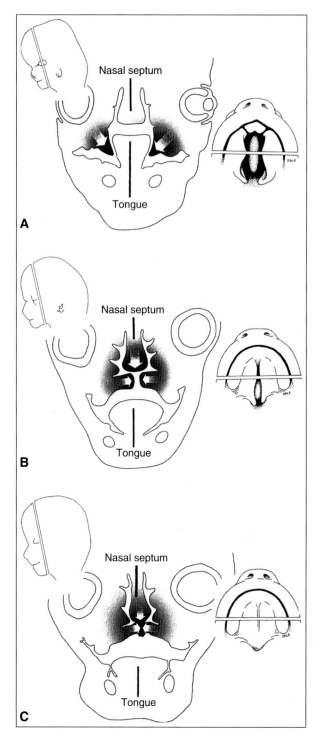

Figure 3-16 Formation of the secondary palate. **A,** At 7 weeks the palatine shelves are forming from the maxillary processes and are directed downward on each side of the developing tongue. **B,** At 8 weeks the tongue has been depressed and the palatine shelves are elevated but not fused. **C,** Fusion of the shelves and the nasal septum is completed.

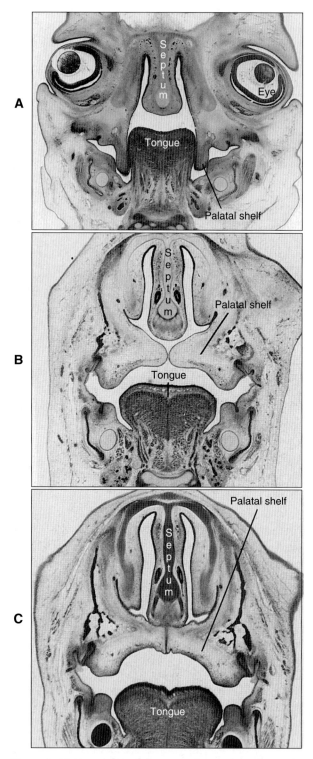

Figure 3-17 Formation of the secondary palate. Coronal sections through human embryos at approximately **(A)** 7 weeks, **(B)** 8 weeks, and **(C)** 9 weeks. The initial disposition of palatine shelves on each side of the tongue is shown in **A,** their elevation coincident with depression of the tongue in **B,** and their final fusion with each other and with the nasal septum in **C.** *(From Diewert VM: Am J Anat 167:495, 1983.)*

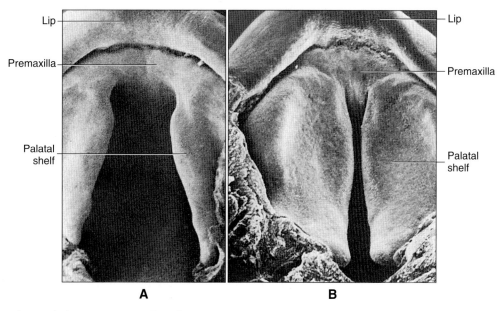

Figure 3-18 Palatine shelves in (**A**) 7-week and (**B**) 8-week human embryo corresponding approximately to Figures 3-15, *A* and *B*, and 3-16, *B*. *(From Waterman RE, Meller SM: Anat Rec 180:111, 1974.)*

complex, and the lower lip is positioned behind the upper one. The head is folded onto the developing thoracic region, and the tongue occupies an elevated position between the palatine shelves (Figure 3-19, *A* and *B*). By 9 weeks the upper facial complex has lifted away from the thorax and thus permits the tongue and lower jaw to grow forward so that the lower lip now is positioned in advance of the upper lip and the tongue is situated below the palatine shelves (Figure 3-19, *C* and *D*).

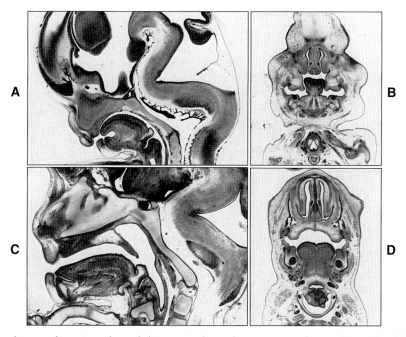

Figure 3-19 Sagittal and coronal sections through human embryos between 7 and 9 weeks. **A,** The folded head has the upper lip in front of the lower, with the tongue elevated. **B,** Palatine shelves are positioned on each side of the tongue. **C,** At 9 weeks the head is raised so that the tongue not only is lowered but also has grown forward. The lower lip is now slightly in front of the upper. **D,** In this coronal section the palatine shelves have fused over the lowered tongue. *(From Diewert V: Contribution of differential growth of cartilages to changes in craniofacial morphology. In Dixon AD, Sarnat BG, editors: Factors and mechanisms influencing bone growth, New York, 1982, Alan R. Liss.)*

For fusion of the palatine shelves to occur and (for that matter) fusion of any other processes, elimination of the epithelial covering of the shelves is necessary. As the two palatine shelves meet, adhesion of the epithelia occurs so that the epithelium of one shelf becomes indistinguishable from that of the other, and a midline epithelial seam that consists of two layers of basal epithelial cells forms. This midline seam must be removed to permit ectomesenchymal continuity between the fused processes. Even though the epithelial cells of the seam continue to divide, growth of the seam fails to keep pace with palatal growth so that the seam first thins to a single layer of cells and then breaks up into discrete islands of epithelial cells (Figure 3-20). The basal lamina surrounding these cells then is lost, and the epithelial cells lose their epithelial characteristics and assume fibroblast-like features. In other words, epithelial cells transform into mesenchymal cells; that is, they undergo an *epitheliomesenchymal transformation (transition)*. This is a fundamental embryonic process that also is implicated in the invasive behavior of epithelial neoplastic cells. During craniofacial development, such a transformation is a prerequisite for neural crest cell migration (see Chapter 2) and also may be implicated in cementoblast differentiation (see Chapter 9).

FORMATION OF THE TONGUE

The tongue begins to develop at about 4 weeks. The pharyngeal arches meet in the midline beneath the primitive mouth. Local proliferation of the mesenchyme then gives rise to a number of swellings in the floor of the mouth (Figure 3-21; see also Figure 3-9). First, a swelling (the *tuberculum impar*) arises in the midline in the mandibular process and is flanked by two other bulges, the *lingual swellings*. These lateral lingual swellings quickly enlarge and merge with each other and the tuberculum impar to form a large mass from which the mucous membrane of the anterior two thirds of the tongue is formed. The root of the tongue arises from a large midline swelling developed from the mesenchyme of the second, third, and fourth arches. This swelling consists of a *copula* (associated with the second arch) and a large *hypobranchial eminence* (associated with the third and fourth arches). As the tongue develops, the hypobranchial eminence overgrows the copula, which disappears. The posterior part of the fourth arch marks the development of the epiglottis.

The tongue separates from the floor of the mouth by a down-growth of ectoderm around its periphery, which subsequently degenerates to form the lingual sulcus and gives the tongue mobility. The muscles of the tongue have a different origin; they arise from the occipital somites, which have migrated forward into the tongue area, carrying with them their nerve supply, the twelfth cranial (*hypoglossal*) nerve (Figure 3-22).

This unusual development of the tongue explains its innervation. Because the mucosa of the anterior two thirds of the tongue is derived from the first arch, it is supplied by the nerve of that arch, the fifth cranial (trigeminal) nerve; whereas the mucosa of the posterior third of the tongue, derived from the third arch, is supplied by the ninth cranial (glossopharyngeal) nerve. As previously explained, the motor supply to the muscles of the tongue is the twelfth cranial nerve.

The development of the tongue and palate and the formation of the oral cavity are diagrammed in Figure 3-23, which illustrates midline sagittal sections through the developing embryo at progressively later stages of gestation.

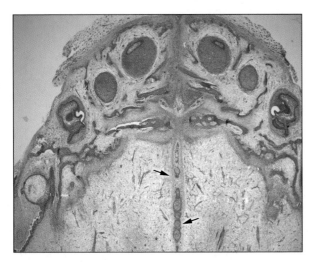

Figure 3-20 Ventrodorsal histologic section of the forming maxilla, from a human embryo, passing through the developing teeth and fusing palatal shelves. Remnants of the surface epithelium of the shelves (*arrows*) are visible along the line of fusion. (Courtesy M. Seccani Galassi.)

DEVELOPMENT OF THE SKULL

The skull can be divided into three components: (1) the *cranial vault*, (2) the *cranial base*, and (3) the *face* (Figure 3-24). Membranous bone, formed directly in mesenchyme with no cartilaginous precursor, forms the cranial vault and face (Figure 3-25) while the cranial base undergoes endochondral ossification (Figure 3-26). Some of these membrane-formed bones may develop secondary cartilages to provide rapid growth.

For skull development, standard texts on embryology should be consulted. This text considers in detail only the development of the jaws.

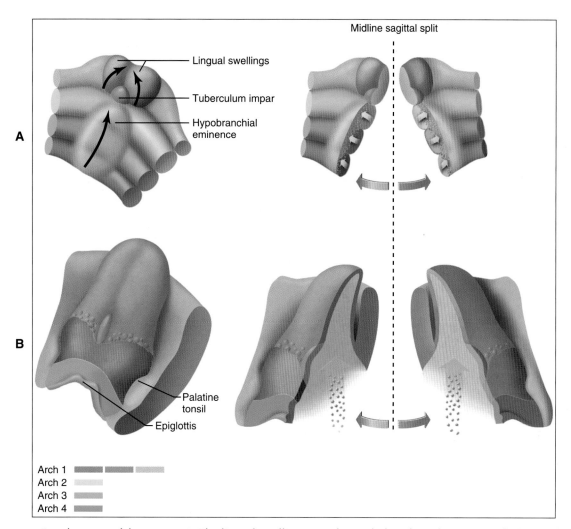

Figure 3-21 Development of the tongue. **A,** The lingual swellings, together with the tuberculum impar, which arise from the first arch, will form the anterior two thirds of the tongue. The hypobranchial eminence overgrows the second arch. **B,** Final disposition of the tongue and the relative contributions of the first to fourth arch. The arrow depicts the route of incoming occipital myotomes that form the tongue muscle.

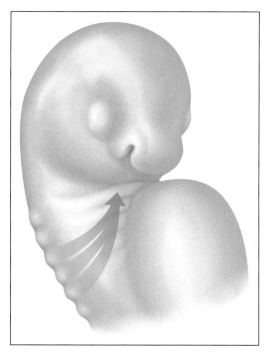

Figure 3-22 Occipital somites migrating forward into the floor of the mouth to form the tongue musculature.

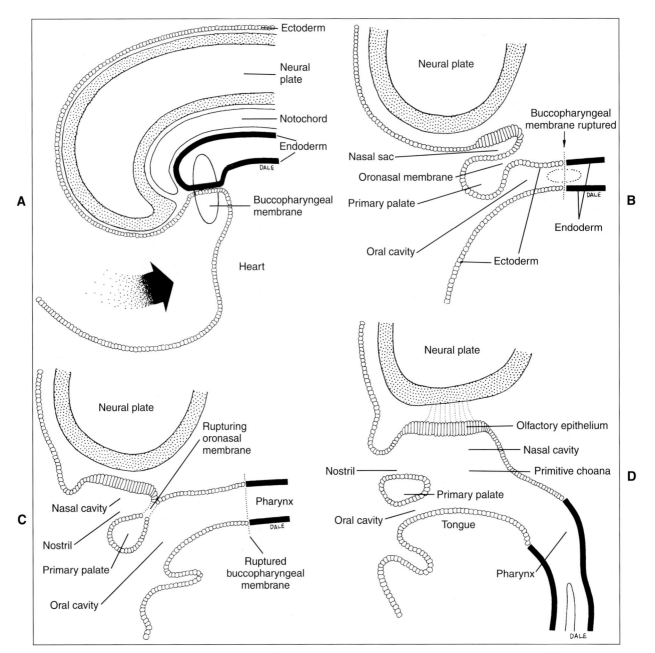

Figure 3-23 Summary of the development of the oral cavity as seen in midsagittal section. **A,** Head fold and formation of the stomatodeum, or oral cavity. **B,** Formation of the nasal pit and primary palate. **C,** How continuity is established between the presumptive nasal and oral cavities. **D** and **E,** Final anatomy of the nasal and oral cavities established by development of the secondary palate.

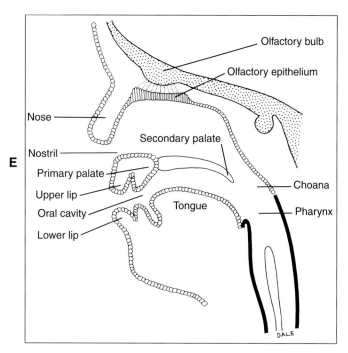

Figure 3-23, cont'd

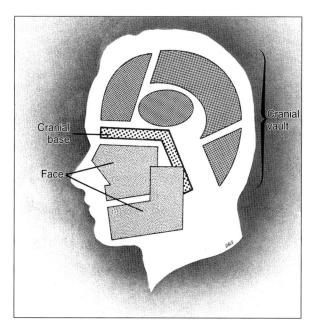

Figure 3-24 Subdivisions of the skull.

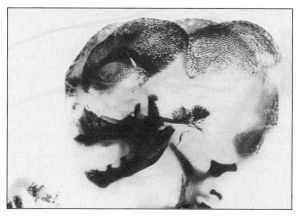

Figure 3-25 A 14-week cleared human embryo in which the mineralized bone has been stained with alizarin red. *(Courtesy V.M. Diewert, photographed from the University of Washington collection.)*

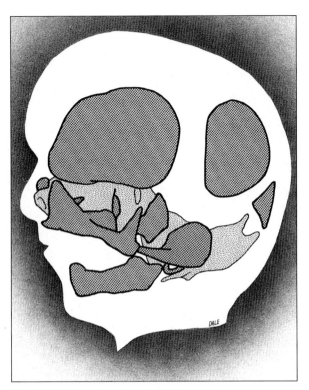

Figure 3-26 Diagram showing the cranial bones formed by intramembranous (*lighter shading; cranial vault, face*) and by endochondral (*darker shading; cranial base*) ossifications.

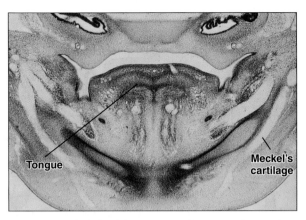

Figure 3-27 Slightly oblique coronal section of an embryo demonstrating almost the entire extent of Meckel's cartilage. (*From Diewert VM:* Am J Anat *167:495, 1983.*)

DEVELOPMENT OF THE MANDIBLE AND MAXILLA

The mandible and the maxilla form from the tissues of the first branchial arch, the mandible forming within the mandibular process and the maxilla within the maxillary process.

MANDIBLE

The cartilage of the first arch (Meckel's cartilage) forms the lower jaw in primitive vertebrates. In human beings, Meckel's cartilage has a close positional relationship to the developing mandible but makes no contribution to it. At 6 weeks of development this cartilage extends as a solid hyaline cartilaginous rod, surrounded by a fibro-cellular capsule, from the developing ear region (otic capsule) to the midline of the fused mandibular processes (Figure 3-27). The two cartilages of each side do not meet at the midline but are separated by a thin band of mesenchyme. The mandibular branch of the trigeminal nerve (the nerve of the first arch) has a close relationship to Meckel's cartilage, beginning two thirds of the way along the length of the cartilage. At this point the

mandibular nerve divides into lingual and inferior alveolar branches, which run along the medial and lateral aspects of the cartilage, respectively. The inferior alveolar nerve further divides into incisor and mental branches more anteriorly.

On the lateral aspect of Meckel's cartilage, during the sixth week of embryonic development, a condensation of mesenchyme occurs in the angle formed by the division of the inferior alveolar nerve and its incisor and mental branches. At 7 weeks, intramembranous ossification begins in this condensation, forming the first bone of the mandible (Figure 3-28). From this center of ossification, bone formation spreads rapidly anteriorly to the midline and posteriorly toward the point where the mandibular nerve divides into its lingual and inferior alveolar branches. This spread of new bone formation

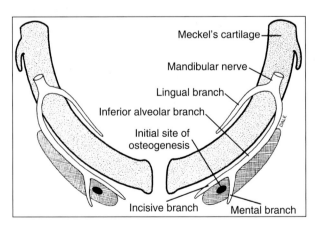

Figure 3-28 Site of initial osteogenesis related to mandible formation. Bone formation extends from this anteriorly and posteriorly along Meckel's cartilage.

occurs anteriorly along the lateral aspect of Meckel's cartilage, forming a trough that consists of lateral and medial plates that unite beneath the incisor nerve. This trough of bone extends to the midline, where it comes into approximation with a similar trough formed in the adjoining mandibular process. The two separate centers of ossification remain separated at the mandibular symphysis until shortly after birth. The trough soon is converted into a canal as bone forms over the nerve, joining the lateral and medial plates.

Similarly, a backward extension of ossification along the lateral aspect of Meckel's cartilage forms a gutter, later converted into a canal that contains the inferior alveolar nerve. This backward extension of ossification proceeds in the condensed mesenchyme to the point where the mandibular nerve divides into the inferior alveolar and lingual nerves. From this bony canal, extending from the division of the mandibular nerve to the midline, medial and lateral alveolar plates of bone develop in relation to the forming tooth germs so that the tooth germs occupy a secondary trough of bone. This trough is partitioned, and thus the teeth come to occupy

individual compartments, which finally are enclosed totally by growth of bone over the tooth germ. In this way the body of the mandible essentially is formed (Figure 3-29).

The ramus of the mandible develops by a rapid spread of ossification posteriorly into the mesenchyme of the first arch, turning away from Meckel's cartilage (Figure 3-30). This point of divergence is marked by the lingula in the adult mandible, the point at which the inferior alveolar nerve enters the body of the mandible.

Thus by 10 weeks the rudimentary mandible is formed almost entirely by membranous ossification, with little or no direct involvement of Meckel's cartilage (Figures 3-31 and 3-32). Meckel's cartilage has the following fate (see Table 3-1): its most posterior extremity forms the incus and malleus of the inner ear and the spheno-malleolar ligament. From the sphenoid to the division of the mandibular nerve into its alveolar and lingual branches, the cartilage is lost totally, but its fibrocellular capsule persists as the sphenomandibular ligament. From the lingula forward to the division of the alveolar nerve into its incisor and mental branches, Meckel's cartilage degenerates (see Figure 3-32). Forward from this point to the midline, some evidence exists that the cartilage might make a small contribution to the mandible by means of endochondral ossification.

The further growth of the mandible until birth is influenced strongly by the appearance of three secondary (growth) cartilages and the development of muscular attachments: the condylar cartilage, which is most

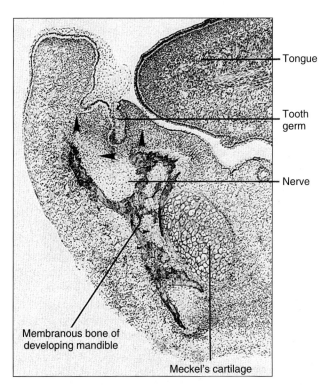

Figure 3-29 Photomicrograph of a coronal section through an embryo showing the general pattern of intramembranous bone deposition associated with formation of the mandible. The relationship among nerve, cartilage, and tooth germ is evident. Arrowheads indicate the future directions of bone growth to form the neural canal and lateral and medial alveolar plates. Compare this with the development of the maxilla (Figure 3-35).

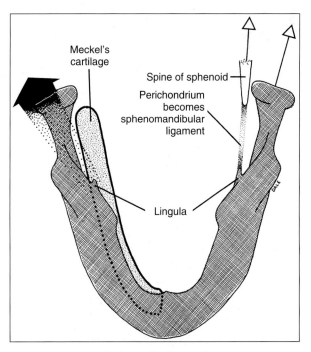

Figure 3-30 Spread of mandibular ossification away from Meckel's cartilage at the lingula.

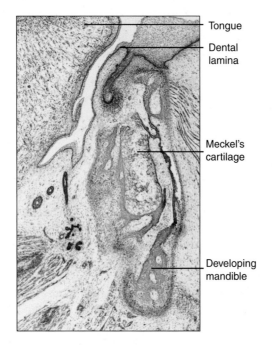

Tongue

Dental
lamina

Meckel's
cartilage

Developing
mandible

Figure 3-31 Photomicrograph of a sagittal section through the developing jaw of an embryo showing how bone forms around Meckel's cartilage as it forms the body of the mandible.

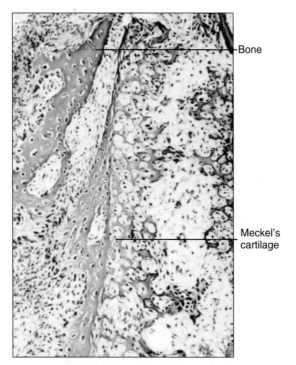

Bone

Meckel's
cartilage

Figure 3-32 Photomicrograph of the degeneration of Meckel's cartilage. As the cartilage is degraded, the space previously occupied by cartilage becomes filled with new bone. This is not an example of endochondral ossification, which involves deposition of bone on mineralized cartilage.

important; the coronoid cartilage; and the symphyseal cartilage. These cartilages are called *secondary* cartilages, to distinguish them from the *primary* Meckel's cartilage; they have a different histologic structure from the primary cartilages in that their cells are larger and less intercellular matrix is formed.

The condylar cartilage appears during the twelfth week of development and rapidly forms a cone-shaped or carrot-shaped mass that occupies most of the developing ramus (Figure 3-33). This mass of cartilage is converted quickly to bone by endochondral ossification (see Chapter 6), so that at 20 weeks only a thin layer of cartilage remains in the condylar head. This remnant of cartilage persists until the end of the second decade of life, providing a mechanism for growth of the mandible, in the same way as the epiphyseal cartilage does in the limbs.

The *coronoid* cartilage appears at about 4 months of development, surmounting the anterior border and top of the coronoid process. Coronoid cartilage is a transient growth cartilage and disappears long before birth.

The *symphyseal* cartilages, two in number, appear in the connective tissue between the two ends of Meckel's cartilage but are entirely independent of it. They are obliterated within the first year after birth. Small islands of cartilage also may appear as variable and transient structures in the developing alveolar processes.

Thus the mandible is a membrane bone, developed in relation to the nerve of the first arch and almost entirely independent of Meckel's cartilage. The mandible has neural, alveolar, and muscular elements (Figure 3-34), and its growth is assisted by the development of secondary cartilages.

MAXILLA

The maxilla also develops from a center of ossification in the mesenchyme of the maxillary process of the first arch. No arch cartilage or primary cartilage exists in the maxillary process, but the center of ossification is associated closely with the cartilage of the nasal capsule. As in the mandible, the center of ossification appears in the angle between the divisions of a nerve (that is, where the anterosuperior dental nerve is given off from the inferior orbital nerve). From this center, bone formation spreads posteriorly below the orbit toward the developing zygoma and anteriorly toward the future incisor region (Figure 3-35). Ossification also spreads superiorly to form the frontal process. As a result of this pattern of bone deposition, a bony trough forms for the infraorbital nerve. From this trough a downward extension of bone forms the lateral alveolar plate for the maxillary tooth germs. Ossification also spreads into the palatine process to form the hard palate. The medial alveolar plate develops from the junction of the palatal process and the main body of the forming maxilla. This plate, together with its lateral

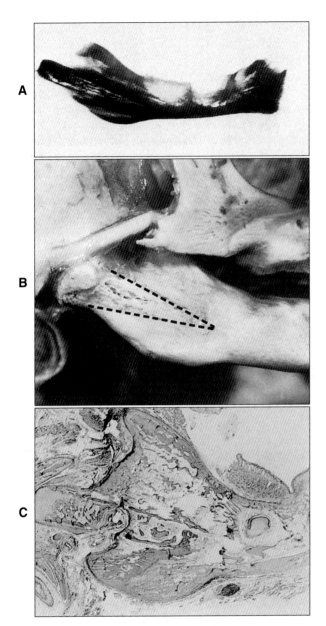

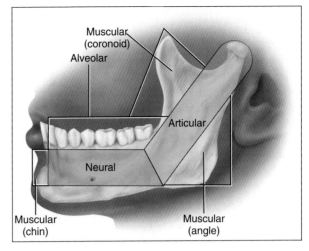

Figure 3-34 Differing developmental blocks for the mandible.

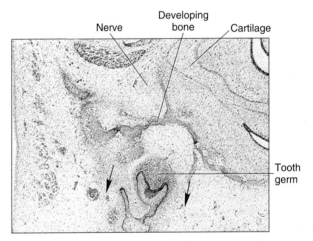

Figure 3-35 Coronal section through an embryo showing the general pattern of membranous bone deposition associated with formation of the maxilla. The relationship between cartilage, nerve, and tooth germ is evident. Arrows indicate the future directions of bone growth to form the lateral and medial alveolar plates. Compare this with the developing mandible in Figure 3-31.

Figure 3-33 Condylar cartilage. **A,** A radiograph of the mandible of a midterm fetus shows the carrot-shaped wedge of new bone that has formed from the condylar cartilage. **B,** The new bone as seen in a dried fetal mandible. **C,** Histologic examination of the same shows the distinction between cartilaginous and intramembranous ossification. *(A and B from Scott JH, Dixon AD:* Anatomy for students of dentistry, *London, 1979, Churchill Livingstone; C from Chi JG, Lee SK:* Sequential atlas of human development, *Seoul, South Korea, 1992, Medical Publishing.)*

counterpart, forms a trough of bone around the maxillary tooth germs, which eventually become enclosed in bony crypts in the same way as described for the mandible.

A secondary cartilage also contributes to the development of the maxilla. A *zygomatic,* or *malar,* cartilage

appears in the developing zygomatic process and for a short time adds considerably to the development of the maxilla. At birth the frontal process of the maxilla is well marked, but the body of the bone consists of little more than the alveolar process containing the tooth germs and small though distinguishable zygomatic and palatal processes. The body of the maxilla is relatively small because the maxillary sinus has not developed. This sinus forms during the sixteenth week as a shallow groove on the nasal aspect of the developing maxilla. At birth the sinus is still a rudimentary structure about the size of a small pea.

COMMON FEATURES OF JAW DEVELOPMENT

This account of jaw development shows that in their development the mandible and maxilla have much in common. Both begin from a single center of membranous ossification related to a nerve, both form a neural element related to the nerve, and both develop an alveolar element related to the developing teeth. Finally, both develop secondary cartilages to assist in their growth.

DEVELOPMENT OF THE TEMPOROMANDIBULAR JOINT

The temporomandibular joint is an articulation between two bones initially formed from membranous centers of ossification. Before the condylar cartilage forms, a broad band of undifferentiated mesenchyme exists between the developing ramus of the mandible and the developing squamous tympanic bone. With formation of the condylar cartilage, this band is reduced rapidly in width and is converted into a dense strip of mesenchyme. The mesenchyme immediately adjacent to this strip breaks down to form the joint cavity, and the strip becomes the articular disk of the joint.

The complicated changes that occur during embryogenesis between the fourth and eighth weeks of development have been described. They lead to, among other things, the formation of the face, mouth, and tongue and their associated structures. After 8 weeks, development is essentially a matter of growth.

CONGENITAL DEFECTS

The development of an individual is a complicated and delicately balanced process; malfunctions produce congenital defects. The genetic basis of some of these defects has been discussed previously. Environmental factors, including teratogens (agents causing congenital defects), also must be considered. The timing of environmental factors can be critical. If a teratogen exerts its effect during the first 4 weeks of life, when the embryo is developing rapidly, the teratogen usually damages so many cells that death of the embryo occurs. However, if only a few cells are damaged, normal proliferation is great enough that minor damage is eliminated readily. Probably, many teratogenic agents acting in this first phase of development are not appreciated because the embryo dies and is miscarried. A possible exception is alcohol, the effects of which are manifested in the so-called fetal alcohol syndrome, which does not necessarily kill the early embryo but stunts its repair potential. During the next stage of development,

between 4 and 8 weeks, when histodifferentiation and organ differentiation are taking place, teratogenic agents are most likely to produce malformation. The subsequent growth phase is not as susceptible to teratogenic agents.

Not surprisingly, therefore, most teratogenic agents leading to facial and dental malformations exert their effects during the period of morphogenesis and histodifferentiation within the embryo. These malformations include the various types of clefts, which can be understood readily from knowledge of embryology: the oblique facial cleft (results from lack of fusion between the maxillary process and lateral nasal process), the median cleft lip (harelip; lack of fusion between the two

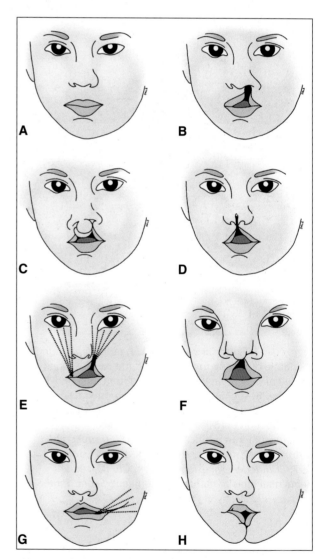

Figure 3-36 Types of facial clefts. **A,** Normal. **B,** Unilateral cleft lip. **C,** Bilateral cleft lip. **D,** Median cleft lip. **E,** Oblique facial cleft. **F,** Median cleft (frontonasal dysplasia). **G,** Lateral facial cleft. **H,** Mandibular cleft.

medial nasal processes), bilateral cleft lip (lack of fusion between the maxillary process and median nasal process), microstomia (which is an excessive merging of the mandibular and maxillary processes), the converse or macrostomia (resulting from failure of the maxillary and mandibular processes to fuse), and the rare mandibular cleft (Figures 3-36 and 3-37).

Clefts have different causes. Those of the lip and anterior maxilla result from defective development of the embryonic primary palate. Often when such clefts occur, the distortion of facial development prevents the palatine shelves from making contact when they swing into the horizontal position; thus clefts of the primary palate often are accompanied by clefts of the secondary (hard and soft) palate. Facial clefts usually result from a deficiency of mesenchyme in the facial region, caused by failure of the neural crest to migrate or failure of the facial mesenchyme to proliferate.

When clefts of the palate occur with no corresponding facial cleft, the cause is different (see Figure 3-37, G).

Such palatal clefts may result from (1) failure of the shelves and septum to contact each other because of a lack of growth or because of a disturbance in the mechanism of shelf elevation, (2) failure of the shelves and septum to fuse after contact has been made because the epithelium covering the shelves does not break down or is not resorbed, (3) rupture after fusion of the shelves has occurred, or (4) defective merging and consolidation of the mesenchyme of the shelves. The extent of clefting reflects the time when the processes involved in closure of the secondary palate have been affected. Full clefting results from interference at the start of closure and partial clefting later as the process proceeds posteriorly.

The types of environmental factors affecting the embryo can be classified into five groups: (1) infectious agents, (2) x-ray radiation, (3) drugs, (4) hormones, and (5) nutritional deficiencies. The classic example of an infectious agent causing a congenital defect is the rubella virus, which induces German measles. Among the

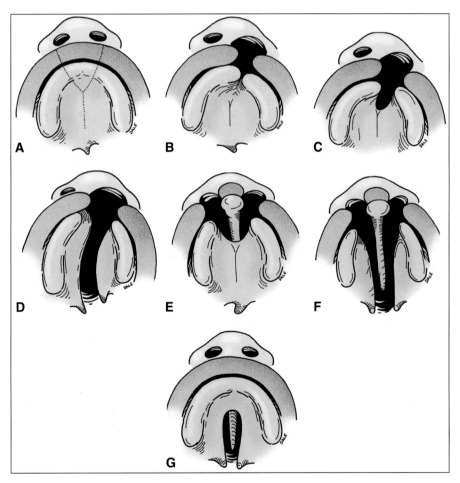

Figure 3-37 Palatal clefts seen from a ventral view. **A,** Normal. **B,** Cleft of lip and alveolus. **C,** Cleft of lip and primary palate. **D,** Unilateral cleft lip and palate. **E,** Bilateral cleft lip and primary palate. **F,** Bilateral cleft lip and palate. **G,** Cleft palate only.

widespread malformations that result from this infection of the mother are cleft palate and deformities of the teeth. The teratogenic effect of x-ray radiation is well understood, and many defects, including cleft palate, can result from the irradiation of pregnant women. In addition to affecting the embryo directly, x-ray radiation also may affect the germ cells of the fetus, causing genetic mutations that lead to congenital malformations in succeeding generations. Cortisone injected into mice and rabbits causes a high percentage of cleft palates in the offspring. The same is also true for nutritional deficiencies, especially vitamin deficiencies. Although vitamin deficiencies have been shown to be teratogenic in experimental animals, this effect has not been demonstrated in human beings.

RECOMMENDED READING

Brugmann SA, Tapadia MD, Helms JA: The molecular origins of species-specific facial pattern, *Curr Top Dev Biol* 73:1, 2006.

Creuzet S, Couly G, LeDouarin NM: Patterning the neural crest derivatives during development of the vertebrate head: insights from avian studies, *J Anat* 207:447, 2005.

Langman J: *Langman's medical embryology: human development—normal and abnormal*, ed 6, Baltimore, 1990, Williams & Wilkins.

Moore KL, Persaud TV: *The developing human: clinically orientated embryology*, ed 7, Philadelphia, 2003, Saunders.

Cytoskeleton, Junctions, Fibroblasts, and Extracellular Matrix

Arthur R. Hand and Antonio Nanci

CHAPTER OUTLINE

The various cells, tissues, and organs that compose the oral cavity and related structures are complex entities that exhibit unique developmental and functional characteristics. They, however, have several structural and functional features in common with other cells and tissues in various parts of the body. This chapter focuses on the cytoskeleton and cellular junctions of oral tissue cells and on the fibroblast and the extracellular matrix it produces. This chapter is intended to provide an overview of the subject area, and the reader is referred to a cell biology textbook, such as the one indicated in the recommended reading section, for more detailed coverage the characteristics that oral tissues share with their counterparts in other organs. The specific roles of oral tissue cells in their formation, growth, maintenance, and function are described fully in the following chapters.

CYTOSKELETON

Cells possess a cytoskeleton that provides a structural framework for the cell, facilitates intracellular transport, supports cell junctions and transmits signals about cell contact and adhesion, and permits motility. The three structural elements of the cytoskeleton are *microfilaments*, *intermediate filaments*, and *microtubules*. All are dynamic structures assembled from protein subunits and disassembled as cellular activities and external influences on the cell change.

Microfilaments are 6 to 8 nm in diameter and consist of globular *actin* molecules polymerized into long filaments (Figure 4-1). Microfilaments form tracks for the movement of *myosin* and serve as intracellular "muscles" concerned with the maintenance of cell shape, movement, and contractility. Microfilament networks, along with actin-binding and actin-bundling proteins, are found in association with adhesive cell junctions, as a "web" beneath cell membranes, especially the apical membrane, and as the structural "core" of microvilli and filopodia. Actin interacts with the other two components of the cytoskeleton.

Intermediate filaments are approximately 10 nm in diameter and have a diverse protein composition. They are not contractile but are important in the maintenance of cell shape and contact between adjacent cells and the extracellular matrix. In cells of mesenchymal origin such as fibroblasts and osteoblasts, intermediate filaments are polymers of the protein *vimentin* (Figure 4-2). In epithelial cells, intermediate filaments consist of *cytokeratins*. The filaments form bundles, called *tonofilaments*, that anchor on desmosomes (see Figure 4-2 *B* and *C*). Cytokeratins are a multigene family of proteins made up

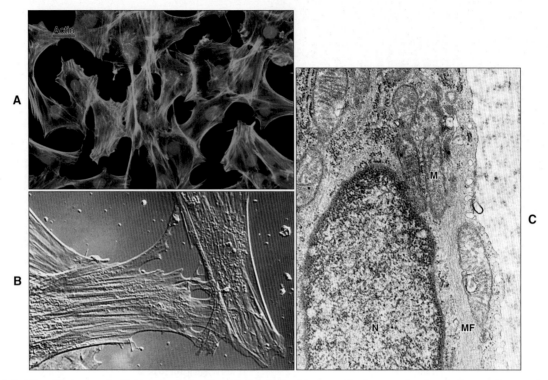

Figure 4-1 Microfilaments. **A,** Cultured osteogenic cells labeled with an antibody to actin, the main protein constituting microfilaments, using the fluorescence technique (nuclei are stained using DAPI [4,6-diamino-2-phenylindole] and appear blue). **B,** Nomarski differential interference contrast image of microfilament bundles in the cytoplasm of cultured fibroblasts from the pig periodontal ligament. Nomarski images are produced by using the interference conditions generated by optical-path-length differences of two beams of coherent light. The microfilament bundles appear as elongated, raised lines. **C,** Electron micrograph of microfilaments in the cytoplasm of a fibroblast. *MF,* Microfilaments; *M,* mitochondria; *N,* nucleus. (**A** *courtesy P. Tambasco de Oliveira;* **B** *courtesy Jane Aubin.)*

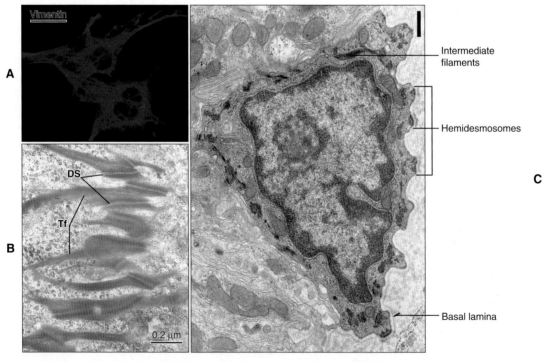

Figure 4-2 A, Intermediate filaments in cultured osteogenic cells stained for vimentin by the immunofluorescence method. **B** and **C,** Electron micrographs of intermediate filaments; these form discrete bundles, called tonofilaments *(Tf),* that insert into desmosomes *(DS)* or distribute around the periphery of a cell. **C,** Basal cell of a salivary gland excretory duct; hemidesmosomes form attachments to the basal lamina surrounding the duct.

of basic and more acidic proteins. Cytokeratins occur as linked acidic and basic pairs with differing combinations in different types of epithelia. Their expression patterns have been used to determine the relationship between cell types and as an indication of the origin of various tumors.

Microtubules are tubular or cylindrical structures with an average diameter of 25 nm (Figure 4-3). Microtubules are composed of the protein *tubulin* arranged in rings stacked end to end, making up the tubules. Microtubules provide internal support for the cell; are the basis of motility for certain organelles, such as cilia; act as guide paths and part of the motor mechanism for the movement of secretory vesicles and other organelles; and serve to position certain organelles within the cell.

INTERCELLULAR JUNCTIONS

When cells come into contact with one another, and sometimes with the extracellular matrix, specialized junctions may form at specific sites on the contacting cell membranes. These specialized junctions may be classified into several different categories as follows:

1. Occluding (tight) junctions (zonula occludens)
2. Adhesive junctions

a. Cell-to-cell
   i. *Zonula adherens*
   ii. *Macula adherens* (desmosome)
b. Cell-to-matrix
   i. Focal adhesions
   ii. Hemidesmosomes
3. Communicating (gap) junctions

The term *zonula* describes a junction that completely encircles the cell; *macula* indicates a junction that is more circumscribed in extent (e.g., patchlike). Junctions may occur in certain combinations. A *junctional complex*, present between cells of a simple or pseudostratified epithelium, usually consists of a tight junction, a *zonula adherens*, and a desmosome (Figure 4-4). On the molecular level, intercellular junctions typically consist of three components: a *transmembrane adhesive protein*, a *cytoplasmic adapter protein*, and a *cytoskeletal filament*. These three components differ depending on the type of junction.

In occluding, or tight junctions (Figure 4-5, A; see also Figure 4-4), the opposing cell membranes are held in close contact by the presence of transmembrane adhesive proteins arranged in anastomosing strands that encircle the cell. The intercellular space essentially is obliterated at the tight junction. The transmembrane adhesive proteins—which include *occludin*, members of the *claudin* family, and in some tissues, *junctional adhesion*

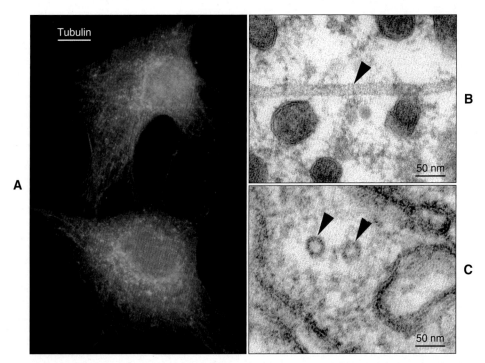

Figure 4-3 Microtubules. **A,** Fluorescent micrograph of cultured osteogenic cells labeled with an antibody to tubulin, the main protein of microtubules. **B** and **C,** Electron micrographs of portion of a longitudinally oriented (**B**) microtubule and cross-sectioned (**C**) microtubules *(arrowheads).*

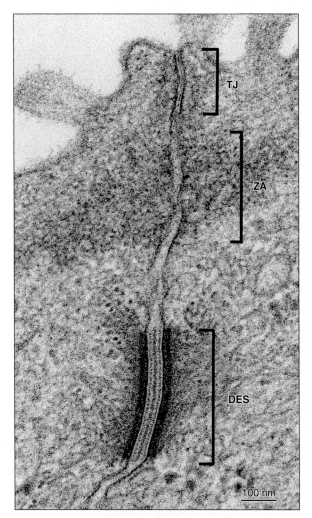

Figure 4-4 Electron micrograph of a junctional complex between epithelial cells of a salivary gland. In the tight junction (zonula occludens; *TJ*), located at the boundary of the apical and lateral cell membranes, the intercellular space is obliterated. In the adherens junction (zonula adherens, *ZA*), the cell membranes are separated by approximately 20 nm, and a dense mat of microfilaments is present in the cytoplasm. In the desmosome *(DES)*, the cell membranes are parallel and separated by approximately 25 nm, and a central dense line is present in the intercellular space. Intermediate filaments insert into dense plaques on the cytoplasmic surface of the desmosome.

molecule—interact homotypically with the same proteins on the adjacent cell. Several cytoplasmic proteins associate with the intracellular portions of the transmembrane proteins; these include cell polarity–related proteins, vesicular transport–related proteins, kinases, transcription factors, and a tumor suppressor protein. In addition, some of the cytoplasmic proteins of the tight junctions bind to actin filaments. Tight junctions control the passage of material through the intercellular spaces (e.g., from the interstitium to the lumen of a gland). They also have an important role as a "fence" to

define and maintain the two major domains of the cell membrane, the apical and basolateral surfaces. The "tightness" of the junction to water and ions (especially cations) is related to the specific claudin(s) present and is correlated with the number of strands of transmembrane proteins. For example, tight junctions joining salivary gland secretory cells have only two or three junctional strands and are relatively permeable to water, whereas those joining salivary gland striated duct cells may have six to nine strands and are relatively impermeable to water. The permeability of tight junctions in some tissues may be regulated by certain neurotransmitters and hormones.

Adhesive junctions hold cells together or anchor cells to the extracellular matrix. In contrast to tight junctions, the intercellular space in cell-cell adhesive junctions is maintained at approximately 20 nm. Adhesive junctions also are important in cellular signaling. Their cytoplasmic components may interact with the cytoskeleton, triggering changes in cell shape or motility, or with certain tumor suppressor molecules, or they may act as nuclear transcription factors or coactivators. In some instances, the loss of cell-cell or cell-matrix contact may lead to apoptosis (programmed cell death), whereas in others, loss of contact may lead to loss of cell polarity and differentiation or unregulated cell proliferation. In cell-cell adhesive junctions the principal transmembrane proteins are members of the *cadherin* family. Cadherins are calcium ion–dependent proteins that interact homotypically with cadherins on the adjacent cell. The cytoplasmic adapter proteins are members of the *catenin* family. Catenins interact with the cytoplasmic domain of the transmembrane cadherin molecule, with the cytoskeleton, and with a number of other proteins, including kinases, and tumor suppressor molecules that are associated with adhesive junctions. In the zonula adherens (see Figures 4-4 and 4-5, *B*), the cadherin family member is E-cadherin, α- and β-catenin are the cytoplasmic adapters, and actin filaments are the cytoskeletal component. The catenins and actin filaments are concentrated on the cytoplasmic side of the cell membrane at the zonula adherens to form a dense web that is continuous with the terminal web of actin at the apical (and sometimes the basal) end of the cells. Another transmembrane adhesive protein present in the adherens junction is *nectin*, a member of the immunoglobulin superfamily. Nectin has an important role during junction formation, establishing the initial adhesion site and recruiting E-cadherin and other proteins to the junction. Other cytoplasmic proteins associated with the zonula adherens include *p120 catenin*, a signaling molecule associated with E-cadherin that is important in stabilizing the junction; *afadin*, which links nectin to the actin cytoskeleton; *vinculin* and *α-actinin*, which are actin-binding proteins; and *ponsin*, which links afadin and vinculin (see Figure 4-5, *B*).

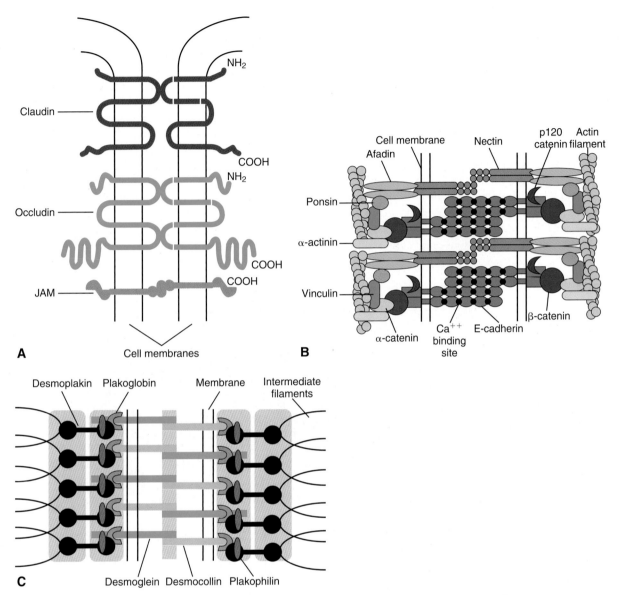

Figure 4-5 Diagrams showing molecular structures of intercellular junctions. **A,** Tight junction. **B,** adhering junction. **C,** desmosome. *JAM,* Junctional adhesion molecule.

In the desmosome (see Figures 4-4 and 4-5, C), the cadherins are *desmoglein* and *desmocollin*. The interaction of these transmembrane proteins with those from the adjacent cell results in a dense line in the middle of the intercellular space at the desmosome. The catenins are *desmoplakin*, plakoglobin, and *plakophilin*, which form an electron-dense plaque on the cytoplasmic side of the desmosome. This plaque serves as an attachment site for the cytoskeletal components, which in the case of the desmosome are intermediate filaments.

Cell-matrix junctions have a structural organization similar to that of cell-cell adhesive junctions, but they use different molecular components and attach the cell to the extracellular matrix. In focal adhesions the transmembrane component is a member of the *integrin*

family of adhesion molecules. Integrins are heterodimers of different alpha and beta subunits that occur in different combinations with specificity for various extracellular matrix molecules. The cytoplasmic adapter proteins, which include the actin-binding proteins α-actinin, vinculin, and *talin*, link the transmembrane integrins to the actin cytoskeleton. Binding of the integrin to *collagen*, laminin, fibronectin, and other extracellular matrix proteins results in recruitment and remodeling of the actin cytoskeleton. Ligand binding by integrins also leads to the recruitment and activation of various intracellular signaling molecules, including guanine nucleotide–binding proteins and several protein kinases.

Hemidesmosomes link the cell to the basal lamina and, through additional extracellular molecules, to the rest of the extracellular matrix. The transmembrane adhesive molecules present in hemidesmosomes (Figure 4-6) are the integrin $\alpha_6\beta_4$, which binds specifically to the basal lamina glycoprotein laminin, and *collagen XVII* (also identified as *BP180*). Like a desmosome, the cytoplasmic adapter proteins, *bullous pemphigoid antigen 230* (BP230) and *plectin*, form a dense plaque on the cytoplasmic surface of the hemidesmosome, which functions as an attachment site for intermediate filaments.

Gap junctions are plaquelike regions of the cell membrane where the intercellular space narrows to 2 to 3 nm and transmembrane proteins of the *connexin* family form aqueous channels between the cytoplasm of adjacent cells (Figure 4-7). These proteins have specific tissue and cellular distributions and confer differing permeability properties to the gap junctions. Six connexin molecules form a *connexon*, which has a central channel approximately 2 nm in diameter (see Figure 4-7, *D*). The connexons in one cell pair with connexons in the adjacent cell to create a patent channel. Small molecules such as ions and signaling molecules can move readily from one cell to another. Gap junctions electrically couple cells and allow for a coordinated response to a stimulus by the cells that are interconnected.

Cell-cell and cell-matrix junctions have important roles in the differentiation, development, and function of normal cells, tissues, and organs. However, the functions of these junctions may be altered or disrupted by genetic abnormalities of junctional or cytoskeletal proteins or by autoimmune diseases in which circulating

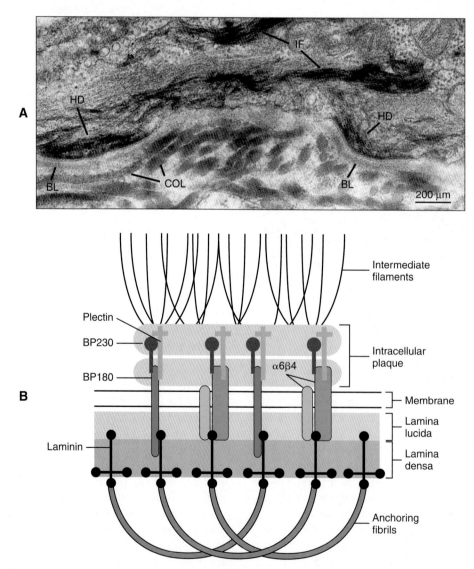

Figure 4-6 A, Electron micrograph of hemidesmosomes (*HD*) of a basal epithelial cell from a rat salivary gland excretory duct. *BL,* Basal lamina; *COL,* collagen fibrils; *IF,* intermediate filaments. **B,** Diagram of a hemidesmosome.

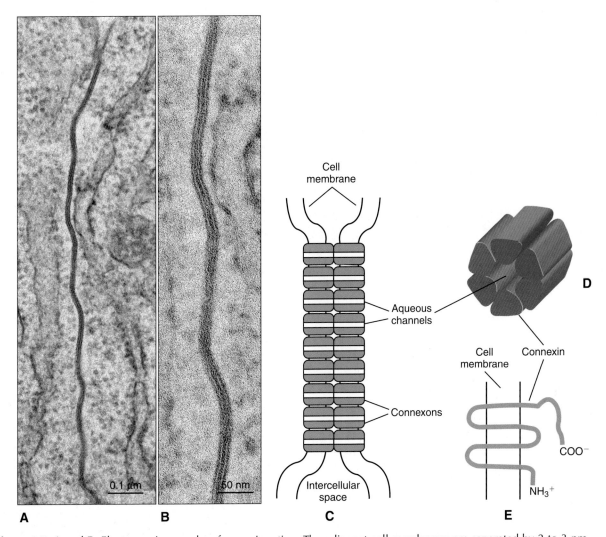

Figure 4-7 A and **B**, Electron micrographs of a gap junction. The adjacent cell membranes are separated by 2 to 3 nm. Indistinct regions in the junction result from the varying orientation of the membranes in the section. **C** to **E**, Diagrams of gap junction structure. **C**, View corresponding to thin-section electron micrographs. **D**, A single connexon consists of six connexin molecules. **E**, A connexin molecule has four transmembrane domains, and the N- and C-terminal domains are located in the cytoplasm.

antibodies to junctional proteins are present. Mutations of connexin genes have been identified as the bases for certain types of deafness, congenital cataracts, a demyelinating disease (Charcot-Marie-Tooth), and oculodentaldigital dysplasia, a disease that exhibits craniofacial abnormalities, syndactyly, conductive hearing loss, and hair and nail abnormalities. Several types of *epidermolysis bullosa*, a blistering skin disorder, have been shown to be caused by mutations of the genes for various desmosomal, hemidesmosomal, and intermediate filament proteins. In addition, some forms of the disease are caused by mutations of the genes for extracellular matrix proteins involved in cell-matrix adhesion. *Pemphigus vulgaris* and *pemphigus foliaceus*, blistering diseases of the oral mucosa and skin, respectively, are caused by autoantibodies to desmoglein-3 and desmoglein-1, the cadherin in desmosomes. Another blistering skin

disease, *bullous pemphigoid*, results from the presence of autoantibodies to the hemidesmosomal components collagen XVII (BP180) and BP230.

EPITHELIUM–CONNECTIVE TISSUE INTERFACE

All epithelia are separated from the underlying connective tissue by a layer of extracellular matrix organized as a thin sheet immediately adjacent to the epithelial cells. This is the *basal lamina*, which is a product of the epithelium and connective tissue. The basal lamina, along with hemidesmosomes, attaches the epithelium to the underlying connective tissue, functions as a filter to control the passage of molecules between the epithelium and connective tissue, and acts as a barrier to cell

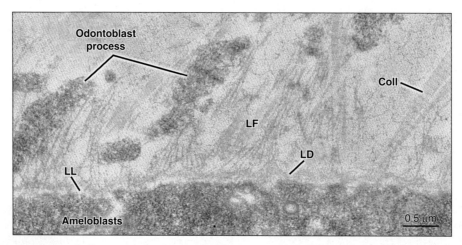

Figure 4-8 Electron micrograph illustrating the three components—the lamina lucida *(LL)*, lamina densa *(LD)*, and lamina fibroreticularis *(LF)*—forming the basal lamina associated with epithelial cells, here interposed between differentiating ameloblasts and odontoblasts. *Coll*, Collagen fibrils.

migration. The basal lamina also has important signaling functions, which are essential for epithelial differentiation and the development and maintenance of cell polarity.

The basal lamina has an overall thickness of 50 to 100 nm and consists of two structural components, the *lamina lucida*, adjacent to the basal cell membrane, and the *lamina densa*, between the lamina lucida and the connective tissue (Figure 4-8). In epithelia, there is a third layer, the *lamina fibroreticularis*, closely associated with the lamina densa. The main constituents of the basal lamina are *type IV collagen*, which forms a "chicken-wire" network; the adhesive glycoprotein *laminin*; and a *heparan sulfate proteoglycan*. *Fibronectin*, an adhesive glycoprotein, *type III collagen* (reticular fibers), *type VII collagen* (anchoring fibrils), and other types of collagen all made by fibroblasts are present in the lamina fibroreticularis and help maintain the attachment of the basal lamina to the underlying connective tissue.

FIBROBLASTS

Fibroblasts are the predominant cells of connective tissue. They are responsible for the formation and maintenance of the fibrous components and the ground substance of connective tissue.

CELLULAR ORGANIZATION

Fibroblasts usually are recognized by their association with collagen fiber bundles (Figures 4-9 and 4-10). The resting fibroblast is an elongated cell with little cytoplasm and a dark-staining, flattened nucleus containing condensed chromatin (see Figure 4-9, A). Active fibroblasts have an oval, pale-staining nucleus and a

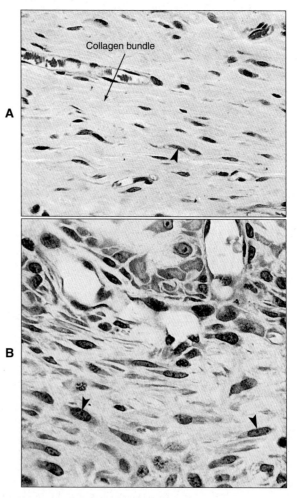

Figure 4-9 Light microscope images. **A,** Inactive fibroblasts can be identified by their relationship to collagen bundles, their dark-staining, usually elongated nuclei *(arrowhead)*, and their sparse cytoplasm. **B,** Active fibroblasts *(arrowheads)* have larger, less densely stained nuclei and clearly visible cytoplasm.

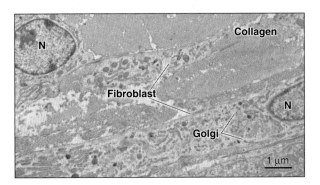

Figure 4-10 In electron micrographs, fibroblasts typically lie adjacent to collagen fibrils and have elongated cell bodies. The quantity and density of heterochromatin in nuclei *(N)* is indicative of their activity; active fibroblasts have less heterochromatin, and it is also less condensed. Protein synthetic organelles are more abundant in active fibroblasts and the Golgi complex, in particular, is more extensive in these cells.

greater amount of cytoplasm (see Figure 4-9, *B*). The degree of synthetic and secretory capacity of fibroblasts is evidenced by the amount of rough endoplasmic reticulum, secretory granules, and mitochondria, and the extent of the Golgi complex in their cytoplasm (Figure 4-10).

CONTRACTION AND MOTILITY

Fibroblasts exhibit motility and contractility, which are important during connective tissue formation and remodeling and during wound repair. The actin cytoskeleton of fibroblasts allows them to move through the ground substance. In certain tissues, fibroblasts have significant contractile properties and are called *myofibroblasts*.

JUNCTIONS

In most connective tissues, fibroblasts are separated from one another by the extracellular matrix components; therefore, intercellular junctions are not present. Exceptions are embryonic tissue, in which gap junctions occur frequently, and the periodontal ligament, in which fibroblasts frequently exhibit cell-to-cell contacts of the adherens type. Fibroblasts also form specialized focal contacts with components of the extracellular matrix (Figure 4-11). In such a focal contact, also called a *fibronexus*, a dense plaque may be present on the cytoplasmic side of the cell membrane, and intracellular actin filaments are linked by a transmembrane αβ integrin complex to extracellular fibrils of the adhesive glycoprotein fibronectin.

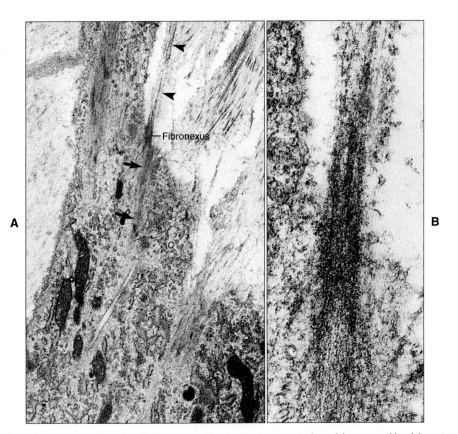

Figure 4-11 A and **B,** Electron micrographs illustrating a fibronexus in a periodontal ligament fibroblast. Intracellular filaments of actin *(arrows)* are linked to extracellular filaments of fibronectin *(arrowheads)* via transmembrane integrin receptors. *(From Garant PR, Cho MI, Cullen MR: J Periodontal Res 17:70-79, 1982.)*

HETEROGENEITY

Although fibroblasts of different tissues have similar appearances, distinguishable mainly as active or quiescent, considerable heterogeneity exists within fibroblast populations. This heterogeneity is manifested as differences in their synthetic products, rates of synthesis and turnover, response to regulatory molecules, proliferation rates, and others. For example, it has been estimated that collagen in the periodontal ligament has a turnover rate approximately 8 times that of collagen in the skin and about twice that of gingival collagen.

AGING

Fibroblasts originate from mesenchymal cells. Once differentiated, they can replicate by mitosis. An inverse correlation has been found between the age of a donor and the number of divisions that cultured fibroblasts can undergo before they become senescent. The exact cause of this replicative senescence is unknown. Fibroblasts from long-lived species can divide more times than fibroblasts from short-lived species, suggesting a genetic component. Many studies have demonstrated a relationship between the gradual loss of telomere DNA at the ends of the chromosomes that occurs during each mitotic cycle and the onset of senescence. Other studies suggest that the accumulation of oxidative

damage to DNA and proteins also contributes to senescence. Fibroblasts that become senescent remain viable but exhibit changes in metabolism and gene expression that suggest an aging phenotype (e.g., a decrease in the production of extracellular matrix proteins and an increase in the production of degradative enzymes). Altogether, these changes result in many of the signs associated with human aging (e.g., skin fragility and loss of elasticity and decreased capacity for wound healing).

SECRETORY PRODUCTS OF FIBROBLASTS

Fibroblasts can synthesize and secrete a variety of extracellular molecules. These include the components of the fibrous elements of the extracellular matrix, the components of the amorphous ground substance, and a number of biologically active molecules, such as proteinases, cytokines, and growth factors.

COLLAGENS

The collagen superfamily contains at least 27 types of collagens that together constitute the most abundant proteins found in the body (Table 4-1). All collagens are composed of three polypeptide alpha chains coiled

TABLE 4-1   The Collagens

TYPE	GENE NAME	CHAINS	SUPRAMOLECULAR ASSEMBLY	CHARACTERISTIC FEATURES	TISSUE DISTRIBUTION	MAJOR FUNCTION
Fibril-Forming Collagens						
I	COL1A1, COL1A2	$[\alpha1(I)]_3$, $[\alpha1(I)]_2\alpha2(I)$	Fibrils 300 nm	Most abundant collagen	Abundant in skin, bone, dentin, cememtum, tendons, ligaments, and most connective tissue	Provides tensile strength to connective tissue
II	COL2A1	$[\alpha1(II)]_3$	Fibrils 300 nm	Forms heterofibrils with Col IX and XI	Cartilage, vitreous humor, intervertebral disk	Provides tensile strength to connective tissue
III	COL3A1	$[\alpha1(III)]_3$	Fibrils 300 nm	Abundant in elastic tissues	Embryonic connective tissue, pulp, skin, blood vessels, lymphoid tissue (reticular fibers)	Provides tensile strength to connective tissue
V	COL5A1, COL5A2, COL5A3	$[\alpha1(V)]_2\alpha2(V)$	Fibrils 390 nm	Forms core of type I fibrils; Binds to DNA, heparan sulfate, thrombospondin, heparin, and insulin	Basal laminae, blood vessels, ligaments, skin, dentin, periodontal tissues	Provides tensile strength
		$\alpha1(V)\alpha2(V)\alpha3(V)$ $[\alpha1(V)]_3$			Placenta; Present in tumor cells	

TABLE 4-1 The Collagens—cont'd

TYPE	GENE NAME	CHAINS	SUPRAMOLECULAR ASSEMBLY	CHARACTERISTIC FEATURES	TISSUE DISTRIBUTION	MAJOR FUNCTION
XI	COL11A1, COL11A2	$\alpha1(XI)\alpha2(XI)\alpha3(XI)$	Fibrils	Forms core of type II fibrils	Cartilage, vitreous humor, placenta	Provides tensile strength, controlling lateral growth of type II fibrils
XXIV	COL24A1	$[\alpha1(XXIV)]_3$	Fibrils	Displays structural features unique to invertebrate fibrillar collagens	Bone, cornea	Regulation of type I fibrillogenesis
XXVII	COL27A1	$[\alpha1(XXVII)]_3$	Fibrils	Presence of triple helix imperfections	Cartilage, eye, ear, lungs	Association with type II fibrils (?)
Microfibril-Forming Collagens						
VI	COL6A1, COL6A2, COL6A3	$\alpha1(VI)\alpha2(VI)\alpha3(VI)$	Beaded filaments 150 nm	Highly disulfide cross-linked	Ligament, skin, cartilage, placenta	Bridging between cells and matrix
Transmembrane Collagens						
XIII	COL13A1	$[\alpha1(XIII)]_3$	Linear	Single transmembrane domain and a large, mainly collagenous ectodomain	Epidermis, hair follicle, cell surfaces, focal adhesions, intercalated disks	Cell-matrix, cell-cell adhesion
XVII	COL17A1	$[\alpha1(XVII)]_3$	Linear		Hemidesmosomes	Cell attachment to matrix
XXIII	COL23A1	$[\alpha1(XXIII)]_3$	Linear	Single-pass hydrophobic transmembrane domain	Heart, retina, metastatic tumor cells	Cell-matrix interaction
XXV	COL25A1	$[\alpha1(XXV)]_3$	Linear	Extracellular domain deposited in β-amyloid plaques	Neurons	Neuron adhesion
Multiplexin (Endostatin-Forming Collagens)						
XV	COL15A1	$[\alpha1(XV)]_3$	Linear	Contains antiangiogenic factor	Epithelial and endothelial basement membranes, internal organs (adrenal gland, pancreas, and kidney)	Stabilizes skeletal muscle cells and microvells
XVIII	COL18A1	$[\alpha1(XVIII)]_3$		Contains antiangiogenic factor	Epithelial and endothelial basements membranes, liver, lung, and kidney	Eye development; anchors vitreal collagen fibrils, determining the retinal structure and the closure of the neural tube
Fibril-Associated Collagens with Interrupted Triple Helices (FACIT)						
IX	COL9A1, COL9A2, COL9A3	$\alpha1(IX)\alpha2(IX)\alpha3(IX)$	200 nm	Interacts with glycosamino-glycans in cartilage	Cartilage, vitreous humor	Attaches functional groups to surface of type II fibrils
XII	COL12A1	$[\alpha1(XII)]_3$			Widespread in many connective tissue (type I—containing tissues)	Modulates fibril interactions
XIV	COL14A1	$[\alpha1(XIV)]_3$		Associated with type I	Widespread in many connective tissue	Modulates fibril interactions
XVI	COL16A1	$[\alpha1(XVI)]_3$		Numerous interruptions in the triple helix may make this molecule elastic or flexible	Endothelial, perineural, muscle, some epithelial basal laminae, cartilage, and placenta	Associates with heterotypic II/IX/XI fibrils and fibrillin-1 filaments

Continued

TABLE 4-1   The Collagens—cont'd

TYPE	GENE NAME	CHAINS	SUPRAMOLECULAR ASSEMBLY	CHARACTERISTIC FEATURES	TISSUE DISTRIBUTION	MAJOR FUNCTION
XIX	COL19A1	$[\alpha 1 (XIX)]_3$			Endothelial, perineural, muscle, and some epithelial basal laminae	Muscle differentiation
XX	COL20A1	$\alpha 1 (XX)_3$			Corneal epithelium, skin, cartilage, tendon, heart, lung, liver, skeletal muscle, kidney, pancreas, spleen, testis, ovary, subthalamic nucleus	Associates with fibrils
XXI	COL21A1	$\alpha 1 (XXI)_3$			Widespread in developing connective tissues, abundant in vascular walls	Maintain extracellular matrix integrity
XXII	COL22A1	$\alpha 1 (XXII)_3$			Tissue junctions: myotendinous junction, articular cartilage—synovial fluid, hair follicle—dermis	Cell adhesion ligand, interactions with microfibrils (?)
XXVI	COL26A1	$[\alpha 1 (XXVI)]_3$		Disulfide bonds that form the trimer are made in an N-terminal noncollagenous domain.	Developing and adult testis and ovary	Unknown
Meshwork-Forming Collagens						
IV	COL4A1, COL4A2, COL4A3, COL4A4, COL4A5, COL4A6	$[\alpha 1 (IV)]_2 \alpha 2 (IV)$	Sheetlike network 390 nm	Interactions with type IV, perlecan, laminin, nidogen, integrin	Basal laminae	Structural network of basal laminae together with laminins, proteoglycans, and entactin/nidogen
VIII	COL8A1, COL8A2	$[\alpha 1 (VIII)]_2 \alpha 2 (VIII)$	Hexagonal network 130 nm		Cornea (Descemet's membrane), endothelium	Tissue support, porous meshwork
X	COL10A1	$[\alpha 1 (X)]_3$	Hexagonal network 150 nm		Hypertrophic zone of cartilage growth plate	Calcium binding
Anchoring-Fibril Collagen						
VII	COL7A1	$[\alpha 1 (VII)]_3$	450 nm	Forms bundles made of dimers anchored in anchoring plaques and basal laminae	Epithelium (skin, mucosa)	Strengthens epithelial—connective tissue junction
Protein-Containing Triple Helical Collagen Domains						

around each other to form the typical collagen triple-helix configuration. Common features include the presence of the amino acid glycine in every third position (Gly-X-Y repeating sequence), of hydroxyproline and hydroxylysine, and of noncollagenous domains, and a high proportion of proline residues. Variations among the collagens include differences in the assembly of the basic polypeptide chains, different lengths of the triple helix, interruptions in the helix, and differences in the terminations of the helical domains.

Mesenchymal cells and their derivatives (fibroblasts, chondrocytes, osteoblasts, odontoblasts, and cementoblasts) are the major producers of collagens. Other cell types such as epithelial, endothelial, muscle, and Schwann cells also synthesize collagens, although on a more limited basis in terms of amount and variety of collagen types.

The collagen superfamily is subdivided into the nine subfamilies largely based on their supramolecular assemblies (see Table 4-1):

1. *Fibrillar collagens (types I, II, III, V, XI, XXIV, and XXVII):* These collagens aggregate in a highly organized manner in the extracellular compartment to form fibrils with a typical 64-nm banding pattern. Type I collagen is the most abundant in most connective collagen tissues. Collagen fibrils often are composed of more than one type of collagen. For example, type I collagen fibrils often contain small amounts of types III, V, and XII. Type V collagen is believed to regulate fibril diameter.

2. *Basal lamina collagen (type IV):* Collagen type IV is similar in size to type I collagen but does not assemble as fibrils. It contains frequent nonhelical sequences and aggregates in a sheetlike, chicken-wire configuration. Type IV collagen is a major component of the basal lamina and is a product of epithelial cells.

3. *Fibril-associated collagens with interrupted triple helices (FACIT):* Collagens IX, XII, XIV, XVI, XIX, XX, XXI, XXVI, and XXII consist of chains that have different lengths and contain a variety of noncollagenous domains. They exhibit several interruptions in the triple helix and are found in various locations in different tissues. Several of the FACIT collagens associate with fibrillar collagens and other extracellular matrix components. Of these, type XIX collagen is found in basal laminae, and appears to be important for skeletal muscle cell differentiation. Although sometimes classified as a FACIT, type XXVI collagen seems to lack features of this and other collagen types. Type XXVI is found in the extracellular matrix of the testis and ovary; however, its function and association with other collagens or matrix proteins have not been established.

4. *Network-forming collagens:* Type VIII collagen assembles into a hexagonal lattice, which is believed to impart compressive strength while providing an open, porous meshwork. Type X collagen has a similar size and structure and is largely restricted to the hypertrophic zone of the epiphyseal cartilage growth plate.

5. *Anchoring-fibril collagen:* Collagen VII has unusually large nonhelical ends making up two thirds of the size of the molecule. The C-terminal ends associate to form dimers that subsequently are assembled into the anchoring fibrils that extend from the basal lamina into the underlying connective tissue.

6. *Microfibril-forming collagen:* Type VI collagen, which has large N- and C-terminal globular domains that associate in an end-to-end fashion, forms beaded filaments. Type VI collagen is present in most connective tissues. This collagen has binding properties for cells, proteoglycans, and type I collagen and may serve as a bridge between the cells and the matrix.

7. *Transmembrane collagen types XIII, XVII, XXIII, and XXV:* These collagens are transmembrane proteins with extracellular collagenous domains and a C-terminal noncollagenous domain that functions in cell adhesion. Type XVII collagen is found in hemidesmosomes of basal epidermal cells and attaches the cells to the basal lamina. Type XIII collagen is present in focal adhesion sites of fibroblasts and at cell-matrix interfaces in some epithelia, muscle, and nerves. Type XIII collagen also is present in the cell-cell adhesive specializations. These collagens may interact with other cell surface or extracellular matrix molecules to alter cell behavior.

8. *Multiplexin (endostatin-forming) collagens:* Type XVIII collagen is a component of basal laminae of epithelial and endothelial cells and is believed to stabilize structures of the basal lamina. Type XVIII collagen has multiple interruptions in the central helical domain and a large, unique C-terminal nonhelical domain. This C-terminal domain can be cleaved by extracellular proteases to form endostatin, a potent inhibitor of endothelial cell migration and angiogenesis. In the brain, endostatin may be deposited in the amyloid plaques of Alzheimer's disease. Type XV collagen has a similar structure and a wider distribution, including the papillary dermis. However, its C-terminal endostatin-like domain (restin) has less potent antiangiogenic activity than that of type XVIII collagen. Both collagens have glycosaminoglycan side chains and also can be classified as proteoglycans. The C-terminal domain of type IV collagen also inhibits endothelial cell migration and angiogenesis.

9. *Proteins containing helical collagenous domains:* There is also a highly heterogenous group of proteins that contain collagen domains but have not been defined as collagens.

COLLAGEN SYNTHESIS AND ASSEMBLY

As a secretory protein, fibrous collagen is synthesized as a proprotein (procollagen) in a manner similar to secretory proteins of other cells (Figure 4-12). Messenger RNA directs the assembly of specific amino acids into polypeptide chains on ribosomes associated with the rough endoplasmic reticulum. These initial polypeptide chains are about one and a half times longer than those in the final collagen molecule because they have N- and C-terminal extensions that are important for assembly of the triple-helical molecule. As the chains are synthesized,

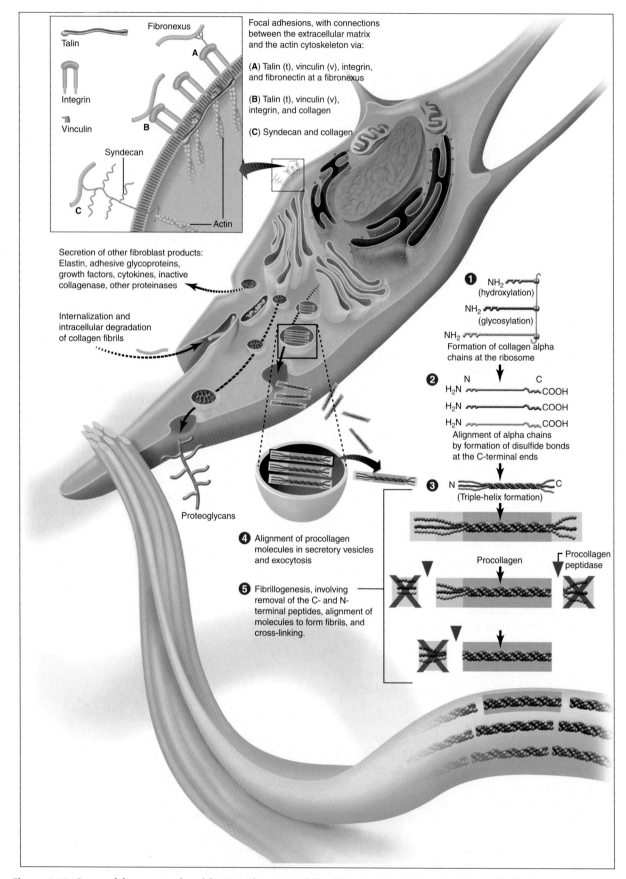

Figure 4-12 Some of the structural and functional aspects of fibroblasts, and formation of collagen fibrils (1-5).

they are translocated into the lumen of the rough endoplasmic reticulum, where several posttranslational modifications occur. The first modification is hydroxylation of many of the proline and lysine residues in the chain, which permits hydrogen bonding with the adjacent chains as the triple helix is assembled. The vitamin C–dependent enzymes *prolylhydroxylase* and *lysylhydroxylase* are required for this step. In vitamin C deficiency, fewer collagen molecules are formed and they are less stable. Tissues with a high collagen content and high rate of turnover of collagen, such as the periodontal ligament, are affected severely; one of the early symptoms of vitamin C deficiency (scurvy) is loosening of the teeth. Through the action of *galactosyltransferase* in the rough endoplasmic reticulum, some of the hydroxylysine residues are glycosylated by addition of galactose.

The three polypeptide chains then are assembled into the triple helix. Proper alignment of the chains is achieved by disulfide bonding at the C-terminal extension, a process catalyzed by the enzyme protein disulfide isomerase. The three chains then twist around themselves to "zip up" the helix. The assembled helix then is transported to the Golgi complex, where glycosylation is completed by the addition of glucose to the O-linked galactose residues. Secretory granules containing the procollagen molecules are formed at the *trans* face of the Golgi complex (see formation of bone collagen in Chapter 6) and are released subsequently by exocytosis at the cell surface.

The formation of typical banded collagen fibrils occurs extracellularly (Figure 4-13). The C-terminal extensions, and at least part of the N-terminal ones,

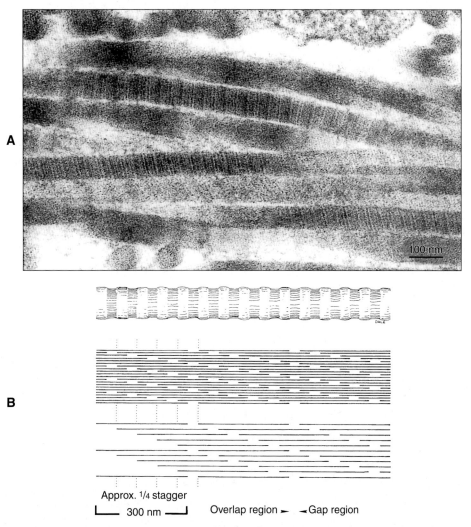

Approx. ¼ stagger

|___ 300 nm ___| Overlap region ► ◄ Gap region

Figure 4-13   A, Transmission electron micrograph of collagen fibrils showing the typical 64-nm banding pattern revealed by the differential binding of heavy metal stains used in such preparations. **B,** Diagram illustrating the arrangement of collagen molecules in a banded collagen fibril. In electron micrographs of negatively stained preparations, densely stained molecules fill the gap regions or holes between the ends of adjacent collagen molecules. In hard tissues (bone, dentin, and cementum), these holes are filled with mineral crystals.

are removed by the action of C- and N-proteinases in the secretory granule as the molecules are about to be secreted and also extracellularly soon after their release. The main C-proteinase is identical to bone morphogenetic protein-1. The shortened collagen molecules align as five-unit, quarter-staggered microfibrils, which then assemble in a parallel fashion, giving rise to a regular series of gaps or holes within the fibril. These gaps are the location of the initial deposits of mineral associated with the collagen fibrils in bone, dentin, and cellular cementum. After the fibrils are assembled, the remaining portions of the N-terminal extensions are removed by procollagen peptidase. The oxidation of some lysine and hydroxylysine residues by the extracellular enzyme *lysyl oxidase*, forming reactive aldehydes, results in intermolecular cross-links that further stabilize the fibrils. The newly deposited fibrils are of small diameter and length. As the tissues mature, the fibrils may increase in diameter (by a much as tenfold) and length to further strengthen the tissue.

Inherited Diseases Involving Collagens

Several mutations occur in collagen genes, resulting in a variety of different phenotypes depending on the affected collagen. Some of the more common mutations include *osteogenesis imperfecta*, or brittle bone disease, caused by mutations of the type I collagen genes and often including dental abnormalities; several types of *Ehlers-Danlos syndrome* (hyperextensible skin, hypermobile joints, and tissue fragility), resulting from mutations in the type I, type III, or type V collagen genes; *Stickler's syndrome*, caused by mutations in the type II or type XI collagen genes and characterized by retinal detachments,

cataracts, hearing loss, joint problems, cleft palate, and facial and dental abnormalities; *Alport's syndrome*, nephrosis caused by defects of the basal lamina in the kidney glomerulus and sensorineural hearing loss because of mutations in certain type IV collagen genes; and different forms of *epidermolysis bullosa*, a separation of the epidermis and dermis, caused by mutations of the type VII or type XVII collagen genes. Other mutations in collagen genes causing less common diseases have been identified, and it is likely that additional mutations that cause or contribute to other human diseases will be discovered.

ELASTIN

Elastin is a rubberlike protein produced by fibroblasts and smooth muscle cells. Its formation follows a pathway similar to that described for collagen, with final assembly into sheets (laminae) or fibers occurring outside the cell. The elastic properties of elastin result from numerous intermolecular cross-links between lysine groups, formed by the enzyme lysyl oxidase, and its highly hydrophobic nature. To form an elastic fiber, the glycoproteins *fibrillin-1*, *fibrillin-2*, and several *microfibril-associated glycoproteins* are secreted first and assembled into microfibrils. The microfibrils then provide a scaffold for assembly of elastic fibers (Figure 4-14). As the elastin accumulates, the microfibrils are displaced peripherally, resulting in a core of elastin surrounded by a sleeve of microfibrils. Mutations in the fibrillin-1 gene result in *Marfan syndrome*, the second most common inherited connective tissue disease.

Microfibrils may exist in the absence of elastin, in which case they may be called *oxytalan* fibers. During elastic

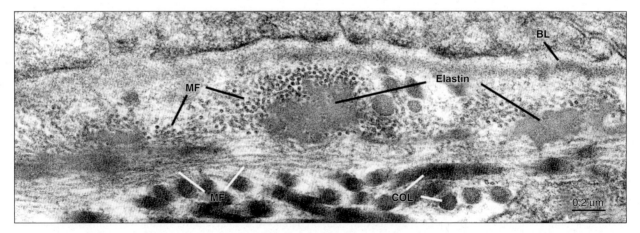

Figure 4-14 Electron micrograph of elastic fibers adjacent to epithelial cells of a salivary gland excretory duct. Elastin has a dense, amorphous appearance; numerous longitudinal and cross-sectioned microfibrils *(MF)* surround the elastin. *BL,* Basal lamina; *COL,* collagen fibrils.

fiber formation, the ratio of microfibrils to elastin is greater than in mature elastic fibers; these developing elastic fibers have been called *elaunin* fibers.

PROTEOGLYCANS

The ground substance of the extracellular matrix appears amorphous in the microscope but contains a complex mixture of macromolecules with important functions. These macromolecules interact with cells and the fibrous components of the matrix and are involved in adhesion and signaling events. The ground substance also is highly hydrated, providing a mechanism for regulating tissue water content and the diffusion of nutrients, waste products, and other molecules. Fibroblasts synthesize two main classes of macromolecules making up the ground substance: *proteoglycans* and *glycoproteins*.

Proteoglycans are a large group of extracellular and cell surface–associated molecules that consist of a protein core to which *glycosaminoglycan* chains are attached. Glycosaminoglycans are long chains of repeating disaccharide units consisting of a hexosamine and uronic acid. Depending on the combination of hexosamine and uronic acid, several different glycosaminoglycans are recognized. The large number of carboxyl and sulfate groups in glycosaminoglycans makes them acidic (negatively charged). They readily bind various proteins and other molecules, and their hydrophilic nature allows them to bind large amounts of water.

Hyaluronic acid is a large glycosaminoglycan present in most connective tissues and is especially abundant in embryonic tissues and cartilage. With its bound water, hyaluronic acid forms a viscous hydrated gel. In cartilage, hyaluronic acid forms a large aggregate with 50 to 100 molecules of the proteoglycan monomer *aggrecan* (Figure 4-15). This aggregated proteoglycan, with its bound water, accounts for the resistance of cartilage to compressive forces. A similar aggregating proteoglycan, *versican*, is present in many connective tissues. Nonaggregating proteoglycans, typically containing one to a few glycosaminoglycan chains, include *decorin*, fibromodulin, perlecan, agrin, glypican, syndecan, and CD44. Decorin and fibromodulin bind to collagen and probably function in regulating the growth and/or diameter of collagen fibrils (Figure 4-16). Perlecan and agrin are heparan sulfate proteoglycans of basal laminae and bind to several matrix glycoproteins. Perlecan is present in almost all basal laminae and in cartilage, whereas agrin is found in high concentrations in basal lamina at specific sites, for example, the neuromuscular junction and the kidney glomerulus. Glypican is a lipid-anchored membrane proteoglycan, and syndecan and CD44 are transmembrane proteoglycans that bind

cells to collagen, fibronectin, hyaluronic acid, and other matrix molecules.

An important property of cell surface and matrix proteoglycans is their ability to bind growth factors, cytokines, and other biologically active molecules. At the cell surface, membrane-associated proteoglycans such as syndecan and glypican are capable of binding members of the fibroblast growth factor and transforming growth factor β families, hepatocyte growth factor, and others and presenting them to their specific receptors on the surface of the same cell. In some cases, proteoglycans modulate the activity of the bound growth factor; in other cases, they are essential coreceptors for the growth factor. Through interactions of the cytoplasmic domain of its core protein with cytoskeletal elements, kinases, and other proteins, syndecan is involved in transmembrane signaling. In the extracellular matrix, growth factors bound to proteoglycans constitute a reservoir of active molecules that can exert their effects on nearby cells. In matrices that are remodeled continually, such as that of bone, bound growth factors may be released during matrix turnover.

GLYCOPROTEINS

Several glycoproteins are found in the ground substance; a number of these have adhesive properties. One of their primary functions is to bind cells to extracellular matrix elements.

Fibronectin is a major extracellular matrix and plasma glycoprotein synthesized by hepatocytes and fibroblasts. Fibronectin consists of two disulfide-linked polypeptide chains that have several structural domains capable of reacting with cells and extracellular matrix components such as heparin, collagen, and fibrin. Through these linkages, fibronectin is involved in the attachment, spreading, and migration of cells.

Tenascin is a large molecule with a six-arm, star-shaped structure. Tenascin is synthesized at specific times and locations during embryogenesis and is present in adult connective tissues, but with a more restricted distribution. Tenascin binds to fibronectin and to proteoglycans, particularly the cell surface proteoglycan syndecan. Tenascin blocks the binding capacity of syndecan, thereby allowing cells to move more freely. The migratory pathway for neural crest cells is forecast by the expression of tenascin along that pathway. Tenascin also is present in developing cartilage.

Thrombospondin is expressed in a number of tissues and is synthesized by several cell types. Thrombospondin has a trimeric or pentameric structure and functions at the cell surface and in the extracellular matrix to promote cell attachment, spreading, and migration. Thrombospondin also is important for the proper organization of collagen fibrils in the skin and cartilage.

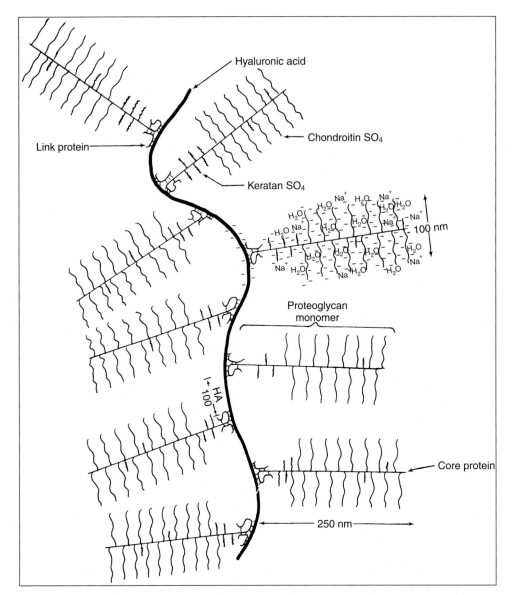

Figure 4-15 Diagram of a proteoglycan aggregate. Aggregating proteoglycans are abundant in cartilage. Fibrous connective tissues contain similar aggregating proteoglycans and smaller nonaggregating proteoglycans. These smaller proteoglycans are similar in structure to the proteoglycan monomers shown in this figure; some may have only one or two glycosaminoglycan chains. *(From Daniel JC. In Meyer J, Squier CA, Gerson SJ et al, editors:* The structure and function of oral mucosa, *New York, 1984, Pergamon Press.)*

GROWTH FACTORS AND CYTOKINES

Fibroblasts, particularly those activated and responding to some type of stimulation, such as inflammation or mechanical forces, secrete a number of growth factors, cytokines, and inflammatory mediators. The repertoire of factors varies depending on the location and type of fibroblast but may include interleukin-1, interleukin-6, and interleukin-8, tumor necrosis factor α, prostaglandin E_2, platelet-derived growth factor, insulin-like growth factor-1, transforming growth factor β, vascular endothelial growth factor, fibroblast growth factor 2, hepatocyte growth factor, and keratinocyte growth factor. These molecules, principally acting locally in a paracrine or autocrine fashion, have important roles in developmental processes, wound healing, and tissue remodeling.

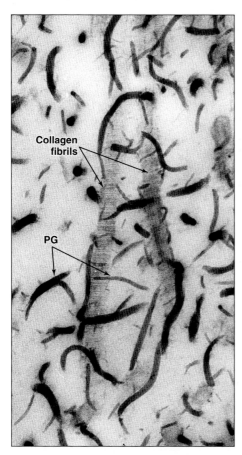

Figure 4-16 Collagen fibrils in loose connective tissue surrounded and connected by small and large proteoglycans *(PG)*. The proteoglycans are stained densely because of special tissue preparation procedures. *(From Erlinger R, Willerhausen-Zönnchen B, Welsch U: J Periodontal Res 30:108-115, 1995.)*

EXTRACELLULAR MATRIX DEGRADATION

In addition to their important function in the synthesis and assembly of the extracellular matrix, fibroblasts also participate in the remodeling of connective tissues through the degradation of collagen and other extracellular matrix molecules and their replacement by newly synthesized molecules. These processes are essential for certain aspects of normal embryonic development, tissue morphogenesis, and remodeling and also occur during wound repair, inflammatory diseases, and tumor growth and metastasis. Two mechanisms for the degradation of collagen have been recognized: (1) the secretion by cells of enzymes that sequentially degrade collagen and other matrix molecules extracellularly, and (2) the selective ingestion of collagen fibrils by fibroblasts and their intracellular degradation.

The collagen triple helix is highly resistant to proteolytic attack. The *matrix metalloproteinase* (MMP) family is a large family of proteolytic enzymes that includes *collagenases* (MMP-1, MMP-8, and *MMP-13*), gelatinases (MMP-2 and *MMP-9*), metalloelastase (MMP-12), stromelysins (MMP-3, MMP-10, and *MMP-11*), and *matrilysins* (MMP-7 and *MMP-26*). In addition to these secreted enzymes, several membrane-type (MT) MMPs exist. MT-MMPs have transmembrane domains and extracellular active sites. These enzymes are capable of degrading collagen and other matrix macromolecules into small peptides extracellularly (Figure 4-17). The MMPs are synthesized and secreted by fibroblasts, inflammatory cells, and some epithelial and tumor cells. Extracellular degradation often occurs in inflammatory lesions or when large amounts of collagen

---

TOPICS FOR CONSIDERATION   Intercellular Communication

Cell-cell and cell-matrix signaling are crucial factors for the development, maintenance, and function of tissues and organs. Adjacent cells may communicate via cell-cell contact at specialized intercellular junctions, whereas cells separated by variable distances may communicate by the secretion of hormones, cytokines, growth factors, or other substances. Cells also communicate with their extracellular matrix by means of cell-surface receptors of the integrin family. Fibroblasts use all of these mechanisms to communicate with adjacent cells and their surrounding environment.

Fibroblasts respond to and produce a wide variety of factors that influence their behavior, as well as the behavior of other cells. These may include factors involved in normal developmental or physiologic processes in addition to a variety of substances released by different cells during infections, tumorigenesis, and other pathologic processes. Because of the heterogeneity of fibroblast populations, cells located in different tissues and organs may exhibit different responses or may be unresponsive to a specific factor. The inflammatory mediators released by cells of the immune system in individuals with gingival and periodontal disease are of particular significance in dentistry. Interactions of the signals generated by receptors for these factors are responsible for the control of fibroblast gene expression, proliferation,

Continued

TOPICS FOR CONSIDERATION   Intercellular Communication—cont'd

apoptosis, and cytoskeletal dynamics. The factors known to have significant effects on gingival and periodontal fibroblasts include the proinflammatory cytokines interleukin-1 (IL-1), IL-6, IL-8, tumor necrosis factor α (TNF-α), and interferon-γ, the antiinflammatory cytokines IL-4 and IL-10, and the growth factors granulocyte-macrophage colony-stimulating factor (GM-CSF), transforming growth factor β (TGF-β), fibroblast growth factor-2 (FGF-2), and platelet-derived growth factor (PDGF). Additionally, several components of periodontal bacteria that may be released in diseased tissues have effects on fibroblasts. These components include lipopolysaccharide, phosphorylated dihydroceramides and phosphatidylethanolamine, lipid A-associated protein, bacterial fimbriae, and various bacterial surface proteins. Fibroblasts respond to these bacterial products by releasing IL-1, IL-6, IL-8, TNF-α, monocyte chemotactic protein-1, and prostaglandins.

These factors have a wide range of effects on fibroblasts. For example, IL-1 and TNF-α increase the secretion of prostaglandins, which are proinflammatory mediators that promote tissue destruction. They also promote synthesis and release of matrix metalloproteinases that degrade extracellular matrix components. The various growth factors induce fibroblast proliferation and increase the synthesis of extracellular matrix components. PDGF also is a chemotactic agent, and FGF-2 promotes cell migration. TGF-β and GM-CSF promote synthesis of alpha smooth muscle actin and induce the differentiation of fibroblasts to myofibroblasts. In contrast, interferon-γ has antifibrotic effects, decreasing alpha smooth muscle actin expression and inhibiting cell proliferation.

Many of these cytokines and growth factors also play important roles in the process of wound healing. Platelets in the blood clot release PDGF, TGF-β, and insulin-like growth factor-1, which attract neutrophils, macrophages, mast cells, fibroblasts, and endothelial cells to the wound site, forming a granulation tissue. Epidermal growth factor (also released by platelets),

insulin-like growth factor-1, and keratinocyte growth factor (FGF-7; released by fibroblasts) promote proliferation and migration of epithelial cells to cover the wound site. TGF-β, FGF-2 and GM-CSF induce fibroblast proliferation, extracellular matrix secretion, and differentiation into myofibroblasts, which are important for wound contraction. The fibrotic response strengthens the wound but also results in scar formation. In normal healing, myofibroblasts are eliminated by apoptosis, and the scar is reduced through gradual remodeling of the connective tissue. In some individuals, the healing process is prolonged, with continued growth factor stimulation of fibrous tissue formation and decreased extracellular matrix degradation, resulting in formation of a hypertrophic scar or keloid. Interestingly, certain early embryonic tissues heal without scarring. Differences in the inflammatory response and the resulting combination of cytokines and growth factors in embryonic wounds from those present in more mature tissues probably account for the scarless healing. For example, embryonic wound sites contain lower levels of the TGF-β1 and TGF-β2 isoforms, which promote a fibrotic response, and higher levels of the TGF-β3 isoform, which reduces extracellular matrix deposition and scarring. Wounds and incisions of the oral mucosa typically heal without scarring; whether this reflects cytokine and growth factor profiles similar to those found during embryonic healing or is due to other mechanisms is unknown.

Current research efforts are focused on further defining the role of growth factors and cytokines in normal and diseased tissues and during wound healing. An increased knowledge of the multiple mechanisms that cells use to communicate with one another will facilitate development of new therapeutic approaches to treat periodontal disease and improve tissue healing.

Arthur R. Hand
Department of Craniofacial Sciences
University of Connecticut Health Center
Farmington, Connecticut

---

must be degraded rapidly. Several mechanisms are used to regulate this process, which is necessary to avoid indiscriminate degradation of matrix components at other times. Some of the normal components of serum, such as α$_2$-*macroglobulin*, inhibit MMPs. The MMPs are secreted as inactive precursors (proenzymes) and must be cleaved proteolytically themselves to become active. MT-MMPs, which are activated intracellularly before insertion into the membrane, can activate certain MMPs such as gelatinase A (MMP-2) and

collagenase 3 (MMP-13). Activated gelatinases, along with other extracellular proteinases, in turn can activate collagenases and other soluble MMPs. Finally, many cells secrete inhibitors of MMPs, called *tissue inhibitors of metalloproteinases*. Fibroblasts secrete the activators and the inhibitors of MMPs, which allow these cells to participate in regulating extracellular degradation.

Intracellular degradation is considered the most important mechanism for the physiologic turnover and remodeling of collagenous connective tissue (Figure 4-18).

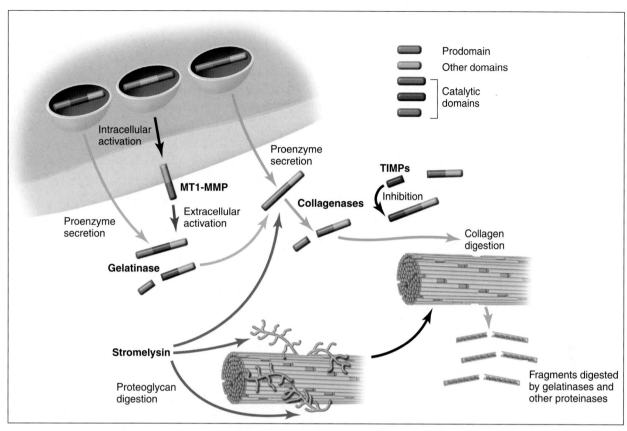

Figure 4-17 Sequence of events in the extracellular degradation of collagen fibrils. Fibroblasts, inflammatory cells, epithelial cells and tumor cells produce soluble and/or membrane-type matrix metalloproteinases (MMPs). The prodomain of membrane-type MMPs (MT-MMP) is cleaved intracellularly by a furin-like enzyme, and the active enzyme is inserted into the cell membrane. Soluble MMPs are secreted as inactive proenzymes. The prodomains of gelatinase A (MMP-2) and stromelysin 1 (MMP-3) are cleaved by MT1-MMP or other extracellular proteinases; the activated stromelysin and gelatinase then can activate collagenases (e.g., MMP-1 and MMP-13). Stromelysin also digests proteoglycans and other matrix glycoproteins. The activated collagenases cleave the collagen molecules of the fibril into two smaller fragments, which may be further digested by gelatinases and other proteinases. MT1-MMP also can digest collagen fibrils and other extracellular matrix molecules. Collagenases and other MMPs are inhibited by tissue inhibitors of metalloproteinases (*TIMPs*), which bind to the active site of the enzyme.

This process involves recognition of the fibrils to be degraded, possibly through binding to fibroblast integrin receptors; partial digestion of the fibrils into smaller fragments, probably by gelatinase A (MMP-2); phagocytosis of the fragments; formation of a phagolysosome; and intracellular digestion of the collagen fragments within the acidic environment of the phagolysosome by lysosomal enzymes, particularly the *cathepsins*. Little is known about how these processes are regulated and carried out.

SUMMARY

Cells interact with and respond to their neighbors and to their environment in many ways. These interactions include the formation of specialized cell-cell and cell-matrix junctions and the synthesis and secretion of a variety of products to create and maintain the cellular environment. Cell-cell and cell-matrix junctions are involved in cell adhesion, organization of the cytoskeleton, intercellular and intracellular signaling, and development and maintenance of the differentiated state. The proteins, glycoproteins, and proteoglycans of the extracellular matrix function in cell-matrix adhesion and signaling; regulate diffusion of nutrients, waste products and soluble signaling molecules; impart connective tissues with their characteristic properties of tensile and compressive strength and elasticity; and in certain tissues provide the appropriate conditions for the nucleation and growth of mineral crystals.

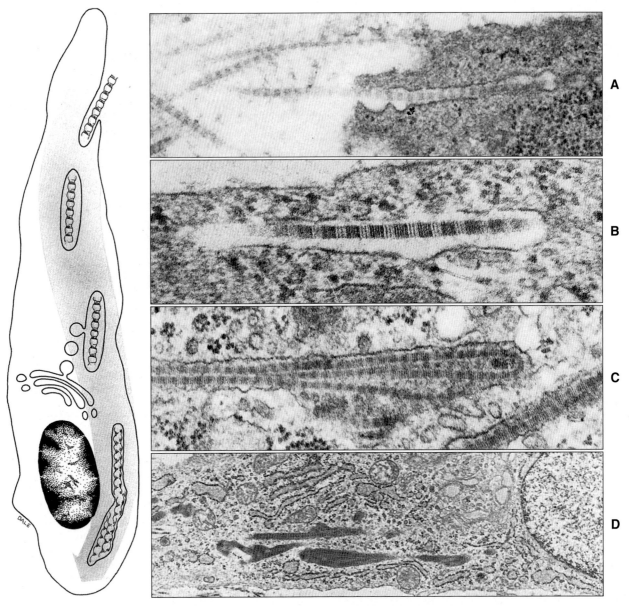

Figure 4-18 Intracellular degradation of collagen by fibroblasts. **A,** Ingestion of extracellular collagen fibrils. **B,** Formation of phagosome. **C,** Initial fusion of lysosomes with collagen-containing phagosome. **D,** Advanced stages of intracellular collagen degradation in dense lysosomal structures. *(**B** from Ten Cate AR, Deporter DA, Freeman E: Am J Orthod 69:155-168, 1976.)*

RECOMMENDED READING

Cattaruzza S, Perris R: Approaching the proteoglycome: molecular interactions of proteoglycans and their functional output, *Macromol Biosci* 6:667, 2006.

Erez N, Bershadsky A, Geiger B: Signaling from adherens-type junctions, *Eur J Cell Biol* 84:235, 2005.

Kottke MD, Delva E, Kowalczyk AP: The desmosome: cell science lessons from human diseases, *J Cell Sci* 119:797, 2006.

Laird DW: Life cycle of connexins in health and disease, *Biochem J* 394:527, 2006.

Nagase H, Visse R, Murphy G: Structure and function of matrix metalloproteinases and TIMPS, *Cardiovasc Res* 69:562, 2006.

Pollard TD, Earnshaw WC: *Cell biology*, Philadelphia, 2004, Saunders.

Schneeberger EE, Lynch RD: The tight junction: a multifunctional complex, *Am J Physiol* 286:C1213, 2004.

Development of the Tooth and Its Supporting Tissues

Chapter 3 explained how the stomatodeum, or primitive oral cavity, is formed. Under a light microscope the newly formed stomatodeum can be seen to be lined by a primitive two- or three-cell—thick layered epithelium covering an embryonic connective tissue that, because neural crest cells have migrated in it, is termed *ectomesenchyme*.

This chapter discusses the histologic aspect of tooth development and the coming together of the different tissues that form the tooth and its surrounding tissues. However, to better understand *morphogenesis*, the molecular signals that control cell growth, migration, and ultimately cell fate and differentiation also must be considered. For every developmental event, whether of limb, kidney, or tooth, a complex and intricate cascade of gene expression takes place to direct the cells to the right place and onto the proper differentiation pathway. Because hundreds of genes likely are expressed for each developmental pathway, this chapter covers only the most important signaling molecules and pathways so far described.

The molecular aspect of tooth development is interesting in that it shares many similarities with development of a number of other organs (e.g., lung and kidney) and that of the limb. Thus the tooth organ represents an advantageous system in which to study not only its own development but also developmental pathways in general. Interestingly, many of these pathways all result from epithelial-mesenchymal interactions in which essentially the same molecular mediators are implicated. In the case of mammalian tooth development, most molecular analyses have been done in the mouse because it is readily amenable to genetic analysis and manipulations (knockout and transgenic animals).

PRIMARY EPITHELIAL BAND

Chapter 3 explains how, after about 37 days of development, a continuous band of thickened epithelium forms around the mouth in the presumptive upper and lower jaws. These bands are roughly horseshoe shaped and correspond in position to the future dental arches of the upper and lower jaws (Figures 5-1 and 5-2, A and B). The formation of these thickened epithelial bands is the result not so much of increased proliferative activity

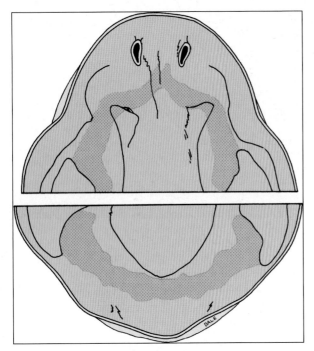

Figure 5-1 Schematic representation of the early oral cavity showing the internal surface of the upper and lower jaws, and illustrating the position of the primary epithelial band. *(Adapted from Nery EB, Kraus BS, Croup M: Arch Oral Biol 15:1315, 1970.)*

within the epithelium as of a change in orientation of the mitotic spindle and cleavage plane of dividing cells (Figure 5-2, C). Each band of epithelium, called the *primary epithelial band*, quickly gives rise to two subdivisions: the *dental lamina*, which forms first, and the *vestibular lamina*, which forms shortly afterward and which is positioned just in front of the dental lamina. A key feature of the initiation of tooth development is the formation of localized thickenings or *placodes* within the primary epithelial bands. It is noteworthy that placodes morphologically similar to those of the dental placodes also initiate the development of other ectodermal appendages (see box by Irma Thesleff for a more detailed consideration of placodes and their implication in tooth development and ectodermal dysplasias).

DENTAL LAMINA

On the anterior aspect of the dental lamina, continued and localized proliferative activity leads to the formation of a series of epithelial outgrowths into the ectomesenchyme at sites corresponding to the positions of the future deciduous teeth. At this time the mitotic index, the labeling index, and the growth of the epithelial cells are significantly lower than corresponding indexes in the underlying ectomesenchyme, and ectomesenchymal cells accumulate around the outgrowths. From this

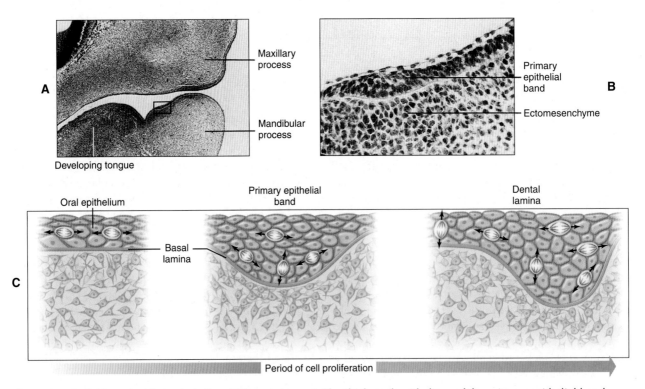

Figure 5-2 Sagittal section through the head of an embryo. **A,** The thickened epithelium of the primary epithelial band. **B,** The same structure at higher magnification. **C,** Schematic representation of the change in plane of cleavage during formation of the band and subsequently of the dental lamina. *(A and B from Nery EB, Kraus BS, Croup M: Arch Oral Biol 15:1315, 1970; C adapted from Ruch JV. In Linde A, editor: Dentin and dentinogenesis, vol 1, Boca Raton, Fla, 1984, CRC Press.)*

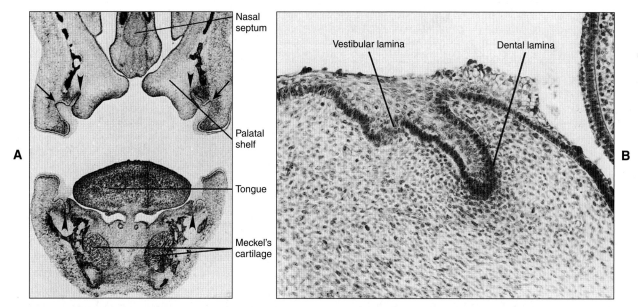

Figure 5-3 Coronal section through the anterior portion of the developing head. **A,** The positions of the dental and vestibular laminae in the four quadrants are marked with arrowheads and arrows, respectively. **B,** The two laminae at higher magnification.

point, tooth development proceeds in three stages: the *bud, cap,* and *bell.* These terms are descriptive of the morphology of the developing tooth germ but do not describe the significant functional changes that occur during development, such as morphogenesis and histodifferentiation. One should note also that because development is a continuous process, clear distinction between the transition stages is not possible. Another problem for the beginning student is that in examining sections of developing teeth, a tooth germ possibly may be sectioned at a particular stage of development in such a way that it mimics another.

VESTIBULAR LAMINA

If a coronal section through the developing head region of an embryo at 6 weeks of development is examined, no vestibule or sulcus can be seen between the cheek and tooth-bearing areas (Figure 5-3). The vestibule forms as a result of the proliferation of the vestibular lamina into the ectomesenchyme soon after formation of the dental lamina. The cells of the vestibular lamina rapidly enlarge and then degenerate to form a cleft that becomes the vestibule between the cheek and the tooth-bearing area.

INITIATION OF THE TOOTH

An intriguing question is how dental development is initiated. When murine (mouse) first arch epithelium is combined with caudal or cranial neural crest in the anterior chamber of the eye, teeth form (Figure 5-4).

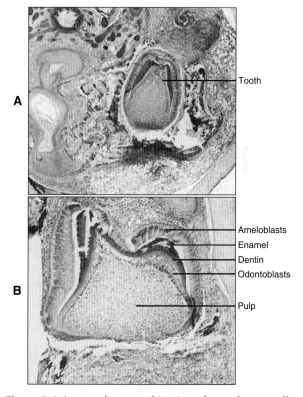

Figure 5-4 Intraocular recombination of neural crest cells and dental epithelium. **A,** Tooth formed from the combination of neural crest cells expanded from the neural folds and mandibular epithelium but not from combination with limb bud epithelium. **B,** Tooth formed from the combination of neural crest expanded from the trunk level and mandibular epithelium. This indicates that tooth formation is initiated by factors residing in the oral epithelium. *(Courtesy A.G.S. Lumsden.)*

TABLE 5-1	Outcome of Various Recombinations of Epithelium and Neural Crest			
COMBINATION	TEETH	BONE	CARTILAGE	NEURAL CREST
Neural crest and mandibular epithelium	+	+	+	+
Neural crest and limb epithelium	–	+	+	+
Neural crest alone	–	–	+	+
Mandibular epithelium alone	–	–	–	–

From Lumsden AGS. In Mederson PFA, editor: *Development and evolutionary biology of the neural crest*, New York, 1987, John Wiley & Sons.

Epithelium from other sources, such as a limb bud or the second arch, does not elicit this response (Table 5-1). However, after the twelfth day of development, first arch epithelium loses this odontogenic potential, which then is assumed by the ectomesenchyme so that the ectomesenchyme can elicit tooth formation from a variety of epithelia. For example, recombination of late first arch ectomesenchyme with embryonic plantar (foot) epithelium changes the developmental direction of the epithelium so that an enamel organ is formed (Figure 5-5). Conversely, if the epithelial enamel organ is recombined with skin mesenchyme, the organ loses its dental characteristics and assumes those of epidermis. What these experiments indicate is that odontogenesis is initiated first by factors resident in the first arch epithelium influencing ectomesenchyme but that with time this potential is assumed by the ectomesenchyme. These experimental findings are mirrored by the expression pattern of transcription and growth factors in these tissues. Some of the genes involved in tooth formation are listed in Box 5-1 and are discussed in the following text (see Table 5-1).

The earliest histologic indication of tooth development is at day 11 of embryogenesis, which is marked by a thickening of the epithelium where tooth formation will occur on the oral surface of the first branchial arch. What are the signals mediating the initial steps in tooth development? To date, the earliest mesenchymal markers for tooth formation are the *Lim*-homeobox domain genes (transcription factors), *Lhx-6* and *Lhx-7*. Both of these genes are expressed in the neural crest–derived ectomesenchyme of the oral half of the first branchial arch as early as day 9. Experimental data demonstrate that the

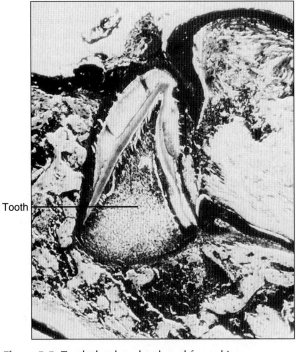

Tooth

Figure 5-5 Tooth that has developed from skin epithelium. Molar ectomesenchyme combined with plantar epithelium to produce this anomaly. *(From Kollar EJ, Baird GR: J Embryol Exp Morphol 24:173, 1970.)*

Box 5-1   Genes Expressed During Tooth Development

Barx BarH1 *homologue in vertebrates (TF)*
Bmp *Bone morphogenetic proteins (SP)*
Dlx *Distaless homologue in vertebrates (TF)*
Fgf *Fibroblast growth factor (SP)*
Gli *Glioma-associated oncogene homologue (zinc finger protein) (TF)*
Hgf *Hepatic growth factor (SP)*
Lef *Lymphoid enhancer-binding factor 1 (TF)*
Lhx *Lim-homeobox domain gene (TF)*
Msx *Msh-like genes in vertebrates (TF)*
Otlx *Otx-related homeobox gene (TF)*
Pax *Paired box homeotic gene (TF)*
Pitx *Transcription factor named for its expression in the pituitary gland*
Ptc *Patched cell-surface receptor for sonic hedgehog (SHH)*
Shh *Sonic hedgehog (SP)*
Slit *Homologous to* Drosophila *slit protein (SP)*
Smo *Smoothed PTC coreceptor for SHH*
Wnt *Wingless homologue in vertebrates (SP)*

TF, Transcription factor; SP, secreted protein.

expression of *Lhx-6* and *Lhx-7* results from a signaling molecule originating from the oral epithelium of the first branchial arch. If second arch mesenchyme is recombined with first branchial arch oral epithelium, *Lhx-6* and *Lhx-7* will be induced. However, if first branchial arch mesenchyme (which expresses *Lhx-6* and *Lhx-7*) is recombined with second branchial arch epithelium, expression of both genes will be down-regulated quickly. A prime candidate for the induction of *Lhx* genes is *Fgf-8* (secreted fibroblast growth factor); this growth factor is expressed at the proper place and time in the first branchial arch and is able to induce *Lhx-6* and *Lhx-7* expression in in vitro experiments.

This explains in rather simple terms the establishment of the oral-aboral axis. The next question in terms of developmental signals is what controls the position and the number of tooth germs along the oral surface? Again from the experimental data available, the signals for these aspects appear to originate from the oral epithelium. *Fgf-8* already has been shown to play a role in the oral-aboral axis and also seems to have a role in determining the positions where the tooth germs will form. The *Pax-9* gene is one of the earliest mesenchymal genes that define the localization of the tooth germs. *Pax-9* gene expression colocalizes with the exact sites where tooth germs appear. *Pax-9* is induced by *Fgf-8* and is repressed by bone morphogenetic proteins (*BMP-2* and *BMP-4*). *Fgf-8*, *Bmp-2*, and *Bmp-4* are expressed in nonoverlapping areas, with *Pax-9* being expressed at sites where *Fgf-8* but not *Bmp* is. Of course, a number of other genes also are expressed (e.g., *Otlx-2*, *Dlx-2*, *Msx-1*, *Msx-2*, and *Lef-1*) in oral epithelium at the same time. Whether they directly regulate the expression of *Fgf-8* or *Bmps* is not clear at this time. Signaling molecules often regulate the expression of transcription factors that turn out to regulate the expression of those same signaling molecules. Little is known about the regulatory mechanisms of signaling molecules, and untangling the network or regulatory events can be difficult. At least 12 transcription factors are expressed in odontogenic mesenchyme, and some have redundant roles. To date, more than 90 genes have been identified from the oral epithelium, dental epithelium, and dental mesenchyme during the initiation of tooth development. The reader is directed to the *Gene Expression in Tooth* web page (*http://bite-it.helsinki.fi*) for a more up-to-date and complete list. The level of complexity becomes evident quickly in that generating a single knockout mutant often is not sufficient to determine the role played by specific genes, especially when they are members of a large family. For example, *Dlx-1* and *Dlx-2* show a tooth phenotype only in double knockout mutants, and not all the teeth are affected. This may be explained by the compensatory action of other *Dlx* genes (e.g., *Dlx-5* and *Dlx-6*). Thus the evidence from experimental embryology,

recombinant DNA technology, and immunocytochemistry indicates that first arch epithelium is essential for the initiation of tooth development.

In mice, expression of *Shh* is localized to the presumptive dental ectoderm at E11 and is thus another good signaling candidate for tooth initiation (Figure 5-6). *Shh* knockout mice have little development of the facial processes, and thus any role in tooth initiation cannot be identified from these. Mutations in *Gli* genes that are downstream mediators of *Shh* action suggest a role in early tooth development because *Gli2*$^{-/-}$ and *Gli3*$^{-/-}$ double mutant embryos do not produce any recognizable tooth buds. Addition of *Shh*-soaked beads to oral ectoderm can induce local epithelial cell proliferation to produce invaginations that are reminiscent of tooth buds. *Shh* thus appears to have a role in stimulating epithelial cell proliferation, and its local expression at the sites of tooth development implicates *Shh* signaling in tooth initiation.

Lef-1 is a member of the high-mobility group family of nuclear proteins that includes the T-cell factor proteins, known to be nuclear mediators of *Wnt* signaling. *Lef-1* is first expressed in dental epithelial thickenings and during bud formation shifts to being expressed in the condensing mesenchyme. In *Lef-1* knockout mice, all dental development is arrested at the bud stage; recombination assays, however, have identified the requirement for *Lef-1* in the dental epithelium as occurring earlier, before bud initiation. Ectopic expression of *Lef-1* in the oral epithelium also results in ectopic tooth formation.

Expression of several genes in ectomesenchyme marks the sites of tooth germ initiation. These include *Pax-9* and *Activin-A*, both of which are expressed beginning around E11 in mice within small localized groups of cells corresponding to where tooth epithelium will invaginate to form buds. In the case of *Pax-9*, antagonistic

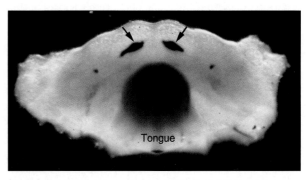

Figure 5-6 Expression of sonic hedgehog *(Shh)* in an isolated mouse embryonic jaw primordium at E11.5 showing expression in the dental epithelium at the future sites of tooth formation *(arrows)*.

interactions between *Fgf-8* and *Bmp-4*, similar to those found to regulate *Barx-1* expression, from oral ectoderm have been shown also possibly to act to localize *Pax-9* expression. *Activin-A* expression is not regulated by the same mechanism, suggesting that such *FGF-8—BMP-4* interactions may not have a direct role in tooth initiation.

Once the ability to initiate tooth development has been acquired by ectomesenchyme, dental papillary cells maintain it. Thus if early tooth germs are cultured for an extended period, the cells dedifferentiate, and the morphology of the germs is lost completely; yet if these dedifferentiated epithelial and ectomesenchymal cells are harvested and recombined in vivo, they form a tooth (the program for tooth formation is not lost). Of particular interest in this regard is that if mouse tooth ectomesenchyme is combined with chick epithelium, tooth genes are induced in the mesenchyme by the epithelium, and teethlike structures develop. Avian oral epithelium has maintained the competence to form a dental organ, a competence last expressed some 100,000 years ago.

TOOTH TYPE DETERMINATION

The determination of specific tooth types at their correct positions in the jaws is referred to as *patterning* of the dentition. The determination of crown pattern is a remarkably consistent process. Although in some animals teeth are all the same shape (homodont), in most mammals they are different (heterodont), falling into three families: incisiform, caniniform, and molariform. Two hypothetical models have been proposed to explain how these different shapes are determined, and evidence exists to support both. The first is the *field model*, which proposes that the factors responsible for tooth shape reside within the ectomesenchyme in distinct graded and overlapping fields for each tooth family (Figure 5-7). The fact that each of the fields expresses differing combinations of patterning homeobox genes supports this theory. The *clone model* proposes that each tooth class is derived from a clone of ectomesenchymal cells programmed by epithelium to produce teeth of a given pattern (Figure 5-8). In support of this contention, isolated presumptive first molar tissues have been shown to continue development to form three molar teeth in their normal positional sequence. Possibly both models can be combined, for temporal factors may play a role. For instance, the coded pattern of homeobox gene expression in the ectomesenchyme might be expressed following an epithelial signal, as was the case for tooth initiation. Furthermore, as with tooth initiation, ectomesenchyme eventually assumes the dominant role in crown pattern formation. Recombination of molar

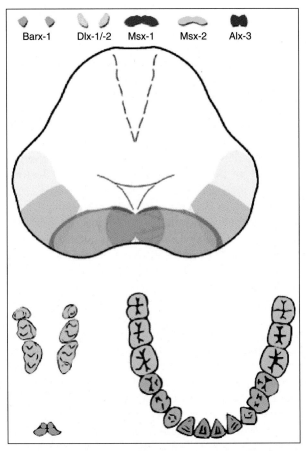

Figure 5-7 Odontogenic homeobox code model of dental patterning. Epithelial FGF8 and BMP4 expressed during early initiation induce the mesenchymal expression of a number of homeobox-containing genes in the underlying mesenchyme as overlapping domains that provide the spatial information necessary to determine tooth type. **A,** Domains of *Barx-1* and *Dlx-1/-2* expression overlap in the mesenchyme of the presumptive molar region, whereas domains of *Msx-1*, *Msx-2*, and *Alx-3* overlap in presumptive incisor mesenchyme. **B,** Mouse dental pattern. Incisors deriving from *Msx-1/Alx-3* expressing cells; molars deriving from *Barx-1/Dlx-1/-2* expressing cells. **C,** Human dental pattern. Premolars and canines can be derived from the same odontogenic code as that observed in mice by virtue of the overlapping domains of gene expression. Thus canines and premolars may be derived from cells expressing *Dlx-1/-2* and *Msx-1*, for example. *(From McCollum MA, Sharpe PT:* Bioessays *23:481, 2001.)*

papilla with incisor dental organ results in molar development; conversely, recombination of incisor papilla with molar dental organ results in incisor development (Figure 5-9).

The *homeobox code* (field) model for dental patterning is based on observations of the spatially restricted expression of several homeobox genes in the jaw primordia

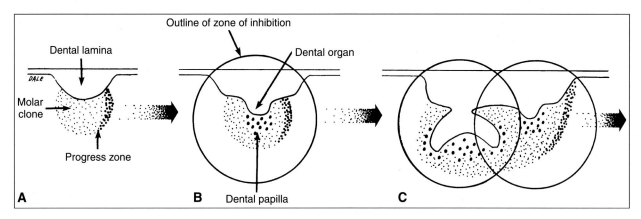

Figure 5-8 Clone theory. **A,** The molar clone ectomesenchyme has induced the dental lamina to begin tooth development. The clone and dental lamina progress posteriorly. **B,** When a clone reaches the critical size, a tooth bud is initiated at its center. The next tooth bud, **C,** is not initiated until the progress zone of the clone escapes the influence of a zone of inhibition surrounding the tooth bud. *(From Osborn JW, Ten Cate AR: Advanced dental histology, ed 3, Oxford, UK, 1983, Elsevier.)*

ectomesenchyme cells before E11. The early expression of *Msx-1* and *Msx-2* homeobox genes before the initiation of tooth germs is restricted to distal, midline ectomesenchyme in regions where incisors (and canine in human beings), but not multicuspid teeth, will develop; whereas *Dlx-1* and *Dlx-2* are expressed in ectomesenchyme cells where multicuspid teeth, but not incisors (or canines), will develop. These expression domains are broad and do not exactly correspond to specific tooth types. Rather, they are considered to define broad territories. Expression of *Barx-1* overlaps with *Dlx-1* and *Dlx-2* and corresponds closely to

ectomesenchymal cells that will develop into molars in mice. The homeobox code model proposes that the overlapping domains of these genes provide the positional information for tooth type morphogenesis.

Support for this model comes from the dental phenotype of *Dlx-1⁻/⁻* and *Dlx2⁻/⁻* double-knockout mice in which development of maxillary molar teeth is arrested at the epithelial thickening stage. As predicted by the code model, incisor development is normal in these mice; normal development of mandibular molars (not predicted by the code) results from functional redundancy with other *Dlx* genes such as *Dlx-5* and

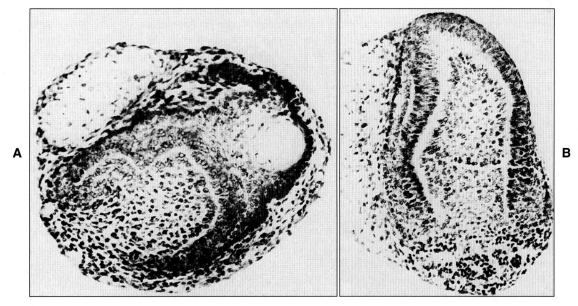

Figure 5-9 Recombination of dental epithelium and ectomesenchyme. **A,** Incisor epithelium combined with molar papilla results in a molariform tooth. **B,** Molar epithelium combined with incisor papilla results in an incisiform tooth. *(From Kollar EJ, Baird GR: J Embryol Exp Morphol 21:131, 1969.)*

Dlx-6 that are expressed in ectomesenchyme in the mandibular primordium.

Further functional support for the code model comes from misexpression of *Barx-1* in distal ectomesenchyme cells, which results in incisor tooth germs developing as molars. *Barx-1* expression is localized to proximal ectomesenchyme (molar) by a combination of positive and negative signals from the oral ectoderm. *FGF-8* localized in proximal ectoderm induces *Barx-1* expression, whereas *BMP-4* in the distal ectoderm represses *Barx-1* expression. Expression of *Barx-1* experimentally induced in distal (presumptive incisor) ectomesenchyme by inhibition of *BMP* signaling has the effect of repressing *Msx* gene expression, which is induced in distal ectomesenchyme by *BMP-4*. The transformation of incisors into molars thus may require a combination of loss of "incisor" genes (*Msx*) and gain of "molar" genes (*Barx-1*).

INSTRUCTIVE SIGNALS FOR PATTERNING

Recombinations of incisor and molar epithelium with mesenchyme from E10 to E14 mouse embryos showed that when molar epithelium was recombined with incisor mesenchyme, a molar tooth formed, and when incisor epithelium was recombined with molar mesenchyme, an incisor formed. This led to the conclusion that the epithelium was responsible for determining the type and shape of a tooth. Other recombinations at E13-E16, however, produced different results, in which molar epithelium recombined with incisor mesenchyme resulted in incisor teeth and incisor epithelium recombined with molar mesenchyme resulted in molar teeth. Further experiments used tissue from the hairless (plantar) surface of the foot in combination with dental tissues. At E14 or E15, dental epithelium, when recombined with foot mesenchyme, showed no tooth development; however, when plantar epithelium was combined with dental mesenchyme, then tooth development occurred.

The apparent conflict produced by these experiments of whether the ectoderm or ectomesenchyme provides the instructive information for patterning now has been resolved by studying the temporal regulation of homeobox gene expression in ectomesenchyme by ectodermal signals. Removal of the ectoderm from E10 mandibular arch explants results in loss of expression of ectomesenchymal homeobox gene expression within 6 hours, indicating that expression requires signals produced by the ectoderm. Expression can be restored by implantation of beads soaked in fibroblast growth factor 8 (FGF-8), a factor expressed in oral ectoderm at this time. Expression of *Dlx-1*, *Dlx-2*, *Msx*, and *Barx-1* is seen around the implanted beads regardless of their position

in the explant, indicating that all ectomesenchymal cells at this time are competent to respond to FGF-8. When this experiment was repeated at E10.5, ectomesenchymal gene expression again was lost following removal of ectoderm, but this time implantation of FGF-8 beads only restored expression in the original domains. Thus at E10.5 ectomesenchymal cell competence to express homeobox genes in response to FGF-8 has become restricted to those cells that expressed the gene at E10. By E11, removal of ectoderm had no effect on ectomesenchymal gene expression, showing that by this stage expression is independent of ectodermal signals. These results provide a molecular understanding of the control of dental patterning and an explanation for the conflicting recombination results. The distoproximal (incisor-molar) spatial domains of homeobox gene expression (homeobox code) are produced in response to spatially restricted ectodermal signals acting on pluricompetent ectomesenchymal cells. Recombinations carried out before E10.5 therefore will show the instructive influence of ectoderm on tooth shape, whereas those carried out after E10.5 will show an instructive influence of ectomesenchyme because by this stage expression is independent of ectodermal signals.

REGIONALIZATION OF ORAL AND DENTAL ECTODERM

Because regionally restricted expression of signaling protein genes in oral ectoderm controls dental initiation and patterning, it follows that the mechanisms that control the regional restriction of ectodermal signals need to be understood. During insect segmentation, interactions between *HH* and wingless signaling are involved in ectodermal cell boundary specification. Several *Wnt* genes are expressed during tooth development and one, *Wnt-7b*, has a reciprocal expression pattern to *Shh* in oral ectoderm. *Wnt-7b* is expressed throughout the oral ectoderm except for presumptive dental ectoderm where *Shh* is expressed. Misexpression of *Wnt-7b* in presumptive dental ectoderm results in loss of *Shh* expression and failure of tooth bud formation. This shows that WNT-7B represses *Shh* expression in oral ectoderm and thus the boundaries between oral and dental ectoderm are maintained by an interaction between WNT and SHH signaling similar to ectodermal boundary maintenance in segmentation in insects.

BUD STAGE

The bud stage is represented by the first epithelial incursion into the ectomesenchyme of the jaw (Figure 5-10). The epithelial cells show little if any change in shape or

TOPICS FOR CONSIDERATION   Dental Placodes: Roles in Tooth Formation and in Ectodermal Dysplasia Syndromes

A key feature of the initiation of tooth development is the formation of ectodermal placodes. They appear as localized thickenings of the oral epithelium within the primary epithelial band, which is a line of thickened epithelium at the site of the future dental arches in the embryonic maxilla and mandible. The placodes so far have been studied in detail only in mice, where they appear at the sites of incisors and first molars. Mice have only one incisor and three molars in each jaw quadrant, and so they lack the canines and premolars. Because no placodes have been observed in the oral epithelium for the second and third molars, which apparently form successively from the preceding molar, it is believed that the dental placodes initiate the formation of each tooth family. Whether the canines and premolars are initiated from their own placodes remains to be demonstrated.

It is noteworthy that placodes morphologically similar to those of the dental placodes also initiate the development of other organs that form as appendages of the ectoderm.[1] These include hairs and nails, as well as glands such as mammary, salivary, sweat, and sebaceous glands. It has become evident that the basic mechanisms and genes involved in the formation and function of placodes are similar in all ectodermal organs.

Interactions between the surface epithelium and underlying mesenchyme have key functions in the formation of placodes. The molecular signals mediating these interactions belong to several conserved signal families, and they regulate important genes in the epithelium and mesenchyme. This leads to the formation of the epithelial thickening and underlying mesenchymal cell condensation. Studies mainly on hairs and feathers have identified FGFs and Wnts as activators of placode formation and BMPs as inhibitors.[2] The balance of stimulatory and inhibitory signals is important in the initiation of the placode,

and the fine-tuning of signaling affects the pattern of the organs. The mechanisms whereby teeth are patterned in the jaws are poorly understood at present, but the available evidence indicates that the conserved signal pathways also play important roles determining the positions of teeth.

The current knowledge on the molecular mechanisms of dental placode formation has derived largely from studies on syndromes called *ectodermal dysplasias*. These syndromes are defined as conditions in which two or more types of ectodermal organs are affected. Many ectodermal dysplasia patients have dental defects that typically include multiple missing teeth (oligodontia) and small and misshapen teeth. Many genes have been identified in which mutations cause ectodermal dysplasias. Taking the similarities particularly in the early development of various ectodermal organs, it is not surprising that these genes regulate placode formation and function.

Mutations in the transcription factor p63 cause the *EEC* (ectrodactyly-ectodermal dysplasia-clefting) *syndrome* featured by ectodermal dysplasia and by ectrodactyly (split hands and feet) and cleft lip and palate.[3] A typical patient has a severe dental phenotype with multiple missing and misshapen teeth. The deletion of p63 function in mice leads to a lack of ectodermal organs, and the mice die at birth. The development of teeth, hair, and other ectodermal organs is arrested in the embryos before placode development. Also, the dental placodes are completely absent, but a normal horseshoe-shaped primary epithelial band forms. The function of p63 is necessary for FGF, BMP, and Notch1 signaling, indicating that placode formation requires the interplay of many different signal pathways.[4]

The positional cloning of genes behind *HED* (*hypohidrotic ectodermal dysplasia*), led to the discovery of a novel TNF (tumor necrosis factor) pathway

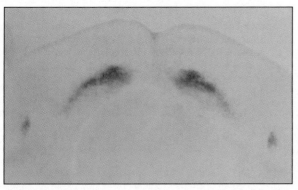
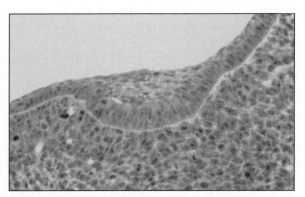

The placodes of incisors and molars in the lower jaw of an E12 mouse embryo. Visualized by the localized expression of the signal molecule sonic hedgehog.

Continued

TOPICS FOR CONSIDERATION   Dental Placodes: Roles in Tooth Formation and in Ectodermal Dysplasia Syndromes—cont'd

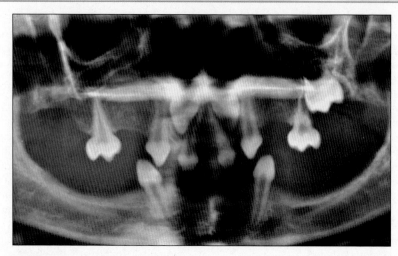

Oligodontia (severe hypodontia) in a patient with hypohidrotic ectodermal dysplasia (loss of function of the signal molecule ectodysplasin regulating placode formation).

and the ectodysplasin (Eda) pathway, which has turned out to be an important stimulator of placode development.[5] The characteristic features of HED are oligodontia (see the figure), thin and sparse hair, and severe lack of sweat glands, but other ectodermal defects such as in nails and salivary glands are also common.

The role of the Eda pathway in the development of teeth and other ectodermal organs has been analyzed in detail in mice. In the mouse model for X-linked HED, the *Tabby* mouse lacks Eda and has a tooth phenotype characterized by lack of third molars and sometimes incisors, as well as by misshapen crowns of the first molars. The *Tabby* mouse also lacks the first wave of hair follicles and has defects in many ectodermal glands. Transgenic mice overexpressing Eda in the ectoderm also have been informative in elucidating the role of the Eda pathway and the pathogenesis of the ectodermal defects. The accumulated information indicates that Eda signaling is required for the formation and growth of placodes. The Eda receptor Edar is expressed in all ectodermal placodes, and when it is overactivated, the placodes grow larger than normal. This results in stimulated organ development seen as extra teeth, aberrant cusp morphology in molars, longer hairs, increased sweat excretion, and extra mammary glands.[6] The supernumerary teeth form in front of the molars and may represent premolars, which were lost early during rodent evolution. Interestingly, the injection of Eda protein to pregnant *Tabby* mice rescues the hair and tooth phenotype of their offspring.[7] Hence, it appears that the stimulation of placode formation at an early stage is sufficient to rescue the development of the organs. This finding obviously may lead to novel possibilities to prevent human X-linked HED.

In conclusion, it is evident that placode formation is a key event in tooth development. The size of a placode may be a critical determinant for tooth formation by determining the number of cells that will generate a tooth family. Hence, a smaller than normal placode may lead to missing and/or smaller teeth and a large placode to supernumerary and/or larger teeth, respectively.

Irma Thesleff, DDS, PhD
Professor, Research Director
Institute of Biotechnology
University of Helsinki
Helsinki, Finland

REFERENCES

1. Pispa J, Thesleff I: Mechanisms of ectodermal organogenesis, *Dev Biol* 262:195-205, 2003.
2. Jung HS, Francis-West PH, Widelitz RB et al: Local inhibitory action of BMPs and their relationships with activators in feather formation: implications for periodic patterning, *Dev Biol* 196:11-23, 1998.
3. Celli J, Duijf P, Hamel BCJ et al: Heterozygous germline mutations in the p53 homolog p63 are the cause of EEC syndrome, *Cell* 99:143-153, 1999.
4. Laurikkala J, Mikkola ML, James M et al: P63 regulates multiple signalling pathways required for ectodermal organogenesis and differentiation, *Development* 133:1553-1563, 2006.
5. Mikkola M, Thesleff I: Ectodysplasin signaling in development, *Cytokine Growth Factor Rev* 14:211-224, 2003.
6. Mustonen T, Pispa J, Mikkola ML et al: Stimulation of ectodermal organ development by ectodysplasin-A1, *Dev Biol* 259:123-136, 2003.
7. Gaide O, Schneider P: Permanent correction of an inherited ectodermal dysplasia with recombinant EDA, *Nat Med* 9:614-618, 2003.

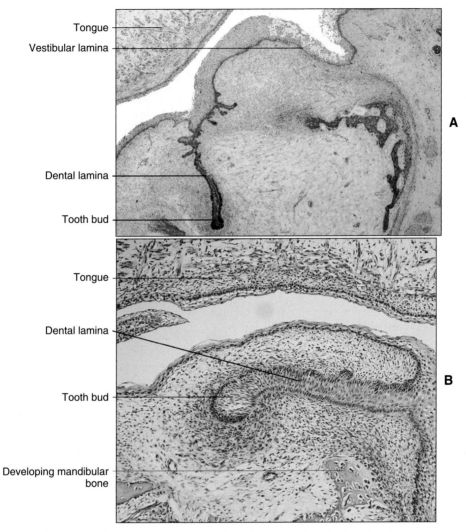

Tongue
Vestibular lamina

Dental lamina

Tooth bud

A

Tongue

Dental lamina

Tooth bud

Developing mandibular
bone

B

Figure 5-10 Bud stage of tooth development seen in coronal section (**A**) and sagittal section (**B**).

function. The supporting ectomesenchymal cells are packed closely beneath and around the epithelial bud.

BUD-TO-CAP TRANSITION

The transition from bud to cap marks the onset of morphologic differences between tooth germs that give rise to different types of teeth. *Msx-1* is expressed with *Bmp-4* in the mesenchymal cells that condense around tooth buds. *Msx-1*⁻/⁻ embryos have tooth development arrested at the bud stage, and *Bmp-4* expression is lost from the mesenchyme, suggesting that *Msx-1* is required for *Bmp-4* expression. *Bmp-4* is able to maintain *Msx-1* expression in wild-type tooth bud mesenchyme, indicating that *Bmp-4* induces its own expression via *Msx-1*. Tooth development can be rescued in *Msx-1*⁻/⁻ embryos by addition of exogenous BMP-4.

Bmp-4 expressed in the bud mesenchyme is required to maintain *Bmp-2* and *Shh* expression in the epithelium. Loss of *Bmp-4* expression in *Msx-1* mutants is accompanied by loss of *Shh* expression at E12.5, which can be restored by exogenous BMP-4. Blocking SHH function with neutralizing antibodies also results in loss of *Bmp-2* expression, suggesting *Shh* and *Bmp-2* may be in the same pathway and that down-regulation of *Bmp-2* in *Msx-1* mutants may be downstream of the loss of SHH.

The loss of SHH signaling at different stages of tooth development has identified distinct time-dependent requirements for SHH. Blocking SHH signaling using neutralizing antibodies or forskolin shows that at E11-E12 SHH is required for dental epithelium proliferation to form tooth buds, whereas blocking at E13 affects tooth bud morphology, but these buds still can form teeth. Genetic disruption of *Shh* signaling from E12.5 by *Cre*-mediated excision of targeted *Shh* null alleles

---

TOPICS FOR CONSIDERATION   Human and Mouse Tooth Genetics

Although studies on tooth development in mice have been useful and have led to the identification of genes controlling many different aspects of development, some important differences between rodent and human tooth development are becoming clear. These differences are most striking when tooth abnormalities caused by mutations in the same genes are compared in human beings and mice. The homeobox gene *Pax-9* is expressed in the mesenchyme of all mouse tooth buds. Mice lacking one copy of the *Pax-9* gene have normal teeth, but mice lacking both copies develop no teeth. Mutations in the human *PAX-9* gene can result in molar hypodontia, but this occurs when only one copy of the gene is mutated. Similarly, mice lacking both copies of *Cbfa1 (Runx2)* have severely abnormal teeth. Human beings with only one mutated copy of *CBFA-1 (RUNX-2)* have cleidocranial dysplasia.

One possible explanation for these differences is that abnormalities in tooth number in human beings predominantly affect the permanent dentition, whereas the deciduous teeth are only rarely affected. Mice have only one set of teeth that are most probably the equivalent of human deciduous teeth in their development. Little currently is known about the genes involved in formation of permanent teeth. Thus an important future direction will be to understand the genes involved in the development of permanent teeth in human beings.

Paul T. Sharpe
*Department of Craniofacial Development
Dental Institute, Guy's Hospital
King's College London
London, England*

---

results in a disruption of molar tooth morphology, but cytodifferentiation appears normal, suggesting that *Shh* has a major role at the cap stage of development.

Another homeobox gene with a role in the bud-to-cap transition is *Pax-9*. *Pax-9* is expressed in bud stage mesenchyme and also earlier in domains similar to *Activin-βA* and *Msx-1* in patches of mesenchyme that mark the sites of tooth formation. *Pax-9⁻/⁻* mutant embryos have all teeth arrested at the bud stage. Despite being coexpressed, early *Activin-βA* expression is not affected in *Pax-9⁻/⁻* embryos, and *Pax-9* expression is not affected in *Activin-βA⁻/⁻* embryos. These two genes are essential for tooth development to progress beyond the bud stage and thus appear to function independently; however, changes occur in expression of other genes such as *Bmp-4*, *Msx-1*, and *Lef-1* in *Pax-9⁻/⁻* tooth bud mesenchyme.

CAP STAGE

As the epithelial bud continues to proliferate into the ectomesenchyme, cellular density increases immediately adjacent to the epithelial outgrowth. This process, classically referred to as a *condensation* of the ectomesenchyme, results from a local grouping of cells that have failed to produce extracellular substance and have thus not separated from each other (Figure 5-11). As the tooth bud grows larger, it drags along with it part of the dental lamina; so from that point on the developing tooth is tethered to the dental lamina by an extension called the *lateral lamina*. At this early stage of tooth development, identifying the formative elements of the tooth and its supporting tissues is already possible.

The epithelial outgrowth, which superficially resembles a cap sitting on a ball of condensed ectomesenchyme, is referred to widely as the *dental organ* but actually should be called the *enamel organ*, because it eventually will form the enamel of the tooth. Henceforth, the term *enamel organ* is used.

The *enamel niche* is an apparent structure in histologic sections, created because the dental lamina is a

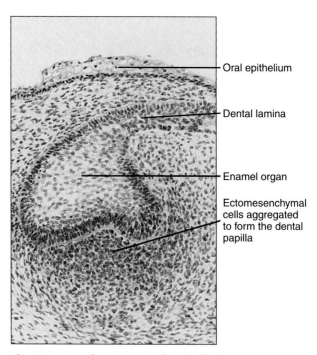

Oral epithelium

Dental lamina

Enamel organ

Ectomesenchymal cells aggregated to form the dental papilla

Figure 5-11 Early cap stage of tooth development. A condensation of the ectomesenchyme associated with the epithelial cap is identified easily.

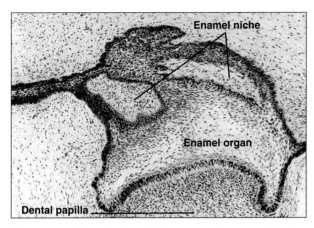

Figure 5-12 Enamel niche. This structure is created by the plane of section cutting through a curved lateral lamina so that mesenchyme appears to be surrounded by dental epithelium.

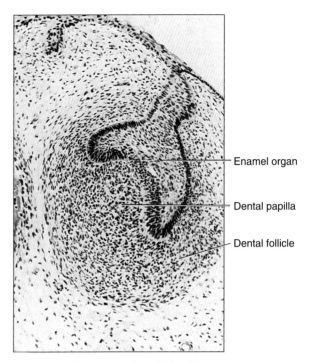

Figure 5-13 Cap stage of tooth development. The epithelial enamel organ sits over a ball of ecto-mesenchymal cells, the dental papilla that extends around the rim of the enamel organ to form the dental follicle.

sheet rather than a single strand and often contains a concavity filled with connective tissue. A section through this arrangement creates the impression that the tooth germ has a double attachment to the oral epithelium by two separate strands (Figure 5-12).

The ball of condensed ectomesenchymal cells, called the *dental papilla*, will form the dentin and pulp. The condensed ectomesenchyme limiting the dental papilla and encapsulating the enamel organ—the *dental follicle* or *sac*—gives rise to the supporting tissues of the tooth. Because the enamel organ sits over the dental papilla like a cap, this stage of tooth development is known as the *cap stage* (Figure 5-13).

The enamel organ, dental papilla, and dental follicle together constitute the dental organ or tooth germ. Early in the ontogeny (life history) of the tooth, those structures giving rise to the dental tissues (enamel, dentin-pulp, and supporting apparatus of the tooth) can be identified as discrete entities. Important developmental changes begin late in the cap stage and continue during the transition of the tooth germ from cap to bell. Through these changes, termed *histodifferentiation*, a mass of similar epithelial cells transforms itself into morphologically and functionally distinct components. The cells in the center of the enamel organ synthesize and secrete glycosaminoglycans into the extracellular compartment between the epithelial cells (Figure 5-14). Glycosaminoglycans are hydrophilic and so pull water into the enamel organ. The increasing amount of fluid increases the volume of the extracellular compartment of the enamel organ, and the central cells are forced apart. Because they retain connections with each other through their desmosomal contacts, they become star shaped (Figure 5-15). The center of the enamel organ thus is termed the *stellate reticulum*.

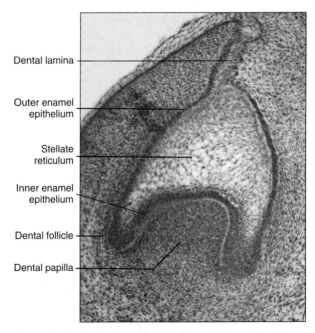

Dental lamina

Outer enamel epithelium

Stellate reticulum

Inner enamel epithelium

Dental follicle

Dental papilla

Figure 5-14 Beginning of histodifferentiation within the enamel organ forming the stellate reticulum. The peripheral epithelial cells are differentiating into the inner and outer enamel epithelia.

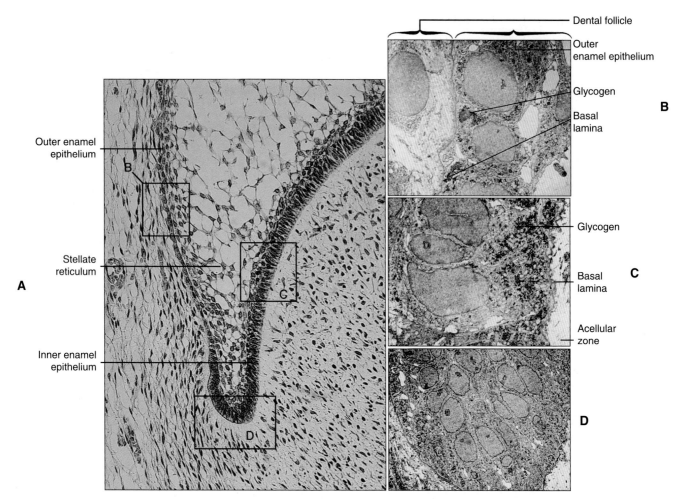

Figure 5-15 Fine structure of a tooth germ at the early bell stage. **A,** The histodifferentiated enamel organ in the region of the cervical loop as seen with light microscopy. **B,** The outer enamel epithelium; its cells are separated from the follicle by a basal lamina. Their cytoplasm contains few organelles, accumulations of glycogen, and a large nucleus. **C,** The short columnar cells of the inner enamel epithelium. The cells are separated from the acellular zone of the dental papilla by a basal lamina. **D,** The cervical loop region of the enamel organ; the difference between the follicle and the acellular zone in **C** is apparent. The latter area has few collagen fibrils in the extracellular compartment, where dentin formation eventually will occur. *(Electron micrographs from Egawa I: Shikwa Gakuho 70:803, 1970.)*

ENAMEL KNOT

Enamel knots are clusters of nondividing epithelial cells visible in sections of molar cap stage tooth germs (Figure 5-16). The enamel knot precursor cells can be detected first at the tip of the tooth buds by expression of the *p21* gene, followed shortly after by *Shh*. By the cap stage, when the enamel knot is visible histologically, it expresses genes for many signaling molecules including *Bmp-2, Bmp-4, Bmp-7, Fgf-4, Fgf-9, Wnt-10b, Slit-1*, and *Shh* (Figure 5-17). Three-dimensional reconstructions of the expression of these genes have revealed highly dynamic spatial and temporal nested patterns in the

enamel knot as it extends between the inner and outer enamel epithelia as the *enamel cord* (Figure 5-18). One possibility is that both these structures may be related anatomically to the site where the lateral lamina attaches to the enamel organ cap. On the whole, receptors for the enamel knot signals are localized in the epithelial cells surrounding the enamel knot. Each tooth germ has a single primary enamel knot at the cap stage, and as these disappear, secondary enamel knots appear at the tips of the future cusps in molars. *Fgf-4* and *Slit-1* may be the best molecular markers for enamel knot formation because these are the only two genes that have been observed in primary and secondary knots.

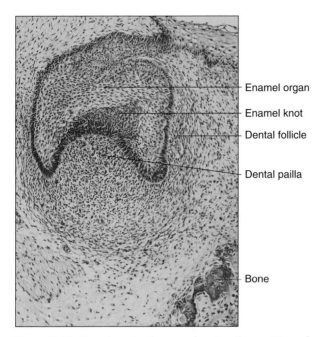

Figure 5-16 Cap stage tooth germ showing the position of the enamel knot.

The exact physical role of the enamel knot is not yet established, but changes in its morphology in tooth germs of spontaneous mouse mutants with abnormal molar cusp formation such as *Tabby (Eda)*, *downless (dl)*, and *Crinkled (Edaar)* have started to reveal some detail of this remarkable structure. The current view is that the enamel knot represents an organizational center, which orchestrates cuspal morphogenesis. The enamel knot shares many similarities with the apical ectodermal ridge of developing limbs: both consist of nondividing cells, both express *Fgfs*, *Bmps*, and *Msx-2*, and both act as signaling centers.

BELL STAGE

Continued growth of the tooth germ leads to the next stage of tooth development, the bell stage (Figure 5-19), so called because the enamel organ comes to resemble a bell as the undersurface of the epithelial cap deepens. During this stage, the tooth crown assumes its final shape (morphodifferentiation), and the cells that will

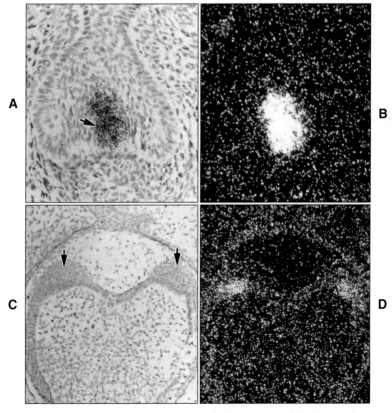

Figure 5-17 Expression of *Fgf-4* visualized by radioactive in situ hybridization technology; silver grains seen with conventional light microscopy **(A, C)** and darkfield microscopy **(B, D).** Expression occurs in the enamel knot *(arrows)* at the cap **(A, B)** and bell **(C, D)** stages of tooth development, indicating a relationship to crown pattern formation. *(From Thesleff I, Vaahtokari A, Partanen AM: Int J Dev Biol 39:35, 1995.)*

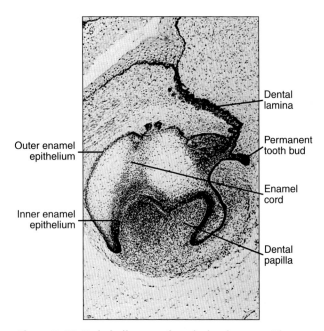

Figure 5-18 Early bell stage of tooth development. The enamel organ seems to be divided by the enamel cord.

be making the hard tissues of the crown (*ameloblasts* and *odontoblasts*) acquire their distinctive phenotype (histodifferentiation).

At the periphery of the enamel organ the cells assume a low cuboidal shape and form the *outer enamel epithelium* (see Figure 5-15, A). The cells bordering on the dental papilla assume a short columnar shape and are

characterized by high glycogen content (see Figure 5-15, B); together they form the *inner enamel epithelium*. The outer and inner enamel epithelia are continuous; the inner epithelium begins at the point where the outer epithelium bends to form the concavity into which the cells of the dental papilla accumulate. The region where the inner and outer enamel epithelia meet at the rim of the enamel organ is known as the *zone of reflexion* or *cervical loop* (see Figure 5-15, A); this point is where the cells continue to divide until the tooth crown attains its full size and which, after crown formation, gives rise to epithelial component of root formation. In the bell stage, some epithelial cells between the inner enamel epithelium and the stellate reticulum differentiate into a layer called the *stratum intermedium*. The cells of this layer soon are characterized by an exceptionally high activity of the enzyme alkaline phosphatase (see Figure 5-19, B). Although these cells are histologically distinct from the cells of the inner enamel epithelium, both layers work synergistically and have been considered as a single functional unit responsible for the formation of enamel.

FINE STRUCTURE OF THE ENAMEL ORGAN AT THE EARLY BELL STAGE

The fine structure of the tooth germ at the bell stage (see Figure 5-15) is uncomplicated but must be understood to appreciate the changes occurring to prepare for the

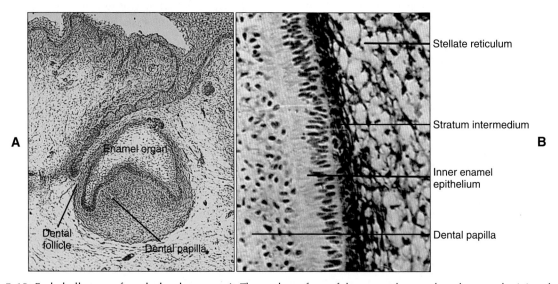

Figure 5-19 Early bell stage of tooth development. **A,** The undersurface of the enamel organ has deepened, giving the organ its bell shape. The dental papilla and dental follicle are evident. The tooth germ appears to have separated from the dental lamina and the permanent tooth bud, but this appearance is caused by the plane of section. **B,** The distribution of alkaline phosphatase in the early tooth germ is shown. Enzyme activity is demonstrated by the black precipitate localized largely in the stratum intermedium.

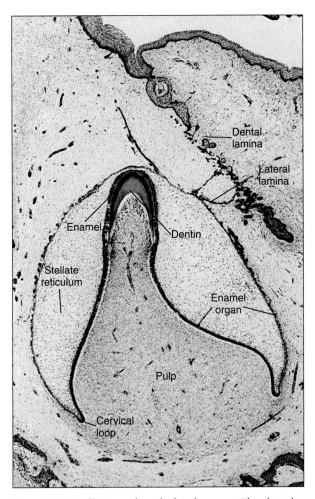

Figure 5-20 Bell stage of tooth development. The dental lamina is disintegrating, so the tooth now continues its development divorced from the oral epithelium. The crown pattern of the tooth has been established by folding of the inner enamel epithelium. This folding has reduced the amount of stellate reticulum over the future cusp tip. Dentin and enamel have begun to form at the crest of the folded inner enamel epithelium.

formation of the dental hard tissues enamel and dentin. The enamel organ is supported by a basal lamina around its periphery. The outer enamel epithelial cells are low cuboidal and have a high nuclear/cytoplasmic ratio (little cytoplasm). Their cytoplasm contains free ribosomes, a few profiles of rough endoplasmic reticulum, some mitochondria, and few scattered tonofilaments. Junctional complexes join adjacent cells.

The star-shaped cells of the stellate reticulum are connected to each other, to the cells of the outer enamel epithelium, and to the stratum intermedium by desmosomes. Their cytoplasm contains all of the usual organelles, but these are distributed sparsely. The cells of the stratum intermedium are connected to each other and to the cells of the stellate reticulum and inner enamel epithelium also by desmosomes. Their cytoplasm also contains the usual complement of organelles and tonofilaments. The cells of the inner enamel epithelium have a centrally placed nucleus and a cytoplasm that contains free ribosomes, a few scattered profiles of rough endoplasmic reticulum, mitochondria evenly dispersed, some tonofilaments, a poorly developed Golgi complex situated toward the stratum intermedium, and a high glycogen content.

DENTAL PAPILLA AND FOLLICLE

The dental papilla is separated from the enamel organ by a basal lamina from which a mass of fine aperiodic fibrils extends into an *acellular zone* (see Figure 5-15, A and C). These fibrils correspond to the lamina fibroreticularis of the basal lamina, and there the first secreted enamel matrix proteins accumulate (see Chapter 7). The cells of the dental papilla appear as undifferentiated mesenchymal cells, having an uncomplicated structure with all the usual organelles. A few fine scattered collagen fibrils occupy the extracellular spaces. The dental papilla is referred to as the tooth *pulp* when the first

---

TOPICS FOR CONSIDERATION   Tooth Agenesis

From an evolutionary genetic standpoint, mammalian dentition is considered a segmental or sequentially arranged organ system in which specific numbers of teeth are distributed in defined locations along the linear axes of the jaws. For developmental biologists, the model of tooth development offers a useful paradigm for studying patterning and morphogenesis or the determination of position, size, shape, and number during organogenesis.

As discussed in this chapter, the process of tooth development is under strict genetic control, suggesting that inherited forms of tooth agenesis are caused by a disruption in one or more of the molecular processes that regulate tooth formation. Notwithstanding the

evolutionary changes that account for differences between the heterodont dentitions of mice and human beings, there appears to be a remarkable conservation in biochemical and developmental pathways that control the initiation of tooth development in different vertebrate species. Therefore, inheritable disorders such as tooth agenesis in human beings provide unique opportunities to observe the clinical effects of different changes in a given signaling molecule and are also crucial to the discovery of novel genes that are important in tooth development.

In human beings, tooth agenesis is classified as a clinically heterogeneous condition that affects various

Continued

combinations of teeth. Tooth agenesis is the most common developmental anomaly in human beings, reported to occur in 2% to 10% of the population excluding third molars. Third molar agenesis is more prevalent and is reported to occur in approximately 25% of the population. This disorder is most often bilaterally symmetrical and affects permanent dentition at a much higher rate than primary teeth. Interestingly, teeth that are present are smaller in size; the lateral incisor frequently appears peg-shaped or conical. Tooth agenesis can be syndromic, nonsyndromic, or acquired. The nonsyndromic form of tooth agenesis can be sporadic or familial. Familial tooth agenesis typically is inherited in an autosomal dominant manner, but autosomal recessive and X-linked forms also have been reported. As noted for other inherited traits, variable expressivities are also evident in twins concordant for tooth agenesis, implying a role for genetic modifiers or dietary and other environmental factors.

Genes implicated in epithelial-mesenchymal interactions by studies in the mouse are strong candidates for human genetic conditions involving teeth anomalies. This is well illustrated in the case of mutations in the *RIEG* gene that is associated with Rieger's syndrome. The latter is an autosomal dominant condition that manifests as hypodontia and anomalies in the eye and umbilicus. The mouse ortholog of *RIEG* is referred to as *Pitx-2* or *Otlx-2* and is expressed in presumptive tooth epithelium as early as embryonic day 8.5 (E8.5). *MSX-1* was the first tooth-signaling molecule associated with human nonsyndromic premolar agenesis in a single large family. Genetic analysis revealed an Arg239Pro missense mutation within the DNA-binding homeodomain of *MSX-1* that was associated with the congenital absence of second premolars and third molars. Elegant biochemical and functional assays further determined that this mutation results in a functional loss of *MSX-1* function and that the mechanism of haploinsufficiency and not dominant-negative activity causes selective tooth agenesis in this family. More recently, another large family with a similar pattern of tooth agenesis was shown to have a nonsense (Ser104Stop) mutation in exon 1 of *MSX-1*. Affected members also had cleft lip, cleft palate, or both conditions. Previously work has shown that cleft palate and cleft lip are in linkage disequilibrium with *MSX-1*, suggesting that allelic heterogeneity involving *MSX-1* may predispose to orofacial clefting. A nonsense mutation in the homeodomain of *MSX-1* that resulted in a truncated MSX-1 protein was discovered recently in a family with Witkop's syndrome, in which premolar and incisor agenesis and nail hypoplasia are present.

Another defect involving the patterning of human dentition is the solitary median maxillary central incisor (SMMCI) caused by the premature fusion of enamel knots in the midline region and that is seen commonly in holoprosencephaly. A new missense mutation, I111F, in sonic hedgehog *(Shh)* recently was shown to be specific for the isolated SMMCI phenotype. Molecules such as *Shh* are thus critical for the initial outgrowth of the dental lamina. An alternate explanation is that SMMCI is a secondary defect that is linked with midline abnormalities.

Knowledge about the genetic cause of posterior tooth agenesis was expanded with the recent discoveries of mutations within the coding region of *PAX-9*. *PAX-9* belongs to the *Pax* family of paired box-containing genes that influence embryonic patterning and organogenesis. In each of these independent kindred, point mutations that resulted in a defective PAX-9 protein were associated with a pattern of tooth agenesis that selectively involved posterior teeth. This suggests a central role for PAX-9 in human tooth development. Because *MSX-1* and *PAX-9* mutations have been associated with a posterior pattern of tooth premolar agenesis, it is likely that the two genes share overlapping functions in the patterning of dentition. The exclusion of *PAX-9* and *MSX-1* in other families with premolar and molar agenesis implies that other genes, yet to be identified, contribute to selective tooth agenesis.

Evidence is mounting in support of the important partnership between Pax9 and Msx1 within the Bmp4 signaling pathway. Recent studies have shown that Pax9 directly transactivates the Msx1 promoter and that the two proteins interact synergistically to modulate the activity of the Bmp4 promoter. This contribution is significant because it is expected to provide the entry point into identifying other genes involved in the Bmp4 cascade that are potential candidate genes for human tooth agenesis.

More recently, *AXIN2*, a Wnt-signaling receptor was identified as responsible for a nonsyndromic form of tooth agenesis. Compared with a fairly mixed pattern of tooth agenesis seen in individuals with a nonsense mutation in AXIN2, the phenotypes reported in *MSX1*— and *PAX9*—affected families are more restricted to posterior dentition. Despite these exciting advances, only a sketchy understanding of the molecular pathways that influence the patterning of human dentition is currently available. Compelling questions still remain about the genetic cause and molecular pathogenesis of tooth agenesis. Further research that will provide a better fundamental understanding of how transcription factors achieve their context-dependent or tissue-specific functions can be anticipated. Therefore, what is learned will be equally applicable to research in emerging areas of tooth bioengineering and regenerative dental medicine.

Rena N. D'Souza
Department of Biomedical Sciences
Baylor College of Dentistry
Texas A&M Health Science Center
Dallas, Texas

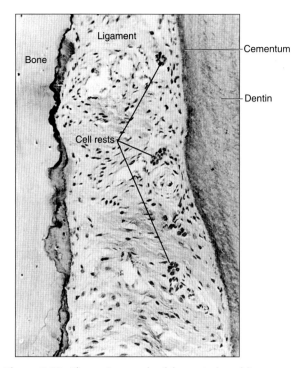

Figure 5-29 Photomicrograph of the periodontal ligament showing the epithelial cell rests of Malassez (remnants of the Hertwig's epithelial root sheath) situated along cementum.

the crown of the tooth. The central cells in this mass degenerate, forming an epithelial canal through which the crown of the tooth erupts (Figure 5-30). In this way, tooth eruption is achieved without exposing the surrounding connective tissue and without hemorrhage.

As the tooth pierces the oral epithelium, another significant development occurs: The dentogingival junction forms from epithelial cells of the oral epithelium and the reduced enamel epithelium (Figure 5-31). The importance of this junction already has been stressed (its histologic appearance is discussed in detail in Chapter 12).

FORMATION OF SUPPORTING TISSUES

While roots are forming, the supporting tissues of the tooth also develop. At the bell stage the tooth germ consists of the enamel organ, dental papilla, and dental follicle; this last component is a fibrocellular layer investing the dental papilla and enamel organ. The supporting tissues of the tooth form from the dental follicle. As the root sheath fragments, ectomesenchymal

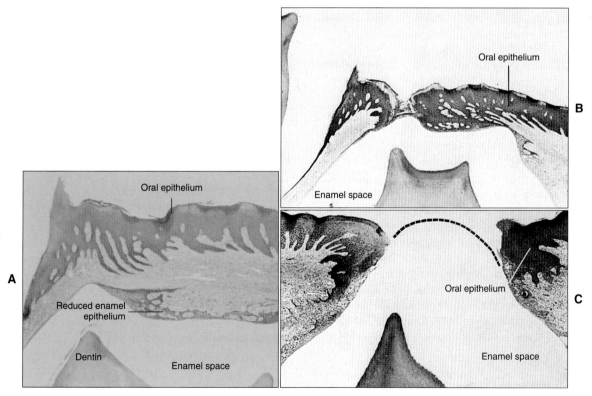

Figure 5-30 Erupting tooth. **A,** As the tooth approaches the oral epithelium, the enamel organ and oral epithelium are supported by the same connective tissue. **B,** The connective tissue is lost, and the two epithelia fuse along the lateral aspect of the tooth crown. The enamel organ over the tooth breaks down to form an epithelium-lined canal through which the tooth erupts. **C,** Epithelial continuity is maintained at all times; the dotted line represents the enamel surface.

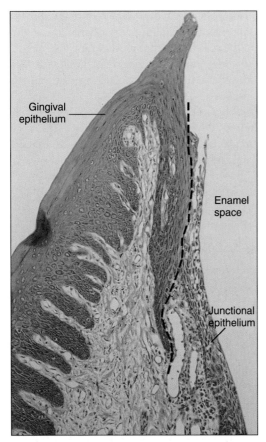

Figure 5-31 Formation of the dentogingival junction from the oral and dental epithelia. The dotted line separates junctional epithelium from oral epithelium.

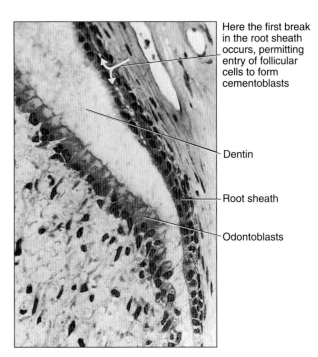

Figure 5-32 Fragmentation of the root sheath and the initial formation of cementum. Follicular cells migrate through a break in the epithelium (*arrow*) to lie against the surface of newly formed dentin.

cells of the dental follicle penetrate between the epithelial fenestrations and become apposed to the newly formed dentin of the root (Figure 5-32). In this situation these cells differentiate into cementum-forming cells (or cementoblasts). Chapter 9 also discusses the possibility that some cells from Hertwig's epithelial root sheath may transform directly into cementoblasts. These cells elaborate an organic matrix that becomes mineralized and in which collagen fiber bundles of the periodontal ligament become anchored. The cells of the periodontal ligament and the fiber bundles also differentiate from the dental follicle. Some recent evidence indicates that the bone in which the ligament fiber bundles are embedded also is formed by cells that differentiate from the dental follicle.

DEVELOPMENTAL QUESTIONS

Many important developmental questions still are unanswered. What is the molecular biology of root development? What is the role of nerves, and how important is angiogenesis for tooth development? These subjects have yet to receive important attention although they are central to understanding fully how teeth develop.

Because many of the genes involved in tooth development are also important for other developing organs or structures, few mutations have been identified that were specific for the teeth. The majority of human mutations causing teeth defects are syndromes with hypodontia. Only a few syndromes occur for which the mutations are known: *MSX-1* and *PAX-9* cause oligodontia; Rieger's syndrome is caused by a mutation in *PITX-2* (eye- and umbilical cord—associated defects) ectodysplasin, and its receptors have been shown to carry mutations causing tooth defects. Obviously, a proper understanding of the signals controlling development can help in understanding the organ and its function (in this case the tooth) and pathologic conditions associated with that organ or structure.

The developing tooth offers an attractive model to study morphogenesis and pattern formation, which in many ways is similar to the developing vertebrate limb. Multiple signaling molecules were found to be expressed in both systems (e.g., *Msx-1* and *Msx-2*, *Fgf-8* and *Fgf-10*, *Bmp-4*, *Shh*, and *Dlx-3* and *Dlx-5*), offering an interesting perspective on the conservation of signaling

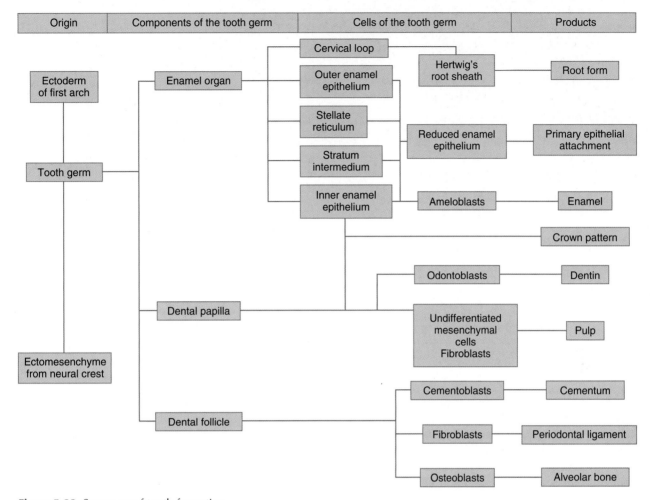

Figure 5-33 Summary of tooth formation.

molecules in the development of different structures. Therefore, any knowledge gained from tooth development also will benefit other developing systems, and vice versa.

In conclusion, this chapter has described the formation of the teeth and their supporting tissues in straightforward terms as summarized in Figure 5-33. Many of the more important aspects of tooth development are discussed in greater detail in subsequent chapters.

RECOMMENDED READING

Lisi S, Peterkova R, Peterka M et al: Tooth morphogenesis and pattern of odontoblast differentiation, *Connect Tissue Res* 44(suppl 1):167, 2003.

Maas P, Bei M: The genetic control of early tooth development, *Crit Rev Oral Biol Med* 8:4, 1997.
Miletich I, Sharpe PT: Normal and abnormal dental development, *Hum Mol Genet* 12(rev issue 1):69, 2003.
Thesleff I: The genetic basis of tooth development and dental defects, *Am J Med Genet A* 140(23): 2530-2535, 2006.

Bone

Bone is a mineralized connective tissue consisting by weight of about 28% type I collagen and 5% noncollagenous, structural matrix proteins such as bone sialoprotein, osteocalcin, osteonectin, osteopontin, and proteoglycans; growth factors and serum proteins also are found in bone (see Table 1-1). This organic matrix is permeated by substituted hydroxyapatite ($Ca_{10}[PO_4]_6[OH]_2$), which makes up the remaining 67% of bone (Figure 6-1). The mineral is in the form of small plates, most of which lodge in the holes and pores of collagen fibrils.

The structural organization and composition of bone reflects the activity of the cells involved in the formation of the organic matrix. Bone from different anatomic sites, developmental stages, and species exhibits different bulk biochemical properties, organizations, and relative proportions of collagenous and noncollagenous components.

Variations also exist at the microenvironmental level in the proportion of noncollagenous matrix proteins; indeed, regions containing a paucity or an abundance of these proteins can be found next to each other, reflecting local tissue dynamics.

In addition to its obvious functions of support, protection, and locomotion, bone constitutes an important reservoir of minerals. Systemically, hormonal factors control the bone physiology; locally, mechanical forces (including tooth movement), growth factors, and cytokines also have regulatory functions. Evidence also is increasing that there is central nervous system control of bone formation mediated by a neuroendocrine mechanism. Bone resists compressive forces best and tensile forces least. Bone also resists forces applied along the axis of its fibrous component; fractures of bone thus occur most readily because of tensile and slicing stresses.

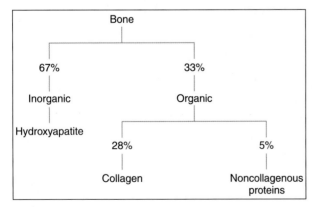

Figure 6-1 Chemical composition of bone.

GROSS BONE HISTOLOGY

Bones have been classified as long or flat based on their gross appearance. Long bones include the bones of the limbs (e.g., tibia, femur, radius, ulna, and humerus). Flat bones include all skull bones plus the sternum, scapula, and pelvis.

Characteristic of all bones are a dense outer sheet of *compact* bone and a central, medullary cavity. In living bone the cavity is filled with red or yellow bone marrow that is interrupted, particularly at the extremities of long bones, by a network of bone trabeculae (*trabecular*, *cancellous*, or *spongy* bone are the terms used to describe

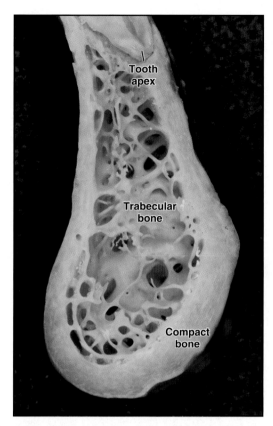

Figure 6-2 Body of the mandible. The outer layer of compact bone and an inner supporting network of trabecular bone can be distinguished clearly.

this network; Figure 6-2). These two types of bone behave differently and have different metabolic responses.

Mature or adult bones, whether compact or trabecular, are histologically identical in that they consist of microscopic layers or lamellae. Three distinct types of layering are recognized: circumferential, concentric, and interstitial (Figures 6-3 to 6-5). *Circumferential* lamellae enclose the entire adult bone, forming its outer and inner perimeters. *Concentric* lamellae make up the bulk of compact bone and form the basic metabolic unit of bone, the *osteon* (also called the *haversian system*). The osteon is a cylinder of bone, generally oriented parallel to the long axis of the bone. In the center of each is a canal, the *haversian canal*, which is lined by a single layer of bone cells that cover the bone surface; each canal houses a capillary. Adjacent haversian canals are interconnected by *Volkmann canals*, channels that, like haversian canals, contain blood vessels, thus creating a rich vascular network throughout compact bone. *Interstitial* lamellae are interspersed between adjacent concentric lamellae and fill the spaces between them. Interstitial lamellae are actually fragments of preexisting concentric lamellae from osteons created during remodeling that can take a multitude of shapes.

Surrounding the outer aspect of every compact bone is connective tissue membrane, the *periosteum*, which has two layers. The outer layer of the periosteum consists of a dense, irregular connective tissue termed the *fibrous layer* (see Figure 6-5). The inner layer of the periosteum, next to the bone surface, consists of bone cells, their precursors, and a rich microvascular supply. The internal surfaces of compact and cancellous bone are covered

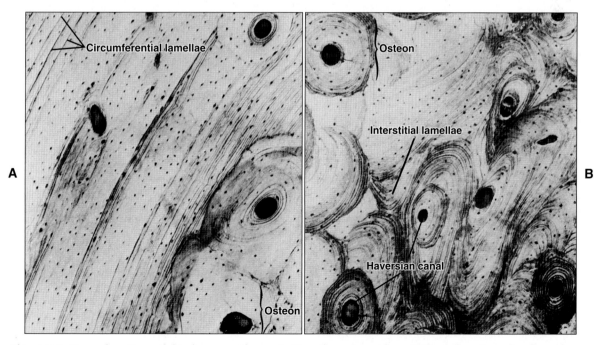

Figure 6-3 Ground sections of dried compact bone. **A,** Near the outer surface. **B,** Central portion of compact bone.

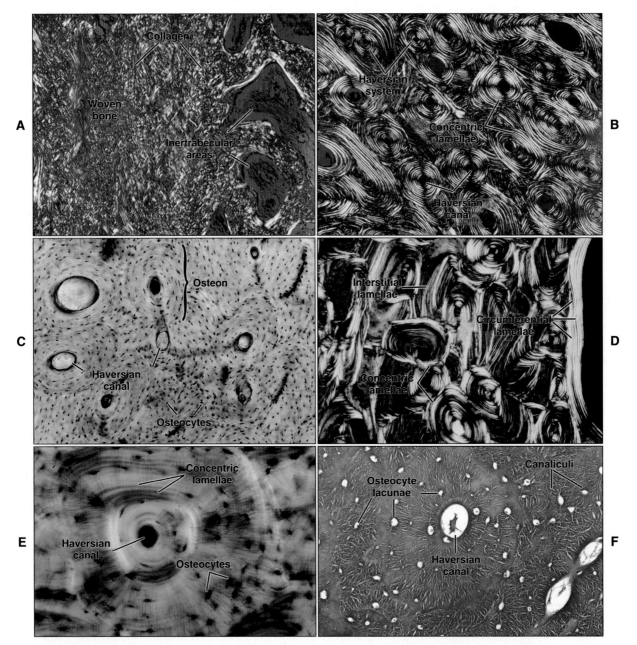

Figure 6-4 The organization of collagen and the various lamellae are seen readily using phase-contrast microscopy (**A, B, D**). **A,** Embryonic (woven) bone is characterized by randomly oriented collagen fibrils. **B** to **F,** Collagen fibrils in lamellar bone assume a layered organization. The osteon is the basic organizational unit in lamellar bone and is particularly evident in compact bone. It consists of concentric lamellae that form a cylinder of bone with a vascular canal—the haversian canal—at its center. Numerous osteocytes are entrapped in these lamellae. These cells reside in lacunae and their processes in interconnecting canaliculi that form an extensive network for the diffusion of nutrients and the transduction of local bone status. Interstitial lamellae are interspersed between osteons; these represent fragments of preexisting concentric lamellae. Circumferential lamellae enclose the outer and inner aspects of bone.

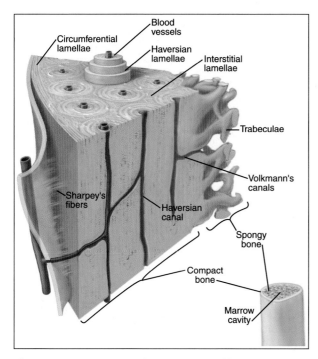

Figure 6-5 Organizational components of bone. *(From Pollard TD, Earnshaw WC:* Cell biology, *Philadelphia, 2002, Saunders).*

by *endosteum.* However, this layer is not well demarcated and consists of loose connective tissue containing osteogenic cells and that physically separates the bone surface from the marrow within. In general, the periosteal surface of bone is more active in bone formation than the endosteal one.

The descriptors used to describe the physical characteristics of bone are summarized in Table 6-1.

BONE CELLS

Different cells are responsible for the formation, resorption, and maintenance of osteoarchitecture. Two cell lineages are present in bone, each with specific functions: (1) *osteogenic cells,* which form and maintain bone, and (2) *osteoclasts,* which resorb bone (Figures 6-6 to 6-8). Osteogenic cells have a variable morphology, including osteoprogenitors, preosteoblasts, osteoblasts, osteocytes, and bone lining cells representing different maturational stages. The differentiation sequence from osteoprogenitor to preosteoblast does not show any distinctive morphologic features, and much research interest is focused on finding molecular markers for the various stages of the osteogenic life cycle.

OSTEOBLASTS

Osteoblasts are mononucleated cells that synthesize collagenous and noncollagenous bone matrix proteins; some of these constituents first accumulate as an uncalcified matrix called *osteoid* that is composed mainly of collagen that will act as a scaffold for the deposition of the apatite crystals of bone. Osteoblasts arise from pluripotent stem cells, which are of mesenchymal origin in the axial and appendicular skeleton and of ectomesenchymal origin (neural crest cells that migrate in mesenchyme) in the head. Although osteoblasts are differentiated cells, both preosteoblasts and osteoblasts can undergo mitosis during prenatal development and occasionally during postnatal growth. Both cell types exhibit high levels of alkaline phosphatase on the outer surface of their plasma membrane (Figure 6-9).

TABLE 6-1	Bone Terminology	
APPEARANCE	BONE TYPE	EXAMPLE
Gross appearance	Flat	Skull, pelvis, scapula
	Long	Axial skeleton
Macroscopic appearance	Compact	Mature bone; flat bones and shaft of long bones
	Spongy/cancellous/trabecular	Early embryonic bone; interior of extremities of long bones
Development/formation	Intramembranous	Direct transformation of mesenchyme
	Endochondral	From a cartilage model
Regions	Diaphysis	Shaft
	Metaphysis	Transitional portion of the shaft leading to the growth plate zone
	Epiphysis	Extremities of long bones
Microstructure	Embryonic/woven	Irregular collagen network
	Lamellar	Collagen arranged in concentric layers
Disposition of lamellae	Circumferential	Found on periosteal and endosteal surfaces
	Osteonic	Concentric lamellae forming osteons
	Interstitial	Residual fragments between osteons
Types of osteons	Primary	The first formed haversian systems (osteons) consisting of poorly organized lamellae
	Definitive	Higher orders of osteons formed after remodeling of primary osteons

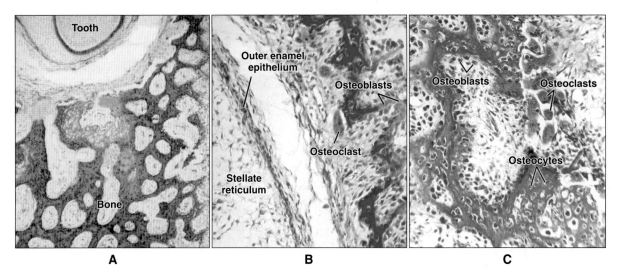

Figure 6-6 Light microscopic views of mandibular bone from an embryo. **A,** The bone forms by intramembranous ossification and initially assumes a trabecular organization. **B,** Plump-looking osteoblasts line forming bone surfaces. **C,** The abundance of large osteocytes entrapped in the bone and the presence of numerous osteoclasts indicates that the bone trabeculae are being formed and turned over rapidly. *PDL,* Periodontal ligament space.

Functionally, the enzyme is believed to cleave organically bound phosphate (see Topics for Consideration, p. 127). The liberated phosphate likely contributes to the initiation and progressive growth of bone mineral crystals. However, the function of alkaline phosphatase in bone-forming cells is likely complex and is not yet defined completely.

Osteoblasts are plump, cuboidal cells (when very active) or slightly flattened cells that are primarily responsible for the production of the organic matrix of bone (Figure 6-10; see also Figures 6-7 and 6-8). Type I collagen

is the dominant component of the matrix, which also contains small amounts of type V collagen and proteoglycans and several noncollagenous proteins. Osteoblasts exhibit abundant and well-developed protein synthetic organelles. At the light microscopic level the Golgi complex characteristically appears as a clear, paranuclear area that can be defined easily following cytochemical reactions for Golgi-resident enzymes (see Figures 6-8, A, and 6-10, A and B). The collagen type I molecule is formed and assembled, as in fibroblasts and odontoblasts

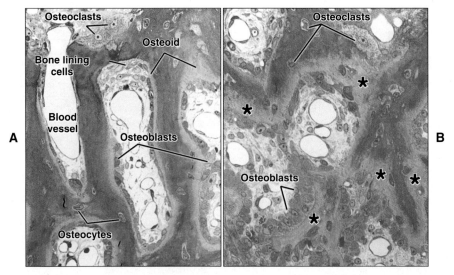

Figure 6-7 **A** and **B,** Mandibular bone soon after birth. By this time the bone has undergone substantial turnover and appears more compact (compare with Figure 6-6). Bone-forming surfaces are covered by plump osteoblasts or flattened, less active cells. Quiescent areas are covered by bone lining cells. Osteocytes are present within the calcified matrix and in some cases within osteoid *(asterisks)*. Osteoclasts usually are found opposite actively forming bone surfaces.

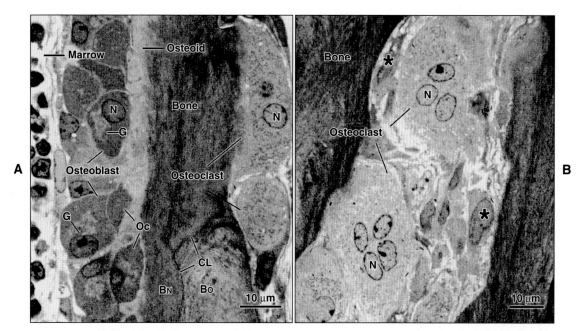

Figure 6-8 Immunohistochemical preparation of bone labeled for osteopontin. The dark, granular precipitates denote the site where this noncollagenous matrix protein is localized. **A,** Bone trabecula being formed along one surface by osteoblasts and resorbed by osteoclasts on the other. Osteoblasts form a layer of cuboidal cells, with an eccentric nucleus *(N)* and a large paranuclear Golgi complex *(G;* which appears as a clear cytoplasmic region) apposed to osteoid. Some of the osteoblasts are entrapped in osteoid as osteocytes *(Oc)*. Osteopontin is not distributed uniformly throughout the calcified bone matrix; one site where osteopontin is concentrated is in cement lines *(CL)* at the interface between old *(Bo)* and new *(BN)* bone. **B,** Osteoclasts are large, multinucleated cells that often work as groups to resorb bone. Mononucleated cells accompany them; some of these mononucleated cells *(asterisks)* eventually differentiate into osteoblasts to produce new bone on the resorbed surface.

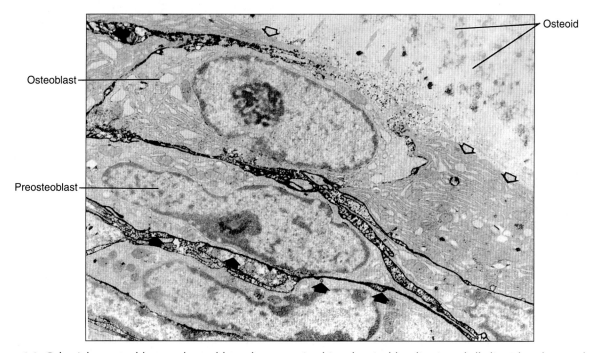

Figure 6-9 Calvarial preosteoblasts and osteoblasts demonstrating histochemical localization of alkaline phosphatase along the plasma membrane *(solid arrows)*. The amount of enzyme on the secretory surface *(open arrows)* of the osteoblasts is significantly less or is absent. *(Courtesy L. Watson.)*

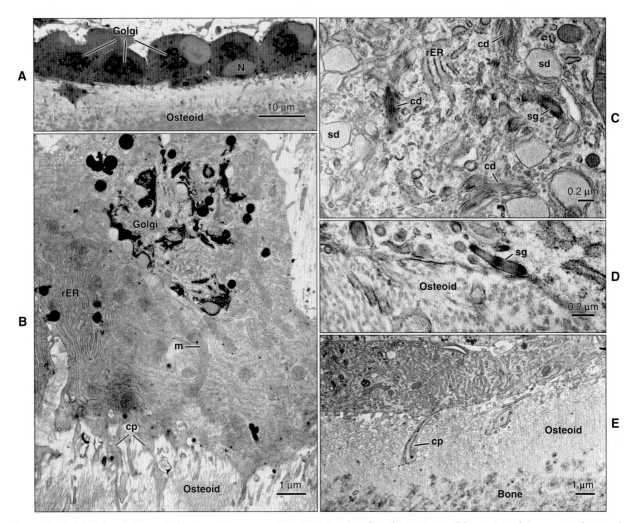

Figure 6-10 Light level **(A)** and electron microscope **(B** to **D)** micrographs of active osteoblasts. **A** and **B** are cytochemical preparations for pH-dependent phosphatase activity in the Golgi complex. **B** to **D,** These cells contain an extensive Golgi complex surrounded by abundant rough endoplasmic reticulum *(rER)* profiles. **C,** The Golgi saccules exhibit spherical *(sd)* and cylindrical *(cd)* distentions characteristic of collagen-producing cells. The linear pattern visible in the cylindrical distentions results from the assembly of the free polypeptides present in spherical distentions into triple-helical procollagen molecules. **D,** The cylindrical distentions bud off from the Golgi complex to form secretory granules *(sg)*. These collagen-containing granules are typically elongated structures with regions of increased electron density. **E,** As osteoblasts reduce their synthetic activity, they flatten, and protein synthetic organelles, particularly the Golgi complex, become reduced. *cp,* Cell process; *m,* mitochondria; *N,* nucleus.

(see Chapters 4 and 8), within the spherical and cylindrical distentions of the Golgi complex (see Figure 6-10, C). The typical elongated, electron-dense, collagen-containing secretory granules release their contents primarily along the surface of the cell apposed to forming bone. These molecules assemble extracellularly as fibrils to form the osteoid layer (see Figure 6-10, D and E). Some debate still continues as to whether the noncollagenous proteins are contained within the collagen secretory granules or in a distinct population of granules. Irrespective of this aspect, noncollagenous proteins also are released mainly along the surface of osteoblasts apposed to osteoid and diffuse from the osteoblast surface toward the mineralization front where they participate in regulating mineral deposition. Near the mineralization front, mineralization foci can be seen within osteoid, and certain noncollagenous proteins, such as bone sialoprotein and osteopontin, accumulate within them (Figure 6-11).

In addition to structural matrix proteins, osteoblasts, their precursors, or both secrete a number of cytokines and growth factors that help regulate cellular function and bone formation. These include several members of the bone morphogenetic protein (BMP) superfamily such as BMP-2, BMP-7, and transforming growth factor β, in addition to the insulin-like growth factors (IGF-I and IGF-II), platelet-derived growth factor, and fibroblastic

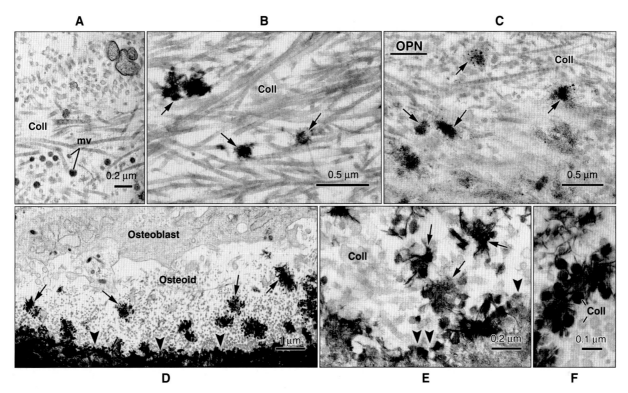

Figure 6-11 **A** to **E,** *Osteoid*, a term generally used in light microscopy, is a layer of nonmineralized matrix that gradually transforms into mineralized bone, a transformation that takes place at the mineralization front *(arrowheads)*. With an electron microscope, **(A)** matrix vesicles *(mv)* sometimes can be seen among the nonmineralized collagen fibrils *(Coll)*, and **(C** to **E)** mineralization foci *(arrows)* are found within osteoid near the mineralization front. **C,** Immunolabeling *(black dots)* reveals the presence of osteopontin *(OPN)*, among other noncollagenous proteins, in these foci. **F,** The linear profiles among the calcified collagen fibrils are mineral crystals.

growth factor. Although the timing of secretion and the complex interactions of these growth factors remain to be clarified, the combinations of IGF-I, transforming growth factor β, and platelet-derived growth factor increase the rapidity of bone formation and bone repair and are being considered for dental therapy. For instance, these combinations may be used to speed healing and bone growth after periodontal surgery or to prevent periodontal disease by the early treatment of periodontal pockets (see Chapter 14). Similarly, these factors may be used to enhance osseous integration after placement of dental implants.

The hormones most important in bone metabolism are parathyroid hormone (PTH), 1,25-dihydroxyvitamin D, calcitonin, estrogen, and the glucocorticoids. The actions of parathyroid hormone and vitamin D are dual, enhancing bone resorption at high (pharmacologic) concentrations but supporting bone formation at lower (physiologic) concentrations. Calcitonin and estrogen inhibit resorption, whereas the glucocorticoids inhibit resorption and formation (but primarily formation). The hormones affecting bone most likely work primarily through altering the secretion of cytokines and growth factors. Evidence is increasing that centrally

mediated mechanisms also are involved in bone metabolism. *Leptin*, a circulating hormone produced by adipocytes that is involved in regulating food intake and body weight, has been proposed also to control bone mass. This hormone acts on the hypothalamus and through involvement of the sympathetic nervous system can promote and inhibit the differentiation of osteoclasts. Some evidence also indicates that leptin also may work locally to promote the differentiation of osteoprogenitor cells and stimulate osteoblasts to make new bone.

Osteoblasts form a cell layer over the forming bone surface and have been proposed to act as a barrier that controls ion flux into and out of bone. Although there are no junctional complexes between cells, gap junctions do form and functionally couple adjacent cells. When bone is no longer forming, osteoblasts flatten substantially, extending along the bone surface (Figure 6-12; see also Figure 6-7, A). These cells, termed *bone lining cells*, contain few synthetic organelles, suggesting that they are less implicated in the production of matrix proteins. Bone lining cells cover most surfaces in the adult skeleton. It has been postulated that bone lining cells retain their gap junctions with osteocytes, creating a network that functions to control mineral homeostasis and ensure bone vitality.

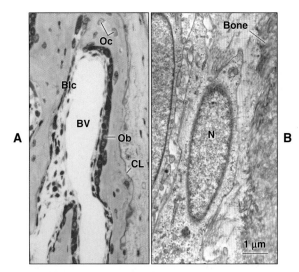

Figure 6-12 A, Light micrograph showing active and quiescent bone surfaces. Plump osteoblasts *(Ob)* line the surface where bone is actively being formed while bone lining cells *(Blc)* cover the quiescent surface. **B,** Electron micrograph of area labeled *Blc* in **A.** Bone lining cells are flattened osteoblasts with poorly developed protein synthetic organelles. *BV,* Blood vessel; *CL,* cement line; *N,* nucleus; *Oc,* osteocyte.

Such quiescent bone surfaces are believed to be the primary site for mineral exchange between blood and bone.

OSTEOCYTES

As osteoblasts form bone, some become entrapped within the matrix they secrete, whether mineralized or unmineralized; these cells then are called *osteocytes* (Figures 6-13 and 6-14; see also Figures 6-4, 6-6, and 6-7). The number of osteoblasts that become osteocytes varies

depending on the rapidity of bone formation; the more rapid the formation, the more osteocytes are present per unit volume. As a general rule, embryonic (woven) bone and repair bone have more osteocytes than does lamellar bone (Figure 6-15; see also Figure 6-6, C).

After their formation, osteocytes become reduced in size. The space in the matrix occupied by an osteocyte is called the *osteocytic lacuna* (see Figures 6-4, *E*; 6-13, *A* and *B*; and 6-14, *B* and *E*). Narrow extensions of these lacunae form enclosed channels, or *canaliculi*, that house radiating osteocytic processes (see Figures 6-4, *F*; 6-13, *C*; and 6-14, *E*). Through these channels, osteocytes maintain contact with adjacent osteocytes and with the osteoblasts (see Figure 6-14, *C*) or lining cells on the bone surfaces. This places osteocytes in an ideal position to sense the biochemical and mechanical environments and to respond themselves or to transduce signals that affect the response of the other cells involved in bone remodeling to maintain bone integrity and vitality, particularly for the repair of microcracks. Failure of any part of this interconnecting system results in hypermineralization (sclerosis) and death of the bone. This nonvital bone then may be resorbed and replaced during the process of bone turnover. Although osteocytes gradually reduce most of their matrix-synthesizing machinery, they still are able to secrete matrix proteins. Osteocytes also have been proposed to participate in the local degradation of bone (osteocytic osteolysis), thus influencing the structure of the perilacunar matrix.

OSTEOCLASTS

Compared with all other bone cells and their precursors, the multinucleated osteoclast is a much larger cell. Because of their size, osteoclasts can be identified easily under the light microscope and often are seen in clusters

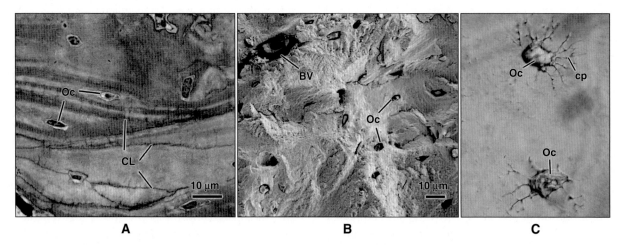

Figure 6-13 Light micrograph of rat mandibular bone **(A)** and scanning electron micrograph of rat tibial bone **(B).** Osteocytes *(Oc),* residing in lacunae, populate the bone. **A,** Abundant cement lines *(CL)* are present in the mandibular bone. **C,** Osteocytes have an extensive network of cell processes *(cp;* Nomarski optics). *BV,* Blood vessel.

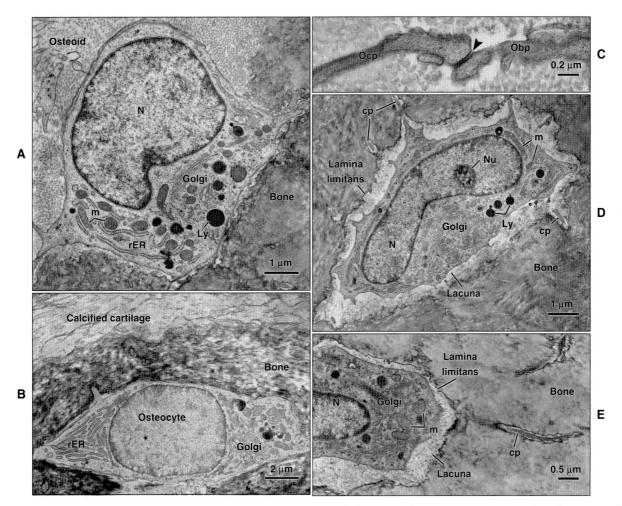

Figure 6-14 Electron micrographs illustrating various osteocyte morphologies. **A,** The osteocyte is entrapped partly in osteoid and bone. **B,** An osteocyte recently surrounded by bone and still near the surface. **C,** Gap junction *(arrowhead)* between an osteoblast process *(Obp)* and an osteocyte process *(Ocp)*. **D** and **E,** Older osteocytes, deep in bone, sit in lacunae delimited by a lamina limitans; these cells have numerous processes *(cp)* that ramify from the cell through bone in canaliculi. Although osteocytes have a reduced matrix-synthesizing machinery, they still are able to synthesize and secrete matrix proteins. They also occasionally exhibit numerous lysosomes *(Ly),* supporting the concept that they may participate in the local degradation of bone. *m,* Mitochondria; *N,* nucleus; *Nu,* nucleolus; *rER,* rough endoplasmic reticulum.

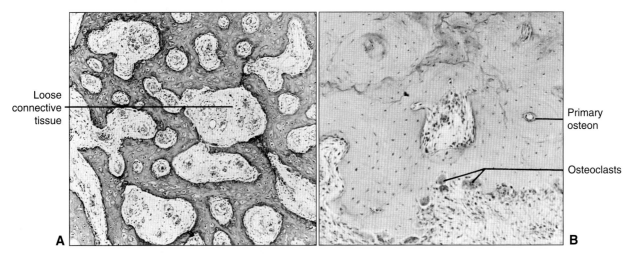

Figure 6-15 A, Light micrograph of woven bone. This bone exhibits high vascularity, soft tissue content, and bone cellularity. **B,** Light micrograph of older alveolar bone. This section exhibits primary osteons, less bone cellularity and loose connective tissue, a forming surface covered by osteoblasts, and a resorbing surface covered by osteoclasts.

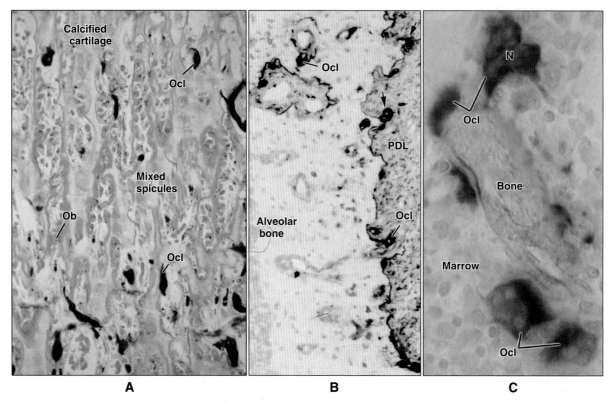

Figure 6-16 Histochemical detection of tartrate-resistant acid phosphatase activity, a marker for osteoclasts *(Ocl)*, in rat tibia **(A)**, alveolar bone **(B)**, and human trabecular bone **(C)**. **A,** Osteoclasts progressively remove the mixed spicules of the primary spongiosa of the growth plate. **B,** Numerous osteoclasts are seen along the surface where the periodontal ligament *(PDL)* attaches and, internally, in vascular channels. **C,** Several nuclei *(N)* are present in osteoclasts. *Ob,* Osteoblasts.

(see Figures 6-6 to 6-8; 6-15, B; and 6-34). The osteoclast is characterized cytochemically by possessing tartrate-resistant acid phosphatase within its cytoplasmic vesicles and vacuoles (Figure 6-16), which distinguishes it from multinucleated giant cells. Different osteoclast morphologies occur; however, unequivocally determining whether the cell is about to initiate or terminate resorption based solely on appearance is difficult.

Typically osteoclasts are found against the bone surface, occupying hollowed-out depressions called *Howship's lacunae* that they have created. Scanning electron microscopy of bone-resorbing surfaces shows that Howship's lacunae are often shallow troughs with an irregular shape (Figure 6-17), reflecting the activity and the mobility of osteoclasts during active resorption.

Under the electron microscope, multinucleated osteoclasts exhibit a unique set of morphologic characteristics (Figures 6-18 to 6-20). Adjacent to the tissue surface, the cell membrane of the osteoclast is thrown into a myriad of deep folds that form a *ruffled border* (see Figures 6-18 and 6-19). At the periphery of this border, the plasma membrane is apposed closely to the bone surface; and the adjacent cytoplasm, devoid of cell organelles, is enriched in actin, vinculin, and talin, proteins associated with integrin-mediated cell adhesion. This *clear* or *sealing zone* not only attaches the cells to the mineralized surface but also (by sealing the periphery of the

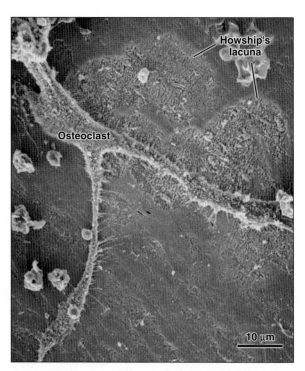

Figure 6-17 Scanning electron micrograph of a Howship's lacuna created by an osteoclast grown on a dentin slice. The cell portion visible on the micrograph is part of the osteoclast moving away from this resorption site to another.

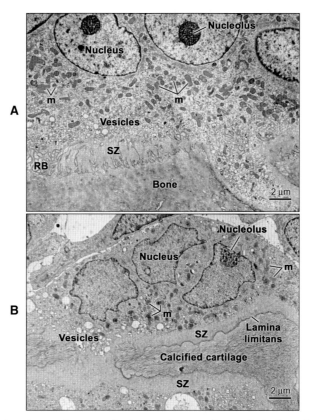

Figure 6-18 Electron micrographs of osteoclasts attached to **(A)** bone and **(B)** calcified cartilage. Osteoclasts are large, multinucleated cells with abundant mitochondria. Attachment occurs via the sealing zone *(SZ)* and resorptive activity along the ruffled border *(RB)*. An electron-dense, interfacial matrix layer *(lamina limitans)* often is observed between the sealing zone and calcified tissue surface. Abundant vesicles in the cytoplasm face the site of resorption.

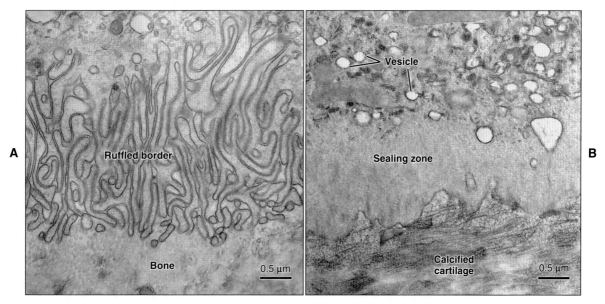

Figure 6-19 High-magnification views of **(A)** the myriad of membrane infoldings making up the ruffled border and **(B)** the sealing zone of osteoclasts. The fine striation and granularity in the sealing zone represents the concentration of contractile proteins in this region.

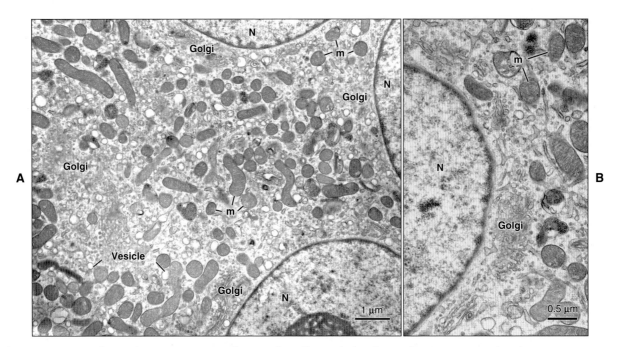

Figure 6-20 Osteoclasts possess numerous Golgi complexes located near the nuclei *(N)*. *m*, Mitochondria.

ruffled border) isolates a microenvironment between them and the bone surface. An electron-dense, interfacial matrix layer (lamina limitans) often is observed between the sealing zone and calcified tissue surface (Figure 6-21, *A*; see also Figure 6-18). Several mechanisms bind the osteoclasts to surfaces; among these, the concentration of arginine-glycine-aspartic acid (RGD)-containing molecules such as *bone sialoprotein* (BSP) and *osteopontin* on bone surfaces (lamina limitans) may facilitate osteo-clast adhesion and formation of the sealing zone by means of an $\alpha_v\beta_3$-mediated mechanism (see Figure 6-21, *A*). The cell organelles consist of many nuclei, each of which is surrounded by multiple Golgi complexes, mitochondria, rough endoplasmic reticulum, and numerous vesicular structures situated between the Golgi complex and resorption surface (see Figures 6-18 to 6-20). For years, osteoclasts have been known to be rich in acid phosphatase and other lysosomal enzymes. These enzymes, however, are not concentrated in the lysosomal structures as in most other cells. Instead, the enzymes are synthesized in the rough endoplasmic reticulum, transported to the Golgi complexes, and moved to the ruffled border in transport vesicles where they release their content into the sealed compartment adjacent to the bone surface, essentially creating an extracellular lysosome (Figure 6-21, *B*). Another feature of osteoclasts is a proton pump associated with the ruffled border that pumps hydrogen ions into the sealed compartment. Thus the sequence of resorptive events is considered to be as follows:

1. Attachment of osteoclasts to the mineralized surface of bone

2. Creation of a sealed acidic microenvironment through action of the proton pump, which demineralizes bone and exposes the organic matrix
3. Degradation of the exposed matrix by the action of released enzymes such as acid phosphatase and cathepsin B
4. Endocytosis at the ruffled border of organic degradation products
5. Translocation of degradation products in transport vesicles and extracellular release along the membrane opposite the ruffled border (*transcytosis*).

REGULATION OF BONE CELL FORMATION

Large numbers of cells must be recruited continuously to maintain the structural integrity of bone. Interference with recruitment mechanisms can cause pathologic conditions. Bone-forming cells have a mesenchymal origin, whereas that of osteoclasts is hematopoietic. Differentiation of both cell types is a multistep process that is stimulated by a unique set of cytokines, growth factors, and hormones that are part of complex signal transduction pathways. Figure 6-22 summarizes current opinion concerning the origin of bone cells.

Two transcription factors have been identified as essential for osteoblast differentiation from mesenchymal stem cells and their function; these are *Runx2* and *Osterix*. The Runx (runt-related) family of transcription factors is an important regulator of cell fate during embryogenesis and tissue differentiation. Only *Runx2* is

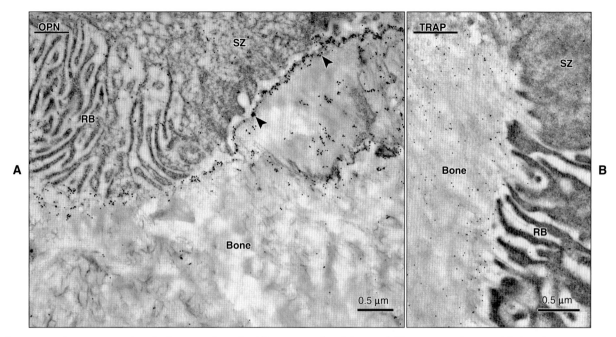

Figure 6-21 Immunocytochemical preparations for **(A)** osteopontin *(OPN)* and **(B)** tartrate-resistant acid phosphatase *(TRAP).* **A,** The bone surface *(arrowheads)* onto which the sealing zone *(SZ)* attaches often shows a concentration of osteopontin *(black dots).* **B,** Enzymes can be detected in the extracellular matrix where resorption is taking place. *RB,* Ruffled border.

involved in osteoblast differentiation, whereas all family members (*Runx1* to *Runx3*) seem to participate in chondrogenesis. *Runx2* acts as a master regulatory switch that mediates the temporal activation and/or repression of cell growth and phenotypic genes as osteoblasts progress through stages of differentiation. *Runx2* triggers the expression of major bone matrix proteins such as BSP, osteopontin, osteocalcin, and collagen type I, and it seems to control the maturation of osteoblasts and their transition into osteocytes. *Osterix*, which contains zinc finger motifs, belongs to the *Specific Protein (SP)* family of transcription factors. Little is known about how *Osterix* regulates osteoblast differentiation and function. *Osterix* may play an important role in directing precursor cells away from the chondrocyte lineage and toward osteoblast lineage. Bone genes are critical for bone formation; mice that do not express *Runx2* or *Osterix* show a complete absence of intramembranous and endochondral ossification. Also, differentiation of osteoblasts during development and remodeling depends on the activity of the Wnt (wingless) signaling pathway. The mechanism whereby this occurs is not fully understood, but there is evidence that the β-catenin pathway and BMP-2 signalling are involved. Finally, various non–bone-specific transcription factors also have been demonstrated to affect osteoblast differentiation and function; these include, among others, genes from the Dlx and Msx families that, as described previously, are involved in embryogenesis and tooth development.

Important advances also can be expected from the realization that pluripotent mesenchymal cells are found in the postnatal bone marrow stroma. Some cells from this stroma can generate a broad range of skeletal tissues, such as cartilage, bone, adipocytes, and hematopoietic stroma. Other stem cells with the capacity to differentiate in osteogenic cells have been found in adipose tissue, the umbilical cord, pulp, and periodontal tissues. Cells from these sources could be induced to form bone, and their use may form the basis for developing novel therapeutic approaches, such as for augmentation of alveolar bone and repair of the temporomandibular articulation.

The multinucleated osteoclasts arise from hematopoietic precursors of the monocyte/macrophage lineage. Stromal cells in the marrow cavity and osteoblasts modulate the differentiation of osteoclasts via secreted molecules and via direct cell-to-cell interaction. The signaling pathway implicating the *receptor-activated nuclear factor κB* (RANK) and its ligand (RANKL) plays a major role in controlling osteoclastogenesis. RANKL, expressed on the plasma membrane of stromal and osteoblastic cells binds to RANK expressed on the plasma membrane of osteoclast progenitors to induce a signaling cascade leading to the differentiation and fusion of osteoclast precursor cells and promoting the survival and activity of mature osteoclasts. Osteoblasts also secreted a soluble decoy for RANKL called *osteoprotegerin* that blocks the interaction between RANKL and RANK and interferes with osteoclast formation.

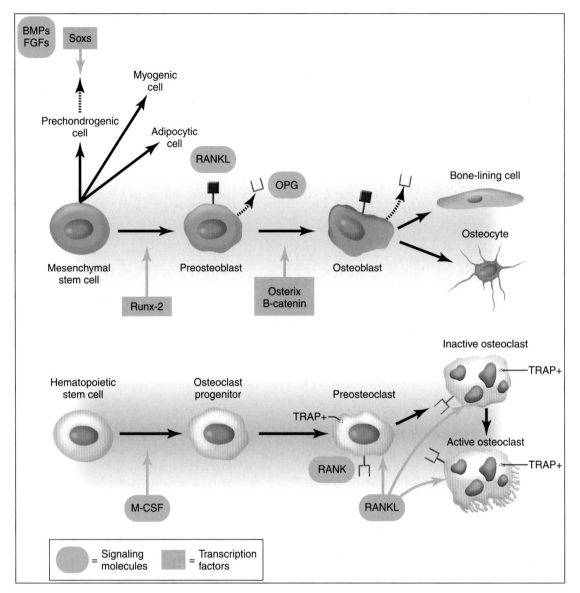

Figure 6-22 Origin of bone cells. *BMPs*, Bone morphogenetic proteins; *FGFs*, fibroblastic growth factors; *M-CSF*, macrophage colony-stimulating factor; *OPG*, osteoprotegerin; *RANK*, receptor-activated nuclear factor κB; *RANKL*, receptor-activated nuclear factor κB ligand; *TRAP*, tartrate-resistant acid phosphatase.

All three—osteoprotegerin, RANKL, and RANK—belong to the *tumor necrosis factor*/receptor superfamily. Several autocrine/paracrine factors influence osteoprotegerin and RANKL production; some of these are proinflammatory cytokines that under normal physiologic conditions help to maintain a proper balance between bone formation and resorption but that in pathologic conditions, such as periodontal diseases, favor bone loss.

Because the bone marrow stroma includes direct progenitors of osteoblasts and regulates the differentiation of osteoclast progenitors, the bone marrow stroma is a tissue of critical importance for skeletal physiology. The main cell type in the bone marrow stroma is a cell with a reticular morphology, which expresses alkaline phosphatase and resides at the abluminal side of sinusoids and arterioles.

BONE DEVELOPMENT

Although histologically one bone is no different from another, bone formation occurs by three main mechanisms: *endochondral*, *intramembranous*, and *sutural*. Endochondral bone formation takes place when cartilage is replaced by bone. Intramembranous bone formation occurs directly within mesenchyme. Bone formation along sutural margins is a special case.

TOPICS FOR CONSIDERATION   Organic-Inorganic Relationships During the Early Phases of the Calcification Process

The mechanism of biologic calcifications and the structures involved in their early phases are still poorly known. Electron microscope studies using approaches that preserve relationships between organic and inorganic components have revealed the presence of organic structures possessing the same ultrastructural morphology as that of the mineral crystals in areas of early calcification. The similarity is so close that the organic structures have been called crystal ghosts.[1,2]

Crystal ghosts can be seen best at early calcification sites (calcification nodules) of cartilage, bone, dentin, and cementum, in which they have the same needlelike or platelike shape as the crystals themselves. Crystal ghosts are also easily detectable in immature enamel, where they show the same ribbonlike shape as the crystals. Crystal ghosts also have been described in calcium oxalate stones and other pathologically calcified tissues. The morphologic similarity between crystals and their ghosts lead to the conclusion that the areas of early calcification consist of organic-inorganic structures (for a review, see Bonucci[3]).

Surprisingly, although these findings suggest that the crystal ghosts have a direct role in inducing calcification, poor attention has been paid to them. This is likely due to the deeply rooted idea that biologic calcifications occur through a physical process of heterogeneous nucleation that in mesenchymal tissues is catalyzed by organic components. According to this theory, early inorganic nuclei are formed from metastable solutions of inorganic ions contained in closed compartments that intrinsic structure of which is epitaxial to apatite nucleation. This means that, on one hand, these compartments are able to accumulate inorganic ions in a metastable equilibrium and that, on the other hand, they contain groups of atoms arranged in such a way as to allow the overgrowth of apatite nuclei according to the apatite reticulum (epitaxy). The nuclei subsequently grow into crystals by the further aggregation of inorganic ions, and the compartments provide the space necessary for their development. This theory leaves no room for crystal ghosts, and their apparently inexplicable presence in areas of early calcification has been explained rather offhandedly by assuming that they are technical artifacts.[4]

The crystal ghost concept, that is, that the early crystals are organic-inorganic structures, has been challenged on the basis that this relationship is not compatible with the atomic lattice that specifically characterizes each crystal according to the laws of mineralogy.[5] Actually, it has long been known that the early crystals display poorly defined, almost amorphous x-ray and electron diffractograms, suggesting that during the earliest phase of their formation, they are not fully crystalline. Moreover, it has been shown that traces of intracrystalline organic material are occluded in mollusk shells, sea urchin spicules, crustacean cuticle, corals, and other organisms, without this altering the crystalline characteristics of the calcified matrix.[6,7] The intracrystalline location of organic material in invertebrate calcified structures is confirmed by immunohistochemical studies, for instance, showing the presence of protein SM30 in spicules of sea urchin larvae.[8]

Although a definitive conclusion on the function of crystal ghosts cannot yet be reached, the following hypothesis can be put forward.[3] Calcifying organic matrices contain acidic, polymeric molecules with acidic groups (phosphate in glycoproteins and/or phospholipids, sulfate in proteoglycans, carboxyl in amino acids such as aspartic acid) that are located in such a way as to link calcium ions according to the apatite reticulum (epitaxy). When these acidic groups are activated (perhaps through their unmasking by the removal of inhibitors), they link inorganic ions and give rise to organic-inorganic, crystal-like structures with shapes that depend on that of the organic component (the crystal ghost) that acts as a template for the whole structure. The removal of the organic component by proteases (a well-known process in mature enamel) eventually leads to the formation of definitive crystals. The glycosylated, sialic acid–rich phosphoprotein called acidic protein-75 or bone acidic glycoprotein (BAG-75), which is a component of fibrillar scaffolds or vesicle-like structures in areas of early calcification in bone and dentin,[9] is an example of acidic molecule possibly involved in early calcification.

The crystal ghost theory assumes that biologic calcifications are initiated by biochemical processes that, in contrast to the theory of heterogeneous nucleation, do not require metastable solutions, compartments, or strictly specific matrix components and can occur in tissues as different as bone and enamel in vertebrates, the shells of mollusks, or the spicules of sea urchin embryos. The theory is still to some extent hypothetical, but it is based on the established, fundamental concept that the early inorganic structures found in the areas of initial calcification are not true crystals formed through a physical process of heterogeneous nucleation; they are organic-inorganic structures the origin of which is a chemical reaction of inorganic ions with the acidic

Continued

groups of a template, as supported by a number of findings. The removal of the organic template eventually permits the maturation of these organic-inorganic structures into true crystals.

REFERENCES

1. Bonucci E, Reurink J: The fine structure of decalcified cartilage and bone: a comparison between decalcification procedures performed before and after embedding, *Calcif Tissue Res* 25:179, 1978.
2. Bonucci E: Crystal ghosts and biological mineralization: fancy spectres in an old castle, or neglected structures worthy of belief? *J Bone Miner Metab* 20:249, 2002.
3. Bonucci E: *Biological calcification: normal and pathological processes in the early stages*, Berlin, 2007, Springer-Verlag.
4. Glimcher MJ: Composition, structure, and organization of bone and other mineralized tissues and the mechanism of calcification. In Greep RO, Astwood EB, editors: *Handbook of physiology: endocrinology*, Washington, 1976, American Physiological Society.
5. Warshawsky H: Organization of crystals in enamel, *Anat Rec* 224:242, 1989.
6. Aizenberg J, Ilan M, Weiner S, Addadi L: Intracrystalline macromolecules are involved in the morphogenesis of calcitic sponge spicules, *Connect Tissue Res* 34:255, 1996.
7. Albeck S, Addadi L, Weiner S: Regulation of calcite crystal morphology by intracrystalline acidic proteins and glycoproteins, *Connect Tiss Res* 35:365, 1996.
8. Seto J, Zhang Y, Hamilton P, Wilt F: The localization of occluded matrix proteins in calcareous spicules of sea urchin larvae, *J Struct Biol* 148:123, 2004.
9. Gorski JP: Acidic phosphoproteins from bone matrix: a structural rationalization of their role in mineralization, *Calcif Tissue Int* 50:391, 1992.

Ermanno Bonucci
*Department of Experimental Medicine
"La Sapienza" University
Rome, Italy*

ENDOCHONDRAL BONE FORMATION

Endochondral bone formation occurs at the extremities of all long bones, vertebrae, and ribs and at the articular extremity of the mandible and base of the skull. Early in embryonic development a condensation of mesenchymal cells occurs. Cartilage cells differentiate from these mesenchymal cells, and a perichondrium forms around the periphery, giving rise to a cartilage model that eventually is replaced by bone. Rapid growth of this cartilage anlage ensues by interstitial growth within its core (as more and more cartilage matrix is secreted by each chondroblast) and by appositional growth through cell proliferation and matrix secretion within the expanding perichondrium.

In the case of long bones, as differentiation of cartilage cells proceeds toward the metaphysis, the cells organize roughly into longitudinal columns. These columns can be subdivided into three functionally different zones: the zone of proliferation, the zone of hypertrophy and maturation, and the zone of provisional mineralization (Figures 6-23 and 6-24). The cells in the zone of proliferation are smaller and somewhat flattened and primarily constitute a source of new cells.

The zone of maturing cartilage is the broadest zone (see Figure 6-23); in this zone, chondrocytes hypertrophy and their secretory machinery changes. In the early stages of hypertrophy the chondrocytes secrete mainly type II collagen, which forms the primary structural component of the longitudinal matrix septum. As hypertrophy proceeds, mostly proteoglycans are secreted, and when chondrocytes reach their maximum size, they secrete type X collagen and noncollagenous proteins that together with partial proteoglycan breakdown create a matrix environment receptive for mineral deposition. Matrix mineralization begins in the zones of mineralization by elaboration of matrix vesicles (Figure 6-25). These vesicles are small, membrane-bound structures that bud off from the cell to form independent units within the longitudinal septa of cartilage (they are not present in the transverse septa). The first morphologic evidence of a crystallite formation occurs in association with the membrane of these vesicles. The matrix vesicle provides a microenvironment in which all the proposed mechanisms for initial mineralization exist (see Topics for Consideration, p. 127). Thus the matrix vescicle contains alkaline phosphatase, pyrophosphatase, calcium-adenosinetriphosphatase, metalloproteinases, proteoglycans, and anionic phospholipids, which can bind to calcium and inorganic phosphate and thereby form calcium-inorganic phosphate phospholipid complexes. The longitudinal cartilage septa thus become calcified.

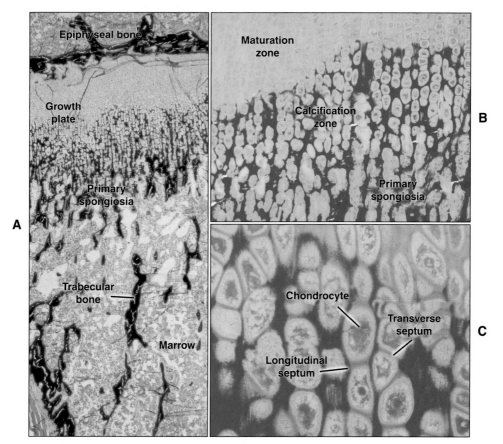

Figure 6-23 **A** to **C,** Light micrographs of endochondral ossification in the rat tibia. Sections were stained with von Kossa's stain for revealing mineral (in black). **C** shows at higher magnification the transition between the maturation and calcification zones of the growth plate cartilage.

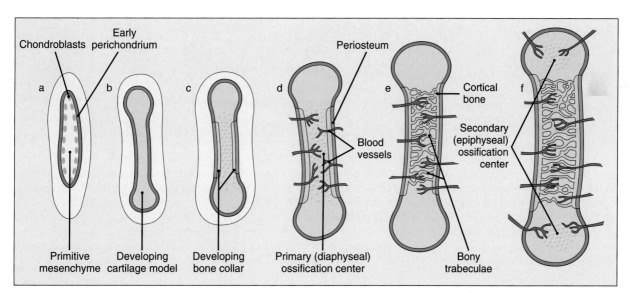

Figure 6-24 Endochondral bone formation. *a,* Chondroblasts develop in primitive mesenchyme and form an early perichondrium and cartilage model. *b,* The developing cartilage model assumes the shape of the bone to be formed, and a surrounding perichondrium becomes identifiable. *c,* At the midshaft of the diaphysis the perichondrium becomes a periosteum through the development of osteoprogenitor cells and osteoblasts, the osteoblasts producing a collar of bone by intramembranous ossification. Calcium salts are deposited in the enlarging cartilage model. *d,* Blood vessels grow through the periosteum and bone collar, carrying osteoprogenitor cells within them. These cells establish a primary (or diaphyseal) ossification center in the center of the diaphysis. *e,* Bony trabeculae spread out from the primary ossification center to occupy the entire diaphysis, linking up with the previously formed bone collar, which now forms the cortical bone of the diaphysis. At this stage the terminal club-shaped epiphyses are still composed of cartilage. *f,* At about term (the precise time varies between long bones), secondary or epiphyseal ossification centers are established in the center of each epiphysis by the ingrowth along with blood vessels of mesenchymal cells, which become osteoprogenitor cells and osteoblasts. *(From Stevens A, Lowe J:* Human histology, *ed 3, London, 2005, Mosby Elsevier.)*

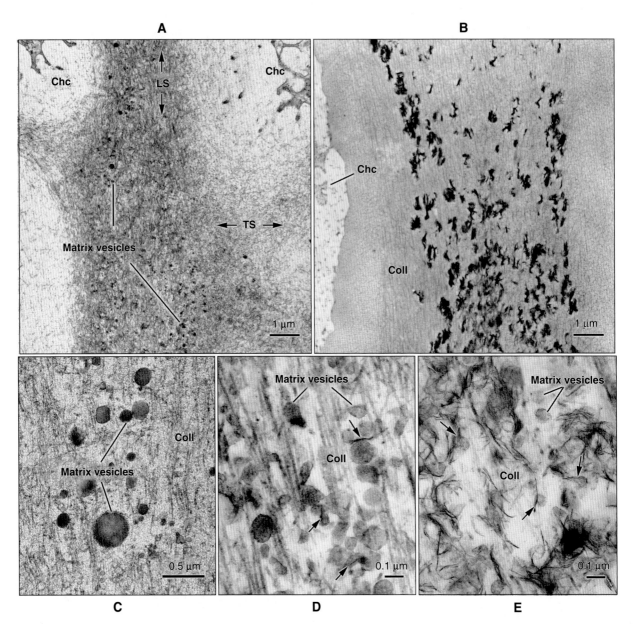

Figure 6-25 Electron micrographs of rat tibia growth plate cartilage illustrating matrix events in **(A)** the zone of maturation and **(B)** the zone of mineralization, and **(C to E)** the progression of matrix vesicles across these two zones. Matrix vesicles are small, membrane-bound structures that bud off from chondrocytes *(Chc)* and that provide a microenvironment favorable for mineral deposition. Crystal formation is believed to initiate in relation to the membrane of the vesicles. These first crystals *(arrows)* encourage the formation of more crystals around them, forming mineralization foci seen in **B** as irregular black deposits within the type II collagen matrix *(Coll)*. These foci gradually increase in size, transforming the organic matrix of the longitudinal septa *(LS)* into calcified cartilage. The transverse septa *(TS)* do not mineralize.

TOPICS FOR CONSIDERATION   Alkaline Phosphatase: Its Role in Skeletal Mineralization

The alkaline phosphatase isozyme expressed in skeletal tissue is one of several members of the mammalian alkaline phosphatase gene family.[1] In human beings, alkaline phosphatases are encoded by four loci traditionally named after the tissues where they are expressed predominantly. The tissue-nonspecific alkaline phosphatase (TNAP) gene *(ALPL)*, located on chromosome 1, is expressed at highest levels in liver, bone, and kidney (hence the alternative name L/B/K alkaline phosphatase) and at lower levels in numerous other tissues. The orthologous TNAP gene in mice is called *Akp2* and is located on mouse chromosome 4. The other three human isozymes—that is, placental (PLAP), placental-like or germ cell (GCAP), and intestinal alkaline phosphatase (IAP)—show a much more restricted tissue expression, hence the general term *tissue-specific alkaline phosphatases*. These isozymes are encoded by three genes *(ALPP, ALPP2,* and *ALPI,* respectively) clustered on human chromosome 2, bands q34-q37, and are closely related to one another, showing 90% and 87% identical nucleotide and amino acid sequences, respectively.

The identification and study of inborn errors of metabolism often provides invaluable clues as to the in vivo function of a molecule. In human beings, only deficiencies in the *ALPL* gene have been observed. No cases of deficiencies in the *ALPP, ALPP2,* or *ALPI* genes have been reported, so the in vivo functions of the PLAP, GCAP, and IAP isozymes remain unclear. However, missense mutations in the human *ALPL* gene lead to the inborn error of metabolism known as hypophosphatasia, and studies of this disease in human beings and in mouse models have provided compelling evidence for the important role that alkaline phosphatase plays in normal skeletal mineralization. Hypophosphatasia represents a rare form of rickets and osteomalacia in which neither calcium nor inorganic phosphate levels in serum are subnormal. This condition is characterized biochemically by very low to mildly subnormal levels of serum alkaline phosphatase activity and elevated concentrations of pyridoxal-5′-phosphate (PLP, a hydrophilic form of vitamin B_6), inorganic pyrophosphate (PP_i), and phosphoethanolamine in serum and urine. The clinical severity of hypophosphatasia in patients varies widely, with perinatal and infantile hypophosphatasia representing the most severe forms and adult and odontohypophosphatasia, the mildest forms. The severity and expressivity of hypophosphatasia depends on the nature of the *ALPL* mutation, and the mapping of hypophosphatasia mutations to specific three-dimensional locations on the alkaline phosphatase molecule has provided clues as to the structural significance of these areas for enzyme structure

and function. Alkaline phosphatases are homodimeric metaloenzymes that contain two Zn^{2+} and one Mg^{2+} ions in the active site and an additional noncatalytic Ca^{2+} ion site. Most mutations causing severe hypophosphatasia map to five crucial regions on the alkaline phosphatase structure, namely, the active site and its vicinity, the active site valley, the homodimer interface, the top flexible surface loop or crown domain, and the Ca^{2+}-binding site.

Functional inactivation of the mouse TNAP gene *(Akp2)* phenocopies the severe infantile hypophosphatasia condition. The $Akp2^{-/-}$ mice display rickets and osteomalacia at about 6 to 10 days after birth; they develop extensive epileptic seizures and suffer from apnea, increased apoptosis in the thymus, and abnormal lumbar nerve roots, and they die shortly after at around postnatal day 12 to 15. Biochemically, these animals show the expected increased serum concentrations of PLP, PP_i, and phosphoethanolamine, all molecules that have been proposed as natural substrates for TNAP. Administration of pyridoxal (a hydrophobic form of vitamin B_6 that can traverse biologic membranes easily) temporarily suppresses the epileptic seizures and reverses the apoptosis in the thymus and the morphology of the lumbar nerve roots. However, the $Akp2^{-/-}$ mice still show a 100% mortality rate before weaning, and their demise often is preceded by epileptic seizures. Vitamin B_6 is an important coenzyme in several biochemical reactions, including the biosynthesis of the neurotransmitters γ-aminobutyric acid, dopamine, and serotonin, and is likely to be important for the normal perinatal development of the central nervous system. $Akp2^{-/-}$ mice have reduced brain levels of γ-aminobutyric acid, and it is also possible that impaired myelination of nerve cells in the brain and nerve roots descending within the dura may be a contributing factor to the development of epileptic attacks in $Akp2^{-/-}$ mice.

Although abnormalities in the metabolism of PLP explain some of the abnormalities of infantile hypophosphatasia, it is not the basis for the rickets and osteomalacia that characterizes this disease. In skeletal tissues, TNAP is confined to the cell surface of chondroblasts and osteoblasts, including the membranes of their shed matrix vesicles. Matrix vesicles are submicroscopic, extracellular, membrane-invested bodies containing calcium and inorganic phosphate (P_i). The first crystals of hydroxyapatite are generated within matrix vesicles in growth plate cartilage, developing bone, and dentin (panel 1 of the figure). This initial phase of hydroxyapatite mineral deposition occurs within the protected microenvironment provided by the membrane

Continued

TOPICS FOR CONSIDERATION   Alkaline Phosphatase: Its Role in Skeletal
Mineralization—cont'd

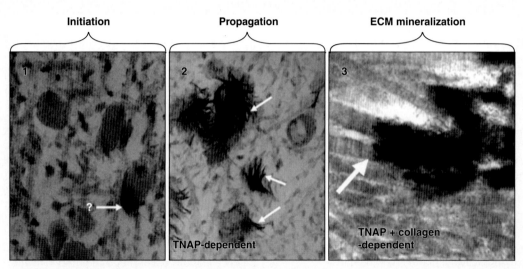

Current model of the sequence of events leading to skeletal calcification. **1,** The first step of mineralization (initiation step) encompasses the deposition of seed crystals of hydroxyapatite. This step appears to be independent of tissue-nonspecific alkaline phosphatase *(TNAP)* function because osteoblast-derived matrix vesicles from patients with hypophosphatasia and from *Akp2-/-* mice still have hydroxyapatite crystals in their interior. **2,** Subsequently, the hydroxyapatite crystals grow beyond the confines of the matrix vesicle membrane (propagation step). Clearly this step depends on the function of TNAP. **3,** Finally, the growing hydroxyapatite crystals continue to expand along collagen fibrils in the extracellular matrix (ECM mineralization). This step depends on the activity of TNAP and on the presence of fibrillar collagens (type I, II, or X).

of matrix vesicles and is followed by a second phase of mineral propagation in which hydroxyapatite protrudes into the matrix surrounding individual matrix vesicles (panel 2 of the figure). By an unknown mechanism, matrix vesicles are greatly enriched in TNAP compared with whole cells and the plasma membrane. It has been proposed that the role of TNAP in the calcifying matrix is to generate the iP_i needed for hydroxyapatite crystallization. TNAP also has been hypothesized to hydrolyze the mineralization inhibitor PP_i to facilitate mineral precipitation and growth. PP_i antagonizes the ability of P_i to crystallize with calcium to form hydroxyapatite and thereby inhibits hydroxyapatite deposition. Therefore, for normal mineralization to proceed, a balance is required between levels of P_i and PP_i. Electron microscopy studies using samples from patients with hypophosphatasia and also from *Akp2-/-* mice have revealed that TNAP-deficient matrix vesicles still contain apatite-like mineral crystals in the interior of the matrix vesicle, and thus it appears that the first step of matrix vesicle–mediated calcification is independent of TNAP function and unaffected in TNAP-deficiency. At this time, it is unclear what exact mechanisms might contribute to achieving the appropriate P_i/PP_i ratio

inside matrix vesicles needed to facilitate the initial deposition of hydroxyapatite crystals. A novel phosphatase, PHOSPHO1, with specificity for phosphoethanolamine and phosphocholine, the two most abundant phosphomonoesters in cartilage, has been proposed to function in this regard. However, hydroxyapatite crystal proliferation and growth is inhibited in the matrix surrounding matrix vesicles, both in patients with hypophosphatasia and in *Akp2-/-* mice. These data suggest that hypomineralization in TNAP-deficient mice results primarily from an inability of initial mineral crystals within matrix vesicles to self-nucleate and to proliferate beyond the protective confines of the matrix vesicle membrane. This failure of the second stage of mineral formation (panel 2 of the figure) may be caused by the lack of P_i generation or by accumulation of an excess of the mineral inhibitor PP_i in the extracellular fluid around matrix vesicles. Recent studies have provided compelling proof that the function of TNAP in bone tissue consists primarily in hydrolyzing PP_i to maintain a proper concentration of this mineralization inhibitor to ensure normal bone mineralization.

The nucleotidetriphosphate pyrophosphohydrolase activity of NPP1 and the transmembrane PP_i-channeling protein ANK are responsible for supplying the larger amount of PP_i to the extracellular spaces. Mice deficient in NPP1 *(Enpp1^{-/-})* or ANK *(ank/ank)*, have decreased levels of extracellular PP_i and display soft tissue ossification that includes the development of hyperostosis, starting at approximately 3 weeks of age, in a progressive process that culminates in ossific intervertebral fusion and peripheral joint ankylosis, as well as Achilles tendon calcification. Interestingly, affecting the function of NPP1 or ANK has been shown to have beneficial consequences on hypophosphatasia by reducing the amounts of extracellular PP_i in the *Akp2^{-/-}* mice. Indeed, the combination of two mutations—that is, [*Akp2^{-/-}; Enpp1^{-/-}*] and [*Akp2^{-/-}; ank/ank*]—led to normalization of extracellular PP_i concentrations and amelioration of hypophosphatasia. Interestingly, the expression of yet another mineralization inhibitor, osteopontin, was highly elevated in *Akp2^{-/-}* mice although it was decreased in the *Enpp1^{-/-}* and the *ank/ank* osteoblasts. Importantly, PP_i and osteopontin levels were corrected in [*Akp2^{-/-}; Enpp1^{-/-}*] and [*Akp2^{-/-}; ank/ank*] double-knockout mice. In vitro experiments on osteoblasts treated with exogenous PP_i revealed an increase in osteopontin expression and decreased NPP1 and ANK expression. These studies provided evidence for a direct regulation of osteopontin expression by NPP1 and ANK, mediated by PP_i, and suggest a model for the concerted action of the molecules that produce, transport, and degrade PP_i. Under normal conditions the concerted action of TNAP, NPP1, and ANK regulate PP_i and osteopontin levels and thus control hydroxyapatite deposition. Hypophosphatasia in the *Akp2^{-/-}* mice arises from deficits in TNAP activity, resulting in an increase in PP_i levels and a concomitant increase in osteopontin levels; the combined inhibitory effect of these molecules leads to hypomineralization.

Interestingly, the rescue of hypophosphatasia abnormalities by abolishing NPP1 function is site-specific and extends to the calvaria, spine, and partially to the metatarsals but not to the long bones in [*Akp2^{-/-}; Enpp1^{-/-}*] double-deficient mice. This is likely due to the relatively higher endogenous levels of NPP1 activity in the cranium, vertebrae, and ligaments compared with long bones. In tissues such as calvaria and vertebrae in which endogenous NPP1 activity is high, the resulting high PP_i concentrations would have an inhibitory effect on mineralization, and thus ablation of NPP1 in a *Akp2^{-/-}* mice would lead to normalization of PP_i concentration and amelioration of the abnormalities in those tissues. However, although PP_i concentrations above 1 mM inhibit mineral deposition, concentrations in the range 0.01 to 0.1 mM have been shown to stimulate mineralization in organ-cultured chick femurs and by isolated rat matrix vesicles. Given that at physiologic pH the K_m of TNAP for PP_i is about 0.5 mM, at this range of physiologic extracellular PP_i concentrations, most PP_i would be hydrolyzed to P_i by TNAP, thus providing P_i for incorporation into nascent mineral. Thus in long bones, PP_i concentrations may not reach the levels required to act as an inhibitor of calcification, and thus no improvement would be observed in those skeletal sites in the [*Akp2^{-/-}; Enpp1^{-/-}*] double-knockout mice. This dichotomy of the effect of PP_i concentrations nicely illustrates the bases for ongoing controversy as to whether it is the P_i-generating activity or the pyrophosphatase activity of alkaline phosphatase that is of most significance in vivo. The answer may well depend on the concentrations of substrates at specific skeletal sites.

Extracellular matrix mineralization is a physiologic process in bones and teeth and also in growth plate cartilage during skeletal growth. Recent data have shown that it is the unique coexpression of TNAP and fibrillar collagen in teeth and bones that primarily restricts calcification to those tissues under normal conditions (panel 3 of the figure). Experiments were conducted using transgenic expressing TNAP in the dermis, a skin layer rich in type I collagen, using the *col1a2* promoter, or in the epidermis, a skin layer that does not contain fibrillar collagen, using the keratin 14 promoter. All *Col1a2-Tnap* mice analyzed developed a dramatic mineralization of their skin extracellular matrix, consisting of hydroxyapatite crystal deposits as measured by electron diffraction and occurring along collagen fibers. In contrast, expression of *K14*-TNAP in keratinocytes, a cell type that does not secrete fibrillar collagen, did not lead to mineralization of the epidermis. Extracellular matrix mineralization also was observed in other locations such as arteries and sclera of the eye, two other tissues rich in type I collagen in which the transgene was expressed. Thus from the foregoing presentation, it is clear that alkaline phosphatase function is not required for the initial deposition of hydroxyapatite crystals inside matrix vesicles but is crucial for the propagation of hydroxyapatite crystal in the second step of matrix vesicle–mediated calcification and for the extensive deposition of hydroxyapatite crystals along collagen fibers in the calcifying matrix.

REFERENCE

1. Millán JL: Mammalian alkaline phosphatases. In *Biology to applications in medicine and biotechnology*, Weinheim, Germany, 2006, Wiley-VCH Verlag.

José Luis Millán
*Burnham Institute for Medical Research
La Jolla, California*

Concurrently, vascularization of the middle of the cartilage occurs. Within the perichondrium in the diaphysis, vascularization is increased, the perichondrium converts to a periosteum, and intramembranous bone begins to form. Centrally, the calcified cartilage disintegrates, and multinucleated cells called *chondroclasts* (identical to osteoclasts) resorb most of the mineralized matrix, making room for further vascular ingrowth. Mesenchymal (perivascular) cells accompany the invading blood vessels, proliferating and migrating onto the remains of the mineralized cartilage matrix. The longitudinal septa are generally all that is left of cartilage,

the horizontal septa having been resorbed completely. The mesenchymal cells differentiate into osteoblasts and begin to deposit osteoid on the mineralized cartilage columns and then mineralize it. As the bone matrix is produced, the mineralized cartilage becomes covered by a circular rim of new bone matrix, together forming *mixed spicules*, which hang in the marrow space (Figure 6-26; see also Figures 6-16, A, and 6-23). Bone matrix surrounds and entraps some of the osteoblasts and these become osteocytes. The network of mixed spicules collectively is termed the *primary spongiosa*. With time, the space created by the invading vascular system develops into red

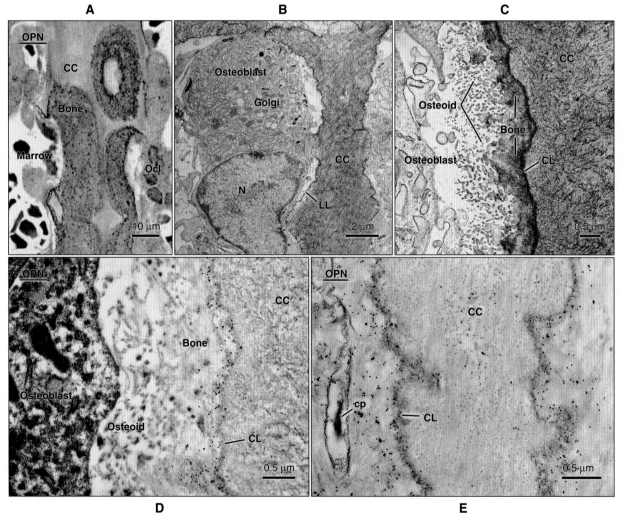

Figure 6-26 Endochondral bone formation. **A,** Light-level micrograph of a mixed spicule consisting of a calcified cartilage core *(CC)* onto which bone is deposited. The black deposits over bone represent immunocytochemical labeling for osteopontin *(OPN)*. **B** and **C** are electron micrographs that illustrate the sequence of bone deposition onto calcified cartilage. Osteoblasts surround the cartilage. First, an electron-dense surface coating appears on the cartilage; this coating is initially termed *lamina limitans (LL)* when osteoblasts are apposed to it and *cement line (CL)* when it is at the interface between bone and calcified cartilage. Subsequently, there is deposition of osteoid, which gradually transforms into calcified bone. **D** and **E** are electron microscope immunocytochemical preparations showing the distribution of osteopontin *(black dots)* in the newly formed bone. *cp,* Cell process; *N,* nucleus; *Ocl,* osteoclast.

bone marrow. As the developing bone grows longer, the marrow continues to expand. Osteoclasts progressively remove the core of mineralized cartilage and the surrounding bone so that cartilage activity becomes restricted to extremities of the developing bone. This process occurs at approximately the same rate as cartilage formation, so that the volume of the primary spongiosa remains relatively constant during growth. Osteoclasts also expand the marrow cavity radially by resorbing bone along the entire endosteal surface.

In some bones (e.g., the tibia, but not the mandible), a secondary invasion of blood vessels into the head (end) of the bone creates a secondary ossification center (see Figure 6-24). This secondary bone growth proceeds in a fashion identical to that occurring in primary bone growth, resulting in a plate of growing cartilage remaining between the diaphysis and the end (epiphysis) of the bone. This plate is termed the *epiphyseal growth plate* (see Figure 6-23). Longitudinal bone growth occurs as a result of cell division and interstitial growth in the plate and ceases when the cartilage cells stop proliferating and the growth plate disappears. In addition, as longitudinal bone growth slows and ceases, so does the expansion of the marrow cavity. The bone-covered cartilage remaining in the primary spongiosa and in the secondary ossification centers is replaced by lamellar bone, thus creating the secondary spongiosa found throughout adult bone. The shaft grows in diameter as osteoblast differentiation and new bone deposition occurs on the periosteal surface while old bone is removed on the endosteal surface by osteoclasts.

INTRAMEMBRANOUS BONE FORMATION

Intramembranous bone formation was first recognized when early anatomists observed that the fontanelles of fetal and newborn skulls were filled with a connective tissue membrane that was replaced gradually by bone during development and growth of the skull. In intramembranous bone formation, bone develops directly within the soft connective tissue. The mesenchymal cells proliferate and condense (Figure 6-27, A). Concurrent with an increase in vascularity at these sites of condensed mesenchyme, osteoblasts differentiate and begin to produce bone matrix (Figure 6-27, B). As the mesenchymal cells differentiate into osteoblasts, they start exhibiting alkaline phosphatase activity (Figure 6-28). This sequence of events occurs at multiple sites within each bone of the cranial vault, maxilla, body of the mandible, and midshaft of long bones.

Once begun, intramembranous bone formation proceeds rapidly. This first embryonic bone is termed *woven bone* (Figure 6-29; see also Figure 6-6). At first the woven

bone takes the form of radiating spicules and trabecules, but progressively these fuse into thin bony plates. In the cranium, more than one plate may fuse to form a single bone. Early plates of intramembranous bone are structurally unsound, not only because of poor fiber orientation and mineralization but also because many islands of soft connective tissue remain within the plates. Soon after plate formation in the skull or the establishment of intramembranous bone formation in the midshaft region, the bone becomes polarized. The establishment and expansion of the marrow cavity turns the endosteal surfaces of bone into primarily a resorbing surface, whereas the periosteum initiates the formation of most of the new bone. However, depending on adjacent soft tissues and their growth, segments of the periosteal surface of an individual bone may contain focal sites of bone resorption. For instance, growth of the tongue, brain, and nasal cavity and lengthening of the body of the mandible require focal resorption along the periosteal surface. Conversely, segments of the endosteum of the same bone simultaneously may become a forming surface, resulting in bone drift.

Woven bone of the early embryo and fetus turns over rapidly. As fetal bones begin to assume their adult shape, continued proliferation of soft connective tissue between adjoining bones brings about the formation of sutures and fontanelles.

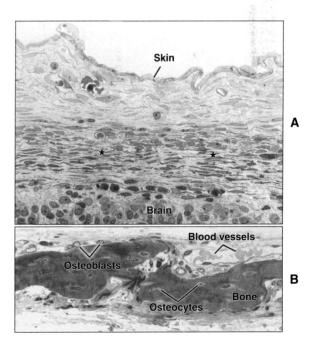

Figure 6-27 Light micrographs of intramembranous bone formation in the rat calvaria. **A,** Ectomesenchymal cells *(asterisks)* condense between the skin and developing brain. **B,** These cells differentiate into osteoblasts that deposit bone directly as woven cancellous bone.

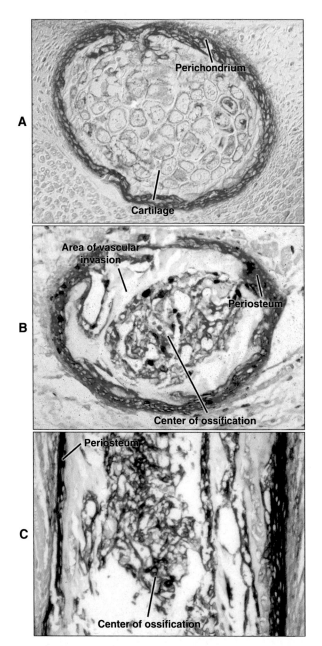

Figure 6-28 Intramembranous bone formation around the cartilage model of digits: **A** and **B,** cross section; **C,** longitudinal section. The preparations are stained for alkaline phosphatase activity, seen here in blue. Such activity is present in the perichondrium and periosteum, as well as in areas of vascular invasion.

From early fetal development to full expression of the adult skeleton, a continual, slow transition occurs from woven bone to lamellar bone. This transition is rapid during late fetal development and the first years of life (Figure 6-29, B; see also Figure 6-15, B) and involves the formation of primary osteons deposited around a blood vessel. The primary osteon tends to be small, with lamellae that are neither numerous nor well delineated.

As more osteons are formed at the periosteal surface, they become more tightly packed so that eventually a higher percentage of compact bone consists of osteons.

Woven bone is characterized by intertwined collagen fibrils oriented in many directions, showing wide interfibrillar spaces. Collagen fibrils in lamellar bone, however, are generally thicker and are arranged in ordered sheets consisting of aligned and closely packed fibrils. It follows from these structural features that the widely spaced collagen meshwork of woven bone will accommodate more noncollagenous matrix proteins.

Just as in the case of calcified cartilage, matrix vesicles are believed to be implicated in the initiation of mineral deposition during intramembranous bone formation. The relative importance of matrix vesicles versus secreted noncollagenous matrix proteins in the control of initial events in mineralization remains unclear, and both may be implicated, independently or in succession. The sporadic observation of matrix vesicles in osteoid (Figure 6-30, A; see also Figure 6-11, A) and their increase in number under some altered physiologic conditions suggest that matrix vesicles may play a predominant role when mineralization needs to be intensely promoted (see Topics for Consideration, pp. 11 and 127).

Among noncollagenous bone matrix proteins, BSP and osteopontin have received particular attention because they are implicated in cellular and matrix events. They are part of a family of proteins (SIBLING: small integrin-binding ligand, N-linked glycoprotein) believed to have evolved from the divergent evolution of a single ancestral gene. Because the site where a protein is present is suggestive of its function, the distribution of these two proteins has been studied extensively. In general, consensus exists that BSP and osteopontin codistribute. They are found in mineralization foci near the mineralization front, accumulate within the spaces between the calcified collagen fibrils, and are associated with cement lines (Figure 6-30). Depending on the antibody used for immunolocalization, osteopontin and occasionally BSP are immunodetected along the surface of osteocyte lacunae and canaliculi (lamina limitans). With respect to mineralization, the consensus of biochemical, functional, and immunolocalization studies is that BSP is a promotor and osteopontin an inhibitor. Surprisingly, mice that do not express the genes for these proteins (knockouts) do not show overt bone alterations, most likely because they are part of a redundant system. Studies are under way to determine how these proteins exert their effects and to characterize functional domains associated with mineral ion deposition, protein-to-protein interactions, and cell binding; such information is important for the creation of therapeutic peptides derived from these proteins.

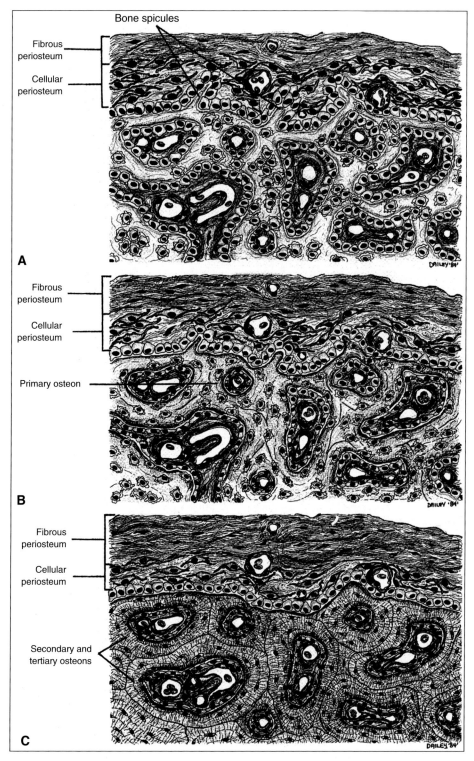

Figure 6-29 Intramembranous bone formation. **A,** Coarse woven bone. The bone is cellular and disorganized. **B,** Immature bone. The bone is less cellular and slightly more organized; some primary osteons are forming. **C,** Mature lamellar bone. The tightly packed osteons create an organized bone matrix; fewer cells and little loose connective tissue are apparent. As remodeling of the bone in its mature state takes place, the periosteal bone surface becomes more regular and eventually will be covered with circumferential lamellae.

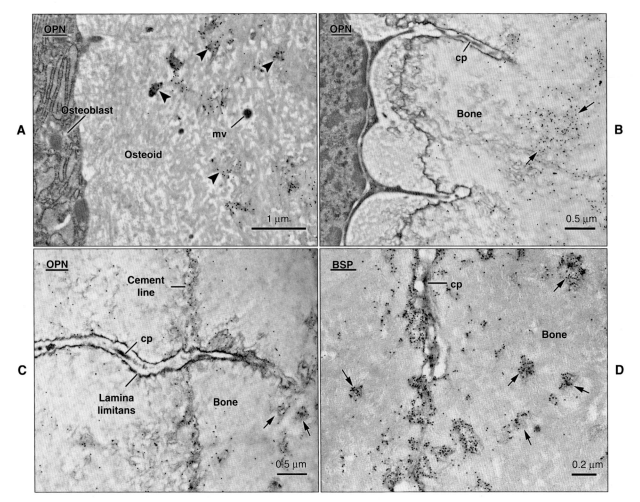

Figure 6-30 Immunocytochemical preparations illustrating the distribution of (**A** to **C**) osteopontin *(OPN)* in rat bone and (**D**) bone sialoprotein *(BSP)* in human bone. Both proteins are essentially found at similar matrix sites, that is, mineralization foci *(arrowheads)*, diffusely or as patches between the calcified collagen fibrils *(arrows)* and cement lines. *cp*, Cell process; *mv*, matrix vesicle.

SUTURAL BONE GROWTH

Sutures play an important role in the growing face and skull. Found exclusively in the skull, sutures are the fibrous joints between bones; however, sutures allow only limited movement. Their function is to permit the skull and face to accommodate growing organs such as the eyes and brain.

Understanding the structure of a suture is based on the knowledge that the periosteum of a bone consists of two layers, an outer fibrous layer and an inner cellular or osteogenic layer. At the suture the outer layer splits, and the outermost leaf runs across the gap of the suture to form a uniting layer with the outermost leaf from the other side. The innermost leaf, together with the osteogenic layer of the periosteum, runs down through the suture along with the corresponding layer from the other bone involved in the joint. The osteogenic layer of

the suture is called the *cambium*, and the inner leaf, the *capsule*. Between these two layers is a loose cellular and vascular tissue (Figure 6-31).

Sutures are best regarded as having the same osteogenic potential as periosteum. When two bones are separated—for example, the skull bones are forced apart by the growing brain—bone forms at the sutural margins, with successive waves of new bone cells differentiating from the cambium. Thus the histologic structure of the suture permits a strong tie between bones while providing a site for new bone formation. The two cambial layers are separated by a relatively inert middle layer so that growth can occur independently at each bony margin.

BONE TURNOVER (REMODELING)

The process by which the overall size and shape of bones is established is referred to as *bone modeling* and extends

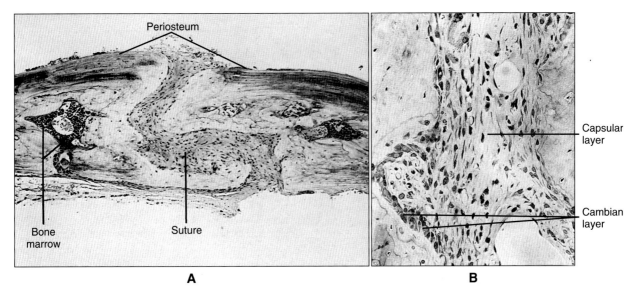

Figure 6-31 Sutural growth. **A,** Low-magnification light micrograph showing that the suture connects two periosteal surfaces. The central marrow cavity is ill-defined. **B,** A higher magnification shows the developing inner osteogenic or cambium layer and the central capsular layer.

from embryonic bone development to the preadult period of human growth. During this phase, bone is being formed rapidly, primarily (but not exclusively) on the periosteal surface. Simultaneously, bone is being destroyed along the endosteal surface at focal points along the periosteal surface and within the osteons of compact bone. Because bones increase greatly in length and thickness during growth, bone formation occurs at a much greater rate than bone resorption. This replacement of old bone by new is called *bone turnover* or *remodeling.* Bone turnover rates of 30% to 100% per year are common in rapidly growing children; most of the bone present today in a child will not be present a year from now. Bone turnover does not stop when adulthood is reached, although its rate slows. Indeed, the adult skeleton is broken down continuously and reformed by the coordinated action of osteoclasts and osteoblasts. In a healthy individual, this turnover is in a steady state; that is, the amount of bone lost is balanced by bone formed. In certain diseases (e.g., osteoporosis) and with age, the resorption exceeds formation, resulting in an overall loss of bone. Bone turnover occurs in discrete, focal areas involving groups of cells called *bone remodeling* or *basic multicellular units.* The sequence of events at these temporary and evolving anatomic sites consists of five phases: activation, resorption, reversal, formation, and resting (Figure 6-32). During the resorption phase, bone is removed and a resorption lacuna is created. Factors produced by osteoclasts, mononuclear reversal cells, or liberated from the resorbed bone matrix trigger the formative phase during which the lacuna then is filled with new bone produced by osteoblasts recruited at

the site. As these osteoblasts mature, they produce more osteoprotegerin and less RANKL, leading to a reduction in RANK/RANKL interactions. This results in an inhibition of osteoclast activity, thereby allowing osteoblasts to refill the resorption lacuna. The formation phase lasts substantially longer than the resorption and reversal phases together. Osteocytes are likely implicated in "sensing" the need for remodeling and transmitting signals via their extensive canalicular network to osteoclast and osteoblast compartments.

The rate of cortical bone turnover is approximately 5% per year, whereas turnover rates of trabecular bone and the endosteal surface of cortical bone can approach 15% per year. The release of mineral ions during bone turnover, together with the concerted action of the kidneys and intestine, is an integral part of the phosphocalcic homeostatis system.

Primary osteons of fetal bone eventually are resorbed by osteoclasts to make room for the expanding marrow cavity or undergo turnover; that is, a primary osteon is replaced by succeeding generations of higher-order osteons (e.g., secondary and tertiary). Each succeeding generation is slightly larger, functionally more mature, and therefore more lamellar (Figure 6-33). Exactly what induces turnover is still poorly understood and likely involves local mechanisms in the bone microenvironment and systemic factors.

As osteoclasts move through compact bone, they create a resorption channel. The leading edge of resorption is termed the *cutting cone* and is characterized by a scalloped array of resorption lacunae (Howship's lacunae), each housing an osteoclast (Figures 6-34 and 6-35). When a

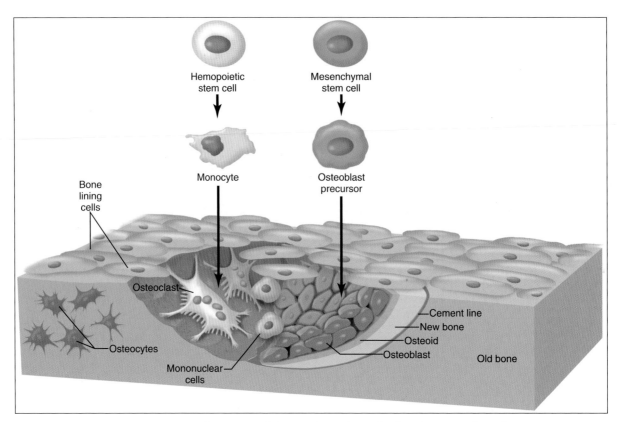

Figure 6-32 Schematic representation of bone remodeling on the surface of trabecular (cancellous) bone as seen in longitudinal sequence. The process occurs through the cooperative activity of various cells that form a temporary functional compartment known as *basic multicellular unit or bone remodeling unit*. The process begins with the activation of osteoclast formation, followed in order by (1) a resorption phase during which osteoclasts remove old bone and create the resorption lacuna, (2) reversal in which mononuclear cells (macrophage-like or osteoblast precursors) deposit a cement line, (3) a formation phase during which new bone is deposited, and finally (4) a resting phase during which osteoblasts become quiescent and become the flattened bone lining cells. These cells are believed to persist as a canopy over the resorption lacuna during the bone remodeling cycle. *(Adapted from Raiz LG:* J Clin Invest *115:3318, 2005.)*

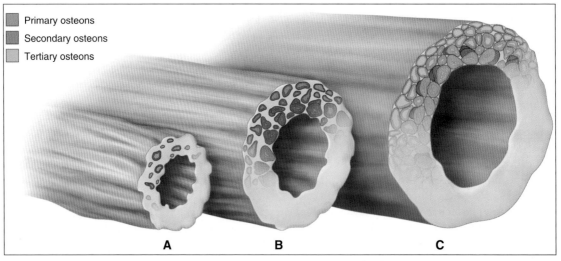

Figure 6-33 Progressive bone growth and turnover. **A,** Young immature bone is thin, with few primary osteons. The periosteal surface is undulating and forms bone rapidly. The endosteal surface is primarily for resorption. **B,** The immature bone thickens. The periosteal surface is not as undulating and secondary osteons are now present. The primary osteons are resorbed, and the fragments are buried by new bone on the periosteal surface. **C,** The bone becomes nearly mature. The bone is thicker still, its periosteal surface is less undulating, and tertiary osteons replace the secondary osteons. Fragments of primary and secondary osteons persist as interstitial lamellae. Eventually, circumferential lamellae smooth out the periosteal surface.

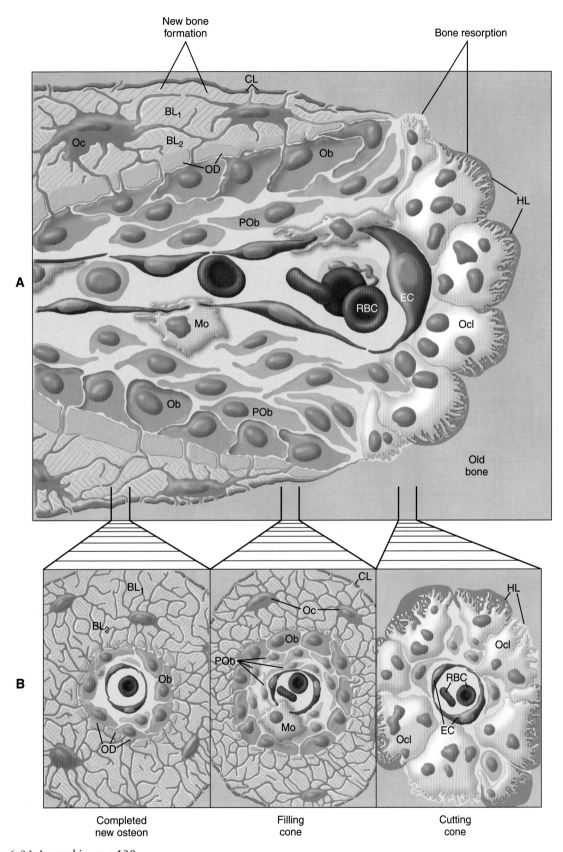

Figure 6-34 Legend is on p.138.

Figure 6-34 Diagrammatic illustration of bone remodeling unit during compact (cortical) bone turnover in (**A**) longitudinal and (**B**) cross section. Turnover of old bone progresses from left to right as osteoclasts continue to resorb and osteoblasts continue to form new bone. Blood-borne monocytes migrate through the endothelial cells and fuse to form osteoclasts, which ream out the old bone, forming a frontal and a circular array of Howship's lacunae. Collectively, they make up what is called the cutting cone. Behind the osteoclasts, uninucleated cells (preosteoblasts) migrate onto the bone surface and differentiate into osteoblasts responsible for forming osteoid that mineralizes to become new bone (filling cone). Some osteoblasts become entrapped in the matrix they produce as osteocytes. A cement line forms at the interface between old and new bone. Collectively, osteoblasts form the filling cone, and as they do, they change the orientation of collagen in succeeding lamellae (BL_1 and BL_2).

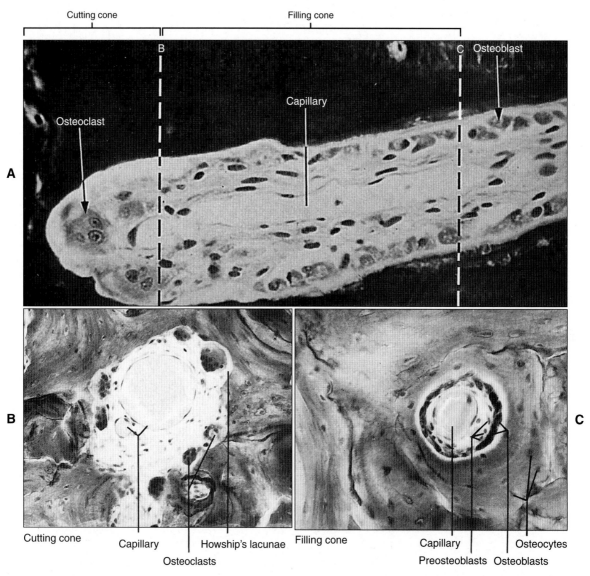

Figure 6-35 Light micrographs showing resorption channels through compact bone in (**A**) longitudinal section and (**B, C**) cross section. **A,** The leading edge of the channel, or cutting cone, contains osteoclasts that resorb the old bone. The portion behind, or filling cone, contains a central capillary and osteoblasts that will deposit bone in concentric lamellae, giving rise to a new osteon. **B,** Several large multinucleated osteoclasts cluster in the cutting cone, each resorbing small packets of bone. The shallow resorption lacunae they create are referred to as Howship's lacunae. **C,** Following resorption, uninucleated osteoblasts ring the eroded bone surface to form new bone onto it.

portion of an earlier osteon is not resorbed, it remains as interstitial lamellae (see Figures 6-3 and 6-4). Behind the cutting cone is a migration of mononucleated cells (macrophages and/or preosteoblasts) onto the roughened surface of the bone channel. As the preosteoblasts differentiate into osteoblasts, they deposit onto the resorbed bone surface a thin "coating" of noncollagenous matrix proteins termed the *cement* or *reversal line*. This layer is composed of at least bone sialoprotein and osteopontin and acts as a cohesive, mineralized layer between the old bone and the new bone that will be formed on top of the cement line by these same osteoblasts (Figure 6-36; see also Figures 6-30, 6-32, and 6-34). The entire area of the osteon where active formation occurs is termed the *filling cone* (see Figures 6-34 and 6-35). As formation proceeds, some osteoblasts become osteocytes. Once formation is complete, the haversian canal contains a central blood vessel and a layer of inactive osteoblasts, the lining cells that communicate by means of cell processes with the embedded osteocytes.

Lamellar cancellous or spongy bone (secondary spongiosa) also turns over (see Figures 6-32 and 6-36). Osteoclasts create resorption cavities on quiescent trabecular surfaces covered by bone lining cells that then are colonized by new osteoblasts that slowly fill in the cavities with new bone as described before. The bone remodeling unit on trabecular bone surfaces can actually be viewed as a resorption channel in compact bone cut in half (compare Figures 6-32 and 6-34).

This account indicates that a considerable amount of internal remodeling by means of resorption and deposition occurs within bone. How such remodeling is controlled is an intriguing problem. A key question is how the osteoclasts become targeted to reach specific sites. As previously stated, osteoblasts, appropriately stimulated by hormones (or perhaps by local environmental changes that occur in situations such as tooth movement), may provide the controlling mechanism for bone resorption. The controlling mechanism that arrests bone resorption also needs to be determined. Such a signal may be hormonal; alternatively, the process of resorption may be self-limiting.

The repeated deposition and removal of bone tissue accommodates the growth of a bone without losing function or its relationship to neighboring structures during the remodeling phase. Thus, for example, a significant increase in size of the mandible is achieved from birth to

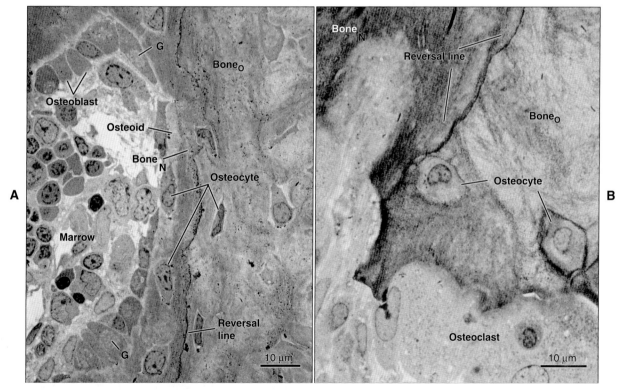

Figure 6-36 Light-level preparations illustrating **(A)** deposition of new bone *(Bone$_N$)* onto the resorbed surface of older bone *(Bone$_O$)* and **(B)** newer and older bone with part of the older bone being resorbed by an osteoclast. The preparations are immunolabeled for osteopontin *(black deposits)*. At the interface between the two layers is a scalloped line, intensely immunoreactive for osteopontin. This scalloped appearance matches the concavities created by osteoclasts during bone resorption. The line is a cement line, or *reversal line*, created during the reversal from the resorptive to the formative phase. The pale regions in the cytoplasm of osteoblasts in **A** represent the Golgi complex *(G)*.

maturity largely by bone remodeling without any loss in function or change in its position relative to the maxilla. Any of the bone present in a 1-year-old mandible most likely is not present in the same bone 30 years later.

RECOMMENDED READING

Bianco P, Riminucci M, Gronthos S et al: Bone marrow stromal stem cells: nature, biology, and potential applications, *Stem Cells* 19:180, 2001.

Cohen MM Jr: Role of leptin in regulating appetite, neuroendocrine function, and bone remodeling, *Am J Med Genet A* 140:515, 2006.

Elefteriou F, Ahn JD, Takeda S et al: Leptin regulation of bone resorption by the sympathetic nervous system and CART, *Nature* 434:514, 2005.

Everts V, Delaissé JM, Korper W et al: The bone lining cell: its role in cleaning Howship's lacunae and initiating bone formation, *J Bone Miner Res* 17:77, 2002.

Gorski JP: Is all bone the same? distinctive distributions and properties of non-collagenous matrix proteins in lamellar vs woven bone imply the existence of different underlying osteogenic mechanisms, *Crit Rev Oral Biol Med* 9:201, 1998.

Karsenty G, Wagner EF: Reaching a genetic and molecular understanding of skeletal development, *Dev Cell* 2:389, 2002.

Klein-Nulend J, Nijweide PJ, Burger EH: Osteocyte and bone structure, *Curr Osteoporo Rep* 1:5, 2003.

Kobayashi T, Kronenberg H: Minireview: transcriptional regulation in development in bone, *Endocrinology* 146:1012, 2005.

Marks SC Jr: The structural basis for bone cell biology, *Acta Med Dent Helv* 2:141, 1997.

Martin TJ, Ng KW: Mechanisms by which cells of the osteoblast lineage control osteoclast formation and activity, *J Cell Biochem* 56:357, 1994.

Parfitt AM: The bone remodeling compartment: a circulatory function for bone lining cells, *J Bone Miner Res* 16:1583, 2001.

Raiz LG: Pathogenesis of osteoporosis: concepts, conflicts, and prospects, *J Clin Invest* 115:3318, 2005.

Roger A, Eastell R: Circulating osteoprotegerin and receptor activator for nuclear factor κB ligand: clinical utility in metabolic bone disease assessment, *J Clin Endocrinol Metab* 90:6323, 2005.

Roodman GD: Osteoclast differentiation and activity, *Biochem Soc Trans* 26:7, 1998.

Salo J, Lehenkari P, Mulari M et al: Removal of osteoclast bone resorption products by transcytosis, *Science* 276:270, 1997.

Young MF: Bone matrix proteins: their function, regulation, and relationship to osteoporosis, *Osteoporos Int* 14(suppl 3):S35, 2003.

Enamel: Composition, Formation, and Structure

Enamel has evolved as an epithelially derived protective covering for teeth. The cells that are responsible for formation of enamel, the ameloblasts, are lost as the tooth erupts into the oral cavity, and hence enamel cannot renew itself. To compensate for this inherent limitation, enamel has acquired a complex structural organization and a high degree of mineralization rendered possible by the almost total absence of organic matrix in its mature state. These characteristics reflect the unusual life cycle of the enamel-forming cells, the *ameloblasts*, and the unique physicochemical characteristics of the matrix proteins that regulate the formation of the extremely long crystals of enamel. This has set enamel apart and has led to the widespread belief that enamel lacks key elements of collagen-based calcified tissues. However, systematic comparisons of the cellular and extracellular matrix events taking place during development reveal fundamental similarities and common themes in the formation of all calcified tissues.

PHYSICAL CHARACTERISTICS OF ENAMEL

Fully formed enamel is the most highly mineralized extracellular matrix known, consisting of approximately 96% mineral and 4% organic material and water. The inorganic content of enamel is a crystalline calcium phosphate (hydroxyapatite) substituted with carbonate ions, which also is found in bone, calcified cartilage, dentin, and cementum. Various ions—strontium, magnesium, lead, and fluoride—if present during enamel formation, may be incorporated into the crystals. The susceptibility of these crystals to dissolution by acid provides the chemical basis for dental caries.

The high mineral content renders enamel extremely hard; this is a property that together with its complex structural organization enables enamel to withstand the mechanical forces applied during tooth functioning. This hardness, which is comparable to that of mild steel,

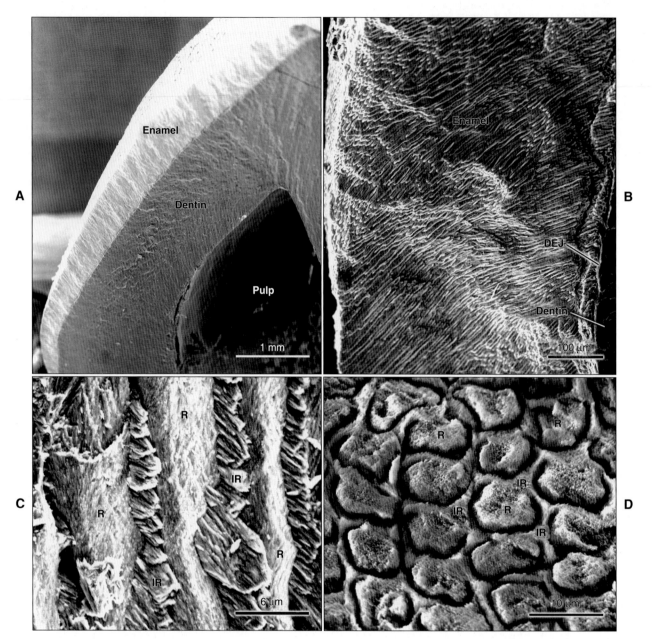

Figure 7-1 Scanning electron microscope views of **(A)** the enamel layer covering coronal dentin, **(B)** the complex distribution of enamel rods across the layer, **(C and D)** and perspectives of the rod-interrod relationship when rods are exposed **(C)** longitudinally or **(D)** in cross section. Interrod enamel surrounds each rod. *DEJ*, Dentinoenamel junction; *IR*, interrod; *R*, rod.

also makes enamel brittle; therefore an underlying layer of more resilient dentin is necessary to maintain its integrity (Figure 7-1, A). If this supportive layer of dentin is destroyed by caries or improper cavity preparation, the unsupported enamel fractures easily.

Enamel is translucent and varies in color from light yellow to gray-white; it also varies in thickness, from a maximum of approximately 2.5 mm over working surfaces to a featheredge at the cervical line. This variation influences the color of enamel because the underlying yellow dentin is seen through the thinner regions.

STRUCTURE OF ENAMEL

Because of the highly mineralized nature of enamel, its structure is difficult to study. When conventional demineralized sections are examined, only an empty

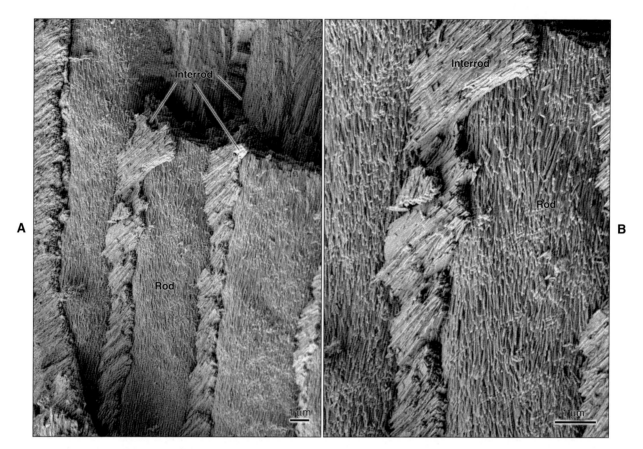

Figure 7-2 A and **B,** High-resolution scanning electron microscope images showing that crystals in rod and interrod enamel are similar in structure but diverge in orientation.

space can be seen in areas previously occupied by mature enamel, because the mineral has been dissolved and the trace organic material has been washed away. However, enough organic material is retained in sections of decalcified developing enamel to reveal some detail of its structure.

The fundamental organizational units of mammalian enamel are the *rods* (prisms) and *interrod enamel* (interprismatic substance; Figure 7-1, *B* to *D*). The enamel rod was first described as hexagonal and prismlike in cross section, and the term *enamel prism* still is used frequently; the term will not be used in this text because rods do not have a regular geometry and hence do not resemble a prism.

Enamel is built from closely packed and long, ribbon-like carbonatoapatite crystals (Figures 7-2 and 7-3) measuring 60 to 70 nm in width and 25 to 30 nm in thickness. The crystals are extremely long; some investigators believe that the length of the crystals actually spans the entire thickness of the enamel layer. The calcium phosphate unit cell has a hexagonal symmetry and stacks up to impart a hexagonal outline to the crystal, which is clearly visible in cross-sectional profile in

maturing enamel (Figure 7-4). However, fully mature enamel crystals are no longer perfectly hexagonal but rather exhibit an irregular outline because they press against each other during the final part of their growth (Figure 7-5). These crystals are grouped together as rod or interrod enamel (see Figures 7-2 and 7-3).

In ground sections the orientation of rods may be misinterpreted because the crystalline nature of enamel leads to optical interference as the light passes through the section, and their outline is difficult to resolve. As a result, when the roughly cylindrical enamel rods are sectioned, cut profiles that line up may be misinterpreted as rods viewed longitudinally, making an assessment of rod direction under the light microscope difficult (Figure 7-6). Use of the electron microscope, with much thinner sections and greater resolving power, has overcome some of these interpretative difficulties.

The rod is shaped somewhat like a cylinder and is made up of crystals with long axes that run, for the most part, in the general direction of the longitudinal axis of the rod (Figure 7-7; see also Figures 7-1, *C* and *D*, 7-2, and 7-3). The interrod region surrounds each rod, and its crystals are oriented in a direction different from those

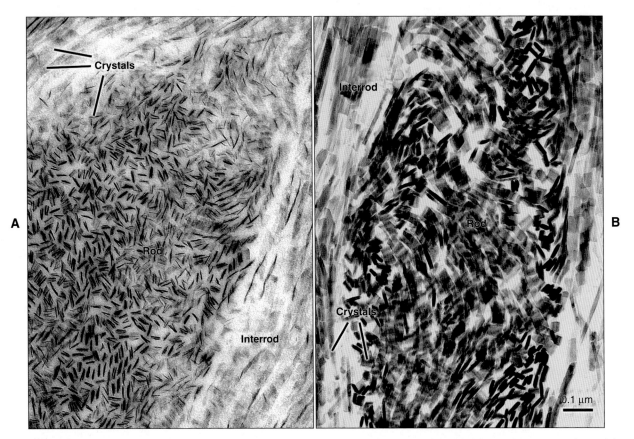

Figure 7-3 Transmission electron microscope images of a rod surrounded by interrod enamel from **(A)** young and **(B)** older forming enamel of a rodent. The crystals that make up the rod and interrod enamel are long, ribbonlike structures that become thicker as enamel matures. They are similar in structure and composition but appear in different planes of sections because they have different orientations.

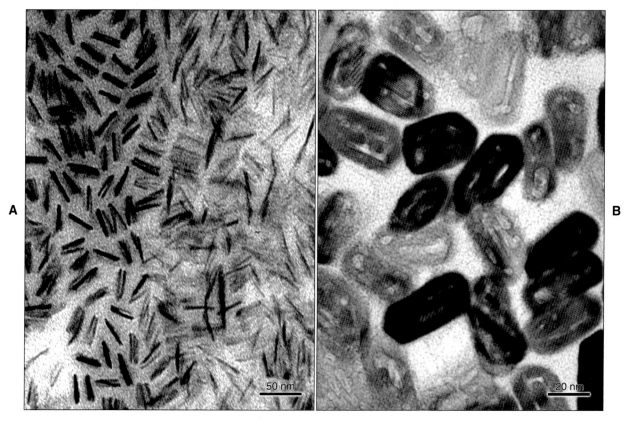

Figure 7-4 Cross-sectional profiles of **(A)** recently formed, secretory stage enamel crystals and **(B)** older ones from the maturation stage. Initially the crystals are thin; as they grow in thickness and width, their hexagonal contour becomes apparent. **B,** The linear patterns seen in older crystals are a reflection of their crystalline lattice.

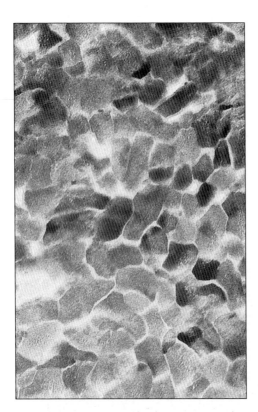

Figure 7-5 Electron micrograph of mature enamel crystals. The outline is irregular as they press against each other. *(Courtesy J.W. Simmelink, V.K. Nygaard, and D.B. Scott.)*

making up the rod (Figure 7-8; see also Figures 7-1, *C* and *D*, 7-2, 7-3, and 7-7). The difference in orientation is significant around approximately three fourths of the circumference of a rod. The boundary between rod and interrod enamel in this region is delimited by a narrow space containing organic material known as the *rod sheath* (Figure 7-9; see also Figures 7-1, *D*, and 7-8); the rod sheath is visualized more clearly in higher mammals (Figure 7-10). Along a small portion of the circumference of the rod the crystals are confluent with those of interrod enamel. In this region, rod and interrod enamel are not separated and there is no space or rod sheath between them (Figure 7-11; see also Figure 7-1, *D*). In sections cut along the longitudinal axis of enamel rods and passing through the narrow region where rod and interrod are confluent, rod crystals can be seen to flare out into the interrod enamel (see Figure 7-8). The cross-sectional outline of these two related components has been compared with the shape of a keyhole. Because the keyhole analogy does not adequately account for some of the variations in the structural arrangement of the enamel components and is not consistent with the pattern of formation of enamel, this terminology has largely been discontinued. The basic organizational pattern of mammalian enamel thus is described more appropriately as cylindrical rods embedded in the interrod enamel.

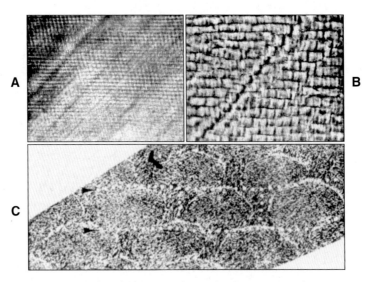

Figure 7-6 Interpretation of rod structure and orientation can be misleading in ground sections examined by light microscopy **(A, B).** When such sections are thinned down and examined in the electron microscope **(C),** what appears to be a longitudinal rod in some cases actually may be crosscut rods. *(From Weber DF, Glick PL: Am J Anat 144:407, 1975.)*

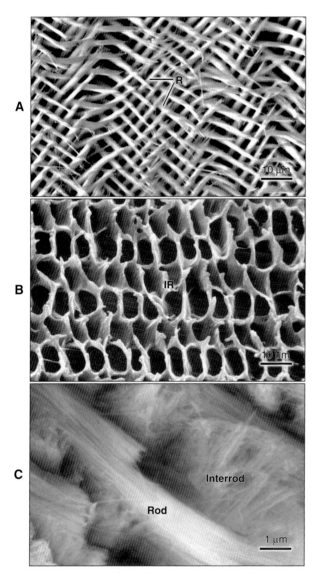

Figure 7-7 Scanning electron microscope images showing various aspects of rat incisor enamel. **A,** The enamel rods *(R)* are arranged in rows with alternating orientations. **B,** The alternating row arrangement is also evident in the interrod *(IR)* cavities that accommodate the enamel rod. **C,** Rod and interrod enamel are made up of thin and long apatite crystals.

AMELOGENESIS

Amelogenesis, or enamel formation, is a two-step process. When enamel first forms, it mineralizes only partially to approximately 30% (Table 7-1). Subsequently, as the organic matrix breaks down and is removed, crystals grow wider and thicker. This process whereby organic matrix and water are lost and mineral is added accentuates after the full thickness of the enamel layer has been formed to attain greater than 96% mineral content.

Ameloblasts secrete matrix proteins and are responsible for creating and maintaining an extracellular environment favorable to mineral deposition. This epithelial cell exhibits a unique life cycle characterized by progressive phenotype changes that reflect its primary activity at various times of enamel formation. Amelogenesis has been described in as many as six phases but generally is subdivided into three main functional stages referred to as the *presecretory, secretory,* and *maturation stages* (Figures 7-12 to 7-14). Classically, ameloblasts from each stage have been portrayed as fulfilling more or less exclusive functions. First, during the presecretory stage, differentiating ameloblasts acquire their phenotype, change polarity, develop an extensive protein synthetic apparatus, and prepare to secrete the organic matrix of enamel. Second, during the secretory stage (also called the formative stage), ameloblasts elaborate and organize the entire enamel thickness, resulting in the formation of a highly ordered tissue. Last, during the maturation stage, ameloblasts modulate and transport specific ions required for the concurrent accretion of mineral. Over the past 10 years or so the cellular activities that occur during each stage have been more extensively defined, and ameloblasts now are considered cells that carry out multiple activities throughout their life cycle and that up-regulate or down-regulate, some or all of them, according to the developmental requirements.

Enamel formation begins at the early crown stage of tooth development and involves the differentiation of the cells of the inner enamel epithelium first at the tips of the cusp outlines formed in that epithelium. The process then sweeps down the slopes of the tooth crown until all cells of the epithelium have differentiated into enamel-forming cells, or ameloblasts. Another feature is notable: when differentiation of the ameloblasts occurs and dentin starts forming, these cells are distanced from the blood vessels that lie outside the inner enamel epithelium within the dental papilla. Compensation for this distant vascular supply is achieved by blood vessels invaginating the outer enamel epithelium and by the loss of the intervening stellate reticulum, which brings ameloblasts closer to the blood vessels (Figure 7-15).

LIGHT MICROSCOPY OF AMELOGENESIS

At the late bell stage, most of the light microscopic features of amelogenesis can be seen in a single section (Figures 7-13 to 7-16). Thus in the region of the cervical loop the low columnar cells of the inner enamel epithelium are clearly identifiable. Peripheral to the inner enamel epithelium lie the stratum intermedium, stellate reticulum, and outer enamel epithelium, the last

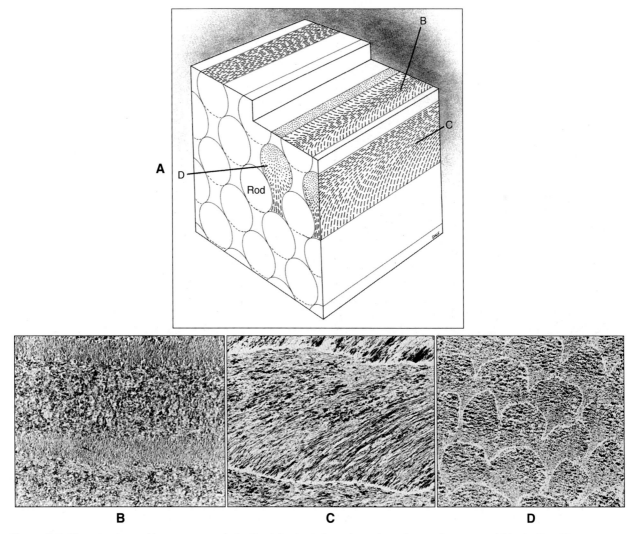

Figure 7-8 Fine structure of human enamel. **A,** Crystal orientation along three faces of an enamel block. **B** to **D,** Transmission electron micrographs of the three faces. *(Courtesy A.H. Meckel.)*

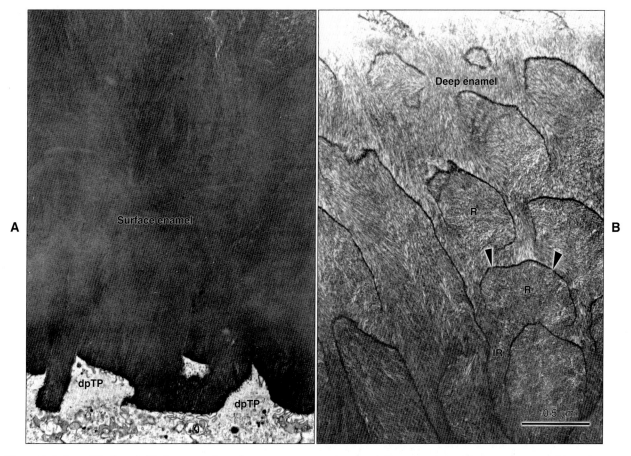

Figure 7-9 A and **B,** Decalcified preparation of cat secretory stage enamel. The organic matrix near the ameloblasts is younger and shows a uniform texture. No rod sheath is discernible in younger enamel near the surface where rods are structured. The distal portion of Tomes' process *(dpTP)* penetrates into the enamel. In deeper areas, near dentin, matrix is older and partly removed. As enamel matures, matrix accumulates at the interface between rod *(R)* and interrod *(IR)* to form the rod sheath *(arrowheads)*.

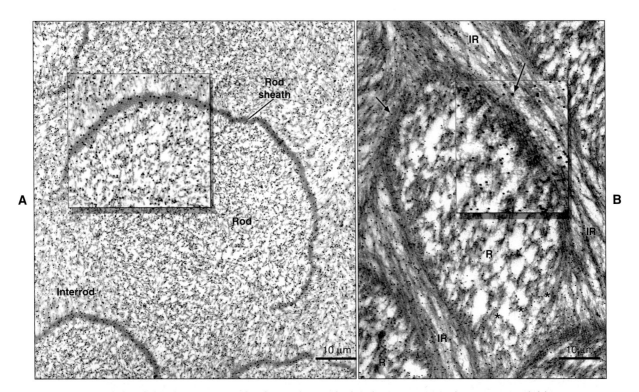

Figure 7-10 The rod sheath has been proposed to be made up of "sheath protein," now known as ameloblastin.
A, However, colloidal gold *(black dots)* immunocytochemical labeling of maturing cat enamel also reveals the presence of amelogenin in the organic matrix that accumulates to form the rod sheath. **B,** Rodents have no well-defined rod sheath; however, decalcified preparations of maturing enamel reveals a concentration of organic matrix *(arrows)* around most of the periphery of the rod *(R)*, except at the zone of confluence *(*)* with interrod *(IR)*. This matrix, like the one at other sites, is immunoreactive for amelogenin. It is thus likely that more than one protein accumulates in the thin space between rod and interrod as enamel matures.

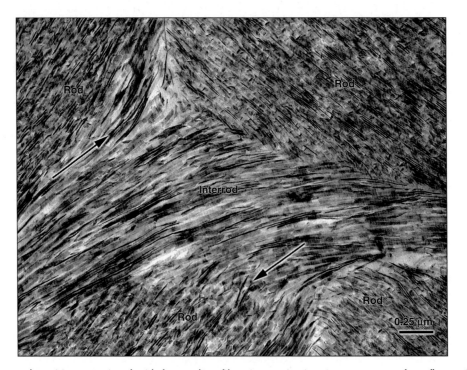

Figure 7-11 Interrod partition associated with four rod profiles. At certain sites *(arrows,* zone of confluence), crystals from interrod enamel enter the rod.

TABLE 7-1	Percentage Wet Weight Composition of Rat Incisor Enamel		
COMPONENT	SECRETORY STAGE (%)	MIDMATURATION (%)	LATE MATURATION (%)
Water	5	3	1
Mineral	29	93	95
Protein	66	4	4

closely associated with the many blood vessels in the dental follicle.

As the inner enamel epithelium is traced coronally in a crown stage tooth germ, its cells become tall and columnar, and the nuclei become aligned at the proximal ends of the cells adjacent to the stratum intermedium. Shortly after dentin formation initiates, a number of distinct and almost simultaneous morphologic changes associated with the onset of amelogenesis occur in the enamel organ. The cells of the inner enamel epithelium, now ameloblasts, begin more actively to secrete enamel proteins that accumulate and immediately participate in the formation of a partially mineralized *initial layer* of enamel (see Figure 7-12, *B*), which does not contain any rods. As the first increment of enamel is formed, ameloblasts move away from the dentin surface. Enamel is identified readily as a deep-staining layer in demineralized hematoxylin-eosin–stained sections (Figure 7-17; see also Figure 7-16). An important event for the production and organization of the enamel is the development of a cytoplasmic extension on ameloblasts, *Tomes' process* (its formation and structure are described later in the chapter), that juts into and interdigitates with the newly forming enamel (see Figures 7-12 and 7-13). In sections of forming human teeth, Tomes' processes give the junction between the enamel and the ameloblast a picket-fence or saw-toothed appearance (see Figure 7-17).

When formation of the full thickness of enamel is complete, ameloblasts enter the maturation stage (see Figures 7-12 and 7-13). Typically this stage starts with a brief transitional phase during which significant morphologic changes occur. These *postsecretory transition* ameloblasts shorten and restructure themselves into squatter maturation cells (see Figure 7-12). Cells from the underlying stratum intermedium, stellate reticulum, and outer enamel epithelium reorganize so that recognizing individual cell layers is no longer possible. Blood vessels invaginate deeply into these cells, without disrupting the basal lamina associated with the outer aspect of the enamel organ to form a convoluted structure referred to as the *papillary layer* (Figure 7-18; see also Figure 7-12).

Finally, when enamel is fully mature, the ameloblast layer and the adjacent papillary layer regress and together constitute the *reduced enamel epithelium* (Figure 7-19). The ameloblasts stop modulating (discussed subsequently), reduce their size, and assume a cuboidal appearance. This epithelium, although no longer involved in the secretion and maturation of enamel, continues to cover it and has a protective function. In the case of premature breaks in the epithelium, connective tissue cells are believed to come into contact with the enamel and deposit cementum on the enamel. During this *protective phase*, however, the composition of enamel can still be modified. For instance, fluoride, if available, still can be incorporated into the enamel of an unerupted tooth, and evidence indicates that the fluoride content is greatest in those teeth that have the longest interregnum between the completion of enamel formation and tooth eruption (at which time, of course, the ameloblasts are lost). The reduced enamel epithelium remains until the tooth erupts. As the tooth passes through the oral epithelium, the part of the reduced enamel epithelium situated incisally is destroyed, whereas that found more cervically interacts with the oral epithelium to form the *junctional epithelium.*

ELECTRON MICROSCOPY OF AMELOGENESIS

Ultrastructural studies of enamel formation by electron microscopy have added greatly to the understanding of this complex process. Such studies often have used the continuously erupting rat incisor as a model because all developmental stages can be found in a single tooth and because it has been demonstrated that the various stages of enamel formation bear an overall similarity to those in human teeth. In continuously erupting rodent incisors, the various stages of amelogenesis are disposed sequentially along the length of the tooth (Figure 7-20). In such a system, position represents developmental time, and one can look predictably at the various stages of amelogenesis by sampling at different positions from the apical end, where cell renewal occurs, to the incisal tip, where occlusal attrition balances the continuous, apically initiated tooth-forming activity.

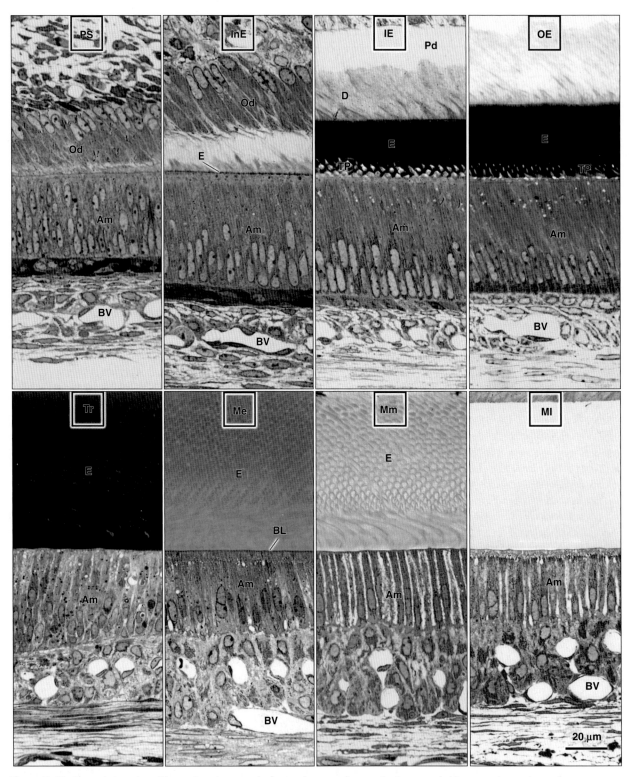

Figure 7-12 Composite plate illustrating the morphologic changes that rat incisor ameloblasts undergo throughout amelogenesis. *Am,* Ameloblasts; *BL,* basal lamina; *BV,* blood vessel; *D,* dentin; *E,* enamel; *IE,* secretory stage inner enamel; *InE,* secretory stage initial enamel; *Me,* early maturation stage; *Ml,* late maturation stage; *Mm,* midmaturation stage; *Od,* odontoblasts; *OE,* secretory stage outer enamel; *Pd,* predentin; *PS,* presecretory stage; *TP,* Tomes' process; *Tr,* maturation stage transition.

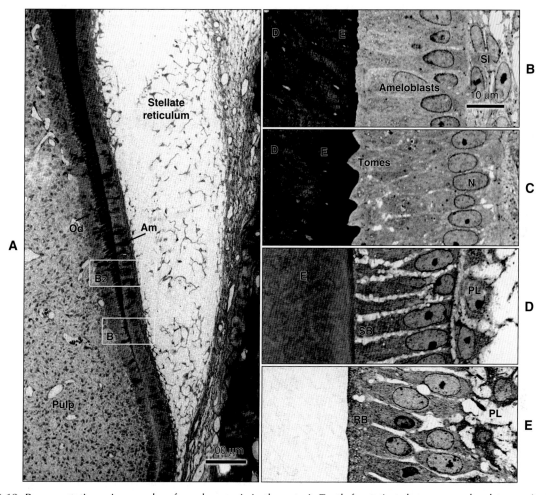

Figure 7-13 Representative micrographs of amelogenesis in the cat. **A,** Tooth formation shows an occlusal-to-cervical developmental gradient so that on some crowns finding most of the stages of the ameloblast life cycle is possible. The panels on the right (**B** corresponds with *B₁* and **C** with *B₂)* are enlargements of the boxed areas in **A. B,** Secretory stage, initial enamel formation. **C,** Secretory stage, inner enamel formation. **D** and **E** are from the incisal tip of the tooth (see Figure 7-14). **D,** Midmaturation stage, smooth-ended ameloblasts. **E,** Late maturation stage, ruffle-ended ameloblasts. *Am,* Ameloblasts; *D,* dentin; *E,* enamel; *N,* nucleus; *Od,* odontoblasts; *PL,* papillary layer; *RB,* ruffled border; *SB,* smooth border; *SI,* stratum intermedium.

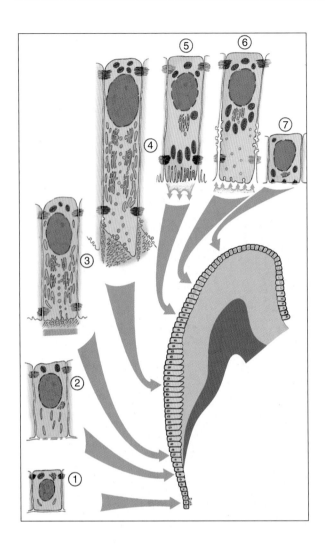

Figure 7-14 The various functional stages in the life cycle of ameloblasts as would occur in a human tooth. *1,* Morphogenetic stage; *2,* histodifferentiation stage; *3,* initial secretory stage (no Tomes' process); *4,* secretory stage (Tomes' process); *5,* ruffle-ended ameloblast of the maturative stage; *6,* smooth-ended ameloblast of the maturative stage; *7,* protective stage.

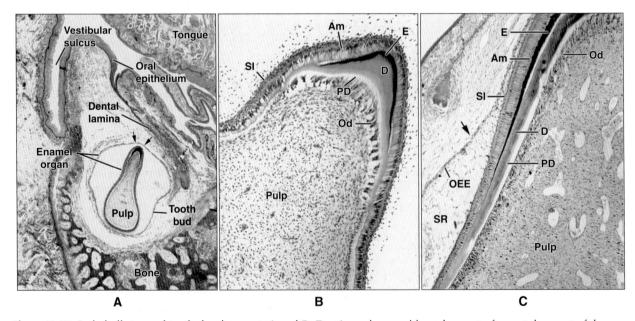

Figure 7-15 Early bell stage of tooth development. **A** and **B,** Dentin and enamel have begun to form at the crest of the forming crown, accompanied by a reduction in the amount of stellate reticulum *(SR)* over the future cusp tip *(arrows* in **A**). **C,** Ameloblast *(Am)* and odontoblast *(Od)* differentiation and formation of enamel *(E)* and dentin *(D)* progress along the slopes of the tooth, in an occlusal to cervical direction. Note the reduction in the amount of stratum intermedium *(SI)* above the arrow where the enamel is actively forming. *PD,* Predentin; *OEE,* outer enamel epithelium. (*B and C courtesy P. Tambasco de Oliveira.*)

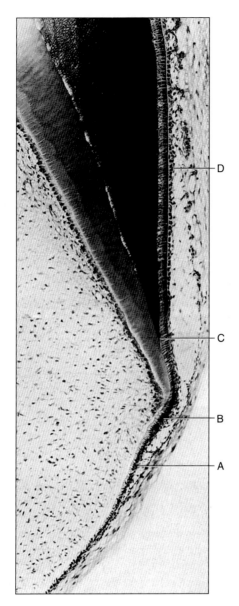

Figure 7-16 Features of amelogenesis as seen through the light microscope. At *A* the inner enamel epithelium consists of short, columnar undifferentiated cells. At *B* these cells elongate and differentiate into ameloblasts that induce the differentiation of odontoblasts and then begin to secrete enamel *(C)*. At *D* ameloblasts are actively depositing enamel matrix.

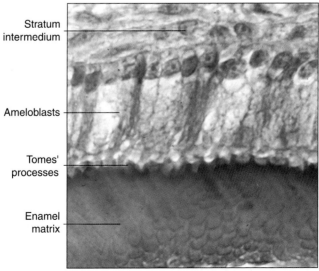

Stratum intermedium

Ameloblasts

Tomes' processes

Enamel matrix

Figure 7-17 Enamel matrix formation as seen with the light microscope. The Tomes' processes of ameloblasts jut into the matrix visible after decalcification, creating a picket-fence appearance.

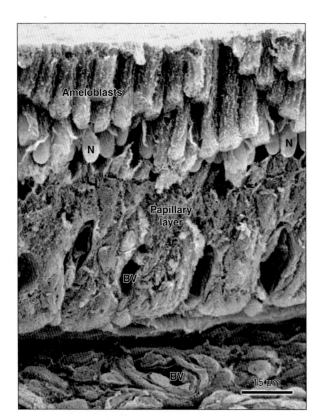

Figure 7-18 Scanning electron microscope view of the enamel organ during the maturation stage. Cells from the stratum intermedium, stellate reticulum, and outer enamel epithelium amalgamate into a single layer. Blood vessels invaginate deeply into this layer to form a convoluted structure referred to as the papillary layer. *BV,* Blood vessel; *N,* nucleus.

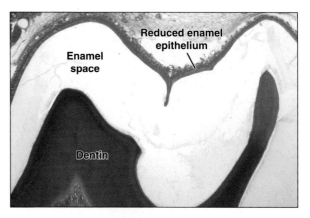

Figure 7-19 When enamel maturation is completed, the ameloblast layer and the adjacent papillary layer together constitute the reduced enamel epithelium. Only an enamel space is visible in this histologic preparation because at this late developmental stage, enamel is heavily calcified and therefore is lost during decalcification.

PRESECRETORY STAGE

Morphogenetic Phase

During the bell stage of tooth development, the shape of the crown is determined. A basal lamina is present between the outer enamel epithelium and the dental follicle and between cells of the inner enamel epithelium and dental papilla (Figures 7-21 and 7-22, A). The cells of the inner enamel epithelium still can undergo mitotic division. They are cuboidal or low columnar, with large, centrally located nuclei and poorly developed Golgi elements in the proximal portion of the cells (facing the stratum intermedium), where a junctional complex occurs. Mitochondria and other cytoplasmic components are scattered throughout the cell.

Differentiation Phase

As the cells of the inner enamel epithelium differentiate into ameloblasts, they elongate and their nuclei shift proximally toward the stratum intermedium. The basal lamina supporting them is fragmented by cytoplasmic projections and disintegrates during mantle predentin formation (see Figure 7-21). In each cell the Golgi complex increases in volume and migrates distally from its proximal position to occupy a major portion of the supranuclear cytoplasm. The amount of rough endoplasmic reticulum increases significantly, and most of the mitochondria cluster in the proximal region, with only a few scattered through the rest of the cell. A second junctional complex develops at the distal extremity of the cell, compartmentalizing the ameloblast into a body and a distal extension called Tomes' process, against which enamel forms (Figure 7-22, *B* and *C*). Thus the ameloblast becomes a polarized cell, with the majority of its organelles situated in the cell body distal to the nucleus. These cells can no longer divide.

Although in the past these differentiating ameloblasts have been regarded as nonsecreting cells, research now clearly demonstrates that production of some enamel proteins starts much earlier than anticipated, even before the basal lamina separating preameloblasts and preodontoblasts is lost (Figure 7-23; see also Figure 7-22, A). Surprisingly, preameloblasts also express dentin sialoprotein, an odontoblast product, albeit transiently. This reciprocal expression of opposing matrix proteins as cells differentiate, as well as the production of typical (ecto)mesenchymal proteins by enamel organ–derived cells at later stages (see Chapter 9), is consistent with the common ectodermal origin (oral epithelium/neural crest) of all hard tissue–forming cells in the craniofacial region.

Adjacent ameloblasts are aligned closely with each other, and attachment specializations, or junctional

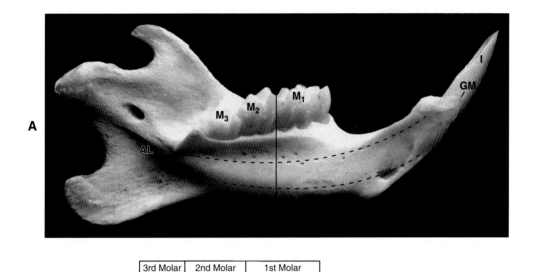

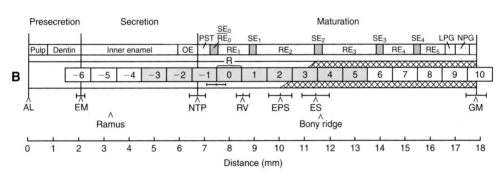

Figure 7-20 A, Mesial view of the left rat hemimandible. The dotted line outlines the approximate position of the incisor within the bone. The solid line perpendicular to the labial surface of the incisor and passing between the first (M_1) and second molar (M_2), demarcates the secretory and maturation stages. Enamel formation progresses sequentially from the apical to the incisal end *(I)* of the tooth. **B,** Schematic representation of the curvilinear length of the labial surface of the incisor from the apical loop *(AL)* to the gingival margin *(GM)*, and mapping of the respective "lengths" occupied by the various stages and regions of amelogenesis. *EM,* Start of enamel matrix secretion; *EPS,* enamel partially soluble during decalcification; *ES,* enamel completely soluble; *LPG,* region where ameloblasts accumulate large pigment granules; *NPG,* region where ameloblasts show no pigment granules; *NTP,* point marking the location of loss of Tomes' process; *OE,* region of outer enamel secretion; *PST,* region of postsecretory transition; *RE,* band of ruffle-ended ameloblasts; *RV,* rods visible; *SE,* band of smooth-ended ameloblasts. *(Adapted from Smith CE, Nanci A: Anat Rec 225:257, 1989).*

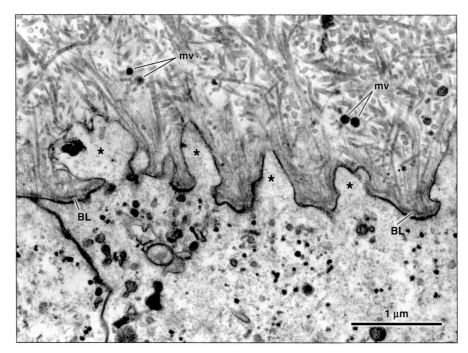

Figure 7-21 Differentiating ameloblasts extend cytoplasmic projections *(*)* through the basal lamina *(BL)*, separating them from the forming mantle predentin. The basal lamina is fragmented and is removed before the active deposition of enamel matrix. *mv,* Matrix vesicle.

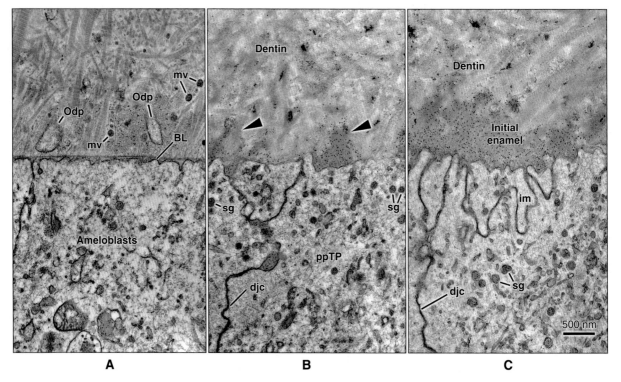

Figure 7-22 Colloidal gold immunocytochemical preparations illustrating the expression of amelogenin by differentiating ameloblasts. **A,** Amelogenin molecules are immunodetected *(black dots)* extracellularly early during the presecretory stage, before the removal of the basal lamina *(BL)* and separating ameloblasts from the developing predentin matrix. Thereafter, enamel proteins **(B)** accumulate first as patches *(arrowheads)* at the interface with dentin and then **(C)** as a uniform layer of initial enamel that in mineralized preparations is seen to contain numerous crystallites. *djc,* Distal junctional complex; *im,* infolded membrane; *mv,* matrix vesicle; *Odp,* odontoblast process; *ppTP,* proximal portion of Tomes' process; *sg,* secretory granule.

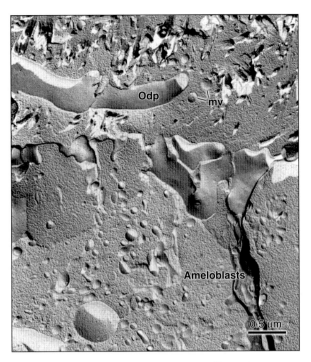

Figure 7-23 Freeze-fracture preparation illustrating a three-dimensional view of presecretory stage ameloblasts, similar to those in Figure 7-22, A, and an odontoblast process *(Odp)* and matrix vesicles *(mv)* in the region of forming mantle predentin where the first enamel proteins are deposited.

complexes, between them maintain the alignment. These complexes encircle the cells at their distal (adjacent to enamel) and proximal (adjacent to the stratum intermedium) extremities. Fine actin-containing filaments radiate from the junctional complexes into the cytoplasm of the ameloblasts and can be distinguished as forming distal and proximal terminal webs (Figure 7-24). These junctional complexes play an important role in amelogenesis by tightly holding together ameloblasts and determining at different times what may, and what may not, pass between them to enter or leave the enamel.

SECRETORY STAGE

The fine structure of secretory stage ameloblasts reflects their intense synthetic and secretory activity. The Golgi complex is extensive and forms a cylindrical organelle surrounded by numerous cisternae of rough endoplasmic reticulum, occupying a large part of the supranuclear compartment (Figures 7-25 to 7-28, A). The messenger RNA for enamel proteins is translated by ribosomes on the membrane of the rough endoplasmic reticulum, and the synthesized proteins then are translocated into its cisternae. The proteins then progress through the Golgi complex for continued posttranslational modification (mainly for nonamelogenins) and are packaged into

membrane-bound secretory granules. These granules migrate to the distal extremity of the cell, that is, into Tomes' process (Figure 7-29, B; see also Figures 7-24, A; 7-27; and 7-28, B). Secretion by ameloblasts is constitutive; that is, it is continuous and secretory granules are not stored for prolonged periods, as is the case for salivary gland acinar cells, for example.

When enamel formation begins, Tomes' process comprises only a proximal portion (Figure 7-30; see also Figure 7-22). The content of secretory granules is released against the newly formed mantle dentin along the surface of the process (see Figure 7-22) to form an initial layer of enamel that does not contain enamel rods. Little if any time elapses between the secretion of enamel matrix and its mineralization. The first hydroxyapatite crystals formed interdigitate with the crystals of dentin (Figure 7-31).

As the initial enamel layer is formed, ameloblasts migrate away from the dentin surface and develop the *distal portion* of Tomes' process as an outgrowth of the *proximal portion.* The proximal portion extends from the distal junctional complex to the surface of the enamel layer, whereas the distal portion penetrates into and interdigitates with the enamel beyond the initial layer (Figure 7-32; see also Figures 7-24, A, and 7-27). The cytoplasm from both portions of Tomes' process is continuous with that of the body of the ameloblast. The rod and interrod configuration of enamel crystals is a property of the ameloblasts and their Tomes' processes. The organizational framework of rod and interrod is similar in all species, but their size and outline vary to reflect the geometry of the cell.

When the distal portion of Tomes' process is established, secretion of enamel proteins becomes staggered and is confined to two sites (Figure 7-32; see also Figure 7-27). The sites where enamel proteins are released extracellularly can be identified by the presence of abundant membrane infoldings (Figure 7-33; see also Figure 7-32). These infoldings are believed to form to accommodate the excess membrane brought about by the rapid fusion of many secretory granules at these sites. Secretion from the first site (on the proximal part of the process, close to the junctional complex, around the periphery of the cell), along with that from adjoining ameloblasts, results in the formation of enamel partitions that delimit a pit (Figure 7-34; see also Figure 7-7, B) in which resides the distal portion of Tomes' process. These partitions are not distinct units and in effect form a continuum throughout the enamel layer called *interrod enamel.* Secretion from the second site (along one face of the distal portion of the Tomes' process) with matrix that participates in formation of the so-called *enamel rod* that later fills the pit. Formation of interrod enamel is always a step ahead because the interrod enamel first must delimit the cavity into which rod enamel is formed. At both sites the enamel is of identical composition, and rod and interrod

Text continued on p. 166

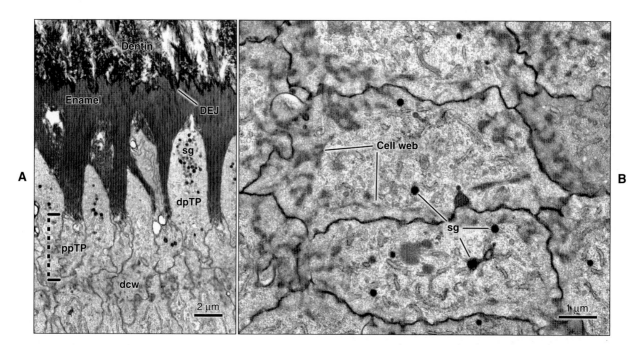

Figure 7-24 A, Differentiated ameloblasts develop a junctional complex at their distal extremity. The cell extension above the complex is Tomes' process and is divided into two parts. The proximal portion of Tomes' process *(ppTP)* extends from the junctional complex to the surface of the enamel layer, whereas the more distal portion *(dpTP)* penetrates into enamel. **B,** Cross-sectional view of ameloblasts at the level of the distal junctional complex. This beltlike complex extends around the entire circumference of the ameloblast and tightly holds the cells together. Bundles of microfilaments *(Cell web)* concentrate and run along the cytoplasmic surface of the complex. *dcw,* Distal cell web; *DEJ,* dentinoenamel junction; *sg,* secretory granule.

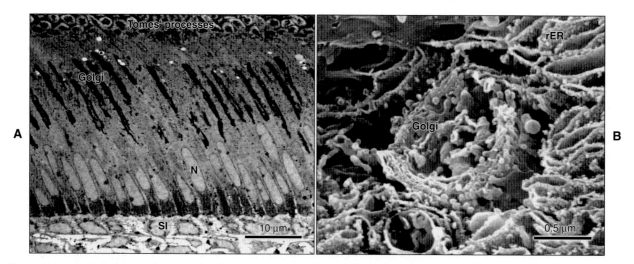

Figure 7-25 A, Cytochemical preparation for an enzyme resident in the Golgi complex showing the extent of this organelle throughout the supranuclear compartment of secretory stage ameloblasts. **B,** Scanning electron microscope image of a cross-fractured ameloblast. The Golgi complex has a cylindrical configuration and is surrounded by rough endoplasmic reticulum *(rER)*. *N,* Nucleus; *SI,* stratum intermedium.

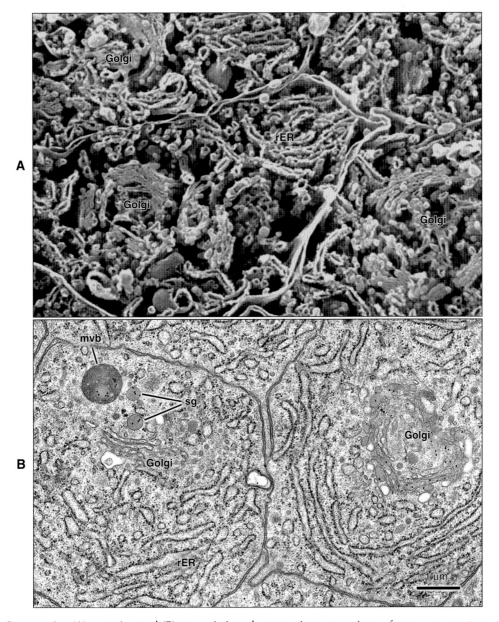

Figure 7-26 Comparative **(A)** scanning and **(B)** transmission electron microscope views of cross-cut secretory stage ameloblasts. The Golgi complex is located centrally and surrounded by cisternae of rough endoplasmic reticulum *(rER)*. The preparation in **B** is immunolabeled *(black dots)* for amelogenin. Labeling is found not only in the Golgi complex and secretory granules *(sg)* but also in organelles involved in protein degradation such as multivesicular bodies *(mvb)*.

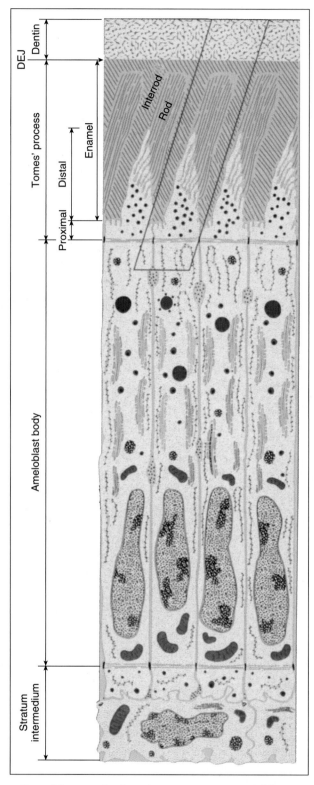

Figure 7-27 Schematic representation of the organization of secretory stage ameloblasts as would be revealed in a section along their long axis. *DEJ,* Dentinoenamel junction.

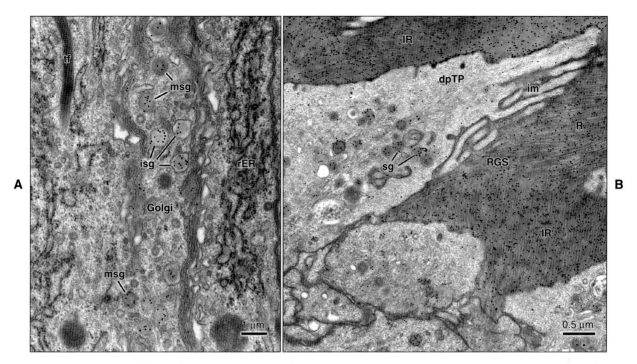

Figure 7-28 Immunocytochemical preparations for amelogenin. **A,** Immature *(isg)* and mature *(msg)* secretory granules are found on the mature face of the Golgi complex. **B,** Secretory granules are translocated into Tomes' process and accumulate near secretory surfaces, recognized by the presence of membrane infoldings *(im)*. *dpTP,* Distal portion of Tomes' process; *IR,* interrod; *R,* rod; *rER,* rough endoplasmic reticulum; *RGS,* rod growth site; *sg,* secretory granule; *tf,* tonofilaments.

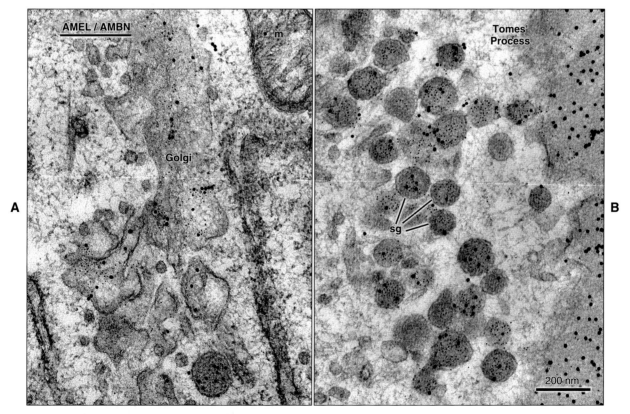

Figure 7-29 Double-labeled immunocytochemical preparations; the fine black dots indicate the presence of ameloblastin *(AMBN),* whereas the larger ones that of amelogenin *(AMEL).* **A,** Both proteins are processed simultaneously in the Golgi complex. **B,** The majority of secretory granules *(sg)* in Tomes' process contains both proteins, indicating that both proteins are cosecreted. *m,* Mitochondria.

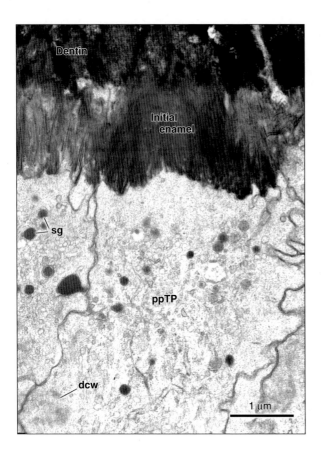

Figure 7-30 When initial enamel forms, the ameloblast only has a proximal portion of Tomes' process *(ppTP)*. The distal portion develops as an extension of the proximal one slightly later when enamel rods begin forming. *dcw,* Distal cell web; *sg,* secretory granules.

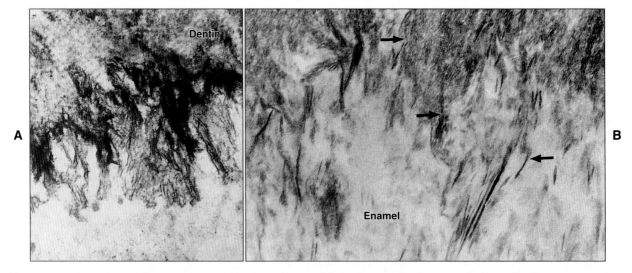

Figure 7-31 Transmission electron micrographs of initial enamel formation. **A,** This micrograph shows the close intermingling of dentin collagen with the ribbonlike crystals of enamel. **B,** A higher magnification shows the apparent continuity between calcified collagen and enamel crystallites. *(From Arsenault LA, Robinson BW:* Calcif Tissue Int *45:111, 1989.)*

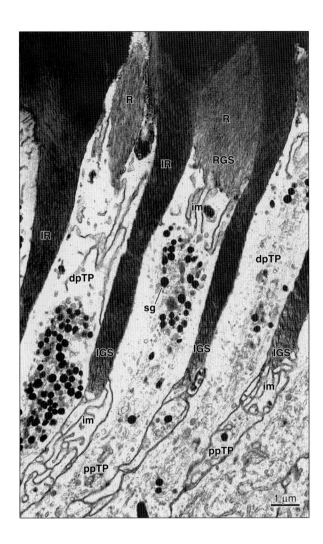

Figure 7-32 Interrod *(IR)* enamel surrounds the forming rod *(R)* and the distal portion of Tomes' process *(dpTP)*; this portion is the continuation of the proximal portion *(ppTP)* into the enamel layer. The interrod *(IGS)* and rod *(RGS)* growth sites are associated with membrane infoldings *(im)* on the proximal and distal portions of Tomes' process, respectively. These infoldings represent the sites where secretory granules *(sg)* release enamel proteins extracellularly for growth in length of enamel crystals that results in an increase in thickness of the enamel layer.

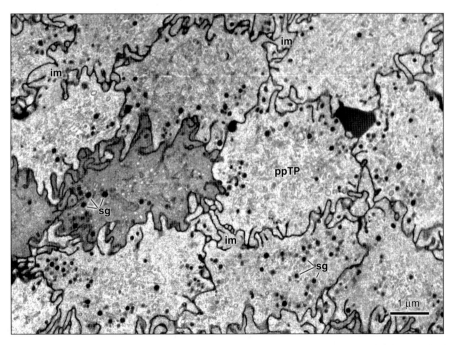

Figure 7-33 Cross-sectional view of the proximal portion of Tomes' process *(ppTP)* of ameloblasts at the level of the interrod secretory surface. Membrane infoldings *(im)* are present around the circumference of a cell and outline the edge of each of the interrod cavities shown in Figure 7-7, *B*. *sg*, Secretory granule.

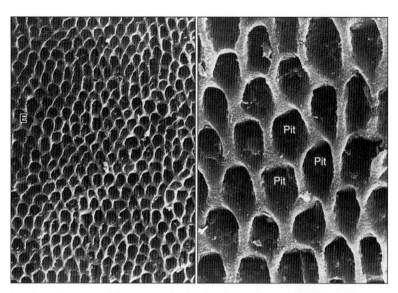

Figure 7-34 Scanning electron micrograph of the surface of a developing human tooth from which ameloblasts have been removed. The surface consists of a series of pits previously filled by Tomes' processes, the walls of which are formed by interrod enamel. *(From Warshawsky H, Josephsen K, Thylstrup A et al: Anat Rec 200:371, 1981.)*

enamel differ only in the orientation of their crystallites (Figure 7-35; see also Figures 7-2, 7-3, and 7-12).

The distal portion of Tomes' process generally is believed to lengthen as the enamel layer thickens and becomes gradually thinner as the rod growing in diameter presses it against the wall of the interrod cavity (see Figure 7-35). The distal Tomes' process eventually is squeezed out of existence, creating a narrow space along most of the circumference between rod and interrod enamel that fills with organic material and, as indicated previously, forms the rod sheath. The secretory surface on the distal portion of Tomes' process faces the region where there is no rod sheath. Rod crystals formed in relation to the secretory surface are created directly against the interrod partition and, consequently, over a narrow area, rod and interrod crystals are confluent (see Figures 7-9, *B*, and 7-35). When the outer portion of the enamel layer is being formed, the shape of the distal portion of Tomes' process is altered, and its orientation to the cell body changes (Figure 7-36; see also Figure 7-12). As a result, enamel rods in the outer third of the enamel layer have a slightly different profile and have a more rectilinear trajectory (Figure 7-37; see also Figure 7-1, *B*). Eventually, the ameloblast becomes shorter and loses its distal portion of Tomes' process; the cell now has the same overall appearance as when it was forming initial enamel (see Figures 7-12 and 7-36). Because rods form in relation to the distal portion of Tomes' process (that no longer exists), the final few enamel increments (final enamel), just as the first few, do not contain any rods (Figure 7-38).

The enamel layer is thus composed of a rod-containing (prismatic) layer sandwiched between thin rodless (aprismatic) *initial* and *final layers*. Notably, the initial, interrod, and final enamel are formed from the same secretory surface—that is, the one on the proximal portion of Tomes' process—and, indeed, are believed to form a continuum.

MATURATION STAGE

Before the tooth erupts in the oral cavity, enamel hardens. This change in physicochemical properties results from growth in width and thickness of preexisting crystals seeded during the formative phase of amelogenesis and not because additional crystals are created de novo (compare Figure 7-4, *A* and *B*). Crystal growth during the maturation stage occurs at the expense of matrix proteins and enamel fluid that are largely absent from mature enamel. Amelogenesis is a rather slow developmental process that can take as long as 5 years to complete on the crowns of some teeth in the permanent dentition in the human being; up to about two thirds of the formation time can be occupied by the maturation stage. Maturation stage ameloblasts seem to carry out small, repeated developmental increments with a cumulative effect of great change.

Although maturation stage ameloblasts generally are referred to as postsecretory cells, they still synthesize and secrete proteins (see Figure 7-36). These ameloblasts still exhibit a prominent Golgi complex, a structural feature consistent with such activity (Figure 7-39). Surprisingly,

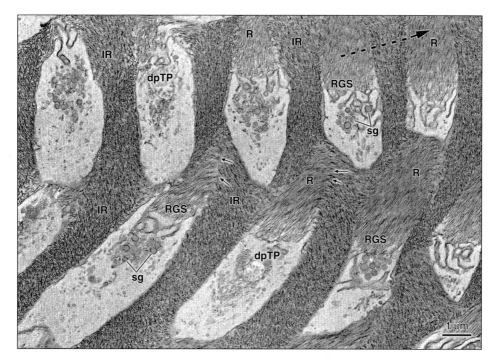

Figure 7-35 In cross section the distal portions of Tomes' processes *(dpTP)* appear as ovoid profiles surrounded by interrod enamel *(IR)*. They decrease in size toward the dentinoenamel junction *(dashed arrow)* as the rod *(R)* grows in diameter. The crystals making up rod blend in with those of interrod enamel (*small arrows*, zone of confluence) at the point where the rod begins forming. *RGS*, Rod growth sites; *sg*, secretory granule.

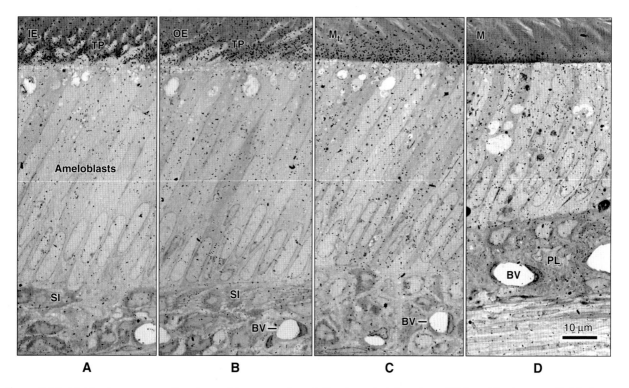

Figure 7-36 Light microscope radioautographic preparations following administration of 3H-methionine to radiolabel secretory products (mainly amelogenins) of ameloblasts. The black silver grains over enamel indicate the presence of newly formed amelogenins. **A** and **B,** As expected, secretory stage ameloblasts actively secrete proteins during inner *(IE)* and outer *(OE)* enamel formation. **C** and **D,** The presence of grains over the surface enamel during the transition phase *(Mt)* and early maturation *(M)* indicates that ameloblasts still produce some enamel matrix proteins during the early part of the maturation stage. **C,** The micrograph is from the beginning of transition; note that the stratum intermedium *(SI)* has started to reorganize to form part of the papillary layer *(PL)*. *BV,* Blood vessel; *TP,* Tomes' process.

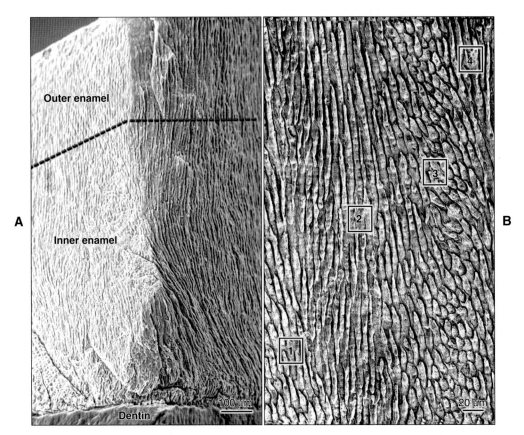

Figure 7-37 A and **B,** Scanning electron microscope illustrations showing the complex trajectory of rods in the inner two thirds of the enamel layer in human teeth. **B,** The rods are organized in groups exhibiting different orientations; this illustration shows four adjacent groups.

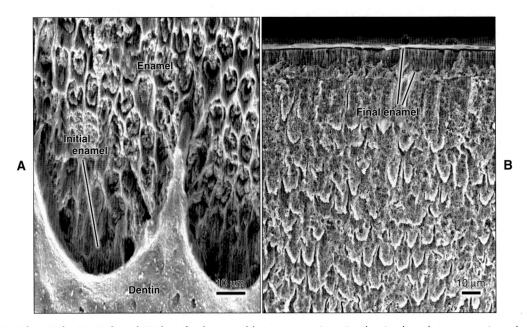

Figure 7-38 The **(A)** first (initial) and **(B)** last (final) enamel layers are aprismatic; that is, they do not contain rods.

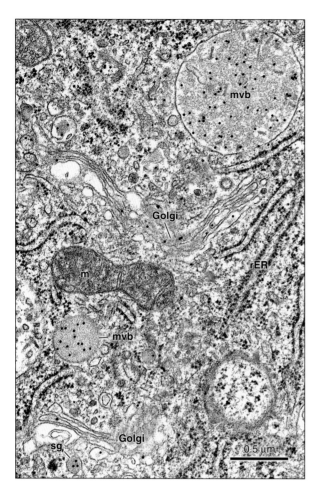

Figure 7-39 As illustrated in this immunocytochemical preparation *(black dots)*, early maturation stage ameloblasts contain amelogenin in their Golgi apparatus, indicating that they still synthesize enamel proteins. Elements of the lysosomal system, such as multivesicular bodies *(mvb)*, are also immunoreactive. *m,* Mitochondria; *rER,* rough endoplasmic reticulum; *sg,* secretory granule.

in some species the ameloblasts still produce enamel proteins, at least during the early part of the stage. Messenger RNA and protein signal for amelogenin and ameloblastin, two enamel proteins described in subsequent text, have been found in maturation ameloblasts. These proteins are immunodetected in protein synthetic and degradative organelles. Although amelogenin signals are found only in the early maturation stage, those for ameloblastin continue to be expressed until much later. The significance of this continued enamel protein production while major matrix removal occurs is unclear.

Transitional Phase

After the full thickness of immature enamel has formed, ameloblasts undergo significant morphologic changes in preparation for their next functional role, that of maturing the enamel. A brief transitional phase involving a reduction in height of the ameloblasts and a decrease in their volume and organelle content occurs (see Figures 7-12 and 7-36). During the maturation stage, ameloblasts undergo *programmed cell death (apoptosis)* (Box 7-1). The particularities of the rat incisor (see the foregoing) have allowed researchers to obtain a quantitative evaluation of the extent of the process in this tooth; approximately 25% of the cells die during the transitional phase, and another 25% die as enamel maturation proceeds. Whether the magnitude of cell loss is the same in human teeth is not known. However, considering the overall similarities in amelogenesis between teeth of continuous and limited eruption, it can be assumed safely that the initial ameloblast population is significantly reduced in all teeth during the maturation phase. Apoptosis also takes place in the enamel knot as part of the morphogenetic events.

Cell death is a fundamental mechanism during embryonic development and throughout the life of an organism. In embryogenesis, cells die at specific times during development to permit orderly morphogenesis. Two major ways by which cell death can occur are *accidental cell death (necrosis)* and programmed cell death (apoptosis). Also now recognized is that programmed cell death can occur without exhibiting the dramatic structural changes typical of apoptosis. The main features of necrosis and apoptosis are summarized in Box 7-1, and the cellular changes associated with apoptosis are schematically illustrated in Figure 7-40. The Bcl-2 family of proteins, comprising antiapoptotic and proapoptotic proteins (Figure 7-41), is a major regulator of apoptosis. Specialized proteinases *(caspases)* also inactivate cellular survival pathways and activate factors that promote death.

Maturation Proper

Next the principal activity of ameloblasts is the bulk removal of water and organic material from the enamel to allow introduction of additional inorganic material. The most visually dramatic activity of these cells is *modulation*, the cyclic creation, loss, and recreation of a highly invaginated ruffle-ended apical surface (the cells alternate between possessing a ruffled border [ruffle-ended] or a smooth border [smooth-ended]; Figure 7-42; see also Figures 7-12 through 7-14). Modulation can be visualized by special stains and occurs in waves traveling across the crown of a developing tooth from least mature regions to most mature regions of the enamel (e.g., in an apical-incisal direction in continuously erupting teeth and cervical-incisal [occlusal] direction in teeth of limited eruption; Figure 7-43). Available evidence suggests that ameloblasts in some species modulate rapidly—as often

Box 7-1   Key Features of Cell Death

Necrosis (Accidental Cell Death)
Cell death that results from irreversible injury to the cell. Cell membranes swell and become permeable. Lytic enzymes destroy the cellular contents, which then leak out into the intercellular space, leading to the mounting of an inflammatory response.

Programmed Cell Death
An active cellular process that culminates in cell death. This process may occur in response to developmental or environmental cues or as a response to physiologic damage detected by the internal surveillance networks of the cell.

Apoptosis
One type of programmed cell death characterized by a particular pattern of morphologic changes. The name comes from the ancient Greek, referring to shedding of the petals from flowers or leaves from trees. Apoptosis is observed in all metazoans, including plants and animals, but the genes encoding proteins involved in apoptosis have yet to be detected in single-celled organisms such as yeasts.

   Apoptotic death occurs in two phases. During the latent phase, the cell looks morphologically normal but is actively making preparations for death. The execution phase is characterized by a series of dramatic structural and biochemical changes that culminate in the fragmentation of the cell into membrane-enclosed apoptotic bodies. Activities that cause cells to undergo apoptosis are said to be proapoptotic. Activities that protect cells from apoptosis are said to be antiapoptotic.

Modified from Pollard TD, Earnshaw WC: *Cell biology,* Philadelphia, 2004, Saunders.

as once every 8 hours—thereby yielding three complete modulations per day. The significance of the modulations is uncertain, but they seem to be related to maintaining an environment that allows accretion of mineral content and loss of organic matrix, in part through alterations in permeability of the enamel organ. One proposal is that the acidification associated with ongoing mineral accretion during maturation causes ruffle-ended ameloblasts to produce bicarbonate ions. This process continuously alkalizes the enamel fluid to prevent reverse demineralization of the growing crystallites and maintain pH conditions optimized for functioning of the matrix degrading enzymes, which prefer slightly acidic to near neutral conditions. Ruffle-ended ameloblasts possess proximal junctions that are leaky and distal junctions that are tight, whereas most smooth-ended

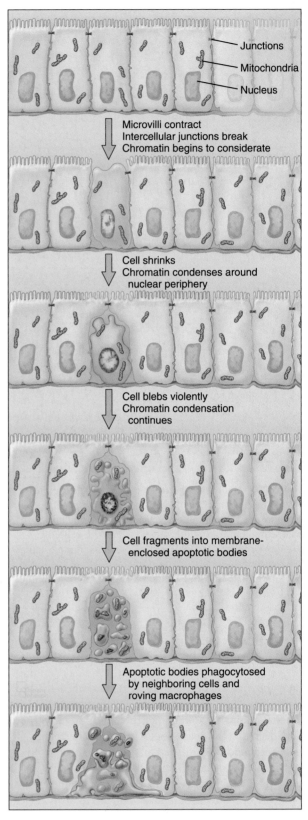

Figure 7-40 Schematic representation of the cellular changes during apoptosis. *(From Pollard TD, Earnshaw WC: Cell biology, Philadelphia, 2004, Saunders.)*

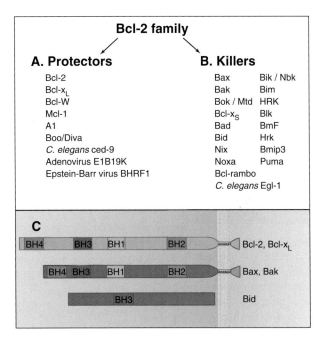

Figure 7-41 The Bcl-2 family of apoptosis regulating proteins. *(From Pollard TD, Earnshaw WC:* Cell biology, *Philadelphia, 2004, Saunders.)*

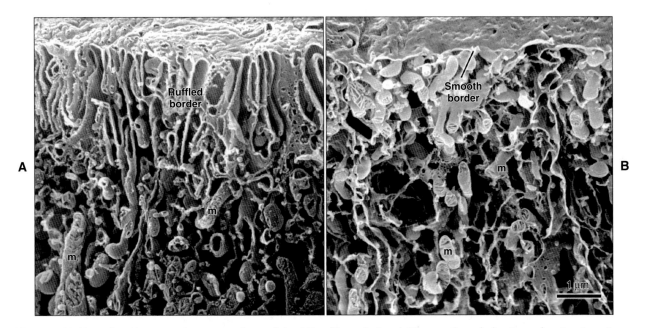

Figure 7-42 Scanning electron microscope views of the **(A)** ruffle-ended and **(B)** smooth-ended apices of maturation stage ameloblasts. *m*, Mitochondria.

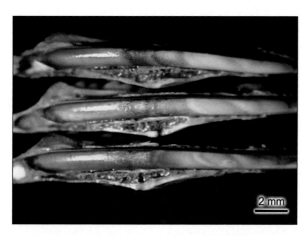

2 mm

Figure 7-43 The modulation cycle of ameloblasts can be visualized by special stains. Indicator dyes were used to detect regional variations in pH along the maturing enamel of rat incisors. The large bands correspond to regions overlaid by ruffle-ended ameloblasts, whereas smaller ones correspond to those associated with smooth-ended cells. *(Courtesy C.E. Smith.)*

ameloblasts have distal junctions that are leaky and proximal ones that are tight (Figure 7-44). Ruffle-ended ameloblasts show considerable endocytotic activity and contain numerous lysosomes, calcium-binding proteins, and membrane-associated calcium-adenosinetriphosphatases that appear to promote the pumping of calcium ions into the maturing enamel. Smooth-ended ameloblasts, however, leak small proteins and other molecules, show little endocytotic activity, and have almost no membrane calcium-adenosinetriphosphatase activity. Interstitial fluids that may leak into the maturing enamel during the smooth-ended phase also may contribute to neutralizing the pH of the enamel fluid.

Data available to date suggest that the calcium ions required for active crystal growth pass through the ruffle-ended ameloblasts (because their distal junctions are tight) but along the sides of the more leaky smooth-ended ameloblasts. Active incorporation of mineral ions into crystals occurs in relation to the ruffle-ended cells. Regarding the withdrawal of organic matrix from maturing enamel, sufficient evidence is now available to indicate that active resorption of intact proteins by ameloblasts is not the main mechanism for the loss of organic matrix observed during enamel maturation. This is attributed largely to the action of bulk-degrading enzymes that act extracellularly to digest the various matrix proteins into fragments small enough to be able to leave the enamel layer. Polypeptide fragments leaving the enamel likely pass between the leaky distal junctions of smooth-ended cells and diffuse laterally among the ameloblasts to be taken up along their basolateral surfaces.

When cells become ruffle-ended, because the proximal junctional complex now in turn becomes leaky, some of the laterally diffusing peptides could disperse throughout the papillary layer and perhaps beyond. Some fragments from the enamel layer also may be taken up by endocytosis across the membrane infoldings of the ruffled border.

Just as ameloblasts complete the transitional phase and begin the first series of modulation cycles, they deposit a basal lamina at their now-flattened apex (no part of Tomes' process is recognizable at this stage). The basal lamina adheres to the enamel surface, and the ameloblasts attach to it by means of hemidesmosomes (Figure 7-45, A). This basal lamina is known to be rich in glycoconjugates, but their nature remains to be determined. Typical basal lamina constituents such as type IV collagen have not yet been demonstrated consistently. However, the basal lamina has been shown to contain laminin-5, a heterotrimer molecule that is essential for the formation of hemidesmosomes. Patients with laminin-5 deficiency show focal enamel hypoplasia, and targeted disruption of laminin-5 function in mice affects the appearance of ameloblasts and enamel formation. Just recently, *amelotin*, a novel ameloblast secretory product that begins to be expressed during postsecretory transition also has been immunolocalized to the basal lamina (Figure 7-45, B). It thus likely represents a unique structure in composition and function; in addition to an adhesive role, the presence of highly glycosylated molecules may confer to the lamina charge-selective properties that could help regulate the movement of material into and out of the enamel layer. Also, the basal lamina is situated such that it could relay to the ameloblasts information about the status of the dynamic enamel compartment.

At this point, recapitulating the many functions that cells of the inner enamel epithelium exhibit during their life cycle is worthwhile: Initially, the cells are involved in establishing the crown pattern of the tooth (morphogenesis); at this time they are small and low columnar with centrally placed nuclei, and they undergo frequent mitoses. Then, the cells undergo morphologic changes, and they become ameloblasts (histodifferentiation). These changes are preparatory to their entering the next phase, active secretion of the enamel matrix, wherein they develop a cell extension called the Tomes' process. The secretory stage is followed by a short transitional phase of cell restructuring leading to enamel maturation proper, wherein the ameloblasts exhibit cyclical variations with ruffle- and smooth-ended borders against the enamel surface; the ruffle-ended cells allowing incorporation of inorganic material, the smooth-ended cells permitting exit of protein fragments and water. The final phase is protection of the newly formed enamel surface until the time of tooth eruption.

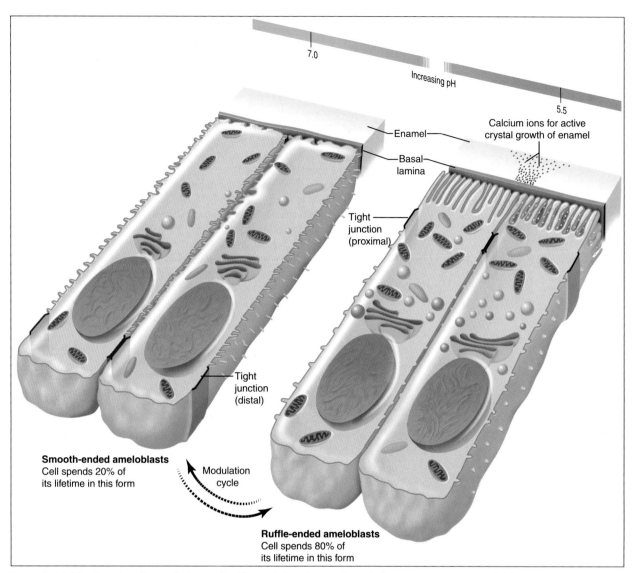

7.0

Increasing pH

5.5

Calcium ions for active
crystal growth of enamel

Enamel

Basal
lamina

Tight
junction
(proximal)

Tight
junction
(distal)

Smooth-ended ameloblasts
Cell spends 20% of
its lifetime in this form

Modulation
cycle

Ruffle-ended ameloblasts
Cell spends 80% of
its lifetime in this form

Figure 7-44 The functional morphology of ruffle-ended and smooth-ended maturation stage ameloblasts.

ENAMEL PROTEINS

The organic matrix of enamel is made from noncollagenous proteins only and contains several *enamel proteins* and enzymes (Table 7-2). Of the enamel proteins, 90% are a heterogeneous group of low-molecular-weight proteins known as *amelogenins*. The remaining 10% consists of *nonamelogenins* such as *enamelin* and *ameloblastin*. The electrophoretic profile of whole enamel homogenates from immature enamel is complex and represents a composite image of newly secreted and partially degraded forms of both categories of proteins. Amelogenins are hydrophobic proteins rich in proline, histidine, and glutamine, showing little posttranslational modifications and with reported molecular weights ranging between

5 and 45 kDa. Their heterogeneity is brought about in three ways. The genes responsible for transcribing amelogenin are found on X and Y chromosomes, and because these two genes are not 100% homologous, a sexual heterogeneity exists at the outset. The functional significance of this sexual dimorphism is not known. Second, the amelogenin gene contains several exons, which can be spliced in numerous ways to produce mature mRNAs that may include all exons or lack some of them, producing as many as nine isoforms. The functional significance of alternatively spliced forms of amelogenins has not yet been fully determined. Third, amelogenins undergo short-term (minor) and long-term (extensive) extracellular processing by proteolytic enzymes into lower-molecular-weight fragments, of which tyrosine-rich amelogenin polypeptide and

TABLE 7-2   Summary of Secreted Proteins Associated with Enamel Formation*

NAME	SYMBOL/GENE LOCATION	FEATURES
Proteins Contributing to Appositional Growth in Thickness of the Enamel Layer		
Amelogenin	AMELX; AMELY	• The protein represents the main protein present in forming enamel; expression stops when enamel reaches full thickness.
	Xp22.3; Yp11.2	• The protein has a relatively low molecular weight (~25 kDa) with few posttranslational modifications.
		• Ameloblasts secrete several versions (isoforms) of the protein arising from active transcription of X- and Y-chromosomes and from alternative splicing of its messenger RNA; most secreted isoforms are truncated relative to hypothetical full length transcript.
		• The N-terminal end of the secreted protein characteristically begins with the amino acid sequence MPLPP—, and the C-terminal end usually finishes with —KREEVD
		• The protein has unusual solubility properties relative to temperature, pH, and calcium ion concentrations; solutions of the protein are capable of transforming into a jelly under physiologic conditions.
		• The protein shows a marked tendency for self-aggregation; it creates unit structures called nanospheres (~20 nm) that themselves aggregate into larger quaternary arrangements including chains and ribbons.
		• The protein inhibits lateral growth (volumetric expansion) of hydroxyapatite crystals.
		LOSS OF FUNCTION: A thin hypoplastic enamel layer is formed that lacks enamel rods.
Ameloblastin	AMBN 4q13.3	• The protein is present in much smaller amounts compared with amelogenin (~10% of matrix); it is found mostly in newly formed (secretory stage) enamel and more so at the outer surface than in deeper areas closest to dentinoenamel junction.
		• The protein is roughly 2.5 times larger in molecular weight than amelogenin (~70 kDa); it has sulfated O-linked sugars.
		• The protein is cleaved rapidly into several fragments soon after it is secreted from ameloblasts; one fragment has calcium-binding properties.
		• Ameloblasts continue to express ameloblastin throughout the maturation stage, although ameloblastin does not appear to cross the basal lamina and enter into the maturing enamel layer.
		• The protein is believed to assist ameloblasts in adhering to the forming enamel surface during the secretory stage.
		LOSS OF FUNCTION: Terminal differentiating ameloblasts detach from the dentin, and enamel formation aborts.
Enamelin	ENAM 4q13.3	• Enamelin is the largest (~186 kDa) and least abundant (>5%) of the enamel matrix proteins.
		• Enamelin is believed to undergo extensive posttranslational modifications; it has N-linked sugars and is phosphorylated.
		• The full-length protein and its largest derivative fragments (to about 89 kDa) created as soon as the protein is secreted are not detected inside forming (secretory stage) enamel; these are present only at the growing enamel surface.
		• Small fragments from enamelin, however, do linger within enamel (e.g., 32 kDa and 25 kDa); these bind strongly to mineral and are inhibitory to crystal growth.
		• The protein is believed to function in part as a modulator for de novo formation of mineral and to promote crystal elongation.
		LOSS OF FUNCTION: To be defined.
Proteins Involved in Postsecretory Processing and Degradation of Amelogenins and Nonamelogenins		
Enamelysin	MMP20	• Enamelysin is a calcium-dependent metalloproteinase of the matrix metalloprotease subfamily; it has some unique structural features.
	11q22.3	• Enamelysin is found primarily in newly formed (secretory stage) enamel.
		• Enamelysin is believed to cleave the hydrophilic C-terminal ends of amelogenins and other internal sites; it is suspected to be responsible for cleaving ameloblastin and enamelin into certain large fragments.
		LOSS OF FUNCTION: Hypomaturation of enamel occurs; MMP20-deficient mice also show thinned enamel.
Enamel matrix serine protease (now called kallikrein4)	KLK4 19q13.4	• Protein is a serine proteinase of the tissue kallikrein subfamily (kallikrein-related peptidase 4); it also is expressed in prostate.
		• Protein is believed to be secreted into enamel that has achieved full thickness once ameloblasts lose their Tomes' processes and start their modulation cycles along the enamel surface.
		• Protein slowly degrades residual amelogenins and fragments from nonamelogenins into small polypeptides.
		LOSS OF FUNCTION: Hypomaturation of enamel occurs.

(*Nonamelogenins* — side label spanning Ameloblastin and Enamelin rows)

*Table prepared by C.E. Smith.

TABLE 7-2 Summary of Secreted Proteins Associated with Enamel Formation—cont'd		
NAME	SYMBOL/GENE LOCATION	FEATURES
Proteins Related to Basal Lamina Covering Maturing and Mature Preeruptive Enamel		
Amelotin	AMTN 4q13.3	• Amelotin is secreted by ameloblasts during and shortly after transition to the maturation stage. • Amelotin resides in the surface basal lamina along with laminin-5 throughout maturation. • Amelotin also is found in the basal lamina located at the surface of junctional epithelium. LOSS OF FUNCTION: To be defined.
Legacy Proteins		
Enamelin		The EDTA-soluble protein described in older literature as "enamelin" turned out to be albumin derived from blood contamination.
Tuftelin		This protein described in older literature has no signal peptide and therefore does not represent a protein intentionally secreted extracellularly.
Amelin/sheathlin		These are older terms for the protein now referred to as ameloblastin.

leucine-rich amelogenin polypeptide are significant because they constitute the bulk of the final organic matrix of maturing enamel.

Ameloblastin and enamelin are the best-studied members of the nonamelogenin family. A 65-kDa sulfated protein also has been described. Nonamelogenins are believed to undergo rapid extracellular processing, and intact molecules do not accumulate in enamel for long periods. Another nonamelogenin called *tuftelin* has been reported, but its role as an enamel matrix protein is questionable because it is present in several tissues and lacks a signal peptide for secretion. The fact that nonamelogenins represent minor components of forming enamel does necessarily imply that they are produced in small amounts but is likely a reflection of their short half-life (i.e., they do not accumulate over time).

Members of at least two general families of *proteinases* are involved in the extracellular processing and degradation of enamel proteins (see Table 7-2). *Enamelysin* (MMP20), an enzyme from the *matrix metalloproteinase* (MMP), family is involved in the short-term processing of newly secreted matrix proteins. Another enzyme from the serine proteinase family, originally termed *enamel matrix serine protease 1* and now called *kallikrein4* (KLK4) functions as a bulk digestive enzyme, particularly during the maturation stage. Loss of function of these enzymes in knockout animals produces hypomineralized enamel and, in the case of enamelysin, a thinner enamel layer.

The focus to date has been on identifying ameloblast products that are secreted into the enamel layer where they would be in a position to have an impact on crystal formation and growth and on structuring the layer. Efforts to find other such molecules recently have led to the identification of novel secretory proteins produced by maturation stage ameloblasts (see Table 7-2). Since at that time the enamel layer is fully formed and structured and any organic matrix present in it undergoes bulk degradation, the novel molecules must have functions not directly related to mineral buildup. Two such proteins have been described recently; these are amelotin and *Apin*, the latter a protein originally isolated from the amyloid of calcifying odontogenic epithelial tumors. As noted previously, amelotin localizes to the basal lamina that forms at the interface between ameloblasts and maturing enamel (see Figure 7-45, *B*). The precise localization of Apin remains to be determined; however, both proteins are coexpressed and are associated with the apical surface of modulating ameloblasts where they may participate in mediating the adhesion of the enamel organ to the enamel surface. As we will see in Chapter 12, these proteins also are expressed in the junctional epithelium where cell adhesion to the tooth surface plays an important role in maintaining periodontal integrity and health.

The extracellular matrix of developing dental enamel is now reasonably well defined in terms of its major protein components. Forming enamel does not exhibit a distinct, unmineralized preenamel layer such as osteoid or predentin, and crystals grow directly against the secretory surfaces of ameloblasts (Figure 7-46). Although the background matrix formed by the marginally soluble amelogenins may provide some physical support, enamel proteins likely do not play any major structuring function as collagen does in bone, dentin, and cellular cementum. Therefore the three-dimensional organization seen in enamel likely results from the direct ordering of the extremely long crystals. Morphologically, the organic matrix of young, forming enamel appears uniform in decalcified histologic preparations; however, immunocytochemical analyses have revealed that enamel proteins are differentially disturbed across the enamel layer (Figure 7-47). Intact or relatively intact nonamelogenin molecules, such as ameloblastin, are concentrated near the cell surface at sites where they are secreted, whereas mostly degradation fragments are found in deeper (older) enamel. The sites where ameloblastin is immunodetected at the highest concentration actually

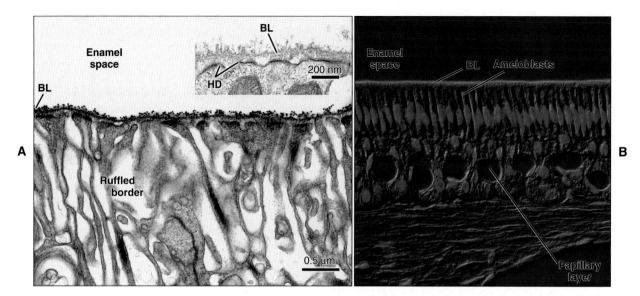

Figure 7-45 A, At the start of the maturation stage, ameloblasts deposit a basal lamina *(BL)* against the enamel surface to which it adheres firmly. Cytochemical detection *(black dots)* of sugar residues using lectins indicates that this structure is rich in glycoconjugates. *Inset,* The cell surface attaches to the basal lamina by means of hemidesmosomes *(HD).* **B,** Immunofluorescence image showing the presence of amelotin in the basal lamina.

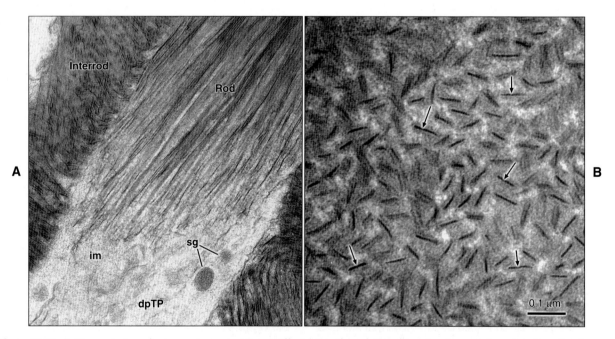

Figure 7-46 A, Transmission electron microscope image illustrating the relationship of rod enamel crystals to a distal portion of Tomes' process *(dpTP)* and surrounding interrod enamel. The elongating extremity of the rod crystals abut the infolded membrane *(im)* at the secretory surface. **B,** In cross section, newly formed crystals appear as small, needlelike structures *(arrows)* surrounded by granular organic matrix. *sg,* Secretory granules.

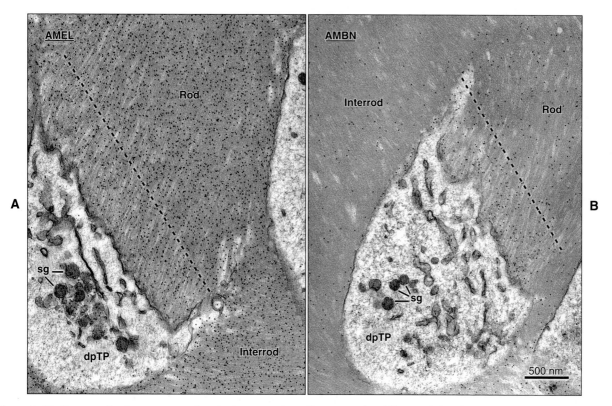

Figure 7-47 Comparative immunocytochemical preparations illustrating the differential distribution of **(A)** amelogenin *(AMEL)* and **(B)** ameloblastin *(AMBN)*, here in relation to a distal portion of Tomes' process *(dpTP)*. Amelogenins are less concentrated in a narrow region near the secretory surface on the process (fewer black dots occur between the cell and the dashed line than beyond), whereas most of the ameloblastin is found in this region. *sg*, Secretory granule.

correspond to the position in enamel where interrod and rod crystals grow in length (enamel growth sites). However, intact and fragmented forms of amelogenin are least concentrated at growth sites and are found abundantly throughout the enamel layer. Amelogenins and ameloblastin are synthesized together and are contained within the same secretory granule (see Figure 7-29). Given that they are cosecreted, their segregation at growth sites is intriguing and may result from microenvironmental conditions, the physicochemical properties of the proteins, or some special attribute of the secretory granule populations. Amelogenins are believed to form supramolecular aggregates called *nanospheres* that surround crystals along their long axis and that are visible on sections of enamel examined under the electron microscope as a granular background material between crystals (see Figure 7-46, *B*). Based on the biochemical characteristics and differential distribution of the various enamel proteins, members of the nonamelogenin family are believed broadly to promote and guide the formation of enamel crystals, whereas amelogenins regulate growth in thickness and width of crystals. Amelogenins prevent crystals from fusing during their formation and must be removed to permit growth.

The expression of matrix proteins at early stages by cells that are not fully differentiated has important functional significance. In particular, the inverted expression of matrix proteins by epithelial and ectomesenchymal cells as they differentiate may be part of the reciprocal epithelial-mesenchymal signaling during tooth morphogenesis and histodifferentiation. The early secretion of amelogenin at a time when odontoblasts have not yet differentiated fully, mantle predentin is not yet discernible, and enamel mineralization has not yet started suggests that this protein is multifunctional. Initially, amelogenins may participate in epithelial-mesenchymal events. Because no overt sign of mineral deposition exists among the initial patches of enamel proteins, any role amelogenin may have in crystal nucleation likely is associated with the temporal expression of specific isoforms, extracellular processing of major isoforms, or the arrival of other proteins such as ameloblastin. When enamel mineralization is ongoing, amelogenin then may function to regulate growth in width and thickness of crystals. The function of certain enamel proteins thus may bear some resemblance to that of noncollagenous bone and cementum proteins, such as bone sialoprotein and osteopontin, which exhibit cellular and matrix activities.

Results from studies using knockout mice (which do not express a given enamel protein) or transgenic mice (overexpressing selected protein or ones with point mutations) now are emerging and will be important in clarifying the functions of the various enamel proteins. Transgenic mice expressing mutated forms of amelogenin and knockout mice exhibit major enamel structural defects that affect overall thickness and enamel rod structure. However, consistent with its proposed role in promoting and sustaining mineral formation, no structured enamel layer is created in the absence of ameloblastin, and the enamel organ detaches from the tooth surface. Mice expressing defective enamelin (point mutations) indicate that this low-abundance protein is also essential for development of a normal enamel layer. In amelogenin and ameloblastin knockout mice, tooth induction and formation proceed apparently normally at the histologic level, raising questions about the suggested potential signaling functions for these proteins. Future investigations will need to address the problem of macromolecular matrix structure in relation to crystal disposition and growth, which will involve determination of the precise relationship in structural terms of one protein species with another. The newer imaging technologies including atomic force microscopy, scanning near field, molecular imaging by cryoelectron microscopy, and nuclear magnetic resonance are likely to be important in understanding these questions and in providing information for the development of biomimetic approaches for treatment of altered enamel.

MINERAL PATHWAY AND MINERALIZATION

The way in which mineral ions are introduced into forming enamel is of interest because it spans the secretory and maturation phases of enamel formation, with the latter demanding a large increase in the influx of mineral. The enamel layer is a secluded environment essentially created and maintained by the enamel organ. The route by which calcium moves from the blood vessels through the enamel organ to reach enamel likely implicates intercellular and transcellular routes. Several years ago, a smooth tubular network, opening onto enamel, was described in secretory stage ameloblasts. It then was speculated that the network might have a role in calcium ion control, similar to the sarcoplasmic reticulum, which it resembles. Recent biochemical findings have led to the proposal that calcium is routed through ameloblasts in high-capacity stores associated with the endoplasmic reticulum, avoiding the cytotoxic effects of excess calcium in the cytoplasm.

No matrix vesicles are associated with the mineralization of enamel, as is the case for collagen-based calcified tissues. In these tissues, matrix vesicles provide a closed environment to initiate crystal formation in a preformed organic matrix. What is observed instead is formation of crystallites directly against mantle dentin and their subsequent elongation against the ameloblast membrane at sites where enamel proteins are released (see Figure 7-46, A) so that no equivalent of predentin or osteoid is ever created. Because there is an apparent continuity between enamel and dentin crystallites, some believe that the first enamel crystallites are nucleated by apatite crystallites located within the dentin (see Figure 7-31).

Although amelogenesis is described correctly as a two-step process involving the secretion of a partially mineralized enamel and its subsequent maturation, studies involving microradiography of thin ground sections and computer enhancement indicate that the mineralization of enamel may involve several stages. These stages result in the creation of an enamel layer that is most highly mineralized at its surface, with the degree of mineralization decreasing toward the dentinoenamel junction until the innermost layer is reached, where mineralization apparently is increased. These changes are represented diagrammatically in Figure 7-48.

In summary, the process of amelogenesis involves cells that secrete enamel proteins, which immediately participate in mineralizing enamel to approximately 30%.

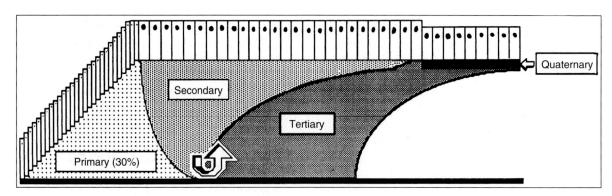

Figure 7-48 Four phases of enamel mineralization. *(Redrawn from Suga S: Adv Dent Res 3:188, 1989.)*

Once the entire thickness of enamel has been formed and structured, it then acquires a significant amount of additional mineral coincident with the bulk removal of enamel proteins and of water to yield a unique layer consisting of more than 95% mineral. This complicated process is under cellular control, and the associated cells undergo significant morphologic changes throughout amelogenesis, reflecting their evolving physiologic activity. In particular, completion of mineralization is characterized by modulation, a process whereby ameloblasts cyclically alternate their appearance several times so that matrix removal and crystal growth can go on efficiently within the secluded enamel space.

STRUCTURAL AND ORGANIZATIONAL FEATURES OF ENAMEL

ROD INTERRELATIONSHIPS

In human teeth, rods tend to be maintained in groups arranged circumferentially around the long axis of the tooth. In general, rods run in a perpendicular direction to the surface of the dentin, with a slight inclination toward the cusp as they pass outward. Near the cusp tip they run more vertically and in cervical enamel mainly horizontally.

TOPICS FOR CONSIDERATION   The Organic Matrix of Enamel: Why Is There So Much Complexity and Protein Diversity in an Environment That Is Essentially Destructive?

One aspect of amelogenesis that remains perplexing is understanding the reason why ameloblasts devote so much time and energy to form a relatively thick layer of organic material that has considerable compositional complexity but no survival potential beyond the point of mineral induction. This complexity includes routine secretion of multiple versions (isoforms) of the same protein that forms the bulk of the organic matrix of developing enamel, amelogenin. All amelogenin isoforms have identical N-terminal and C-terminal sequences but otherwise lack one or more clusters of sequences within the main body of the protein. Ameloblasts in some species (e.g., mouse) potentially can manufacture as many as nine distinct isoforms ranging from a full-length isoform with all exons translated (M194; 194 amino acids) to a highly truncated leucine-rich amelogenin polypeptide (LRAP) isoform having 3 to 4 times fewer amino acids overall. The reasons for this are unknown. In some mammals, including human beings, an additional level of complexity to amelogenin involves a type of sexual dimorphism in which isoforms actively translated from the Y chromosome in males have internal amino acid sequences that differ from those derived from the X chromosome. The last aspect of compositional complexity in the organic matrix of enamel relates to several locally produced "minor" proteins that collectively make up a group commonly referred to as the "nonamelogenins." These proteins currently include ameloblastin, enamelin, and a sulfated protein, which resembles ameloblastin in molecular weight but has predominately N-linked sugars instead of exclusively O-linked sugars postulated for ameloblastin (tuftelin does not appear to be a true enamel matrix protein).

Nonamelogenins typically are short-lived proteins that are fragmented rapidly near the enamel surface into lower-molecular-weight forms that linger for a time in the enamel layer before they disappear. Amelogenin itself is fragmented and destroyed after it is secreted, but this process occurs during a much longer time frame compared with the nonamelogenins.

Currently, no evidence exists to indicate that an unmineralized layer of preenamel exists at any time during the appositional growth phase of enamel development. Therefore, it seems unlikely that extracellular protein assembly and formation of template(s) of the type associated with mineral acquisition in the collagen-based hard tissues occurs in enamel. (It takes time for extracellular polymerization of tropocollagen into cross-linked fibrils that are receptive to mineral deposition.) Consequently, any protein-to-protein interaction important to mineral induction that occurs between amelogenin isoforms, between nonamelogenins, or between any combination of amelogenin and nonamelogenins probably takes place intracellularly or immediately on release of the proteins from the secretory granules of ameloblasts, considering the spatial proximity of the mineralization front to the plasma membrane of ameloblasts along the proximal and distal regions of Tomes' processes where appositional growth occurs. Forming enamel also lacks any significant amounts of mineral-modulating molecules that are characteristic of the collagen-based hard tissues, such as proteoglycans (inhibitors), osteopontin (inhibitor), osteocalcin (inhibitor), and bone sialoprotein (promoter).

These considerations lead to the inevitable conclusion that one or more of the amelogenin

Continued

TOPICS FOR CONSIDERATION   The Organic Matrix of Enamel: Why Is There So
Much Complexity and Protein Diversity in an
Environment That Is Essentially Destructive?—cont'd

isoforms, with or without the nonamelogenins or
fragments derived from extracellular processing of
amelogenin or nonamelogenins, must possess mineral-
promoting activity to cause new crystals to form de
novo near the surface as the enamel layer expands in
thickness (e.g., interrod areas and sites where rods first
form). A promoter mechanism also must be present to
allow continuous growth in the c-axis length of rod
apatite crystals in tandem with ameloblast movement
away from the dentinoenamel junction. Little evidence
presently exists that there is significant mineral-inhibiting
activity in enamel beyond the widely known effect

that bulk amounts of amelogenin exert on slowing
volumetric expansion of apatite. Once appositional
growth of the enamel layer is complete and all
mineral crystals are spatially in place, the matrix
proteins essentially represent "trash" that must be
removed to provide the physical space needed for final
maturation (volumetric expansion) of the rod and
interrod crystals.

Charles E. Smith
Université de Montréal
Montreal, Quebec, Canada

Superimposed on this arrangement are two other patterns that complicate enamel structure. First, each rod, as it runs to the surface, follows an irregular course bending to the right and left in the transverse plane of the tooth (except in cervical enamel, where the rods have a straight course) and up and down in the vertical plane. Second, in approximately the inner two thirds of the enamel layer, adjacent groups of rods intertwine and thus have dissimilar local orientations but a similar general direction. These complex interrelationships produce some of the structural features seen in enamel and must be remembered to interpret enamel structure.

STRIAE OF RETZIUS

The *striae of Retzius* generally are identified using ground sections of calcified teeth. In a longitudinal section of the tooth, they are seen as a series of dark lines extending from the dentinoenamel junction toward the tooth surface (Figure 7-49); in cross section they appear as concentric rings (Figure 7-50). Although striae of Retzius generally are ascribed to a weekly rhythm in enamel production resulting in a structural alteration of the rod, the basis for their production is still not clear. Another proposal suggests that they reflect appositional or incremental growth of the enamel layer. As the crown becomes bigger, new cohorts of cells are added cervically to compensate for the increase in size. These cells undergo a passive decussation as the enamel layer grows in thickness to assume a more coronal position (Figure 7-51). The demarcation between the enamel produced by these cohorts may appear as a line of Retzius, according to some investigators. The *neonatal line*, when present, is an enlarged stria of Retzius that apparently reflects the great physiologic changes occurring at birth. Accentuated incremental lines also are produced by systemic disturbances (e.g., fevers) that affect amelogenesis.

CROSS STRIATIONS

Human enamel is known to form at a rate of approximately 4 μm per day. Ground sections of enamel reveal what appear to be periodic bands or *cross striations* at 4-μm intervals across so-called rods. With the scanning electron microscope, alternating constrictions and expansions of the rods sometimes are visible; close examination reveals that the constrictions are actually gouges in the rod structure (Figure 7-52). Such a pattern could reflect a diurnal rhythmicity in rod formation, the organization of crystallites within the rod, or structural interrelations between rod and interrod enamel. What may seem to be cross striations on longitudinally sectioned rods on ground sections also has been demonstrated to be obliquely sectioned groups of rods (see Figure 7-6). Thus the light microscope may produce an illusion of longitudinally sectioned rods that are really, as demonstrated by electron microscopy, an alignment of obliquely cut rods in horizontal rows.

BANDS OF HUNTER AND SCHREGER

The *bands of Hunter and Schreger* are an optical phenomenon produced by changes in direction between adjacent groups of rods. The bands are seen most clearly in longitudinal ground sections viewed by reflected light

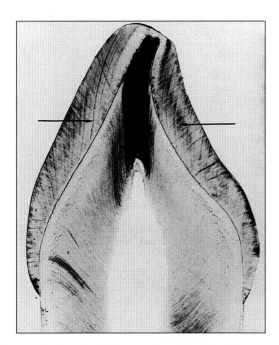

Figure 7-49 Longitudinal ground section showing disposition of the striae of Retzius (*arrows* in the enamel layer).

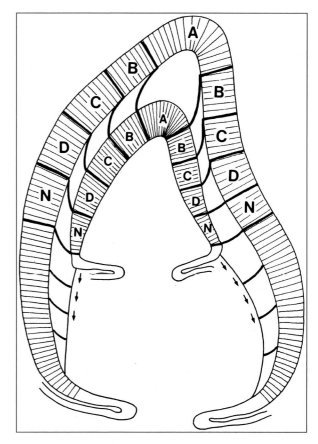

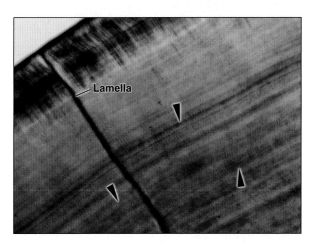

Figure 7-50 Light microscope view of striae of Retzius in a ground section. In cross section the striae appear as a series of concentric, dark lines *(arrowheads)*. An enamel lamella can be seen running from the outer surface to the dentinoenamel junction.

Figure 7-51 Diagram illustrating the increase in crown size and corresponding growth of the enamel organ in a tooth of limited eruption. The ameloblast cohorts are labeled A to N. As the crown becomes larger, these cohorts are displaced apically on the enlarged crown by their own production of enamel. The trajectory followed by rods produced by the cohorts is outlined by the dark lines. The junction between the enamel rods produced by the various cohorts is believed to be responsible for the incremental pattern of enamel and to follow the general direction of the striae of Retzius. New ameloblasts differentiate cervically in the direction of the arrows as the crown grows in size. *(From Warshawsky H. In Butler WT, editor: The chemistry and biology of mineralized tissues, Birmingham, Ala, 1985, Ebsco Media.)*

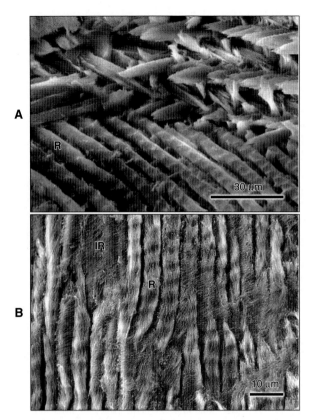

Figure 7-52 In scanning electron microscopy, periodic varicosities and depressions are seen along enamel rods *(R)* in **(A)** rodent and **(B)** human teeth, producing the impression of cross striations along their length. *IR,* Interrod enamel.

and are found in the inner two thirds of the enamel. These bands appear as dark and light alternating zones that can be reversed by altering the direction of incident illumination (Figures 7-53 to 7-55). Scanning electron microscopy clearly reveals the difference in orientation of groups of rods within these zones (see Figures 7-1, *B,* and 7-37, *A).*

GNARLED ENAMEL

Over the cusps of teeth the rods appear twisted around each other in a seemingly complex arrangement known as *gnarled enamel.* One may recall that rods are arranged radially in horizontal planes, each plane surrounding the longitudinal axis of the tooth like a washer. The rods undulate back and forth within the planes. This undulation in vertically directed rods around a ring of small circumference readily explains gnarled enamel.

ENAMEL TUFTS AND LAMELLAE

Enamel tufts and *lamellae* may be likened to geologic faults and have no known clinical significance. They are

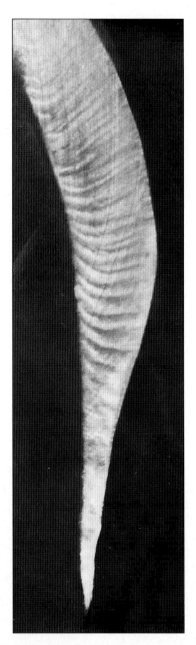

Figure 7-53 Longitudinal section of enamel viewed by incident light. The series of alternating light and dark bands of Hunter and Schreger are apparent.

best seen in transverse sections of enamel (Figure 7-56). Enamel tufts project from the dentinoenamel junction for a short distance into the enamel. They appear to be branched and contain greater concentrations of enamel proteins than the rest of the enamel. Tufts are believed to occur developmentally because of abrupt changes in the direction of groups of rods that arise from different regions of the scalloped dentinoenamel junction. Lamellae extend for varying depths from the surface of enamel and consist of linear, longitudinally oriented defects filled with organic material. This organic material

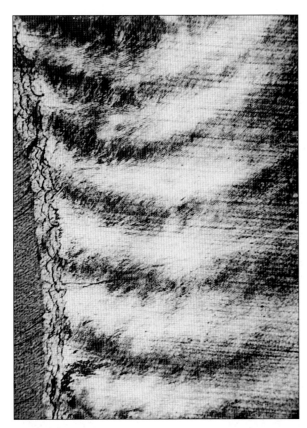

Figure 7-54 Higher-power view of a band of Hunter and Schreger as viewed by incident light.

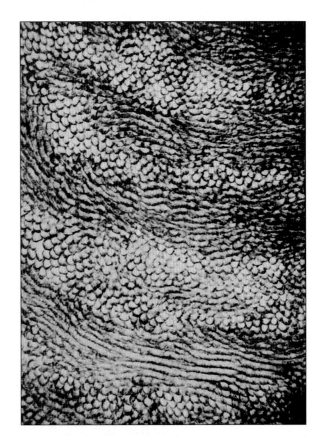

Figure 7-55 Section corresponding to Figure 7-54 viewed under transmitted light. The differing orientation of enamel rods is clearly evident.

may derive from trapped enamel organ components or connective tissue surrounding the developing tooth. Tufts and lamellae are usually best demonstrated in ground sections, but they also can be seen in carefully demineralized sections of human enamel because of their higher protein content. Cracks in the enamel sometimes can be mistaken for lamellae but can be distinguished from the latter because they generally do not contain organic material.

DENTINOENAMEL JUNCTION AND ENAMEL SPINDLES

The junction between enamel and dentin is established as these two hard tissues begin to form and is seen as a scalloped profile in cross section (Figure 7-57; see also Figures 7-24, A; 7-38, A; and 7-56). Before enamel forms, some developing odontoblast processes extend into the ameloblast layer and, when enamel formation begins, become trapped to form *enamel spindles* (Figure 7-58). The electron microscope reveals that crystals of dentin and enamel intermix (Figure 7-59; see also Figure 7-31). The scanning electron microscope

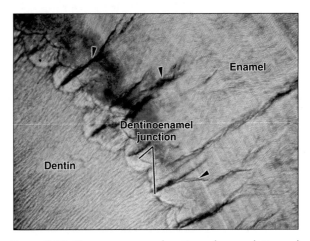

Figure 7-56 Transverse ground section of enamel. Enamel tufts are the branched structures extending from the dentinoenamel junction into the enamel *(arrowheads)*. The junction is seen as a scalloped profile.

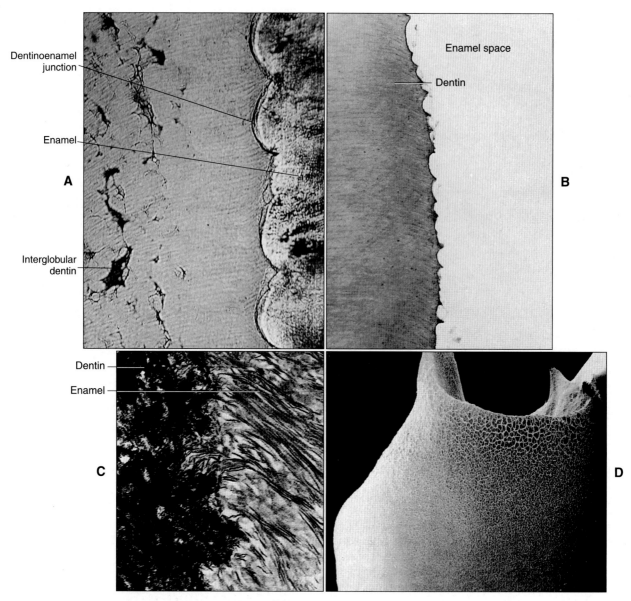

Figure 7-57 Dentinoenamel junction. **A,** Ground section. **B,** Demineralized section after the enamel has been lost. The scalloped nature of the junction when seen in one plane is striking. **C,** A transmission electron micrograph shows the intermingling of dentin and enamel crystals. **D,** A low-power scanning electron micrograph of a premolar from which the enamel has been removed shows that the scalloping is accentuated where the junction is subjected to most functional stress. *(D courtesy W.H. Douglas.)*

reveals the junction to be a series of ridges rather than spikes, which arrangement probably increases the adherence between dentin and enamel; in this regard it is worth noting that the ridging is most pronounced in coronal dentin, where occlusal stresses are the greatest (see Figure 7-38, A). The shape and nature of the junction prevent shearing of the enamel during function.

ENAMEL SURFACE

The surface of enamel is characterized by several structures. The striae of Retzius often extend from the dentinoenamel junction to the outer surface of enamel, where they end in shallow furrows known as *perikymata* (Figures 7-60 to 7-62). Perikymata run in circumferentially horizontal lines across the face of the crown. In addition, lamellae or cracks in the enamel appear as jagged lines in various regions of the tooth surface. The electron microscope shows that the surface structure of enamel varies with age. In unerupted teeth the enamel surface consists of a structureless surface layer (final enamel) that is lost rapidly by abrasion, attrition, and erosion in erupted teeth.

As the tooth erupts, it is covered by a pellicle consisting of debris from the enamel organ that is

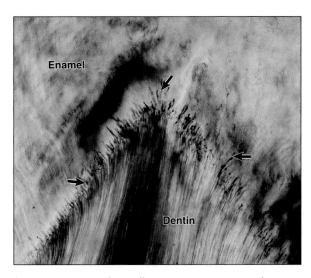

Figure 7-58 Enamel spindles *(arrows)* in a ground section extend from the dentinoenamel junction into the enamel and most frequently are found at cusp tips.

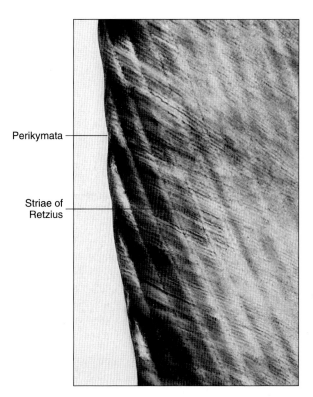

Figure 7-60 Ground section of enamel showing the relationship between the striae of Retzius and surface perikymata. *(Courtesy D. Weber.)*

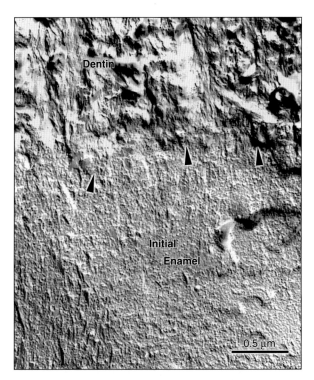

Figure 7-59 Freeze-fracture preparation at the dentinoenamel junction *(arrowheads)*. The distinctive appearance of the collagenous dentin and noncollagenous (initial) enamel layer is notable.

Figure 7-61 Scanning electron micrograph of the labial surface of a tooth, showing the perikymata. *(Courtesy D. Weber.)*

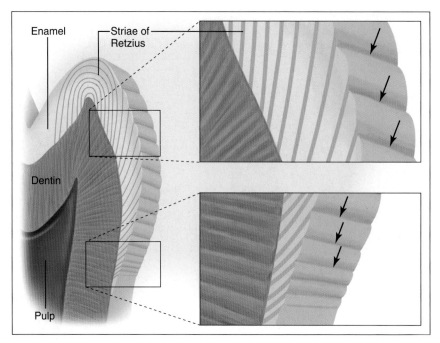

Figure 7-62 The relationship between the striae of Retzius and surface perikymata *(arrows)*. *(From Fejerskov O, Thylstrup A. In Mjör I, Fejerskov O, editors:* Human oral embryology and histology, *Copenhagen, 1986, Munksgaard.)*

lost rapidly. Salivary pellicle, a nearly ubiquitous organic deposit on the surface of teeth, always reappears shortly after teeth have been polished mechanically. Dental plaque forms readily on the pellicle, especially in more protected areas of the dentition.

AGE CHANGES

Enamel is a nonvital tissue that is incapable of regeneration. With age, enamel becomes progressively worn in regions of masticatory attrition. Wear facets increasingly are pronounced in older persons, and in some cases substantial portions of the crown (enamel and dentin) become eroded. Other characteristics of aging enamel include discoloration, reduced permeability, and modifications in the surface layer. Linked to these changes is an apparent reduction in the incidence of caries.

Teeth darken with age. Whether this darkening is caused by a change in the structure of enamel is debatable. Although darkening could be caused by the addition of organic material to enamel from the environment, darkening also may be caused by a deepening of dentin color (the layer becomes thicker with age) seen through the progressively thinning layer of translucent enamel.

No doubt exists that enamel becomes less permeable with age. Young enamel behaves as a semipermeable membrane, permitting the slow passage of water and substances of small molecular size through pores between the crystals. With age the pores diminish as the crystals acquire more ions and as the surface increases in size.

The surface layer of enamel reflects most prominently the changes within this tissue. During aging, the composition of the surface layer changes as ionic exchange with the oral environment occurs. In particular, a progressive increase in the fluoride content affects the surface layer (and that, incidentally, can be achieved by topical application).

DEFECTS OF AMELOGENESIS

In addition to the genetic dysplasias described in the first chapter, many other conditions produce defects in enamel structure. Such defects occur because ameloblasts are cells particularly sensitive to changes in their environment. Even minor physiologic changes affect them and elicit changes in enamel structure that can be seen only histologically. More severe insults greatly disturb enamel production or produce death of the ameloblasts, and the resulting defects are easily visible clinically.

Three conditions affecting enamel formation occur frequently. Defects in enamel can be caused by febrile diseases. During the course of such a disease, enamel formation is disturbed so that all teeth forming at the time become characterized by distinctive bands of malformed enamel. On recovery, normal enamel formation is resumed (Figure 7-63).

Second, defects can be formed by tetracycline-induced disturbances in teeth. Tetracycline antibiotics are incorporated into mineralizing tissues; in the case of enamel, this incorporation may result in a band of brown pigmentation or even total pigmentation. Hypoplasia or absence of enamel also may occur. The degree of damage is determined by the magnitude and duration of tetracycline therapy.

Finally, the fluoride ion can interfere with amelogenesis. Chronic ingestion of flouride ion concentrations in excess of 5 ppm (5 times the amount in fluoridated water supplies) interferes sufficiently with ameloblast function to produce mottled enamel. Mottled enamel is unsightly and often is seen as white patches of hypomineralized and altered enamel. Such enamel, though unsightly, still resists caries.

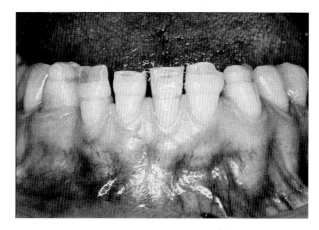

Figure 7-63 Dentition of a patient who had two illnesses at separate times. The enamel defects, separated by normal enamel, are clearly visible.

TOPICS FOR CONSIDERATION   Genetic Basis of Inherited Tooth Defects

Tooth development progresses through initiation, bud, cap, bell, crown formation, and root formation stages; with different molecular processes being critical at different stages. Genetic diseases that disrupt key processes during tooth formation result in dental phenotypes characteristic of when and where the defective gene normally is expressed. Disruptions early in the process lead to familial tooth agenesis or (less often) supernumerary teeth. Disruptions during crown formation lead to inherited defects of dentin (dentinogenesis imperfecta and dentin dysplasia) or enamel (amelogenesis imperfecta). Defects of root formation include taurodontism and cementum agenesis (in hypophosphatasia). Recent advances in the molecular basis of inherited diseases have increased our understanding of normal and pathologic tooth development.

Teeth form as a result of a series of epithelial-mesenchymal interactions. The initiating event appears to be the expression of diffusible signaling molecules (growth factors) by the oral epithelium that stimulates signal transduction in the underlying ectomesenchyme. Transcription factors are induced that drive the expression of downstream genes that guide odontoblast differentiation but that also induce a signaling response that reciprocally coordinates the differentiation of ameloblasts. Failure to execute this genetic program properly leads to an arrest of tooth development. Defects in two transcription factor genes, *MSX1* (4p16.3-p16.1) and *PAX9* (14q12-q13), and in *AXIN2* (17q23-q24), which encodes a protein (conductin) involved in Wnt signaling pathway, exhibit familial tooth agenesis as their primary clinical feature. *AXIN2* mutations also are

associated with colorectal cancer, so identifying the gene causing familial tooth agenesis in a presenting patient could unveil a hidden risk of cancer.

As the developmental program progresses into the late bell and crown formation stages, specialized extracellular matrix proteins are secreted that regulate the formation of dentin and enamel. The major protein in dentin is type I collagen, which is encoded by two genes, *COL1A1* (17q21.31-q22) and *COL1A2* (7q22.1). Two A1 chains fold with one A2 chain to form a collagen triple helix. Defects in these genes cause osteogenesis imperfecta, which has a dentinogenesis imperfecta (DGI) phenotype in about half the cases. Nonsyndromic inherited defects of dentin are classified as dentinogenesis imperfecta types II and III (DGI-II and DGI-III) and dentin dysplasia (DD) types I and II (DD-I and DD-II). Besides type I collagen, the main extracellular dentin proteins are proteolytic cleavage products of dentin sialophosphoprotein (DSPP). Recent genetic studies indicate that defects in *DSPP* (4q21.1) are the predominant cause of DD-II, DGI-II, and DGI-III, leading to the suggestion that these disorders be lumped together as "*DSPP*-associated dentin defects."

Concurrent with the formation of dentin is enamel. The dental enamel of erupted teeth contains only trace amounts of protein, but developing enamel is about 35 percent protein. The bulk of the enamel protein is expressed from the amelogenin gene on the X chromosome (*AMELX*, Xp22). Defects in *AMELX* cause X-linked amelogenesis imperfecta. Females with X-linked amelogenesis imperfecta often display characteristic vertical bands of hypoplastic (thin) enamel. Males are more severely affected, with little or no enamel formed. Besides amelogenin, two other

Continued

TOPICS FOR CONSIDERATION   Genetic Basis of Inherited Tooth Defects—cont'd

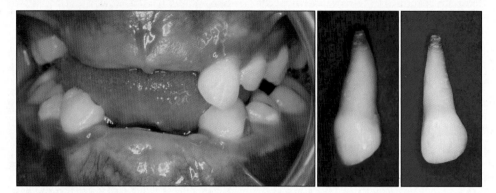

Early exfoliation of fully rooted primary teeth in childhood onset hypophosphatasia. *ALPL* mutations are responsible for the early exfoliation of primary teeth in this patient.

proteins are found in developing enamel: enamelin (*ENAM*, 4q13.3) and ameloblastin (*AMBN*, 4q13.2). Defects in *ENAM* cause autosomal dominant amelogenesis imperfecta. In cases where both *ENAM* alleles are affected, virtually no enamel forms. In the heterozygous condition, horizontal bands of hypoplastic enamel often are observed, especially in the cervical third of the crown. In some cases the cementoenamel junction appears to have moved up the tooth (coronally). In its mildest form, small well-circumscribed enamel pits are observed. No disease-causing mutations have yet been observed in *AMBN*, although ameloblastin null mice lack enamel.

Enamel matrix proteins are secreted along with enamelysin (*MMP20*, 11q22.3). This matrix metalloproteinase cleaves enamel proteins in developing enamel. This matrix metalloproteinase is believed to be the only significant enamel protease during the secretory stage because it is able to generate all of the major amelogenin cleavage products that are observed in secretory stage enamel. The enamel layer in *Mmp20* null mice is thinner and softer than normal and tends to chip away from the underlying dentin. In human beings, *MMP20* mutations cause autosomal recessive pigmented hypomaturation amelogenesis imperfecta.

When secretory ameloblasts enter transition stage, they greatly reduce their secretions of ameloblastin, enamelin, and initiate expression of kallikrein4 (*KLK4*, 19q13.41) and amelotin (*AMTN*, 4q13.3). KLK4 is a serine protease that cleaves amelogenin more aggressively than MMP-20 and is believed to degrade enamel proteins to facilitate their removal, which increases the degree of enamel mineralization. Like *MMP20*, mutations in *KLK4* cause autosomal recessive pigmented hypomaturation amelogenesis imperfecta. Amelotin is a basal lamina protein expressed throughout enamel maturation. No disease state has been discovered that is associated with *AMTN*, but it is believed to play an important role in

cell adherence to enamel. Although four genes (*AMELX, ENAM, MMP20, KLK4*) are known to contribute to the cause of amelogenesis imperfecta, only about a quarter of all amelogenesis imperfecta cases can be linked to these genes, suggesting that many other (unidentified) genes contribute to the pathogenesis of amelogenesis imperfecta.

Root formation occurs after crown formation and is initiated by Herwig's epithelial root sheath, which acts as an epithelial template that shapes the roots. Abnormalities of root number and morphology arise from anomalous root sheath activity. DLX3 (17q21) is a transcription factor involved in root sheath activity. *DLX3* mutations delay the inward invagination of the sheath toward the pulp, resulting in taurodontism, a feature of trichodentoosseous syndrome and some forms of amelogenesis imperfecta. Taurodontism is a malformation of multirooted teeth, characterized by a large crown-to-root ratio. The roots are abnormally short, and the pulp chamber is abnormally large.

Cementum is the mineralized tissue that anchors the collagen fibers that connect the root to bone. Defects in alkaline phosphatase (*ALPL*, 1p36.1-p34) often lead to cementum agenesis in hypophosphatasia. Dentists often diagnose childhood onset hypophosphatasia as fully rooted primary teeth exfoliate early (see the figure).

Jan C-C Hu, DDS, PhD
Department of Orthodontics and Pediatric Dentistry
University of Michigan Dental Research Lab
Ann Arbor, Michigan

James P. Simmer, DDS, PhD
Department of Biologic and Materials Sciences
University of Michigan Dental Research Lab
Ann Arbor, Michigan

CLINICAL IMPLICATIONS

An appreciation of the histology of enamel is important for understanding the principles of fluoridation, acid-etching techniques, and dental caries.

FLUORIDATION

If the fluoride ion is incorporated into or adsorbed on the hydroxyapatite crystal, the crystal becomes more resistant to acid dissolution. This reaction partly explains the role of fluoride in caries prevention, for the caries process is initiated by demineralization of enamel. Obviously, if fluoride is present as enamel is being formed, all the enamel crystals will be more resistant to acid dissolution. The amount of fluoride must be controlled carefully, however, because of the sensitivity of ameloblasts to the fluoride ion and the possibility of producing unsightly mottling. The semipermeable nature of enamel enables topical application to provide a higher concentration of fluoride in the surface enamel of erupted teeth.

The presence of fluoride enhances chemical reactions that lead to the precipitation of calcium phosphate. An equilibrium exists in the oral cavity between calcium and phosphate ions in the solution phase (saliva) and in the solid phase (enamel), and fluoride shifts this equilibrium to favor the solid phase. Clinically, when a localized region of enamel has lost mineral (e.g., a white spot lesion), the enamel may be remineralized if the destructive agent (dental plaque) is removed. The remineralization reaction is enhanced greatly by fluoride.

ACID ETCHING

Acid etching of the enamel surface, or enamel conditioning, has become an important technique in clinical practice. Use of fissure sealants, bonding of restorative materials to enamel, and cementing of orthodontic brackets to tooth surfaces involve acid etching. The process achieves the desired effect in two stages: first, acid etching removes plaque and other debris, along with a thin layer of enamel; second, it increases the porosity of exposed surfaces through selective dissolution of crystals, which provides a better bonding surface for the restorative and adhesive materials.

The scanning electron microscope beautifully demonstrates the effects of acid etching on enamel surfaces. Three etching patterns predominate (Figure 7-64). The most common is *type I*, characterized by preferential

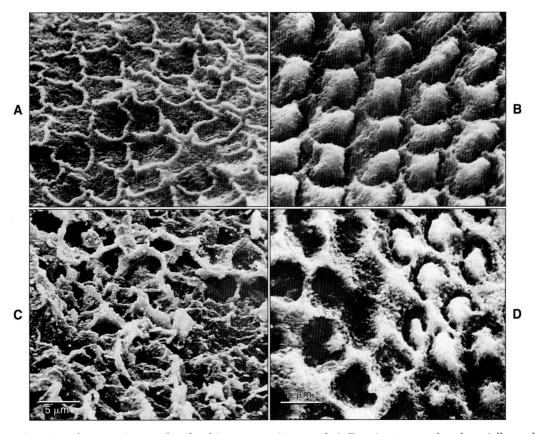

Figure 7-64 Scanning electron micrographs of etching patterns in enamel. **A,** Type I pattern: rod preferentially eroded. **B,** Type II pattern: rod boundary (interrod) preferentially eroded. **C,** Type III pattern: indiscriminate erosion. **D,** Junction between type I and type II etching zones. *(Courtesy L. Silverstone.)*

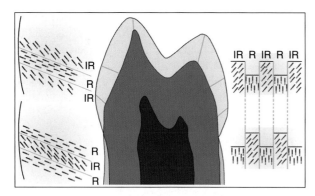

Figure 7-65 Diagrammatic representation of how the difference in general orientation of rod *(R)* and interrod *(IR)* crystals will result in different etching topographies illustrated in Figure 7-64, *A* and *B*. Crystals are more susceptible to dissolution at their extremities than along their sides, such that the ones arriving perpendicular to the surface will be more affected.

removal of rods. In the reverse, *type II*, interrod enamel is removed preferentially and the rod remains intact. Occurring less frequently is *type III*, which is irregular and indiscriminate. Some debate still occurs as to why acid etchants produce differing surface patterns. The most commonly held view is that the etching pattern depends on crystal orientation. Ultrastructural studies of crystal dissolution indicate that crystals dissolve more readily at their ends than on their sides. Thus crystals lying perpendicular to the enamel surface are the most vulnerable. The type I and II etching patterns can be explained easily by noting that crystals reach the enamel surfaces at differing inclinations in the rods compared with the interrod areas (Figure 7-65).

In summary, acid conditioning of enamel surfaces is now an accepted procedure for obtaining improved bonding of resins to enamel. Retention depends mainly on a mechanical interlocking. The conditioning agent removes the organic film from the tooth surface and preferentially etches the enamel surface so that firmer contact is established. In areas with rodless enamel, especially in deciduous teeth, slightly more severe etching is required to obtain adequate mechanical retention.

RECOMMENDED READING

Aoba T, Komatsu H, Shimazu Y et al: Enamel mineralization and an initial crystalline phase, *Connect Tissue Res* 39:129, 1998.

Bartlett JD, Ganss B, Golberg M et al: Protein-protein interactions of the developing enamel matrix, *Curr Top Dev Biol* 74:57, 2006.

Hubbard MJ: Calcium transport across the dental enamel epithelium, *Crit Rev Oral Biol Med* 11:437, 2000.

Margolis HC, Beniash E, Fowler CE: Role of macromolecular assembly of enamel matrix proteins in enamel formation, *J Dent Res* 85:775, 2006.

Nanci A, Smith CE: Matrix-mediated mineralization in enamel and the collagen-based hard tissues. In Goldberg M, Boskey A, Robinson C, editors: *Chemistry and biology of mineralized tissues*, Rosemont, Ill, 1999, American Academy of Orthopaedic Surgeons.

Simmer JP, Hu JC: Expression, structure, and function of enamel proteinases, *Connect Tissue Res* 43:441, 2002.

Smith CE: Cellular and chemical events during enamel maturation, *Crit Rev Oral Biol Med* 9:128, 1998.

Dentin-Pulp Complex

Dentin and pulp sometimes are treated separately in textbooks on dental histology largely because dentin is a hard connective tissue and the pulp is a soft one. However, as explained in Chapter 1, dentin and pulp are related embryologically, histologically, and functionally and therefore are described together in this chapter.

BASIC STRUCTURE OF DENTIN

Dentin is the hard tissue portion of the pulp-dentin complex and forms the bulk of the tooth. Dentin is a bone-like matrix characterized by multiple closely packed *dentinal tubules* that traverse its entire thickness and contain the cytoplasmic extensions of *odontoblasts* that once formed the dentin and then maintain it. The cell bodies of the odontoblasts are aligned along the inner aspect of the dentin, against a layer of *predentin*, where they also form the peripheral boundary of the *dental pulp*.

The dental pulp is the soft connective tissue that occupies the central portion of the tooth. The space it occupies is the *pulp cavity*, which is divided into a coronal portion (or *pulp chamber*) and a radicular portion (the root canal). The pulp chamber conforms to the general shape of the anatomic crown. Under the cusps the chamber extends into pulp horns, which are especially prominent under the buccal cusp of premolar teeth and the mesiobuccal cusp of molar teeth. Their cusps are particularly significant in dental restoration, when they must be avoided to prevent exposure of pulp tissue.

The *root canal* (or root canal system, as it is called in multirooted teeth) terminates at the *apical foramen*, where the pulp and periodontal ligament meet and the main nerves and vessels enter and leave the tooth. In the developing tooth the apical foramen is large

191

and centrally located. As the tooth completes its development, the apical foramen becomes smaller in diameter and more eccentric in position. Sizes from 0.3 to 0.6 μm, with the larger diameter occurring in the palatal root of maxillary molars and the distal root of mandibular molars, are typical of the completed foramen. The foramen may be located at the very end, or anatomic apex, of the root but usually is located slightly more occlusally (0.5 to 0.75 mm) from the apex. If more than one foramen is present on a root, the largest is designated the apical foramen and the others the *accessory foramina.*

Connections between the pulp and the periodontal tissues also may occur along the lateral surface of the root through the lateral canals. Such canals, which may contain blood vessels, are not present in all teeth and occur with differing frequencies in different types of teeth. Occasionally the lateral canals enter the floor of the pulp chamber of multirooted teeth. Because the apical foramen and the lateral canals are areas of communication between the pulp space and the periodontium, they can act as avenues for the extension of disease from one tissue to the other. Hence diseases of the dental pulp can produce changes in the periodontal tissues. More rarely do diseases of the periodontium involve the dental pulp.

COMPOSITION, FORMATION, AND STRUCTURE OF DENTIN

Dentin is first deposited as a layer of unmineralized matrix called predentin that varies in thickness (10 to 50 μm) and lines its innermost (pulpal) portion. Predentin consists principally of collagen and is similar to osteoid in bone; it is easy to identify in hematoxylin-eosin–stained sections because it stains less intensely than mineralized dentin. Predentin gradually mineralizes into dentin as various noncollagenous matrix proteins are incorporated at the *mineralization front.* The thickness of predentin remains constant because the amount that calcifies is balanced by the addition of new unmineralized matrix. Predentin is thickest at times when active dentinogenesis is occurring and diminishes in thickness with age.

Mature dentin is made up of approximately 70% inorganic material, 20% organic material, and 10% water by weight, and 45%, 33%, and 22%, respectively, by volume. The inorganic component of dentin consists of substituted hydroxyapatite in the form of small plates. The organic phase is about 90% collagen (mainly type I with small amounts of types III and V) with fractional inclusions of various noncollagenous matrix proteins and lipids. Although studies have for a long time focused on identifying proteins specific to bone or dentin, it is now clear that bone matrix proteins can be found in dentin and that dentin matrix proteins also are present in bone (see Table 1-1).

The noncollagenous matrix proteins pack the space between collagen fibrils and accumulate along the periphery of dentinal tubules. These proteins make up the following: dentin phosphoprotein/phosphophoryn (DPP), dentin sialoprotein (DSP), dentin glycoprotein (DGP), dentin matrix protein-1 (DMP1), osteonectin/secreted protein acidic and rich in cysteine, osteocalcin, bone sialoprotein (BSP), osteopontin, matrix extracellular phosphoglycoprotein, proteoglycans, and some serum proteins. DPP, DSP, and DGP are expressed as a single molecule at the gene level that then is processed into individual components with distinct physicochemical properties. DPP and DSP represent the major noncollagenous matrix proteins in dentin. DPP is the C-terminal proteolytic cleavage product of dentin sialophosphoprotein (DSPP), DSP is the N-terminal one, and DGP lies in the middle of the molecule. Differentiating odontoblasts also appear to produce, for a short period, enamel proteins such as amelogenin. In addition, differentiating ameloblasts also are believed transiently to produce some dentin proteins.

Collagen type I acts as a scaffold that accommodates a large proportion (estimated at 56%) of the mineral in the holes and pores of fibrils. The noncollagenous matrix proteins regulate mineral deposition and can act as inhibitors, promoters, and/or stabilizers; their distribution is suggestive of their role. For instance, intact proteoglycans appear to be more concentrated in predentin and thus are believed to prevent the premature mineralization of the organic matrix while collagen fibrils mature and attain the correct dimension. DSP and DMP1 are predominantly immunodetected in peritubular dentin (discussed later in the chapter), where they may inhibit its growth and thus prevent occlusion of the tubule. In additional to their codistribution, DSP and DMP1 exhibit similarities in biochemical features; they thus may have redundant or synergistic functions. DSPP mutations result in a variety of dental phenotypes, including dentinogenesis imperfecta III. In both cases, mice that do not express DSPP or DMP1 show enlarged pulp chambers, an increase in the thickness of predentin, and hypomineralization, indicating additional functions to the control of peritubular dentin. Noteworthy is that DSPP and DMP1 are present in bone and dentin as processed fragments and that absence of DMP1 has profound effects on bone.

Dentin is slightly harder than bone and softer than enamel. This difference can be distinguished readily on radiographs on which the dentin appears more radiolucent (darker) than enamel and more radiopaque (lighter) than pulp. Because light can pass readily through the thin, highly mineralized enamel and can be reflected by the underlying yellowish dentin, the crown of a tooth also assumes such coloration. The thicker enamel does not permit light to pass through as readily, and in such teeth the crown appears whiter. Teeth with pulp disease or without a dental pulp often show discoloration of the dentin, which causes a darkening of the clinical crown.

Physically, dentin has an elastic quality that is important for the proper functioning of the tooth because the elasticity provides flexibility and prevents fracture of the overlying brittle enamel. Dentin and enamel are bound firmly at the *dentinoenamel junction* that appears microscopically, as seen in the previous chapter, as a well-defined scalloped border (see Figure 7-57). In the root of the tooth the dentin is covered by cementum, and the junction between these two tissues is less distinct because, in the human being, they intermingle.

TOPICS FOR CONSIDERATION   Dentin and Dentin Sialophosphoprotein

Collagen and dentin sialophosphoprotein (DSPP). Most of the organic material (~85%) secreted into predentin is type I collagen. Collagen triple helices assemble into long fibrils (50 to 200 nm in diameter) that are noted for their tensile strength. The predominant noncollagenous proteins in dentin are generated by proteolysis of DSPP, a large multidomain protein with hundreds of posttranslational modifications.

Inherited dentin malformations. The importance of collagen and DSPP-derived proteins in dentin biomineralization can be inferred from the malformations that are observed in their absence. Inherited dentin malformations are classified into five groups: three types of dentinogenesis imperfecta (DGI) and two types of dentin dysplasia. DGI-I consists of dentin malformations associated with osteogenesis imperfecta. Osteogenesis imperfecta is caused primarily by mutations in the two genes encoding type I collagen: *COL1A1* (17q21.31-q22) and *COL1A2* (7q22.1). Some cases of osteogenesis imperfecta with DGI have been reported in which a collagen gene mutation causes no clinical bony defects but results in dentin defects typical of DGI. DGI-II has the same dental phenotype (opalescent dentin, bulbous crowns, obliterated pulp chambers) as DGI-I, but lacks the nondental (bony) symptoms. DGI-II is caused by mutations in *DSPP* (4q21). Mutations in *DSPP* also can cause DGI-III and dentin dysplasia II. No genes besides *DSPP* have been implicated in the causes of isolated (nonsyndromic) inherited defects of dentin. The overlapping dental phenotypes of collagen and DSPP mutations suggest they act together, at least in part.

The DSPP chimera. DSPP is a chimera, meaning that it is composed of several dissimilar parts. DSPP is cleaved by proteases into these separate parts. The order of the major components is DSP-DGP-DPP, where DSP is dentin sialoprotein, DGP is dentin glycoprotein, and DPP is dentin phosphoprotein (or phosphophoryn). In human beings, DSPP has about 1240 amino acids, but the number varies in different persons because of length polymorphisms in the DPP code, which is highly redundant. The DSPP chimera has only a transient existence. DSPP is cleaved so rapidly following its synthesis that uncleaved DSPP has never been isolated. Based on animal studies, DPP is cleaved off first, generating DSP-DGP (447 amino acids) and DPP (~790 amino acids). In the extracellular matrix, MMP-20 cleaves DSP-DGP into DSP (367 amino acids) and DGP (80 amino acids). DSP and DGP undergo numerous additional cleavages catalyzed by matrix metalloproteinases (MMP-2 and MMP-20). The cleavages occur principally between glycosylation attachment sites. The processing of DSPP is thought to be an activation step (separating domains

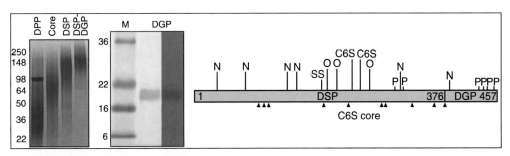

DSPP-derived proteins. DSPP is first cleaved into DSP-DGP and DPP. DSP-DGP splits into DSP and DGP. *Left,* Stains-all gel showing large DSPP-derived proteins isolated from pig dentin during the crown formation stage. DPP (100 kDa) copurifies with a smear of its degradation products. DSP is reduced to a core proteoglycan. *Middle,* Brilliant blue and stains-all gels showing DGP (19 kDa). *Right,* Diagram of pig DSP-DGP posttranslational modifications. *C6S,* Chondroitin 6-sulfate glycan attachment; *N,* N-linked glycosylation; *O,* O-linked glycosylation; *P,* phosphate attachments; *arrowheads,* cleavage sites; *SS,* disulfide bridge in DSP dimers.

Continued

with different structures and functions), but the processing continues and DSPP-derived proteins ultimately are degraded.

DPP is an unusual phosphoprotein. DPP is the most acidic protein ever discovered and has an isoelectric point of 1. DPP has numerous DSS (aspartic acid–serine–serine) repeats, and literally hundreds of its serine residues are phosphorylated. Having a high negative charge, DPP binds large amounts of calcium. In vitro studies show that DPP binds to collagen and is able to initiate hydroxyapatite formation. DPP binds collagen fibrils in "holes" that form between the staggered collagen triple-helices in the fibril assemblies and induces mineralization. One observation that seems inconsistent with this theory is that DPP is degraded as dentin mineralizes, which might not be expected if DPP served a structural role connecting mineral to collagen. Also difficult to understand is how the degradation of DPP could be catalyzed by proteases if it is buried in the mineral.

DSP is a highly glycosylated proteoglycan and can form covalent dimers. Each monomer has two chondroitin 6-sulfate attachments of variable length and about half a dozen N- (glutamine) or O-linked (serine or threonine) glycosylations and a similar number of phosphorylations. The two glycan attachments and the O-linked glycosylations are confined to the middle of the DSP protein (see figure). Proteoglycans consist of a protein core covalently linked to glycosaminoglycan chains. The glycan attachments have large numbers of acidic sulfate and carboxyl groups and tend to associate with and coat collagen fibrils, and these may serve to align and properly space them. Proteoglycans also tend to coat cell surfaces, supporting a potential role for DSP in the formation of peritubular dentin. DGP is a small, phosphorylated glycoprotein of unknown function.

The characterization of DSPP-derived proteins is still in an early stage. These proteins are highly modified following their translation, and these modifications are still only partially characterized. The discovery that *DSPP* as the predominant gene involved in the causes of dentin dysplasia II, DGI-II, and DGI-III has greatly increased interest in its structure and function in dentin biomineralization.

Yasuo Yamakoshi, PhD
University of Michigan Dental Research Lab
Ann Arbor, Michigan

James P. Simmer, DDS, PhD
Department of Biologic and Materials Sciences
University of Michigan Dental Research Lab
Ann Arbor, Michigan

TYPES OF DENTIN

PRIMARY DENTIN

Most of the tooth is formed by *primary dentin*, which outlines the pulp chamber and is referred to as *circumpulpal dentin* (Figure 8-1). The outer layer, near enamel or cementum, differs from the rest of the primary dentin in the way it is mineralized and in the structural interrelation between the collagenous and noncollagenous matrix components. This outer layer is called *mantle dentin*; the term, however, generally is used to refer to the outer layer in coronal dentin.

SECONDARY DENTIN

Secondary dentin develops after root formation has been completed and represents the continuing, but much slower, deposition of dentin by odontoblasts (Figure 8-2). Secondary dentin has a tubular structure that, though less regular, is for the most part continuous with that of the primary dentin. The ratio of mineral to organic material is the same as for primary dentin. Secondary dentin is not deposited evenly around the periphery of the pulp chamber, especially in the molar teeth. The greater deposition of secondary dentin on the roof and floor of the chamber leads to an asymmetrical reduction in its size and shape. These changes in the pulp space, clinically referred to as *pulp recession*, can be detected readily on radiographs and are important in determining the form of cavity preparation for certain dental restorative procedures. For example, preparation of the tooth for a full crown in a young patient presents a substantial risk of involving the dental pulp by mechanically exposing a pulp horn. In an older patient the pulp horn has receded and presents less danger. Some evidence suggests that the tubules of secondary dentin sclerose (fill with calcified material) more readily than those of primary dentin. This process tends to reduce the overall permeability of the dentin, thereby protecting the pulp.

TERTIARY DENTIN

Tertiary dentin (also referred to as reactive or reparative dentin) is produced in reaction to various stimuli, such as attrition, caries, or a restorative dental procedure. Unlike primary or secondary dentin that forms along the entire pulp-dentin border, tertiary dentin is produced

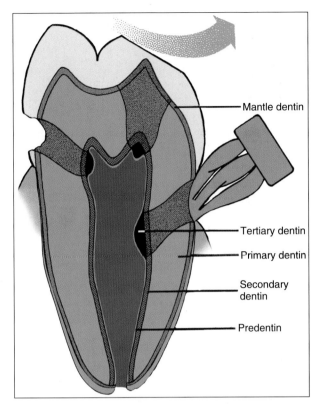

Figure 8-1 Terminology and distribution of dentin.

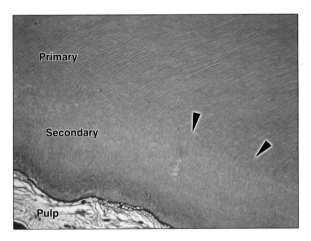

Figure 8-2 Section of dentin. The region where dentinal tubules change direction *(arrowheads)* delimits the junction between primary and secondary dentin.

only by those cells directly affected by the stimulus. The quality (or architecture) and the quantity of tertiary dentin produced are related to the cellular response initiated, which depends on the intensity and duration of the stimulus. Tertiary dentin may have tubules continuous with those of secondary dentin, tubules sparse in number and irregularly arranged, or no tubules at all (Figure 8-3). The cells forming tertiary dentin line its surface or become included in the dentin; the latter case is referred

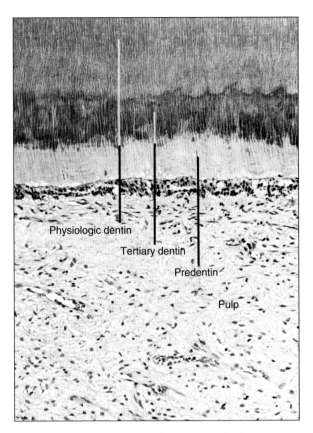

Figure 8-3 Tertiary dentin with a regular tubular pattern and no cellular inclusions. This dentin probably was deposited slowly in response to a mild stimulus.

to as *osteodentin* (Figure 8-4). Tertiary dentin is subclassified as *reactionary* or *reparative dentin*, the former deposited by preexisting odontoblasts and the latter by newly differentiated odontoblast-like cells.

PATTERN OF DENTIN FORMATION

Dentin formation begins at the bell stage of tooth development in the papillary tissue adjacent to the concave tip of the folded inner enamel epithelium (Figure 8-5), the site where cuspal development begins. From that point, dentin formation spreads down the cusp slope as far as the cervical loop of the enamel organ, and the dentin thickens until all the coronal dentin is formed. In multicusped teeth, dentin formation begins independently at the sites of each future cusp tip and again spreads down the flanks of the cusp slopes until fusion with adjacent formative centers occurs. Dentin thus formed constitutes the dentin of the crown of the tooth, or *coronal dentin*.

Root dentin forms at a slightly later stage of development and requires the proliferation of epithelial cells (Hertwig's epithelial root sheath) from the cervical loop of the enamel organ around the growing pulp to initiate

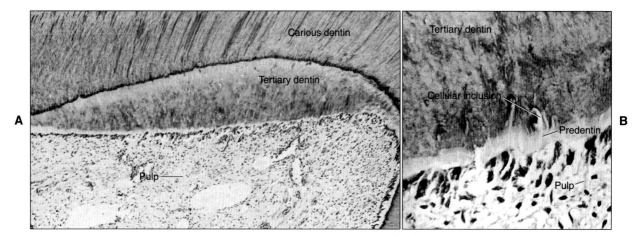

Figure 8-4 **A,** Tertiary (reparative) dentin containing only a few sparse irregular tubules. **B,** At higher magnification, some cellular inclusions can be seen.

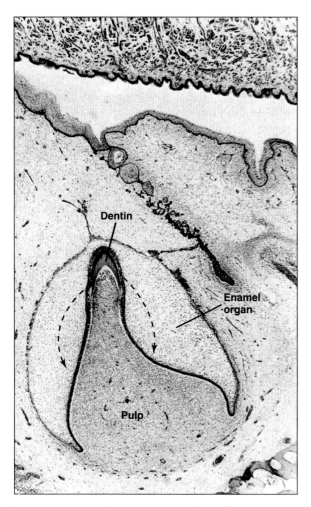

Figure 8-5 Dentin formation during the early bell stage of tooth development. From the apex of the tooth, dentin formation spreads down the slopes of the cusp.

the differentiation of root odontoblasts. The onset of root formation precedes the onset of tooth eruption, and by the time the tooth reaches its functional position, about two thirds of the root dentin will have been formed. Completion of root dentin formation does not occur in the deciduous tooth until about 18 months after it erupts and in the permanent tooth until 2 to 3 years after it erupts. During this period the tooth is said to have an open apex.

Rates of dentin deposition vary not only within a single tooth but also among different teeth. Dentin formation continues throughout the life of the tooth, and its formation results in a gradual but progressive reduction in the size of the pulp cavity.

DENTINOGENESIS

Dentin is formed by cells called *odontoblasts* that differentiate from ectomesenchymal cells of the dental papilla following an organizing influence that emanates from the inner enamel epithelium. Thus the dental papilla is the formative organ of dentin and eventually becomes the pulp of the tooth, a change in terminology generally associated with the moment dentin formation begins.

ODONTOBLAST DIFFERENTIATION

A detailed understanding of how odontoblasts differentiate from ectomesenchymal cells is necessary, not only to understand normal development but also to explain, and eventually be able to influence, their recruitment when required to initiate repair of dentin.

The differentiation of odontoblasts from the dental papilla in normal development is brought about by the expression of signaling molecules and growth factors in the cells of the inner enamel epithelium (see Chapter 5).

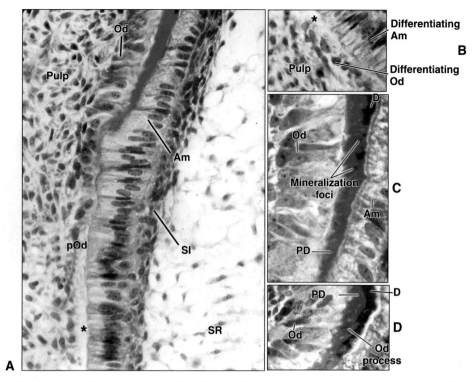

Figure 8-6 Changes in the dental papilla associated with initiation of dentin formation. **A,** An acellular zone *(*)* separates the undifferentiated cells of the dental papilla (preodontoblasts, *pOd*) from the differentiating inner enamel epithelium (ameloblasts, *Am*). **B to D,** Preodontoblasts develop into tall and polarized odontoblasts *(Od)* with the nucleus away from the matrix they deposit at the interface with ameloblasts. The matrix first accumulates as an unmineralized layer, predentin *(PD)*, which gradually mineralizes to form mantle dentin *(D)*. *SI,* Stratum intermedium; *SR,* stellate reticulum.

The dental papilla cells are small and undifferentiated and exhibit a central nucleus and few organelles. At this time they are separated from the inner enamel epithelium by an acellular zone that contains some fine collagen fibrils (Figure 8-6). Almost immediately after cells of the inner enamel epithelium reverse polarity, changes also occur in the adjacent dental papilla. The ectomesenchymal cells adjoining the acellular zone rapidly enlarge and elongate to become preodontoblasts first and then odontoblasts as their cytoplasm increases in volume to contain increasing amounts of protein-synthesizing organelles. The acellular zone between the dental papilla and the inner enamel epithelium gradually is eliminated as the odontoblasts differentiate and increase in size and occupy this zone. These newly differentiated cells are characterized by being highly polarized, with their nuclei positioned away from the inner enamel epithelium.

FORMATION OF MANTLE DENTIN

After the differentiation of odontoblasts (Figure 8-7; see also Figure 8-6), the next step in the production of dentin is formation of its organic matrix. Odontoblasts differentiate in the preexisting ground substance of the dental papilla, and the first dentin collagen synthesized by them is deposited in this ground substance. The first sign of dentin formation is the appearance of distinct, large-diameter collagen fibrils (0.1 to 0.2 μm in diameter) called *von Korff's fibers* (Figures 8-8 to 8-11). These fibers consist of collagen type III associated, at least initially, with fibronectin. These fibers originate deep among the odontoblasts, extend toward the inner enamel epithelium, and fan out in the structureless ground substance immediately below the epithelium. As the odontoblasts continue to increase in size, they also produce smaller collagen type I fibrils that orient themselves parallel to the future dentinoenamel junction (see Figure 8-11). In this way, a layer of mantle predentin appears.

Coincident with this deposition of collagen, the plasma membrane of odontoblasts adjacent to the inner enamel epithelium extends stubby processes into the forming extracellular matrix (Figure 8-12). On occasion one of these processes may penetrate the basal lamina and interpose itself between the cells of the inner enamel epithelium to form what later becomes an *enamel spindle* (see Chapter 7). As the odontoblast forms these

Text continued on p. 201

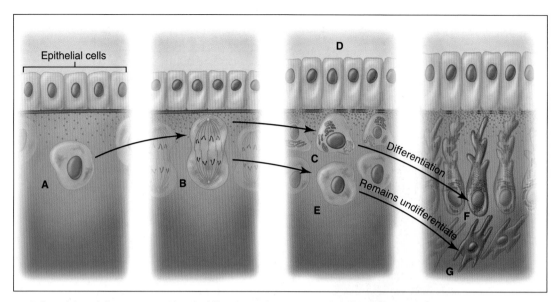

Figure 8-7 Odontoblast differentiation. The undifferentiated ectomesenchymal cell *(A)* of the dental papilla divides *(B)*, with its mitotic spindle perpendicular to the basal lamina *(pink line)*. A daughter cell *(C)*, influenced by the epithelial cells and molecules they produce *(D)*, differentiates into an odontoblast *(F)*. Another daughter cell *(E)*, not exposed to this epithelial influence, persists as a subodontoblast cell *(G)*. This cell has been exposed to all the determinants necessary for odontoblast formation except the last.

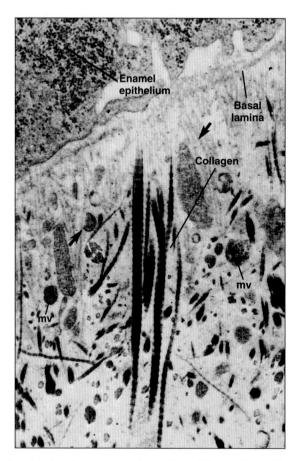

Figure 8-8 Electron micrograph showing the characteristic deposition of first collagen fibers to form coronal mantle predentin. Large-diameter collagen fibers *(Collagen)* intermingle with aperiodic fibrils *(arrows)* associated with the basal lamina supporting the enamel epithelium. *mv,* Matrix vesicle. *(From Ten Cate AR: J Anat 125:183, 1978.)*

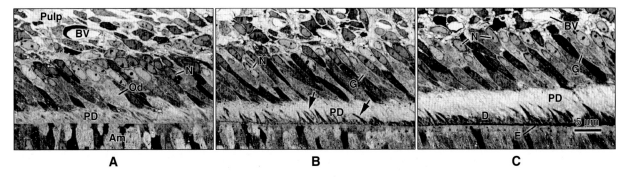

A   **B**   **C**

Figure 8-9 Low-magnification micrographs illustrating the formation of the first layer of (mantle) dentin *(D)* in the rat incisor. **A** to **C,** Differentiated odontoblasts are tall columnar cells tightly grouped in a palisade arrangement. Their nucleus *(N)* is situated basally, the Golgi complex *(G)* occupies much of the supranuclear compartment, and their body is inclined with respect to that of the ameloblasts *(Am)*. **B,** A concentration of large-diameter collagen fibrils *(arrows)* can be seen in the forming predentin *(PD)* matrix near the surface of the ameloblasts. **C,** As this matrix mineralizes, the fibrils become incorporated in the mantle dentin *(D)*. *BV,* Blood vessel; *E,* enamel; *Od,* odontoblasts.

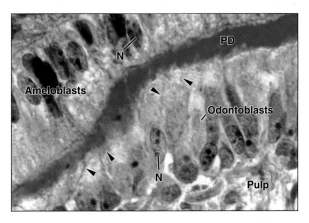

Figure 8-10 Light micrograph of a paraffin section specially stained for collagen. Von Korff's fibers appear as convoluted, threadlike structures *(arrowheads)* that originate deep between odontoblasts.

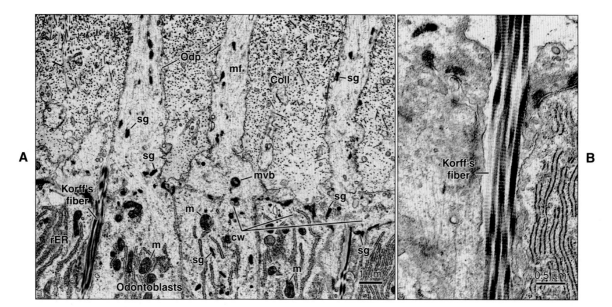

Figure 8-11 Transmission electron microscope images. **A,** The odontoblast process *(Odp)* is the portion of the cell that extends above the cell web *(cw)*. Numerous typical, elongated secretory granules *(sg)*, occasional multivesicular bodies *(mvb)*, and microfilaments *(mf)* are found in the process. The small collagen fibrils *(Coll)* making the bulk of predentin run perpendicularly to the processes and therefore appear as dotlike structures in a plane passing longitudinally along odontoblasts. Bundles of larger-diameter collagen fibrils, von Korff's fibers, run parallel to the odontoblast processes and extend deep between the cell bodies. **B,** At higher magnification, a von Korff's fiber extending between two odontoblasts shows the typical fibrillar collagen periodicity. *m,* Mitochondria; *rER,* rough endoplasmic reticulum.

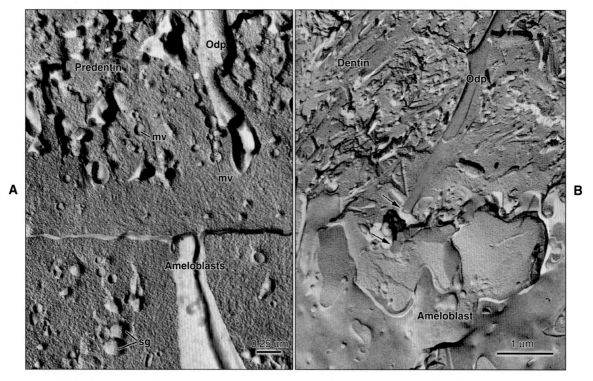

Figure 8-12 Freeze-fracture preparations showing the interface between forming mantle **(A)** predentin and **(B)** dentin and ameloblasts at an early time during tooth formation. **A,** The presence of abundant, well-defined matrix vesicles *(mv)* in the extracellular matrix indicates that mineralization has not yet started. **B,** Odontoblast processes *(Odp)* can establish contact *(arrows)* with ameloblasts, an event believed to be one of the various mechanisms of epithelial-mesenchymal interaction during tooth development. *sg,* Secretory granule.

processes, it also buds off a number of small, membrane-bound vesicles known as *matrix vesicles*, which come to lie superficially near the basal lamina (Figures 8-12, A, and 8-13; see also Figure 8-6, A). The odontoblast then develops a cell process, the *odontoblast process* or *Tomes' fiber*, which is left behind in the forming dentin matrix as the odontoblast moves away toward the pulp (described subsequently). The mineral phase first appears within the matrix vesicles as single crystals believed to be seeded by phospholipids present in the vesicle membrane (see Figure 8-13). These crystals grow

rapidly and rupture from the confines of the vesicle to spread as a cluster of crystallites that fuse with adjacent clusters to form a continuous layer of mineralized matrix (see Topics for Consideration box by Bonucci, Chapter 1). The deposition of mineral lags behind the formation of the organic matrix so that a layer of organic matrix, called *predentin*, always is found between the odontoblasts and the mineralization front. Following mineral seeding, noncollagenous matrix proteins produced by odontoblasts come into play to regulate mineral deposition. In this way coronal mantle dentin is

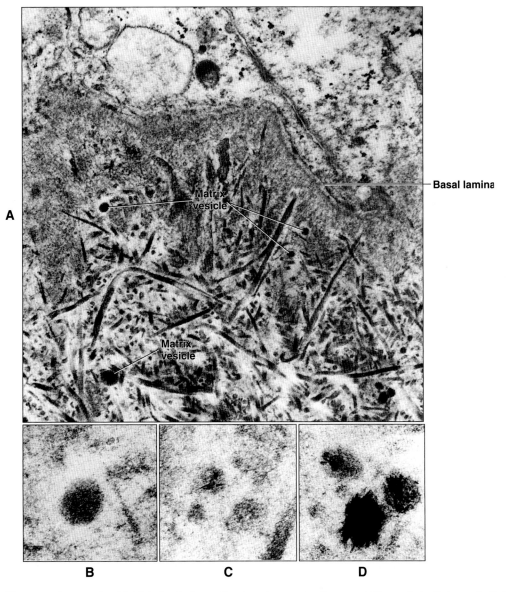

Figure 8-13 Electron micrograph of initial dentin formation in a human tooth germ at the early bell stage. **A,** Collagen fibrils of the first-formed dentin matrix can be seen, along with the basal lamina supporting ameloblasts. Intermingled between the collagen fibrils are matrix vesicles in which initial mineralization of the dentin matrix occurs. **B** to **D** show the occurrence and growth of apatite crystals in these vesicles. *(From Sisca RF, Provenza DV:* Calcif Tissue Res *9:1, 1972.)*

formed in a layer approximately 15 to 20 μm thick onto which then is added the primary (circumpulpal) dentin.

VASCULAR SUPPLY

Chapter 1 stated the requirement for good blood supply during the secretory phase of hard tissue formation. During dentinogenesis, interesting changes have been observed in the rat molar in the distribution and nature of the capillaries associated with the odontoblasts. When mantle dentin formation begins, capillaries are found in the subodontoblast layer, beneath the newly differentiated odontoblast layer. As circumpulpal dentinogenesis is initiated, these capillaries migrate between the odontoblasts, and at the same time their endothelium fenestrates to permit increased exchange. With the completion of dentinogenesis, they retreat from the odontoblast layer, and their endothelial lining once again becomes continuous (Figures 8-14 and 8-15).

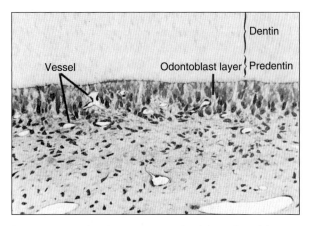

Figure 8-15 Light photomicrograph of the odontoblast layer. This specimen was fixed by perfusion, which forced blood vessels open, thereby better revealing their distribution in the layer.

CONTROL OF MINERALIZATION

Throughout dentinogenesis, mineralization is achieved by continuous deposition of mineral, initially in the matrix vesicle and then at the mineralization front. The question is whether the odontoblast brings about and controls this mineralization. Clearly the cell exerts control in initiating mineralization by producing matrix vesicles and proteins that can regulate mineral deposition and by adapting the organic matrix at the mineralization front so that it receives the mineral deposits.

The problem of how mineral ions reach mineralization sites was reviewed in Chapter 1. In the case of dentinogenesis, some dispute exists because the junctions holding the odontoblasts together in a palisade arrangement are incomplete and thus leaky. Conceptually, simple percolation of tissue fluid supersaturated with calcium and phosphate ions could take place. However, calcium channels of the L type have been demonstrated in the basal plasma membrane of the odontoblast; significantly, when these are blocked, mineralization of the dentin is affected. The presence of alkaline phosphatase activity and calcium adenosinetriphosphatase activity at the distal end of the cell also is consistent with a cellular implication in the transport and release of mineral ions into the forming dentin layer.

PATTERN OF MINERALIZATION

Histologically, two patterns of dentin mineralization can be observed—*globular* and *linear calcification*—that seem to depend on the rate of dentin formation. Globular (or calcospheric) calcification involves the deposition of crystals in several discrete areas of matrix by heterogeneous capture in collagen. With continued crystal growth, globular masses are formed that continue to

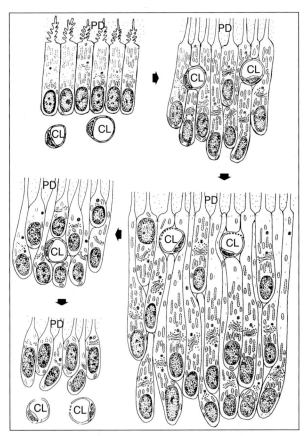

Figure 8-14 The morphologic changes of the peripheral capillaries and odontoblasts in the process of dentinogenesis. *CL,* Capillary; *PD,* predentin. *(From Yoshida S, Ohshima H:* Anat Rec *245:313, 1996.)*

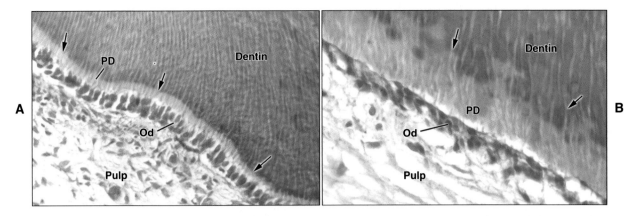

Figure 8-16 Light photomicrographs of the predentin-dentin interface illustrating **(A)** linear and **(B)** globular mineralization fronts *(arrows)*. *Od,* Odontoblasts; *PD,* predentin.

enlarge and eventually fuse to form a single calcified mass. This pattern of mineralization is best seen in the mantle dentin region, where matrix vesicles give rise to mineralization foci that grow and coalesce. In circumpulpal dentin the mineralization front can progress in a globular or linear pattern (Figure 8-16). The size of the globules seems to depend on the rate of dentin deposition, with the largest globules occurring where dentin deposition is fastest. When the rate of formation progresses slowly, the mineralization front appears more uniform and the process is said to be linear.

FORMATION OF ROOT DENTIN

The epithelial cells of Hertwig's root sheath initiate the differentiation of odontoblasts that form root dentin (Figure 8-17). Root dentin forms similarly to coronal dentin, but some differences have been reported. The outermost layer of root dentin, the equivalent of mantle dentin in the crown, shows differences in collagen fiber orientation and organization (Figure 8-18), in part because the collagen fibers from cementum blend with those of dentin (see Chapter 9). Some reports also indicate that the phosphoprotein content of root dentin differs, that it forms at a slower speed, and that its degree of mineralization differs from that of coronal dentin. These possible differences, however, need to be ascertained and simply may reflect the anatomic context of root dentin rather than fundamental differences.

SECONDARY AND TERTIARY DENTINOGENESIS

Secondary dentin is deposited after root formation is completed, is formed by the same odontoblasts that formed primary dentin, and is laid down as a continuation of the primary dentin. As far as is known, secondary dentin

formation is achieved in essentially the same way as primary dentin formation, though at a much slower pace. Secondary dentin can be distinguished histologically from primary dentin by a subtle demarcation line, a slight differential in staining, and a less regular organization of dentinal tubules (see Figure 8-2). Indeed, in some regions tubules may be altogether absent; as the dentin layer becomes thicker, its inner surface is reduced, resulting in the crowding of odontoblasts and the death of some.

Tertiary dentin is deposited at specific sites in response to injury by damaged odontoblasts or replacement cells from pulp. The rate of deposition depends on the degree of injury; the more severe the injury, the more rapid the rate of dentin deposition. As a result of this rapid deposition, cells often become trapped in the newly formed matrix, and the tubular pattern becomes grossly distorted. In addition to its particular structural organization, the composition of tertiary dentin is also distinctive; during its formation, production of collagen, DSP and DMP1 appears to be down-regulated, whereas that of BSP and osteopontin is up-regulated (Figure 8-19).

HISTOLOGY OF DENTIN

When the dentin is viewed microscopically, several structural features can be identified: dentinal tubules, peritubular and intertubular dentin, areas of deficient calcification (called interglobular dentin), incremental growth lines, and an area seen solely in the root portion of the tooth known as the granular layer of Tomes.

DENTINAL TUBULES

Odontoblast processes, similar to osteocyte processes, run in canaliculi that traverse the dentin layer and are

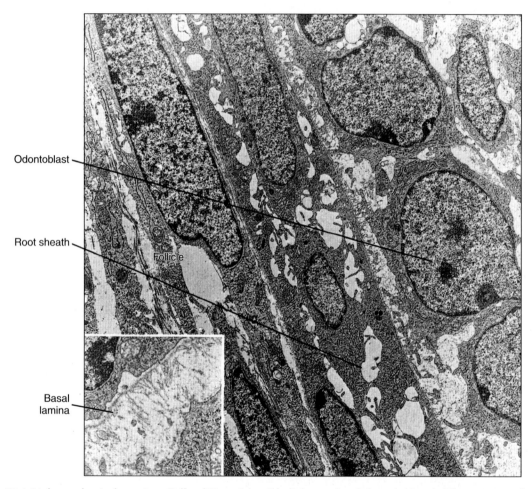

Figure 8-17 Initial root dentin formation. Cells of Hertwig's epithelial root sheath have initiated differentiation of odontoblasts that are about to begin the formation of root dentin. *Inset,* Higher magnification of the milieu in which root dentin matrix will first form. *(From Ten Cate AR:* J Anat *125:183, 1978.)*

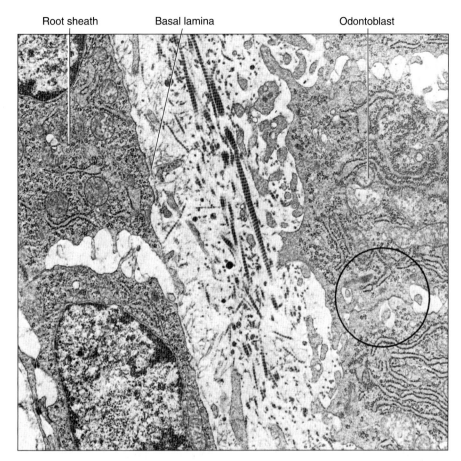

Figure 8-18 Electron micrograph illustrating initial root dentinogenesis. The first collagen fibers of the matrix are aligned parallel to the basal lamina, which supports the root sheath cells and which at this stage is becoming discontinuous. The circled area outlines a junctional complex between two odontoblasts. *(From Ten Cate AR: J Anat 125:183, 1978.)*

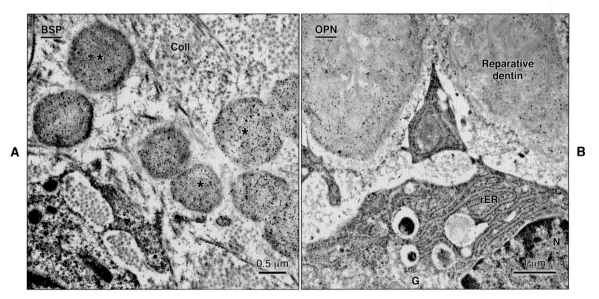

Figure 8-19 As illustrated by these immunogold preparations, reparative dentin is poor in collagen and enriched in noncollagenous matrix proteins, such as bone sialoprotein *(BSP)* and osteopontin *(OPN)*. **A,** In this situation, reparative dentin began formation as globular masses *(*)* among collagen fibrils *(Coll)*. **B,** The globules grew and fused to form larger masses of mineralized matrix. *G,* Golgi complex; *N,* nucleus; *rER,* rough endoplasmic reticulum.

referred to as *dentinal tubules* (Figures 8-20 and 8-21). Dentinal tubules extend through the entire thickness of the dentin from the dentinoenamel junction to the pulp and form a network for the diffusion of nutrients throughout dentin. The configuration of the tubules indicates the course taken by the odontoblasts during dentinogenesis. The tubules follow an S-shaped path from the outer surface of the dentin to the perimeter of the pulp in coronal dentin. This S-shaped curvature is least pronounced beneath the incisal edges and cusps (where the tubules may run an almost straight course; Figure 8-22). These curvatures result from the crowding of and path followed by odontoblasts as they move toward the center of the pulp. Evidence also indicates that some odontoblasts are deleted selectively by apoptosis as they become crowded. In root dentin, little or no crowding results from decrease in surface area, and tubules run a straight course.

The dentinal tubules are tapered structures measuring approximately 2.5 μm in diameter near the pulp, 1.2 μm in the midportion of the dentin, and 900 nm near the dentinoenamel junction. In the coronal parts of young premolar and molar teeth, the numbers of tubules range from 59,000 to 76,000 per square millimeter at the pulpal surface, with approximately half as many per square millimeter near the enamel. This increase per unit volume is associated with crowding of the odontoblasts as the pulp space becomes smaller. A significant reduction in the average density of tubules also occurs in radicular dentin compared with cervical dentin.

Dentinal tubules branch to the extent that dentin is permeated by a profuse anastomosing canalicular system (Figure 8-23). Major branches occur more frequently in root dentin than in coronal dentin (Figure 8-24). The tubular nature of dentin bestows an unusual degree of permeability on this hard tissue that can enhance a

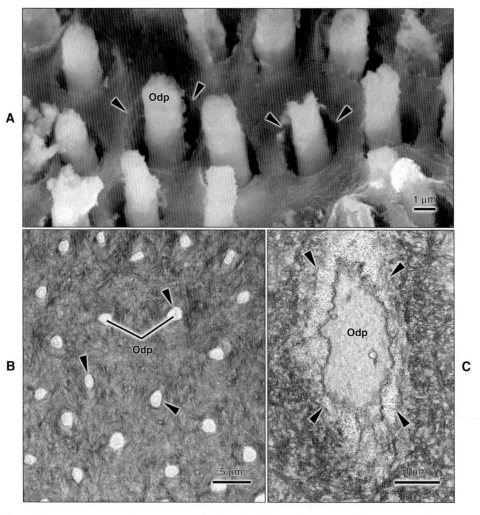

Figure 8-20 Odontoblast processes *(Odp)* run in canaliculi called dentinal tubules *(arrowheads)*. Images from scanning electron microscope **(A)**, light microscope **(B)**, and transmission electron microscope **(C)**.

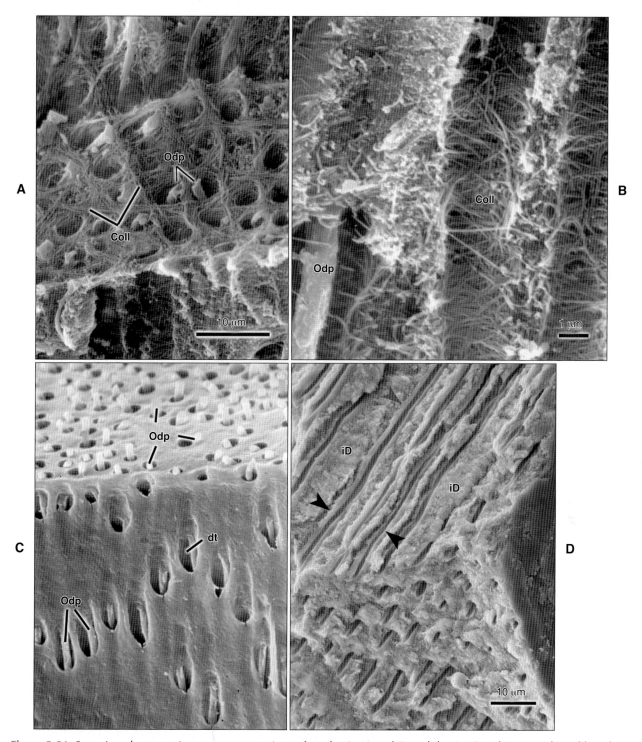

Figure 8-21 Scanning electron microscope preparations of predentin (**A** and **B**) and dentin (**C** and **D**). **A** and **B,** Although no dentinal tubules *(dt)* occur in predentin, each odontoblast process *(Odp)* is surrounded by a meshwork of intertwined collagen fibrils *(Coll)* that outline the future dentinal tubule. As visible in cross-sectional (**A**) and longitudinal (**B**) profile, the fibrils run circumferentially and perpendicular to the process. **C,** In healthy dentin, each tubule is occupied by a process or its ramifications. **D,** The dentinal tubule is delimited by a layer of peritubular dentin *(arrowheads)* that is poor in collagen and more mineralized than the rest of the dentin. The dentin between tubules is referred to as intertubular dentin *(iD)*.

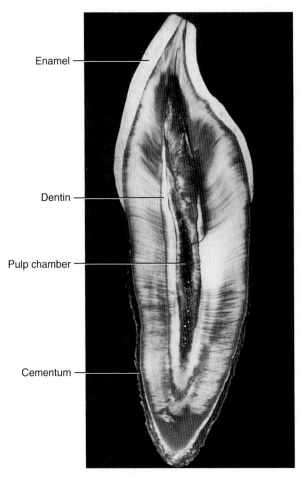

Enamel

Dentin

Pulp chamber

Cementum

Figure 8-22 Ground section showing the S-shaped primary curvature of the dentinal tubules in the crown and their straight course in the root.

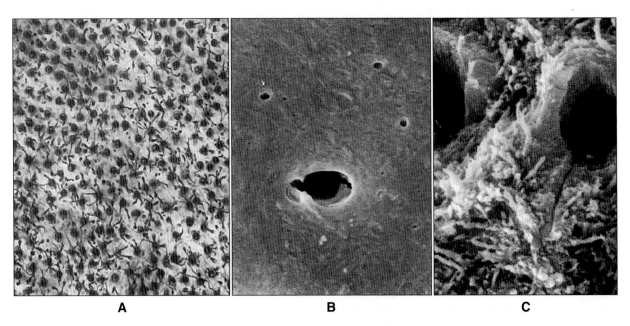

A   **B**   **C**

Figure 8-23 Dentinal tubule branching. **A,** Light microscope cross section of dentin stained with silver nitrate showing the extensive fine branching network of the tubular compartment. **B,** Scanning electron micrograph showing small and larger dentinal tubules that accommodate branches of odontoblast processes of various sizes. **C,** A microbranch extends from a larger dentinal tubule through the peritubular dentin. A thin layer of peritubular dentin also borders the microbranch. (*B and C from Mjor IA, Nordhal I: Arch Oral Biol 41:401, 1996.*)

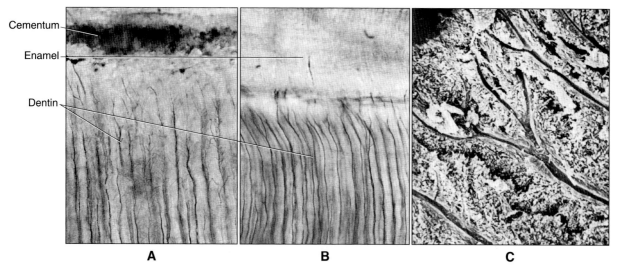

Figure 8-24 Terminal branching of dentinal tubules is more profuse in root dentin (**A**) than in coronal dentin (**B**). **C,** Scanning electron micrograph showing branching.

carious process (Figure 8-25) and accentuate the response of the pulp to dental restorative procedures.

PERITUBULAR DENTIN

Tubules are delimited by a collar of more highly calcified matrix called *peritubular dentin* (see Figure 8-21). The mechanism by which peritubular dentin forms and its precise composition are still not known; peritubular dentin has been shown to be hypermineralized (about 40% more than intertubular dentin) by electron microscopy, electron microprobe analysis, and "soft x-ray" radiographs. Also, peritubular dentin contains little collagen and in rodent teeth appears to be enriched in noncollagenous matrix proteins such as DSP (Figure 8-26) and DMP1. This hypermineralized ring of dentin is readily apparent in human teeth when nondemineralized ground sections cut at right angles to the tubules are examined under the

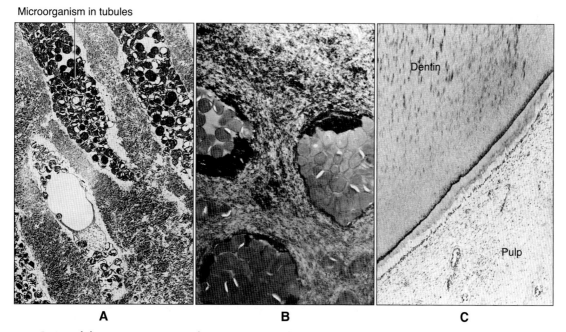

Figure 8-25 Caries of dentin. Transmission electron micrographs showing the natural pathway created for microorganisms by the dentinal tubules in longitudinal section (**A**) and in cross section (**B**). **C,** The microorganisms absorb stain, and in light microscope sections the tubules of carious dentin are seen as dark streaks. (*B courtesy N.W. Johnson.*)

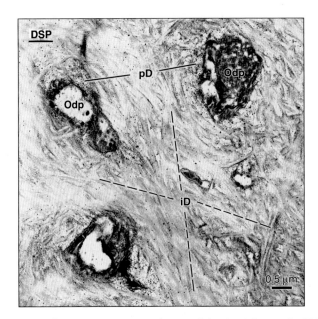

Figure 8-26 Immunogold preparation illustrating an accumulation of dentin sialoprotein *(DSP;* black particles) around odontoblast processes *(Odp)* in certain regions of the rat incisor. Less collagen is present in these areas corresponding to the position of peritubular dentin *(pD)*. The matrix between these areas is the intertubular dentin *(iD)* and constitutes the bulk of the dentin.

light microscope or by scanning electron microscopy (Figure 8-27).

SCLEROTIC DENTIN

Sclerotic dentin describes dentinal tubules that have become occluded with calcified material. When this occurs in several tubules in the same area, the dentin assumes a glassy appearance and becomes translucent (Figure 8-28). The amount of sclerotic dentin increases with age and is most common in the apical third of the root and in the crown midway between the dentinoenamel junction and the surface of the pulp. The occlusion of dentinal tubules with mineral begins in root dentin of 18-year-old

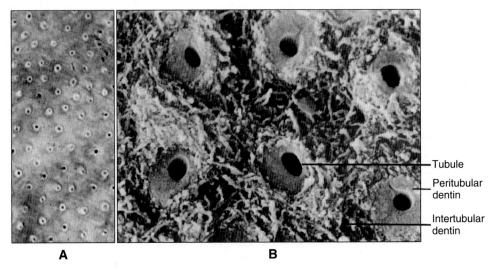

Figure 8-27 Peritubular dentin seen in ground section by **(A)** light microscopy and **(B)** scanning electron microscopy. The dark central spots are empty dentinal tubules surrounded by a well-defined collar of peritubular dentin. *(A from Scott DB, Simmelink JW, Nygaard V: J Dent Res 53:165, 1974.)*

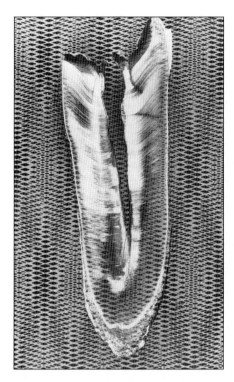

Figure 8-28 Ground section, approximately 100 μm thick, of an old tooth. The section has been placed over a pattern, which can be seen through the apical translucent sclerotic dentin but not through normal dentin.

premolars without any identifiable external influence, hence the assumptions that sclerotic dentin is a physiologic response and that occlusion is achieved by continued deposition of peritubular dentin (Figure 8-29, *A*). However, occlusion of the tubules may occur in several other ways: deposition of mineral within the tubule without any dentin formation (Figure 8-29, *B*), a diffuse mineralization that occurs with a viable odontoblast process still present (Figure 8-29, *C*), and mineralization of the process itself and tubular contents, including intratubular collagen fibrils (Figure 8-29, *D*). Because sclerosis reduces the permeability of dentin, it may help to prolong pulp vitality.

INTERTUBULAR DENTIN

Dentin located between the dentinal tubules is called *intertubular dentin* (see Figures 8-21, *D*, and 8-27). Intertubular dentin represents the primary secretory product of the odontoblasts and consists of a tightly interwoven network of type I collagen fibrils (50 to 200 nm in diameter) in which apatite crystals are deposited. The fibrils are arranged randomly in a plane at roughly right angles to the dentinal tubules. The ground substance consists of noncollagenous proteins proper to calcified tissues and some plasma proteins.

INTERGLOBULAR DENTIN

Interglobular dentin is the term used to describe areas of unmineralized or hypomineralized dentin where globular zones of mineralization (calcospherites) have failed to fuse into a homogeneous mass within mature dentin (Figure 8-30). These areas are especially prevalent in human teeth in which the person has had a deficiency in vitamin D or exposure to high levels of fluoride at the time of dentin formation. Interglobular dentin is seen most frequently in the circumpulpal dentin just below the mantle dentin, where the pattern of mineralization is largely globular. Because this irregularity of dentin is a defect of mineralization and not of matrix formation, the normal architectural pattern of the tubules remains unchanged, and they run uninterrupted through the interglobular areas. However, no peritubular dentin exists where the tubules pass through the unmineralized areas.

INCREMENTAL GROWTH LINES

The organic matrix of primary dentin is deposited incrementally at a daily rate of approximately 4 μm; at the boundary between each daily increment, minute changes in collagen fiber orientation can be demonstrated by means of special staining techniques. Superimposed on this daily increment is a 5-day cycle in which the changes in collagen fiber orientation are more exaggerated. These *incremental lines* run at right angles to the dentinal tubules and generally mark the normal rhythmic, linear pattern of dentin deposition in an inward and rootward direction (Figure 8-31). The 5-day increment can be seen readily in conventional and ground sections as the *incremental lines of von Ebner* (situated about 20 μm apart). Close examination of globular mineralization shows that the rate in organic matrix is approximately 2 μm every 12 hours. Thus the organic matrix of dentin is deposited rhythmically at a daily rate of about 4 μm a day and is mineralized in a 12-hour cycle. As mentioned before, the rate of deposition of secondary dentin is slower and asymmetrical.

Another type of incremental pattern found in dentin is the *contour lines of Owen*. Some confusion exists about the exact connotation of this term. As originally described by Owen, the contour lines result from a coincidence of the secondary curvatures between neighboring dentinal tubules. Other lines, however, having the same disposition but caused by accentuated deficiencies in mineralization, now are known more generally as contour lines of Owen. These are recognized easily in longitudinal ground sections. An exceptionally wide contour line is the neonatal line found in those teeth mineralizing at birth and reflects the disturbance in mineralization created by the physiologic trauma of birth. Periods of illness or inadequate nutrition

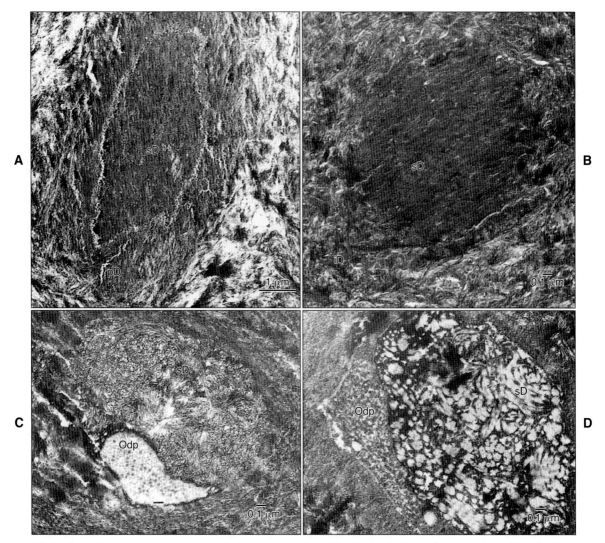

Figure 8-29 Sclerosis of the dentinal tubule, which occurs in different ways. **A,** The tubule is filled with an even deposition of mineral, which has been interpreted as a spread of peritubular dentin. However, at **B,** tubular occlusion has occurred in a similar way, although no peritubular dentin is recognizable. At **C,** diffuse mineralization is occurring in the presence of a viable odontoblast process *(Odp)*. At **D,** mineralization occurs within the odontoblast process and around collagen fibrils deposited within the tubule as a reactionary response. *iD,* Intertubular dentin; *pD,* peritubular dentin; *sD,* sclerotic dentin. (***A** and **D** from Tsatsas BG, Frank RM:* Calcif Tissue Res *9:238, 1972;* **B** *from Frank RM, Nalbandian H:* Handbook of microscopic anatomy, *vol 6,* Teeth, *New York, 1989, Springer Verlag;* **C** *from Frank RM, Voegel JC:* Caries Res *14:367, 1980.)*

also are marked by accentuated contour lines within the dentin.

GRANULAR LAYER OF TOMES

When root dentin is viewed under transmitted light in ground sections (and only in ground sections), a granular-appearing area, the *granular layer of Tomes,* can be seen just below the surface of the dentin where the root is covered by cementum (Figures 8-32 and 8-33). A progressive increase in so-called granules occurs from the cementoenamel junction to the apex of the tooth.

A number of interpretations have been proposed for these structures. This granular appearance was once thought to be associated with minute hypomineralized areas of interglobular dentin. They also were proposed to be true spaces; however, these cannot be seen in hematoxylin-eosin–stained sections or on electron micrographs. Finally, the spaces have been suggested to represent sections made through the looped terminal portions of dentinal tubules found only in root dentin and seen only because of light refraction in thick ground sections. More recent interpretation relates this layer to a special arrangement of collagen and noncollagenous

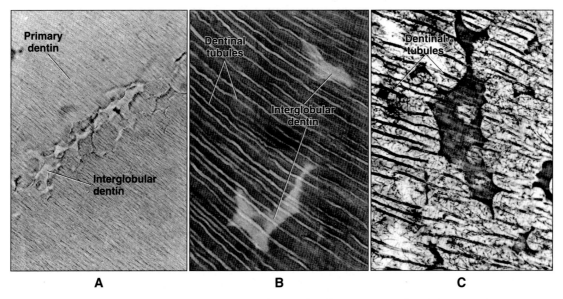

A   B   C

Figure 8-30 Interglobular dentin. **A,** Ground section. **B,** Demineralized section stained with hematoxylin-eosin. **C,** Demineralized section stained with silver nitrate. The spherical borders of the interglobular areas indicate the failure of calcospherite fusion. In **B** the staining of nonmineralized matrix is lighter and in **C** is darker. Dentinal tubules pass through the interglobular dentin, but no peritubular dentin is present in these areas. Silver nitrate staining reveals numerous smaller tubules into which run the branches of the odontoblast process. (**C** *courtesy Dr. Alexanian.*)

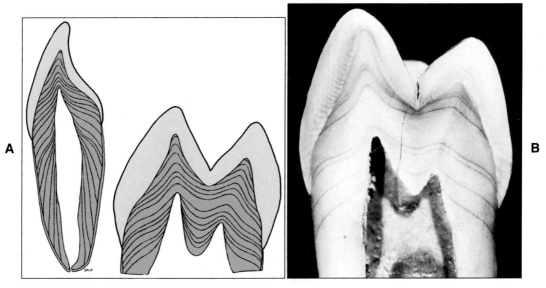

A   B

Figure 8-31 **A,** Pattern of incremental line deposition in dentin. **B,** Tooth section of a person who received tetracycline intermittently. The drug has been incorporated at successive dentin-forming fronts, mimicking incremental line patterns. (**A** *from Kawasaki K:* J Anat *119:61, 1975.*)

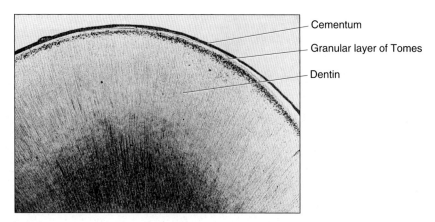

Figure 8-32 Ground section across the root of a tooth. The granular layer of Tomes is visible just beneath the cementum.

matrix proteins at the interface between dentin and cementum (see Chapter 9).

PULP

The dental pulp is the soft connective tissue that supports the dentin. When its histologic appearance is examined, four distinct zones can be distinguished: (1) the *odontoblastic zone* at the pulp periphery; (2) a *cell-free zone of Weil* beneath the odontoblasts, which is prominent in the coronal pulp; (3) a *cell-rich zone*, where cell density is high, which again is seen easily in coronal pulp adjacent to the cell-free zone; and (4) the *pulp core*, which is characterized by the major vessels and nerves of the pulp (Figures 8-34 and 8-35). The principal cells of

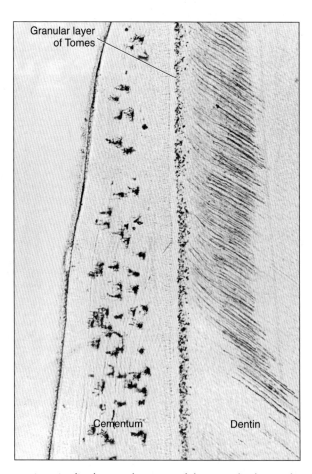

Figure 8-33 Longitudinal ground section of the granular layer of Tomes.

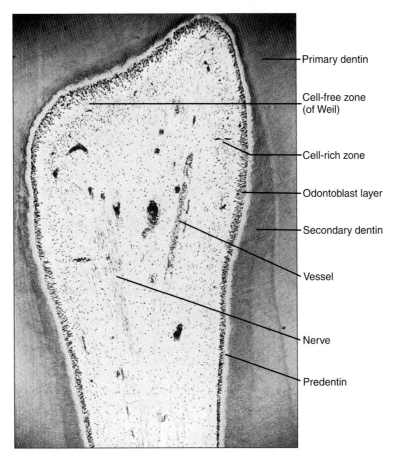

Figure 8-34 Low-power photomicrograph of the dentin-pulp complex of a premolar tooth. Primary and secondary dentin are present in this tooth. The amount of secondary dentin deposition varies, more having occurred on the right than on the left. The cell-free zone (of Weil) beneath the odontoblast layer is clearly visible, as is the cell-rich zone.

the pulp are the odontoblasts, fibroblasts, undifferentiated ectomesenchymal cells, macrophages, and other immunocompetent cells. Interestingly, the tooth pulp has been shown to be a convenient source of multipotent stem cells.

ODONTOBLASTS

The most distinctive cells of the dental pulp, and therefore the most easily recognized, are the odontoblasts. Odontoblasts form a layer lining the periphery of the pulp and have a process extending into the dentin (Figure 8-36, A). In the crown of the mature tooth, odontoblasts often appear to be arranged in a palisade pattern some three to five cells deep. This appearance is an artifact caused by crowding of the odontoblasts as they migrate centripetally and also by a tangential plane of section. The number of odontoblasts corresponds to the number of dentinal tubules and, as mentioned previously, varies with tooth type and location within the pulp space. Although actual cell counts have not been made, the number of dentinal tubules present at the pulp-dentin interface, and therefore the number of odontoblasts, has been estimated in the range of 59,000 to 76,000 per square millimeter in coronal dentin, with a lesser number in root dentin. The odontoblasts in the crown are also larger than odontoblasts in the root. In the crown of the fully developed tooth, the cell bodies of odontoblasts are columnar and measure approximately 50 μm in height, whereas in the midportion of the pulp they are more cuboid and in the apical part more flattened.

The morphology of odontoblasts reflects their functional activity and ranges from an active synthetic phase to a quiescent phase (Figure 8-37). By light microscopy, an active cell appears elongated and can be seen to possess a basal nucleus, much basophilic cytoplasm, and a prominent Golgi zone. A resting cell, by contrast, is stubby, with little cytoplasm, and has a more hematoxophilic nucleus. By electron microscopy, another stage in the life cycle of odontoblasts can be discerned. In addition to the secretory and resting (or aged) states recognizable by light microscopy, defining a transitional stage intermediate between the secretory and resting states also is possible.

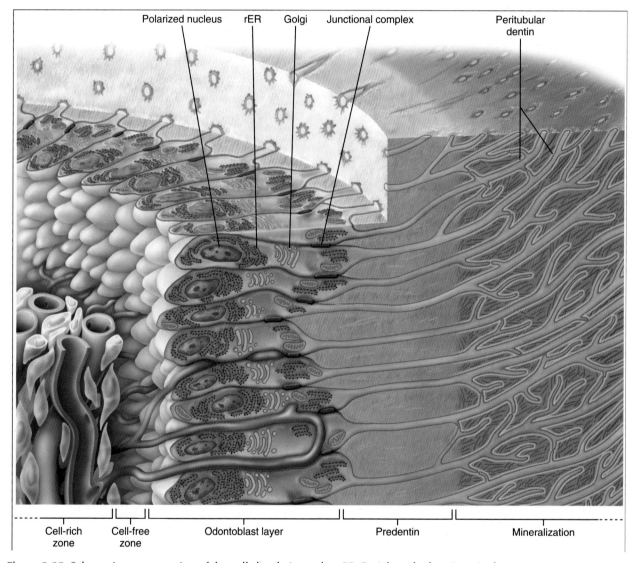

Figure 8-35 Schematic representation of the cells bordering pulp. *rER,* Rough endoplasmic reticulum.

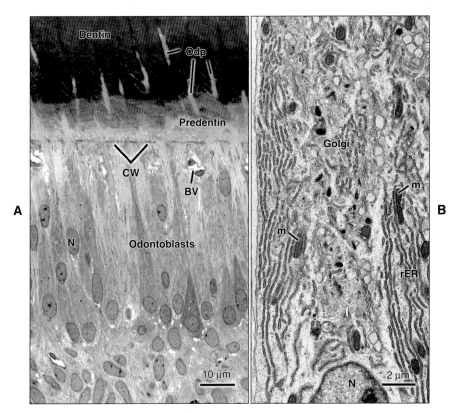

Figure 8-36 A, Low-magnification view of odontoblasts taken by examining the section in the scanning electron microscope. These tall, bowling pin-shaped cells border the pulp and form a tight layer against predentin. Despite the presence of nuclei *(N)* at different levels, there is only one layer of odontoblasts that extend cell processes *(Odp)* across predentin into dentin. Blood vessels *(BV)* are present among the cells. **B,** Transmission electron micrograph; a large portion of the supranuclear compartment of odontoblasts is occupied by an extensive Golgi complex *(Golgi)* surrounded by abundant rough endoplasmic reticulum *(rER)* profiles. *cw,* Cell web; *m,* mitochondria.

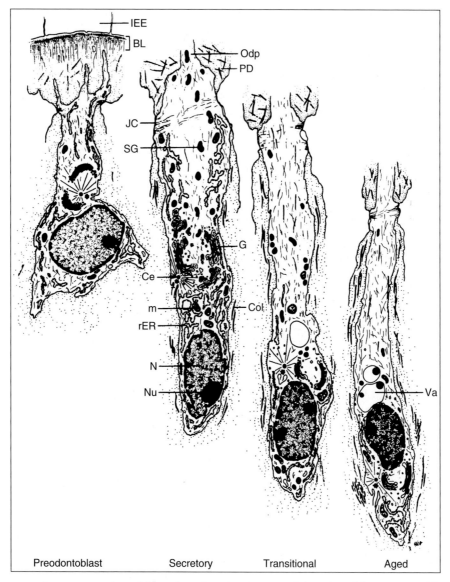

Figure 8-37 Diagrammatic representation of the various functional stages of the odontoblast. *BL*, Basal lamina; *Ce*, centriole; *Col*, collagen; *G*, Golgi complex; *IEE*, inner enamel epithelium; *JC*, junctional complex; *m*, mitochondria; *N*, nucleus; *Nu*, nucleolus; *Odp*, odontoblast process; *PD*, predentin; *rER*, rough endoplasmic reticulum; *SG*, secretory granule; *Va*, vacuole. (*From Couve E:* Arch Oral Biol *31:643, 1986.*)

The organelles of an active odontoblast are prominent, consisting of numerous vesicles, much endoplasmic reticulum, a well-developed Golgi complex located on the dentinal side of the nucleus, and numerous mitochondria scattered throughout the cell body (Figures 8-38 and 8-39; see also Figure 8-36, *B*). The nucleus contains an abundance of peripherally dispersed chromatin and several nucleoli. The pathway for collagen synthesis within the odontoblast and its intracellular and extracellular assembly is similar to that described in the fibroblast (summarized in Figure 4-12). The spherical distentions contain free polypeptides that assemble as a triple helix in the cylindrical distentions to form the procollagen molecule (Figure 8-40; see also Figure 8-39, *B*). The cylindrical distentions bud off as secretory granules that exhibit a characteristic elongated shape and electron density. The secretory granules then are transported toward the odontoblast process, where their content is released (Figure 8-41, *A*). Debate continues as to whether the noncollagenous matrix proteins produced by odontoblasts are packaged within the same secretory granule with collagen or in a distinct granule population. Indeed, immunolabeling for bone sialoprotein and osteocalcin can be found in round granules (Figure 8-42), whereas their presence in the elongated, collagen-containing

ones has not yet been demonstrated. Other membrane-bound granules, similar in appearance to lysosomes, are present in the cytoplasm, as are numerous filaments and microtubules. Decreasing amounts of intracellular organelles reflect decreased functional activity of the odontoblast. Thus the transitional odontoblast is a narrower cell, with its nucleus displaced from the basal extremity and exhibiting condensed chromatin. The amount of endoplasmic reticulum is reduced, and autophagic vacuoles are present and are associated with the reorganization of cytoplasm. Resting, or aged, odontoblasts are smaller cells crowded together. The nucleus of such a cell is situated more apically, creating a prominent infranuclear region in which fewer cytoplasmic organelles are clustered. The supranuclear region is devoid of organelles, except for large, lipid-filled vacuoles in a cytoplasm containing tubular and filamentous structures. Secretory granules are scarce or even absent.

The odontoblast process begins at the neck of the cells just above the apical junctional complex where the cell gradually begins to narrow as it enters predentin (Figure 8-43; see also Figures 8-11, *A*; 8-36, *A*; 8-41, *A*; and 8-42). A major change in the cytologic condition of odontoblasts occurs at the junction between the cell

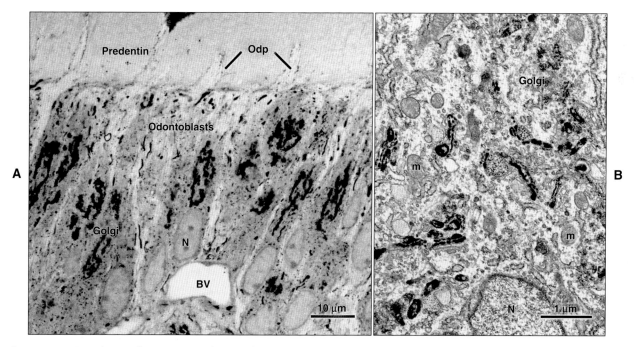

Figure 8-38 Cytochemical preparations for a Golgi-associated phosphatase visualized using scanning (**A**) and transmission (**B**) electron microscopes, illustrating the position and extent of this protein-synthesizing organelle in the supranuclear compartment. Reaction product is found selectively in the intermediate saccules of the Golgi complex. *BV*, Blood vessel; *m*, mitochondria; *N*, nucleus; *Odp*, odontoblast process.

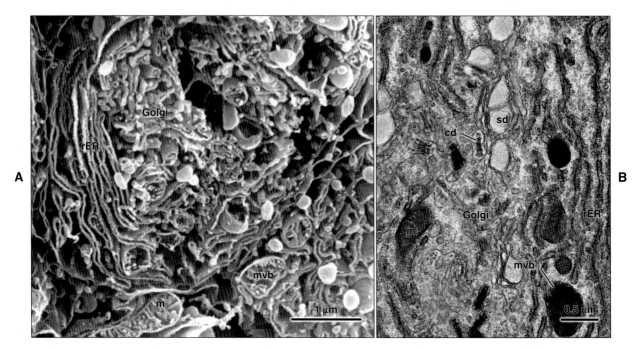

Figure 8-39 **A,** Scanning electron micrograph of a cross-fractured odontoblast at the level of the Golgi complex *(Golgi)*. Rough endoplasmic reticulum *(rER)* surrounds the Golgi complex. **B,** Transmission electron micrograph; Golgi saccules exhibit cylindrical *(cd)* and spherical *(sd)* distentions in which the collagen molecule is assembled. *m,* Mitochondria; *mvb,* multivesicular body.

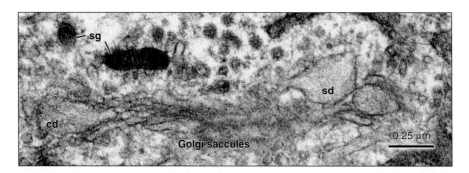

Figure 8-40 Transmission electron micrograph of a Golgi stack. Cylindrical *(cd)* and spherical *(sd)* distentions can be seen at the extremities of the saccules. The procollagen molecule is assembled in the cylindrical distention that, when mature, buds off as atypical elongated and electron-dense collagen-containing secretory granule *(sg)*.

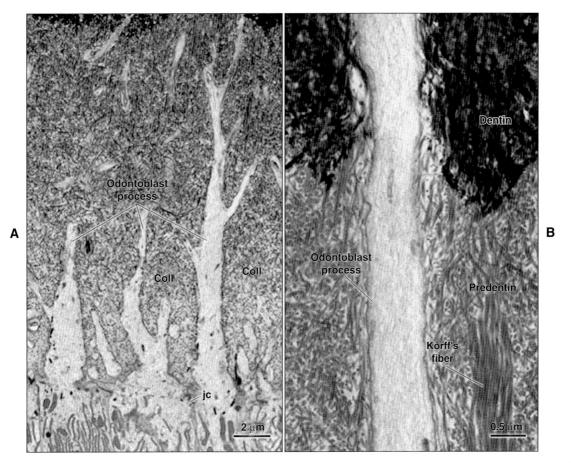

Figure 8-41 Electron micrographs of the odontoblast process. **A,** The process is an arborizing cell extension that extends above the apical junctional complex *(jc)* into predentin and dentin. Numerous collagen-containing secretory granules are found in the process, particularly near its base where the surrounding collagen fibrils *(Coll)* are packed less densely. The fibrils become thicker and more compact toward the dentin. **B,** A process at the predentin-dentin junction. A bundle of larger collagen fibrils, von Korff's fibers, runs parallel to the process. Note the paucity of elongated, collagen-containing secretory granules at this level.

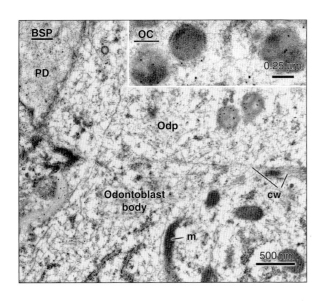

Figure 8-42 Immunogold preparations for bone sialoprotein *(BSP)* and osteocalcin *(OC, inset)*. Round granules are immunoreactive *(black dots)* for these two matrix proteins, suggesting that a secretory granule population may exist, distinct from the elongated collagen-containing ones, that may be responsible for the transport and secretion of noncollagenous dentin matrix proteins. A cell web *(cw)* is associated with the apical junctions and separates the odontoblast body from the process *(Odp)*. *m,* Mitochondria; *PD,* predentin.

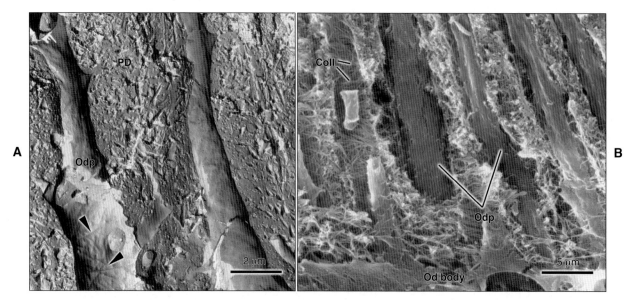

Figure 8-43 Freeze-fracture **(A)** and scanning electron microscope **(B)** preparations illustrating the odontoblast process *(Odp)* near its point of emergence from the cell body. The process is surrounded by the collagen fibrils *(Coll)* of predentin *(PD)*. The fibrils are associated intimately with the process, and in certain areas they imprint the membrane *(arrowheads)*. *Od*, Odontoblast.

body and the process. The process is devoid of major organelles but does display an abundance of microtubules and filaments arranged in a linear pattern along its length (see Figure 8-11, A). Coated vesicles and pits that reflect pinocytotic activity along the process membrane also are present (Figure 8-44).

Junctions occur between adjacent odontoblasts involving gap junctions, occluding zones (tight junctions), and desmosomes. Distally, where the cell body becomes process, the junctions take the form of a junctional complex (see Figure 8-41, A) consisting mostly of adherent junctions interspersed with areas of tight junctions.

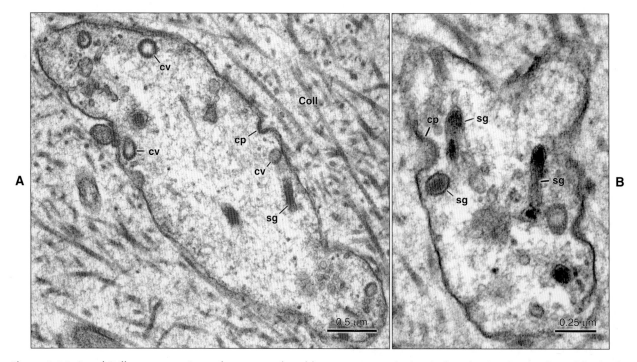

Figure 8-44 **A** and **B** illustrate two views of cross-cut odontoblast processes at the level of predentin, close to the cell body. The processes are surrounded by collagen fibrils *(Coll)* and contain elongated and round secretory granules *(sg)*, coated pits *(cp)*, and vesicles *(cv)* suggestive of intense pinocytotic activity along the cell membrane. **B** is at a higher magnification than **A.**

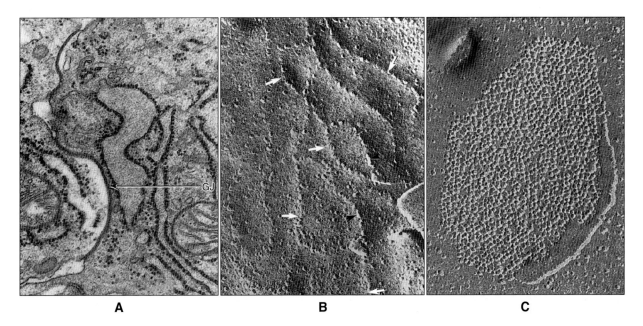

Figure 8-45 Junctions between odontoblasts. **A,** Electron micrograph showing a gap junction *(GJ)*. **B,** Freeze fracture of a tight junction consisting of extensive and branched rows of zipperlike particles *(arrows)*. **C,** Freeze fracture of a gap junction. (**A** and **C** courtesy M. Weinstock; **B** from Arana-Chavez VE, Katchburian E: Anat Rec 248:332, 1997.)

The actin filaments inserting into the adherent junction are prominent and form a *terminal cell web* (see Figures 8-11, A; 8-36, A; and 8-41, A). This junctional complex does not form a zonula, completely encircling the cell, as occurs in epithelia; it is focal, and there is some debate whether it can restrict the passage of molecules and ions from the pulp into the dentin layer. For instance, some molecular tracers have been shown to reach the predentin via the interodontoblastic space, but others are unable to do so. Serum proteins seem to pass freely between odontoblasts and are found in dentin.

Gap junctions occur frequently on the lateral surfaces of odontoblasts and also are found at the base of the cell, where junctions are established with pulpal fibroblasts. The number and location of gap junctions are variable, however, in that they can form, dissolve, and reform rapidly as function dictates (Figure 8-45).

The life span of the odontoblasts generally is believed to equal that of the viable tooth because the odontoblasts are end cells, which means that, once differentiated, they cannot undergo further cell division. This fact poses an interesting problem. On occasion, when the pulp tissue is exposed, repair can take place by the formation of new dentin. This means that new odontoblasts must have differentiated and migrated to the exposure site from pulp tissue, most likely from the cell-rich subodontoblast zone. The differentiation of odontoblasts during tooth development requires a cascade of determinants, including cells of the inner enamel epithelium or Hertwig's root sheath. Epithelial cells, however, are no longer present in the developed tooth, and the stimulus for differentiation of new odontoblasts under these circumstances is thus different and not yet understood.

TOPICS FOR CONSIDERATION   Dentin-Pulp: A Biologic Basis to Restorative Dentistry

The vitality of the dentin-pulp complex plays an important role in the maintenance of a functional dentition. Clinical restorative procedures have long recognized the importance of maintaining tooth vitality while focusing particularly on the cells of the dental pulp. The unique environment of the dental pulp has required special attention to the effects of injury arising from dental caries and other trauma and, especially, the fine balance between the beneficial and harmful effects of inflammatory processes.

The complex events following injury to the dentin-pulp complex are important determinants of the opportunities for regeneration and repair of these tissues. With milder injury, affected odontoblasts may survive

Continued

and be up-regulated to secrete a reactionary type of tertiary dentin at the pulp-dentin interface, thereby increasing the barrier between the injury and the cells of the pulp. Injury of greater intensity can lead to local odontoblast death and if suitable conditions prevail, a new generation of odontoblast-like cells may differentiate and secrete a reparative type of tertiary dentin, thus restoring some of the structural integrity of the tissue. Reparative dentinogenesis provides the basis of dentin bridge formation after pulpal exposure and can be instrumental in maintenance of vitality and tooth survival after more extensive dental injury. The induction of dentin bridge formation during pulp capping highlights the pioneering position of dentistry in regenerative medicine, although until recently the mechanisms responsible for the action of pulp capping agents such as calcium hydroxide have been somewhat empirical.

The mechanisms responsible for reactionary and reparative dentinogenesis have largely remained elusive, and yet these processes offer exciting opportunities for tooth regeneration and tissue engineering. The events of tissue regeneration and repair often recapitulate embryonic development in many organs. Growth factors, especially transforming growth factor βs and bone metalloproteinases morphogenetic proteins, appear to be key signaling molecules in tooth development leading to odontoblast and ameloblast differentiation, and their temporospatial expression in the tooth germ provides precise regulation of events. Expression of members of the transforming growth factor β family and other growth factors by odontoblasts after their differentiation leads to secretion of these molecules into dentin matrix where they become sequestrated through interactions with extracellular matrix components. This provides a new view of dentin matrix, which traditionally has been regarded as a rather inert material. However, the presence of these and other molecules in dentin matrix highlights the bioactive properties of the matrix. Importantly, these bioactive molecules may be released from the dentin matrix in some situations, allowing them to participate in signaling of behavior of odontoblasts and other pulp cells and thus providing an understanding of how reactionary and reparative dentinogenesis may take place. Acid demineralization of the dentin matrix during dental caries may release and expose these bioactive molecules. In addition, treatment of cavities with etchants before restoration also may lead to their release. The tubular structure of dentin allows ready passage of these molecules to interact with receptors on pulp cells during carious demineralization of the tissue. Interestingly, calcium hydroxide recently has been shown to solubilize growth factors from dentin matrix and to influence pulp gene expression,[1] thus providing a possible explanation for the biologic action of this agent in stimulating dentin bridge formation and tissue regeneration.

Although these findings provide a basis for understanding regeneration and repair in the dentin-pulp complex, a number of questions still remain. A key question regards the identity of the progenitor cells giving rise to odontoblast-like cells during reparative dentinogenesis. Various cells, including the subodontoblast cells of the cell-rich layer, undifferentiated mesenchymal cells in the pulp core, fibroblasts, and pericytes, have been suggested as candidates. The cells of the cell-rich layer seem likely candidates because they experience a similar developmental history to odontoblasts except for the final inductive signal for differentiation. Specific dental stem cell populations also have been suggested recently. However, a variety of cell types may participate in dentin regeneration, and their different phenotypes may contribute to the heterogeneity in the structure of the tissues secreted. This emphasizes how regeneration may represent a variety of responses and how the resulting tissues secreted may range from a rather bonelike, atubular mineralized matrix to a tubular matrix resembling physiologic primary dentin. The diversity of tissue structure is also important when we consider sources of stem/progenitor cells for tissue engineering and regeneration applications. Although it has been suggested that these cells might be sourced from exfoliated deciduous teeth[2] and maintained in a tissue bank, questions still remain about their potentiality after expansion and long-term storage. Other noninvasive approaches to sourcing such cells with dentinogenic potential may need to be identified. Discrimination between regeneration and true repair of dentin may be important; the latter implies the need for a more accurate blueprint of normal dentinogenesis, whereby all aspects of the process may be reproduced faithfully for secretion of physiologic-like tubular dentin. The same requirements also may exist for development of tissue engineering approaches in which artificial scaffolds may be used to "build up" the tissue and will need to consider how the nature and architecture of scaffolds influence tissue structure. Controversy exists, however, as to the nature of the matrix that the cells should be "encouraged" to secrete during regeneration and repair. Secretion of an atubular, impermeable bonelike material during regeneration has been suggested as most appropriate because it could avoid some of the tissue permeability problems associated with use of restorative procedures. In contrast, it has been argued that dentin has evolved

TOPICS FOR CONSIDERATION	Dentin-Pulp: A Biologic Basis to Restorative Dentistry—cont'd

to an exquisite level of complexity in its structure, which provides a tubular matrix capable of physiologic function within a demanding and changing environment. The answer to this question may lie in perception of the role of restorative dentistry—simple restoration of structural integrity or restoration of normal physiologic structure to the tissue. Despite such questions, biologic approaches to restorative dentistry offer exciting opportunities to radically change clinical practice in the future. An important challenge with such approaches, however, will be how to control them. Uncontrolled dentin regeneration ultimately will lead to occlusion of the pulp chamber and loss of tooth vitality. Practitioners therefore need to learn how to regulate cellular behavior closely during dentin regeneration and perhaps should look to the regulation of physiologic primary dentinogenesis for answers to this question. Although only limited understanding of the biologic mechanisms responsible for control of odontoblast secretion currently exists, the very close temporospatial regulation of primary dentinogenesis is known to result in a remarkable degree of reproducibility in tooth form and shape. Thus

developing an understanding of the blueprint for physiologic dentinogenesis holds the key for a new biologic era in restorative dentistry.

REFERENCES
1. Graham L, Cooper PR, Cassidy N et al: The effect of calcium hydroxide on solubilisation of bio-active dentine matrix components, *Biomaterials* 27:2865, 2006.
2. Miura M, Gronthos S, Zhao M et al: SHED: stem cells from human exfoliated deciduous teeth, *Proc Natl Acad Sci U S A* 100:5807-5812, 2003.

BIBLIOGRAPHY
Smith AJ: Pulp responses to caries and dental repair, *Caries Res* 36:223, 2002.
Smith AJ, Lesot H: Induction and regulation of crown dentinogenesis: embryonic events as a template for dental tissue repair, *Crit Rev Oral Biol Med* 12:425, 2001.
Tziafas D, Smith AJ, Lesot H: Designing new treatment strategies in vital pulp therapy, *J Dent* 28:77, 2000.

Anthony (Tony) J. Smith, PhD
Unit of Oral Biology
School of Dentistry
University of Birmingham
Birmingham, United Kingdom

The dentinal tubule and its contents bestow on dentin its vitality and ability to respond to various stimuli. The *tubular compartment* therefore assumes significance in any analysis of dentinal response to clinical procedures, such as cavity preparation or the bonding of materials to dentin. The account given so far of the tubule and the odontoblast process has been fairly uncontroversial to help the beginning student understand dentin structure and gain the necessary vocabulary. The student should know that dentin is tubular, that each tubule is (or was once) occupied by an odontoblast process, that the tubule is delimited by a layer of peritubular dentin, and that fluid circulates between dentin and the process. This explanation is simplistic, however, and a number of debatable issues require amplification, especially because the dentin-pulp complex is so crucial to the everyday practice of dentistry. Perhaps the most important issue is the extent of the odontoblast process within the dentinal tubule. Using labeled antibodies against proteins making up the cytoskeleton (actin, vimentin, and tubulin), researchers have shown that the majority of dentinal tubules exhibit these components along their entire extent, up to the dentinoenamel junction. Because these proteins are exclusively intracellular, the presence of a process can be inferred.

Another question concerns the contents of the space between the odontoblast process and the tubule wall, the so-called dentinal fluid. The assumption has been made that the space is filled with fluid (equivalent to tissue fluid), but this is difficult to prove because the demonstration of fluid is achieved only after cavity preparation, which involves tissue damage and the production of exudate containing plasma protein and fibrinogen. What information exists concerning tubule content indicates that proteoglycans, tenascin, fibronectin, the serum proteins albumin, α_2-HS glycoprotein, and transferrin (in ratios differing from those found in serum) may be present, clearly a complex mixture about which much more needs to be learned.

FIBROBLASTS

The cells occurring in greatest numbers in the pulp are fibroblasts (Figures 8-46 and 8-47). Fibroblasts are particularly numerous in the coronal portion of the pulp, where they form the cell-rich zone. The function of fibroblasts is to form and maintain the pulp matrix, which consists of collagen and ground substance. The histologic appearance of these fibroblasts reflects their functional state. In young pulps the fibroblasts are actively synthesizing matrix and therefore have a plump cytoplasm and extensive amounts of all the usual organelles associated with synthesis and secretion. With age the need for synthesis diminishes and the

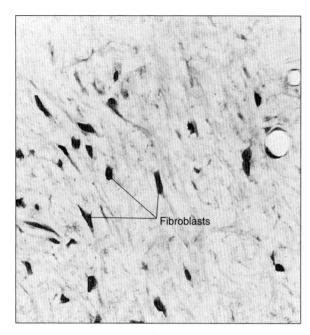

Figure 8-46 Light microscopic appearance of fibroblasts in the dental pulp.

fibroblasts appear as flattened spindle-shaped cells with dense nuclei. Fibroblasts of the pulp also have the capability of ingesting and degrading collagen when appropriately stimulated (see Chapter 4). Apoptotic cell death (see Chapter 7) of pulpal fibroblasts, especially in the cell-rich zone, indicates that some turnover of these cells is occurring. The fine structure of a young pulp is shown in Figure 8-47. Desmosomes are often present between these cells.

UNDIFFERENTIATED ECTOMESENCHYMAL CELLS

Undifferentiated mesenchymal cells represent the pool from which connective tissue cells of the pulp are derived. Depending on the stimulus, these cells may give rise to odontoblasts and fibroblasts. These cells are found throughout the cell-rich area and the pulp core and often are related to blood vessels. Under the light microscope, undifferentiated mesenchymal cells appear as large polyhedral cells possessing a large, lightly stained, centrally placed nucleus. These cells display abundant cytoplasm and peripheral cytoplasmic extensions. In older pulps the number of undifferentiated mesenchymal cells diminishes, along with the number of other cells in the pulp core. This reduction, along with other aging factors, reduces the regenerative potential of the pulp.

MACROPHAGES

Macrophages tend to be located throughout the pulp center. Macrophages appear as large oval or spindle-shaped cells that under the light microscope exhibit a

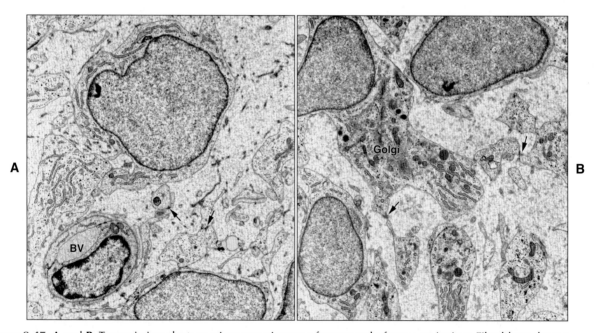

Figure 8-47 **A** and **B,** Transmission electron microscope images of young pulp from a rat incisor. Fibroblasts show a well-developed Golgi complex *(Golgi)* and extensive cell processes that establish desmosomal contacts *(arrows)* with processes of adjacent cells. At this early stage, few collagen fibrils occur, and the extracellular matrix consists mainly of ground substance. *BV,* Blood vessel.

dark-stained nucleus. Occasionally, clear areas can be seen in the cytoplasm, and electron microscopy has shown them to be large lysosomes. Pulp macrophages are involved in the elimination of dead cells, the presence of which further indicates that turnover of dental pulp fibroblasts occurs.

LYMPHOCYTES

In normal pulps, T lymphocytes are found, but B lymphocytes are scarce.

DENDRITIC CELLS

Bone marrow–derived, antigen-presenting dendritic cells (Figure 8-48) are found in and around the odontoblast layer in nonerupted teeth and in erupted teeth beneath the odontoblast layer. They have a close relationship to vascular and neural elements, and their function is similar to that of the Langerhans' cells found in epithelium (see Chapter 12) in that they capture and present foreign antigen to the T cells. These cells participate in immunosurveillance and increase in number in carious teeth, where they infiltrate the odontoblast layer and project their processes into the tubules. Dendritic cells and macrophages have been estimated to constitute some 8% of the total pulpal cell population, with dendritic cells exceeding macrophages.

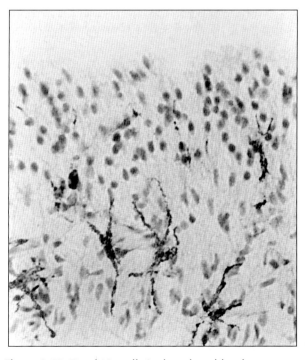

Figure 8-48 Dendritic cells in the odontoblast layer. *(Courtesy G. Bergenholtz.)*

MATRIX AND GROUND SUBSTANCE

The extracellular compartment of the pulp, or matrix, consists of collagen fibers and ground substance. The fibers are principally type I and type III collagen. In young pulps, single fibrils of collagen are found scattered between the pulp cells. Whereas the overall collagen content of the pulp increases with age, the ratio between types I and III remains stable, and the increased amount of extracellular collagen organizes into fiber bundles. The greatest concentration of collagen generally occurs in the most apical portion of the pulp. This fact is of practical significance when a pulpectomy is performed during the course of endodontic treatment. Engaging the pulp with a barbed broach in the region of the apex affords a better opportunity to remove the tissue intact than does engaging the broach more coronally, where the pulp is more gelatinous and liable to tear.

The ground substance of these tissues resembles that of any other loose connective tissue. Composed principally of glycosaminoglycans, glycoproteins, and water, the ground substance supports the cells and acts as the medium for transport of nutrients from the vasculature to the cells and of metabolites from the cells to the vasculature. Alterations in composition of the ground substance caused by age or disease interfere with this function, producing metabolic changes, reduced cellular function, and irregularities in mineral deposition.

VASCULATURE AND LYMPHATIC SUPPLY

The circulation establishes the tissue fluid pressure found in the extracellular compartment of the pulp. Blood vessels enter and exit the dental pulp by way of the apical and accessory foramina. One or sometimes two vessels of arteriolar size (about 150 μm) enter the apical foramen with the sensory and sympathetic nerve bundles. Smaller vessels, without any accompanying nerve bundle, enter the pulp through the minor foramina. Vessels leaving the dental pulp are associated closely with the arterioles and nerve bundles entering the apical foramen. Once the arterioles enter the pulp, an increase in the caliber of the lumen occurs with a reduction in thickness of the vessel wall. The arterioles occupy a central position within the pulp and, as they pass through the radicular portion of pulp, give off smaller lateral branches that extend toward and branch into the subodontoblastic area. The number of branches given off in this manner increases as the arterioles pass coronally so that in the coronal region of the pulp, they divide and subdivide to form an extensive vascular capillary network. Occasionally, U-looping of pulpal arterioles is

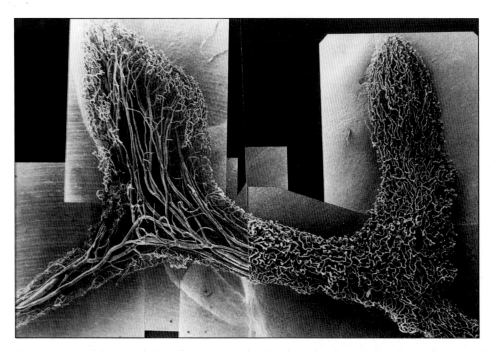

Figure 8-49 Resin cast of the vasculature of a canine molar. On the right, the peripheral vasculature can be seen. On the left, this vasculature has been removed to show the central pulp vessels and their peripheral ramifications. *(Courtesy K. Takahashi.)*

seen, and this anatomic configuration is thought to be related to the regulation of blood flow.

The extensive vascular network in the coronal portion of pulp can be demonstrated by scanning electron microscopy of vascular casts (Figure 8-49). The main portion of the capillary bed is located in the subodontoblastic area and ranges from 4 to 8 μm in diameter. Some terminal capillary loops extend upward between the odontoblasts to abut the predentin if dentinogenesis is

occurring (see Figures 8-14, 8-15, and 8-36, A). Located on the periphery of the capillaries at random intervals are pericytes, the cytoplasm of which forms a partial circumferential sheath about the endothelial wall. These cells are thought to be contractile cells capable of reducing the size of the vessel lumen. Arteriovenous anastomoses also have been identified in the dental pulp. The anastomosis is of arteriolar size, with an endothelium composed of cuboid cells (Figure 8-50) that project toward

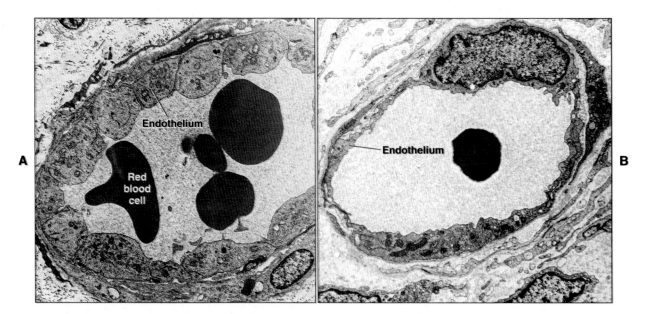

Figure 8-50 Electron micrographs of an arteriovenous shunt in dental pulp. Such a shunt is characterized by a lining of cuboid endothelial cells **(A)** that contrasts with the flattened endothelial lining cells of venules **(B)**.

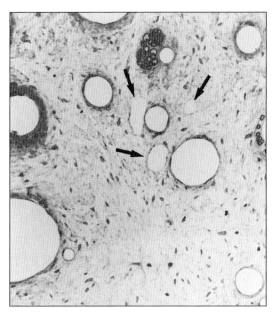

Figure 8-51 Lymphatic vessels *(arrows)* in the dental pulp. *(From Bishop MA, Malhotra M: Am J Anat 187:247, 1990.)*

of which are comparable to those of arterioles, but their walls are much thinner, making their lumina comparatively larger. The muscle layer in the venule walls is intermittent and thin.

Lymphatic vessels also occur in pulp tissue; they arise as small, blind, thin-walled vessels in the coronal region of the pulp (Figure 8-51) and pass apically through the middle and radicular regions of the pulp to exit via one or two larger vessels through the apical foramen. The lymphatic vessels are differentiated from small venules by the presence of discontinuities in their vessel walls and the absence of red blood cells in their lumina.

Sympathetic adrenergic nerves terminate in relation to the smooth muscle cells of the arteriolar walls (Figure 8-52, A). Afferent free nerve endings terminate in relation to arterioles, capillaries, and veins (Figure 8-52, B) and serve as effectors by releasing various neuropeptides that exert an effect on the vascular system.

the lumen. Anastomoses are points of direct communication between the arterial and venous sides of the circulation.

The efferent, or drainage, side of the circulation is composed of an extensive system of venules the diameters

INNERVATION OF THE DENTIN-PULP COMPLEX

The dental pulp is innervated richly. Nerves enter the pulp through the apical foramen, along with afferent blood vessels, and together form the neurovascular bundle. Once in the pulp chamber, the nerves generally follow the same course as the afferent vessels, beginning as large nerve bundles that arborize peripherally as they

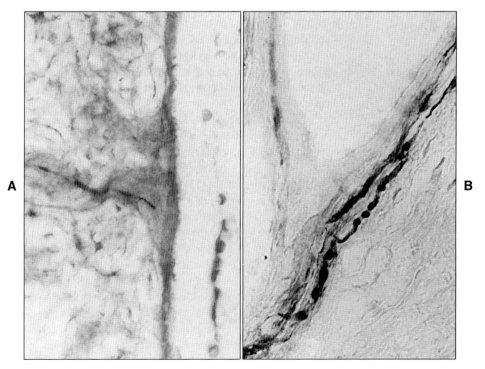

Figure 8-52 A, Free nerve endings terminating in the vascular wall of a capillary. **B,** Varicose nerve endings terminating on an arteriole. *(From Okamura K, Kobayashi I, Matsuo K et al:* Arch Oral Biol *40:47, 1995.)*

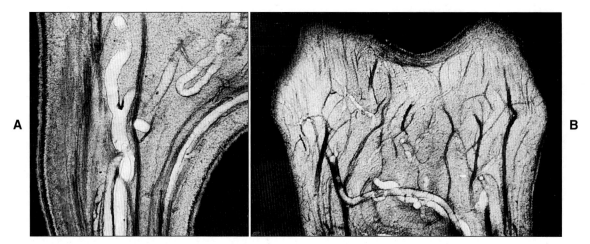

Figure 8-53 Photomicrographs of a tooth showing the general pattern of distribution of nerves and vessels in the root canal **(A)** and in the pulp chamber **(B)**. *(From Bernick S: Oral Surg Oral Med Oral Pathol 33:983-1000, 1972.)*

extend occlusally through the pulp core (Figure 8-53). Each nerve fiber has been estimated to provide at least eight terminal branches. These branches ultimately contribute to an extensive plexus of nerves in the cell-free zone just below the cell bodies of the odontoblasts in the crown portion of the tooth. This plexus of nerves, which is called the *subodontoblastic plexus of Raschkow*, occupies the cell-free zone of Weil and can be demonstrated in silver nitrate–stained sections under the light microscope (Figure 8-54) or by immunocytochemical techniques to discharge various proteins associated with nerves (Figure 8-55). In the root, no corresponding plexus exists. Instead, branches are given off from the

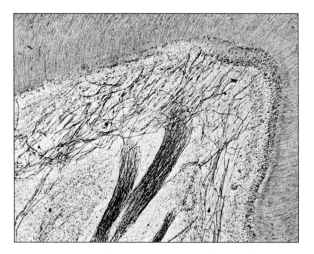

Figure 8-54 Plexus of Raschkow in a silver-stained demineralized section. The ascending nerve trunks branch to form this plexus, which is situated beneath the odontoblast layer. *(From Bernick S. In Finn SB, editor: Biology of the dental pulp organ, Tuscaloosa, 1968, University of Alabama Press.)*

ascending trunks at intervals that further arborize, with each branch supplying its own territory (Figure 8-56).

The nerve bundles that enter the tooth pulp consist principally of sensory afferent nerves of the trigeminal (fifth cranial) nerve and sympathetic branches from the superior cervical ganglion. Each bundle contains myelinated and unmyelinated axons (Figure 8-57). Fine structural investigations of animal tooth pulp have shown increased discontinuities in the investing perineurium as nerves ascend coronally. Furthermore, as the nerve bundles ascend coronally, the myelinated axons gradually lose their myelin coating so that a proportional increase in the number of unmyelinated axons occurs in the more coronal aspect of the tooth.

Although most of the nerve bundles terminate in the subodontoblastic plexus as free, unmyelinated nerve endings, a small number of axons pass between the odontoblast cell bodies (sometimes occupying a groove on the surface of the cell) to enter the dentinal tubules (see Figure 8-55) in proximity to the odontoblast process (Figure 8-58). No organized junction or synaptic relationship has been noted between axons and the odontoblast process. Intratubular nerves characteristically contain neurofilaments, neurotubules, numerous mitochondria, and many small vesicular structures. These characteristics distinguish them from the odontoblast processes that, although they contain microfilaments and microtubules, do not contain mitochondria and accumulated vesicles. The close relationship of these nerves to the odontoblast process is important and is discussed more fully in relation to dentin sensitivity. Intratubular nerve fibrils show significant regional differences in distribution. In human premolars, electron microscopic studies in the pulpal horn and coronal dentin regions have shown that the frequency of nerves decreases from predentin to the mineralizing front

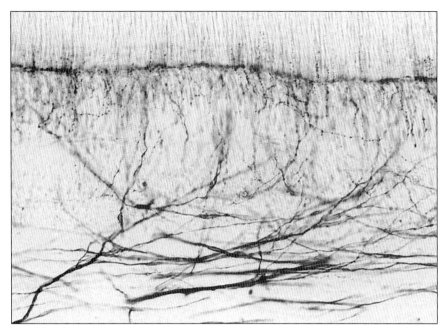

Figure 8-55 Dentin innervation demonstrated by immunocytochemical staining of nerve growth factor receptor (NGFR). NGFR is present in some of the dentinal tubules, suggesting that nerves extend into them. *(From Maeda T, Sato O, Iwanaga T et al: Proc Finn Dent Soc 88[suppl 1]:557, 1992.)*

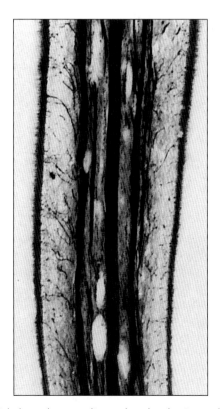

Figure 8-56 Nerves in radicular pulp. Side branches are directed to the dentin, and a plexus of Raschkow is absent. *(From Maeda T: Arch Oral Biol 39:563, 1994.)*

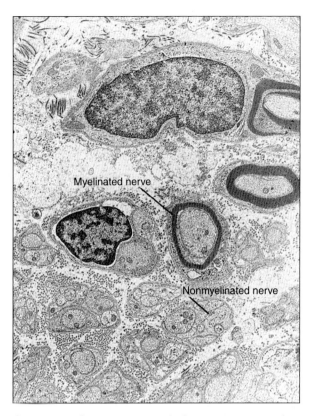

Figure 8-57 Electron micrograph showing a mixture of myelinated and nonmyelinated nerves in pulp.

to dentin. The density of intratubular nerves varies and in some instances can be as high as one for every two tubules in discrete areas of the coronal dentin. Even so and even if they extend deeper into dentin, the number of tubules containing nerve fibers in relation to the overall number of tubules is small. The literature also contains reports of nerves running within predentin at right angles to the tubules, and such loops generally are assumed to represent isolated nerve fibrils from the plexus of Raschkow that are caught up by the advancing process of dentinogenesis (Figure 8-59). However, this description may be too simplified; recent studies examining tangential sections of predentin have indicated that some of these fibers undergo dendritic ramification (Figure 8-60). The functional significance, if any, of this pattern of innervation within the predentin has not been determined.

DENTIN SENSITIVITY

One of the most unusual features of the pulp-dentin complex is its sensitivity. The extreme sensitivity of this complex is difficult to explain, because this characteristic provides no apparent evolutionary benefit. The overwhelming sensation appreciated by this complex is pain, although evidence now indicates that pulpal afferent

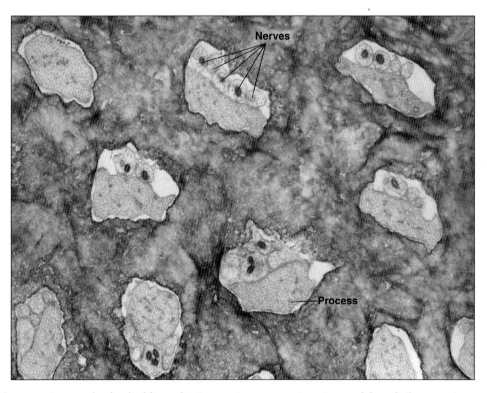

Figure 8-58 Electron micrograph of pulpal horn dentin seen in cross section. Some of the tubules contain a process and multiple fine neural elements. *(Courtesy R. Holland.)*

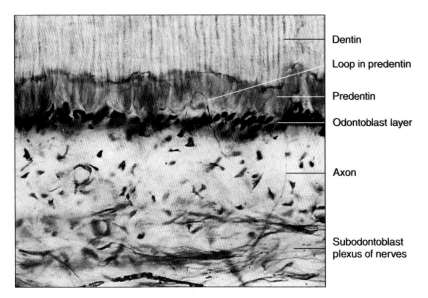

Dentin

Loop in predentin

Predentin

Odontoblast layer

Axon

Subodontoblast plexus of nerves

Figure 8-59 Nerve fibril arising from the plexus of Raschkow is shown passing between the odontoblasts and looping within the predentin. *(From Bernick S. In Finn SB, editor:* Biology of the dental pulp organ, *Tuscaloosa, 1968, University of Alabama Press.)*

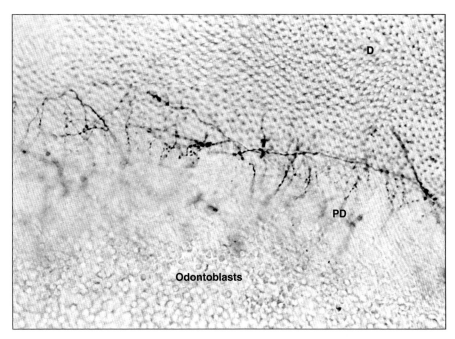

Figure 8-60 Nerve at the predentin-dentin *(PD, D)* junction demonstrated by staining for nerve growth factor receptor in a tangential section. Its extensive ramification is notable. *(From Maeda T, Sato O, Iwanaga T et al:* Proc Finn Dent Soc *88[suppl 1]:557, 1992.)*

nerves can distinguish mechanical, thermal, and tactile stimuli as well (but always as some form of discomfort). Convergence of pulpal afferent nerves with other pulpal afferent nerves and afferent nerves from other orofacial structures in the central nervous system often makes pulpal pain difficult to localize.

Among the numerous stimuli that can evoke a painful response when applied to dentin are many that are related to clinical dental practice, such as cold air or water, mechanical contact by a probe or bur, and dehydration with cotton wool or a stream of air. Of interest is the observation that some products, such as histamine and bradykinin, known to produce pain in other tissues do not produce pain in dentin.

Three mechanisms, all involving an understanding of the structure of dentin and pulp, have been proposed to explain dentin sensitivity: (1) The dentin contains nerve endings that respond when it is stimulated, (2) the odontoblasts serve as receptors and are coupled to nerves in the pulp, and (3) the tubular nature of dentin permits fluid movement to occur within the tubule when a stimulus is applied, a movement registered by pulpal free nerve endings close to the odontoblasts (Figure 8-61).

No debate exists that the pulp is well innervated, especially below the odontoblasts. Nor does any dispute arise that some nerves penetrate a short distance into some tubules in human teeth. The question is whether these intratubular nerves are involved directly in dentin sensitivity. No evidence has been found for nerves in the outer dentin, which is reputedly the most sensitive. Development studies have shown that the plexus of Raschkow and the intratubular nerves do not establish themselves until some time after the tooth has erupted, yet newly erupted teeth are sensitive. In addition, the application of local anesthetics or silver nitrate (a protein precipitant) to exposed dentin does not eliminate dentin sensitivity, and pharmacologic agents that cause pain when applied to skin do not do so when applied to dentin. At present, all that can be stated is that some nerves occur within some tubules in the inner dentin but that dentin sensitivity does not depend solely, if at all, on the stimulation of such nerve endings.

The second possible mechanism to explain dentin sensitivity considers the odontoblast to be a receptor cell. This attractive concept has been considered, abandoned, and reconsidered for many reasons. The point

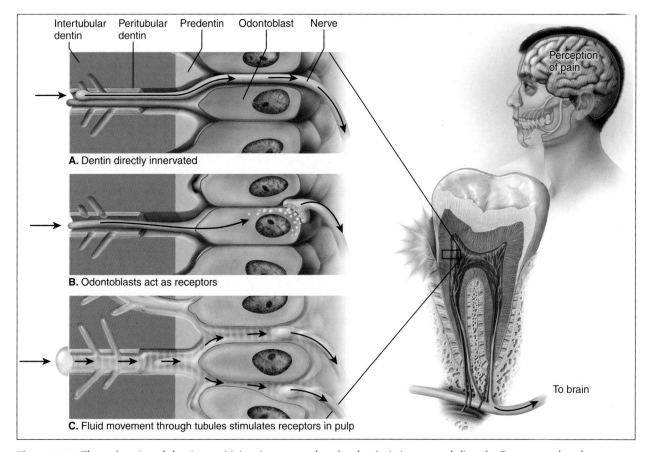

Figure 8-61 Three theories of dentin sensitivity. **A** suggests that the dentin is innervated directly. **B** suggests that the odontoblast acts as a receptor. **C** suggests that the receptors are in the pulp and are stimulated directly or indirectly by fluid movement through the tubules.

once was argued that because the odontoblast is of neural crest origin, it retains an ability to transduce and propagate an impulse. What was missing was the demonstration of a synaptic relationship between the odontoblast and pulpal nerves. That the membrane potential of odontoblasts measured in vitro is too low to permit transduction and that local anesthetics and protein precipitants do not abolish sensitivity also militated against this concept. The fact that odontoblast processes extend to the dentinoenamel junction and the demonstration of gap junctions between odontoblasts (and possibly between odontoblasts and pulpal nerves) are consistent with the direct role of the odontoblast in dentin sensitivity.

The third mechanism proposed to explain dentin sensitivity involves movement of fluid through the dentinal tubules. This *hydrodynamic theory*, which fits much of the experimental and morphologic data, proposes that fluid movement through the tubule distorts the local pulpal environment and is sensed by the free nerve endings in the plexus of Raschkow. Thus when dentin is first exposed, small blebs of fluid can be seen on the cavity floor. When the cavity is dried with air or cotton wool, a greater loss of fluid is induced, leading to more movement and more pain. The increased sensitivity at the dentinoenamel junction is explained by the profuse branching of the tubules in this region. The hydrodynamic hypothesis also explains why local anesthetics, applied to exposed dentin, fail to block sensitivity and why pain is produced by thermal change, mechanical probing, hypertonic solutions, and dehydration.

Attention must be drawn, however, to the fact that dentin sensitivity bestows no benefit on the organism and to the possibility that this sensitivity results from more important functional requirements of the innervated dentin-pulp complex. Increasingly, appreciation is given to the fact that pulpal innervation has a significant role to play in pulpal homeostasis and its defense mechanisms and that this role involves an interplay between nerves, blood vessels, and immunocompetent cells, which have been shown to contact the vascular and neural elements of the pulp. Immunocompetent cells contact vascular endothelium and also have close association with free nerve endings (Figure 8-62). Furthermore, immunocompetent cells express receptors for various neuropeptides. This common biochemical language between the immune, nervous, and vascular systems suggests a functional unit of importance in pulp biology.

PULP STONES

Pulp stones, or denticles, frequently are found in pulp tissue (Figure 8-63). As their name implies, they are

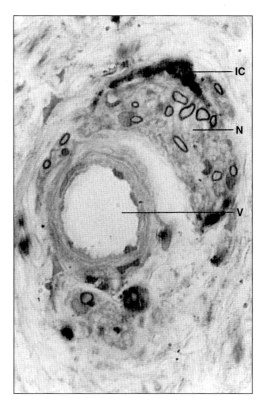

Figure 8-62 Association between immunocompetent cell *(IC)*, vascular *(V)*, and neural elements *(N)*. *(From Yoshiba N, Yoshiba K, Nakamura H et al:* J Dent Res *75:1585, 1996.)*

discrete calcified masses that have calcium-phosphorus ratios comparable to that of dentin. They may be singular or multiple in any tooth and are found more frequently at the orifice of the pulp chamber or within the root canal. Histologically, they usually consist of concentric layers of mineralized tissue formed by surface accretion around blood thrombi, dying or dead cells, or collagen fibers. Occasionally a pulp stone may contain tubules and be surrounded by cells resembling odontoblasts. Such stones are rare and, if seen, occur close to the apex of the tooth. Such stones are referred to as "true" pulp stones as opposed to "false" stones having no cells associated with them.

Pulp stones may form in several teeth and, indeed, in every tooth in some individuals. If during the formation of a pulp stone, union occurs between it and the dentin wall, or if secondary dentin deposition surrounds the stone, the pulp stone is called an *attached stone*, as distinguished from a *free stone* (which is completely surrounded by soft tissue). The presence of pulp stones is significant in that they reduce the overall number of cells within the pulp and act as an impediment to débridement and enlargement of the root canal system during endodontic treatment.

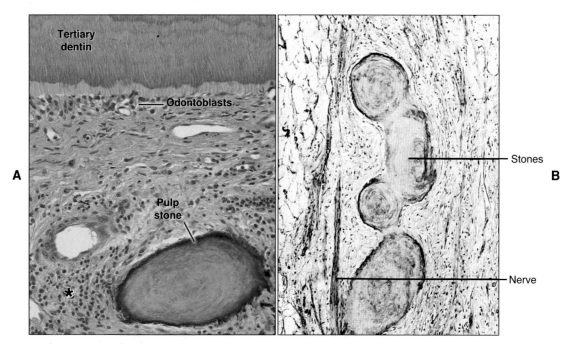

Figure 8-63 A and **B,** Free (false) pulp stones. **A,** The presence of tertiary dentin and a strong mononuclear inflammatory cell infiltrate *(*)* are indicative of a carious lesion. **B,** Multiple stones in an aged pulp. *(**A** courtesy P. Tambasco de Oliveira.)*

AGE CHANGES

The dentin-pulp complex, like all body tissues, undergoes change with time. The most conspicuous change is the decreasing volume of the pulp chamber and root canal brought about by continued dentin deposition (Figure 8-64). In old teeth the root canal is often no more than a thin channel (Figure 8-65); indeed, the root canal on occasion can appear to be obliterated almost completely. Such continued restriction in pulp volume probably brings about a reduction in the vascular supply to the pulp and initiates many of the other age changes found in this tissue.

From about the age of 20 years, cells gradually decrease in number until age 70, when the cell density has decreased by about half. The distribution of the collagen fibrils may change with age, leading to the appearance of fibrous bundles.

With age come a loss and a degeneration of myelinated and unmyelinated axons that correlate with an age-related reduction in sensitivity. Another age change is the occurrence of irregular areas of dystrophic calcification, especially in the central pulp (Figure 8-66). Dystrophic calcifications generally originate in relation to blood vessels or as diffuse mineral deposits along collagen bundles.

That the pulp supports the dentin and that age changes within the pulp are reflected in the dentin has been emphasized. Within dentin the deposition of

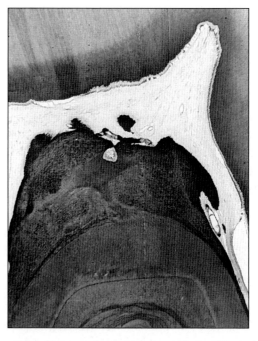

Figure 8-64 Decreased pulp volume with age. The pulp has been reduced considerably by the continued deposition of dentin on the pulp chamber floor. *(From Bernick S, Nedelman CJ: J Endod 1:88, 1975.)*

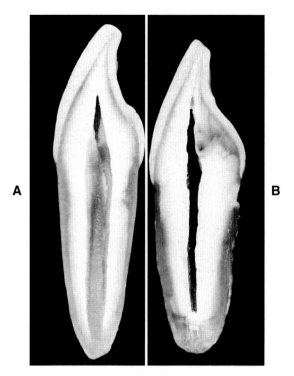

Figure 8-65 Difference in pulp volume between a young tooth (**A**) and an older tooth (**B**).

intratubular dentin continues, resulting in a gradual reduction of the tubule diameter. This continued deposition often leads to complete closure of the tubule, as can be seen readily in a ground section of dentin, because the dentin becomes translucent (or sclerotic). Sclerotic dentin is found frequently near the root apex in teeth from middle-aged individuals (see Figure 8-28). Associated with sclerotic dentin are an increased brittleness and a decreased permeability of the dentin.

Another age change found within dentin is dead tracts (Figure 8-67). Dentinal tubules, on occasion, are emptied by complete retraction of the odontoblast process from the tubule or through death of the odontoblast. The dentinal tubules then become sealed off so that in a ground section air-filled tubules appear by transmitted light as black dead tracts. Dead tracts occur most often in coronal dentin and frequently are bound by bands of sclerotic dentin.

RESPONSE TO ENVIRONMENTAL STIMULI

Many of the age changes in the pulp-dentin complex render it more resistant to environmental injury. For example, the spread of caries is slowed by tubule occlusion. Age changes also accelerate in response to environmental stimuli, such as caries or attrition of enamel. The response of the complex to gradual attrition is to produce more

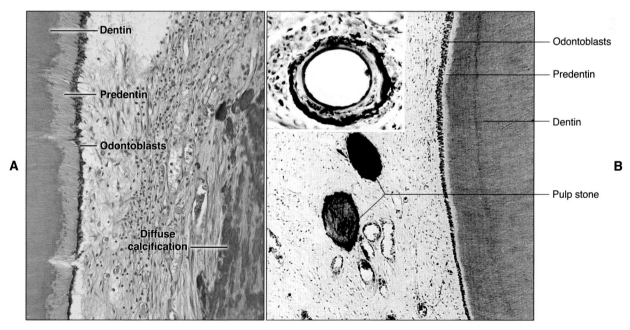

Figure 8-66 A, Diffuse calcification associated with collagen bundles in the center of the pulp chamber. **B,** Pulp stones and dystrophic calcification beginning in a vessel wall *(inset)*. (**A** *courtesy P. Tambasco de Oliveira;* **B** *from Bernick S: J Dent Res 46:544, 1967.)*

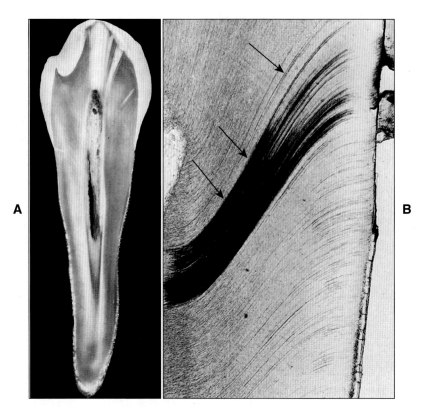

Figure 8-67 Dead tracts *(arrows)* in a ground section of dentin. **A,** Under incident illumination the tracts appear white because light is reflected. **B,** Under transmitted illumination the tracts appear dark because air in them refracts the light.

sclerotic dentin and deposit secondary dentin at an increased rate. If the stimulus is more severe, tertiary dentin is formed at the ends of the tubules affected by the injury.

Age change, however, also lessens the ability of the pulp-dentin complex to repair itself. Injury has been defined as the interference of a stimulus with cellular metabolism. If pulpal injury occurs, the age of the pulp determines its ability to repair the damage. Because cell metabolism is high in young pulps, their cells are prone to injury, which is manifested as altered cell function, but recovery occurs rapidly. If injury is such that the odontoblasts are destroyed, the possibility exists in young pulps for the differentiation of new odontoblasts from the mesenchymal cells of the pulp and the formation of repair dentin. This potential is reduced considerably with age.

RECOMMENDED READING

Brännström M, Aström A: The hydrodynamics of the dentine: its possible relationship to dentinal pain, *Int Dent J* 22:219, 1972.

Butler WT: Dentin matrix proteins, *Eur J Oral Sci* 106:204, 1998.

Linde A: Structure and calcification of dentin. In Bonucci E, editor: *Calcification in biological systems,* Boca Raton, Fla, 1992, CRC Press.

Linde A, Lundgren T: From serum to the mineral phase: the role of the odontoblast in calcium transport and mineral formation, *Int J Dev Biol* 39:213, 1995.

MacDougall M, Dong J, Acevedo AC: Molecular basis of human dentin diseases, *Am J Med Genet A* 140:2536, 2006.

Moses KD: Immunohistochemical study of small integrin-binding ligand, N-linked glycoproteins in reactionary dentin of rat molars at different ages, *Eur J Oral Sci* 114:216, 2006.

Qin C, Baba O, Butler WT: Post-translational modifications of sibling proteins and their roles in osteogenesis and dentinogenesis, *Crit Rev Oral Biol Med* 15:126, 2004.

Ruch JV, Lesot H, Begue-Kirn C: Odontoblast differentiation, *Int J Dev Biol* 39:51, 1995.

Shimono M, Maeda T, Suda H et al, editors: *Dentin/pulp complex,* Tokyo, 1996, Quintessence.

Yamakoshi Y, Hu JC-C, Fukae M et al: Dentin glycoprotein: the protein in the middle of the dentin sialophosphoprotein chimera, *J Biol Chem* 280:17472, 2005.

Periodontium

CHAPTER OUTLINE

The periodontium is defined as those tissues supporting and investing the tooth and consists of cementum, periodontal ligament (PDL), bone lining the alveolus (socket), and that part of the gingiva facing the tooth. Proper functioning of the periodontium is achieved only through structural integrity and interaction between these various tissues. Together, these tissues form a specialized fibrous joint, a *gomphosis*, the components of which are of *ectomesenchymal origin*. The widespread occurrence of periodontal diseases and the realization that periodontal tissues lost to disease can be repaired has resulted in considerable effort to understand the factors and cells regulating the formation, maintenance, and regeneration of the periodontium. This chapter describes the histologic events leading to formation of the supporting tissues (Figure 9-1), except for the dentogingival junction, which is covered under oral mucosa (see Chapter 12).

CEMENTUM

Cementum is a hard, avascular connective tissue that covers the roots of teeth (Figure 9-2). Cementum is classified according to the presence or absence of cells within its matrix and the origin of the collagenous fibers of the matrix. The development of cementum has been subdivided into a *prefunctional stage*, which occurs throughout root formation, and a *functional stage*, which starts when the tooth is in occlusion and continues throughout life. Several varieties of cementum exist; the beginning student, however, needs only to think of two main forms of cementum that have different structural and functional characteristics; namely, *acellular cementum*, which provides attachment for the tooth, and *cellular cementum*, which has an adaptive role in response to tooth wear and movement and is associated with repair of periodontal tissues.

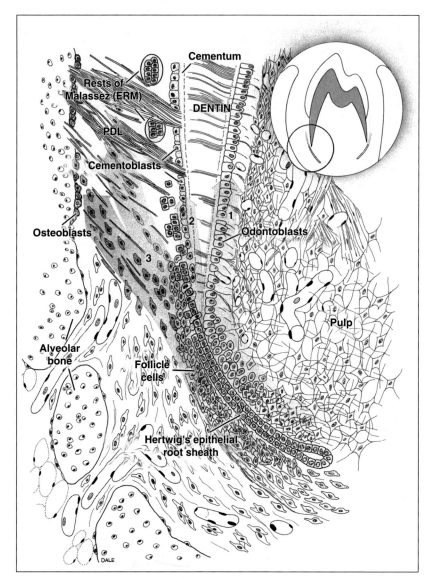

Figure 9-1 Summary of *(1)* the differentiation of odontoblasts from ectomesenchymal cells in the radicular pulp, *(2)* the fragmentation of Hertwig's epithelial root sheath with residual portions forming the epithelial rests of Malassez, and *(3)* the ensuing differentiation of cementoblasts from Hertwig's epithelial root sheath cells or follicle cells, and the follicle contribution to the formation of the fiber bundles of the periodontal ligament *(PDL)* and, possibly, osteoblasts.

BIOCHEMICAL COMPOSITION

Four mineralized tissues are found in the oral cavity, and three of these—enamel, dentin, and cementum—are components of the tooth. Their characteristics and biochemical composition are summarized in Table 1-1. The composition of cementum is similar to that of bone, where proteins unique to cementum have yet to be confirmed. Cementum is approximately 45% to 50% hydroxyapatite (inorganic) and 50% collagen and noncollagenous matrix proteins (organic). Type I collagen is the predominant collagen of cementum and constitutes up to 90% of the organic components in cellular cementum.

Other collagens associated with cementum include type III, a less cross-linked collagen found in high concentrations during development and during repair and regeneration of mineralized tissues, and type XII collagen, a fibril-associated collagen with interrupted triple helices that binds to type I collagen and also to noncollagenous proteins. Type XII collagen is found in high concentrations in ligamentous tissues, including the PDL, and may function in maintaining a mature ligament that can withstand the forces of occlusion. Trace amounts of other collagens, including types V, VI, and XIV, also are found in extracts of mature cementum; however, these may be contaminants from the PDL region, produced by

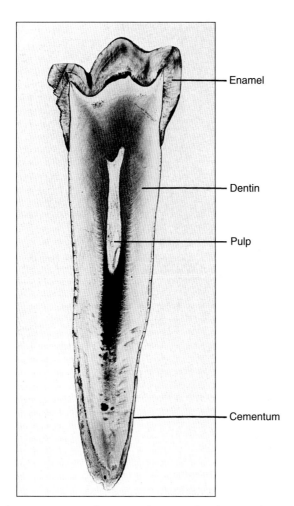

Figure 9-2 Ground section of a premolar showing the distribution of cementum around the root. Increasing amounts of cementum occur around the apex.

— Enamel

— Dentin

— Pulp

— Cementum

PDL fibroblasts associated with collagen fibers inserted into cementum. Noncollagenous proteins identified in cementum also are associated with bone and include the following: alkaline phosphatase, bone sialoprotein, dentin matrix protein 1, dentin sialoprotein, fibronectin, osteocalcin, osteonectin, osteopontin, proteoglycans, proteolipids, tenascin, and several growth factors. Enamel proteins also have been suggested to be present in cementum. Two apparently unique cementum molecules, an adhesion molecule (cementum attachment protein) and an insulin-like growth factor have been identified, but further studies are warranted to confirm the existence and function of these molecules.

INITIATION OF CEMENTUM FORMATION

Although cementum formation takes place along the entire root, its initiation is limited to the advancing root edge (Figure 9-3). At this site, *Hertwig's epithelial root sheath* (HERS), which derives from the coronoapical extension of

the inner and outer enamel epithelium (see Chapter 5), is believed to send an inductive message, possibly by secreting some enamel proteins, to the facing ectomesenchymal pulp cells. These cells differentiate into odontoblasts and produce a layer of predentin (Figure 9-4; see also Figure 9-3). Soon after, HERS becomes interrupted, and ectomesenchymal cells from the inner portion of the dental follicle then can come in contact with the predentin. The next series of events results in formation of cementum on the root surface; however, the specific cells and trigger factors responsible for promoting its formation still are unresolved. Current theories include the following: (1) infiltrating dental follicle cells receive a reciprocal inductive signal from the dentin or the surrounding HERS cells and differentiate into cementoblasts, and (2) HERS cells transform into cementoblasts (a process discussed subsequently). During either of these two processes, some cells within the HERS undergo apoptosis, and some cells from the fragmented root sheath form discrete masses surrounded by a basal lamina, known as *epithelial cell rests of Malassez*, which persist in the mature PDL (Figures 9-5 and 9-6). Evidence is increasing that these rests are not simply residual cells but instead may participate in maintenance and regeneration of periodontal tissues. If some HERS cells remain attached to the forming root surface, they can produce focal deposits of enamel-like material called *enamel pearls*, sometimes in the area of furcation of roots.

ORIGIN OF PERIODONTAL CELLS AND DIFFERENTIATION OF CEMENTOBLASTS

Several fundamental issues still need to be determined to better understand the periodontium, including the following:

1. What are the precursors of cementoblasts and PDL fibroblasts?
2. Do cementoblasts express unique genes products, or are they simply positional osteoblasts?
3. Are acellular and cellular cementum phenotypically distinct tissues?
4. What factors promote cementoblast differentiation?
5. What regulates formation of the PDL versus cementogenesis, thus providing a balance between cementum, PDL, and alveolar bone?

Answers to these questions are important not only to understand normal formation processes but also to envisage novel, targeted therapeutic approaches for periodontal diseases.

The long-standing view is that precursor cells for cementoblasts and PDL fibroblasts reside in the dental follicle and that factors within the local environment

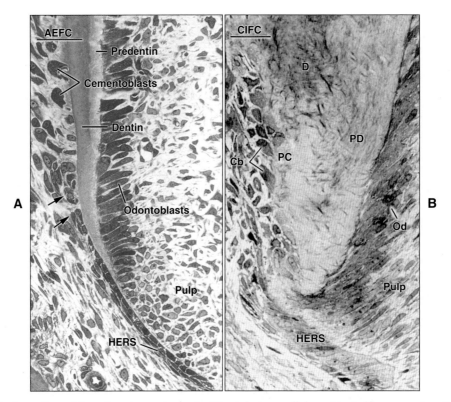

Figure 9-3 Histologic sections of the advancing root edge in **(A)** rat during acellular extrinsic fiber cementum *(AEFC)* formation and **(B)** in human during cellular intrinsic fiber cementum *(CIFC)* formation. In rat, Hertwig's epithelial root sheet *(HERS)* is still present when radicular dentin *(D)* calcifies, and in fact, deposition of acellular cementum starts on mineralized dentin, often in presence of cells with epithelial characteristics *(arrows)*. In human teeth, acellular and cellular cementum are deposited before the surface layer of dentin mineralizes. *Cb,* Cementoblast; *Od,* odontoblasts; *PC,* precementum; *PD,* predentin.

regulate their ability to function as cementoblasts that form root cementum or as fibroblasts of the PDL. Cells involved in regenerating periodontal tissues include stem cells migrating from the vascular region, as well as local progenitor cells. The precise location the progenitor cells and whether there exists a common progenitor or distinct progenitors for each cell type remain to be defined. In addition, there is now increasing evidence that epithelial cells from HERS may undergo epithelial-mesenchymal transformation into cementoblasts during development. Such transformation is a fundamental process in developmental biology that occurs, among other processes, as we have seen during neural crest cell migration and medial edge fusion of the palatal shelves. Structural and immunocytochemical data support the possibility that at least in part cementoblasts are transformed from epithelial cells of HERS. In rodents, initial formation of acellular cementum takes place in the presence of epithelial cells, and some studies have shown that enamel organ–derived cells are capable of producing mesenchymal products such as type I collagen, bone sialoprotein, and osteopontin.

Uncertainty still exists as to whether acellular (primary) and cellular (secondary) cementum are produced by distinct populations of cells expressing spatiotemporal behaviors that result in the characteristic histologic differences between these tissues. This potential cellular and formative distinctiveness is highlighted in mice null for tissue nonspecific alkaline phosphatase gene or rats treated with bisphosphonates. In these animals, acellular cementum formation is affected significantly, whereas cellular cementum appears to develop normally. This suggests differences in cell types or factors controlling development of these two varieties of cementum. In the human counterpart, hypophosphatasia, characterized by low levels of alkaline phosphatase, cementum formation appears to be limited or nonexistent, not exclusive to acellular versus cellular. In contrast, in mice with mutations in genes that maintain extracellular pyrophosphate levels such as *ank* and *PC-1*, resulting in limited levels of pyrophosphate, one sees abundant formation of cellular cementum, even at early stages of root development. These findings suggest an important role for phosphate in controlling the rate of cementum formation.

MOLECULAR FACTORS REGULATING CEMENTOGENESIS

To understand the specific role of phosphate and other molecules, additional studies that focus on defining the

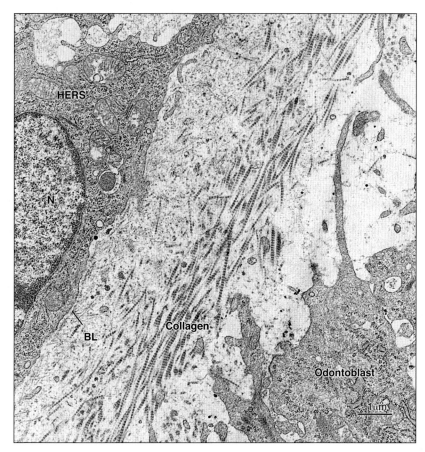

Figure 9-4 Electron micrograph of early root dentinogenesis. The large collagen fibril bundles are first deposited parallel and at a distance from the basal lamina *(BL)* that supports Hertwig's epithelial root sheath *(HERS)*. *N,* Nucleus.

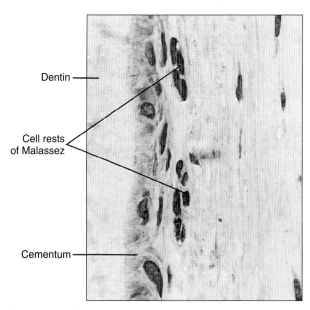

Figure 9-5 Initial cementum formation. The first increment of cementum forms against the root dentin surface. Epithelial cell rests of Malassez (remnants of the root sheath) can be seen within the follicular tissue.

cells and factors controlling development, maintenance, and regeneration of periodontal tissues are required. Some of the factors known to be involved in controlling these events are discussed next and are summarized in Table 9-1.

Bone Morphogenetic Proteins

Bone morphogenetic proteins (BMPs) are members of the transforming growth factor β superfamily that act through transmembrane serine/threonine protein kinase receptors. These signaling molecules have a variety of functions during morphogenesis and cell differentiation, and in teeth they are considered to be part of the network of epithelial-mesenchymal signaling molecules regulating initiation of crown formation. The roles for BMPs in root development, including whether they are implicated in epithelial-mesenchymal signaling, and the signal pathways and transcription factors involved in modulating their behavior remain to be defined. However, several of the BMPs, including BMP-2, BMP-4, and BMP-7, are known to promote differentiation of preosteoblasts and putative cementoblast precursor cells.

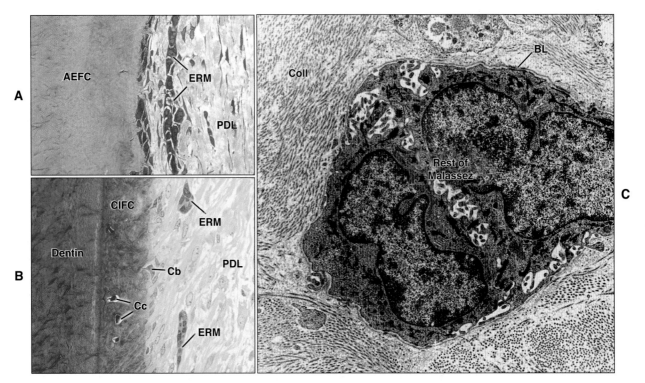

Figure 9-6 Light micrographs taken along the forming root in **(A)** a human tooth and **(B)** a porcine one. Epithelial rests of Malassez *(ERM)* are seen close to the tooth surface. These can appear as long strands or more discrete elongated or spherical groups of cells. The size of the cells and their staining density may vary. **C,** Electron micrograph of an epithelial rest. The scarcity of cytoplasmic organelles and basal lamina *(BL)* surrounding it are notable. *AEFC,* Acellular extrinsic fiber cementum; *Cb,* cementoblast; *Cc,* cementocyte; *CIFC,* cellular intrinsic fiber cementum; *Coll,* collagen fibrils; *PDL,* periodontal ligament.

TABLE 9-1   Some Key Molecules in the Periodontium

	SUGGESTED FUNCTION RELATED TO CEMENTOGENESIS
Growth Factors	
Transforming growth factor β superfamily (including bone morphogenetic proteins)	Reported to promote cell differentiation and subsequently cementogenesis during development and regeneration.
Platelet-derived growth factor and insulin-like growth factor	Existing data suggest that platelet-derived growth factor alone or in combination with insulin-like growth factor promotes cementum formation by altering cell cycle activities.
Fibroblast growth factors	Suggested roles for these factors are promoting cell proliferation and migration and also vasculogenesis—all key events for formation and regeneration of periodontal tissues.
Adhesion Molecules	
Bone sialoprotein	These molecules may promote adhesion of selected cells to the newly forming root. Bone sialoprotein may be
Osteopontin	involved in promoting mineralization, whereas osteopontin may regulate the extent of crystal growth.
Epithelial/Enamel Proteins	Epithelial-mesenchymal interactions may be involved in promoting follicle cells along a cementoblast pathway. Some epithelial molecules may promote periodontal repair directly or indirectly.
Collagens	Collagens, especially types I and III, play key roles in regulating periodontal tissues during development and regeneration. In addition, type XII may assist in maintaining the periodontal ligament space versus continuous formation of cementum.
Gla Proteins	
Matrix Gla protein\Bone Gla protein (osteocalcin)	These proteins contain γ-carboxyglutamic acid, hence the name Gla proteins. Osteocalcin is a marker for cells associated with mineralization—that is, osteoblasts, cementoblasts, and odontoblasts—and is considered to be a regulator of crystal growth. Matrix Gla protein appears to play a significant role in preventing abnormal ectopic calcification.

TABLE 9-1 Some key Molecules in the Periodontium—cont'd

	SUGGESTED FUNCTION RELATED TO CEMENTOGENESIS
Transcription Factors	
Runt-related transcription factor 2 (Runx-2)	As for osteoblasts, these may be involved in cementoblast differentiation.
Osterix	
Signaling Molecules	
Osteoprotegerin	These molecules mediate bone and root resorption by osteoclasts.
Receptor-activated NF-κB ligand	
Receptor-activated NF-κB	

In addition, BMPs have been used successfully to induce periodontal regeneration in a number of experimental models and in certain clinical situations.

Epithelial Factors

Epithelial-mesenchymal interactions are required for formation of the tooth crown, and epithelial factors are implicated. The same two populations of cells involved in crown morphogenesis—that is, dental epithelial and ectomesenchymal cells—also take part in root formation. The possibility that such interactions also are required for development of periodontal tissues and that the some of the same signaling molecules are involved is thus a logical assumption. Prospective candidates include enamel proteins, parathyroid hormone-related protein, and basal lamina constituents. In the case of enamel proteins, the debate centers around the fact that enamel proteins have not been detected consistently along forming roots. However, this does not rule out a transient expression at early stages of root formation where they could influence odontoblast and/or cementoblast differentiation. Along this line, an enamel matrix derivative, consisting predominantly of amelogenin molecules, is used clinically to stimulate repair and regeneration, but its mechanism of action remains to be determined (see Chapter 14).

Major Matrix Proteins with Cell Adhesion Motifs

Bone sialoprotein and osteopontin are multifunctional molecules associated with cementum formation during development and in repair and regeneration of periodontal tissues. They contain the cell adhesion motif arginine–glycine–aspartic acid and thereby are believed to promote adhesion of selected cells onto the newly forming root. Present data further suggest that osteopontin is involved in regulating mineral growth, whereas bone sialoprotein promotes mineral formation on the root surface. The balance between the activities of these two molecules may contribute to establishing and maintaining an unmineralized PDL between cementum and alveolar bone. However, no developmental root anomalies have been reported in knockout mice models, suggesting that other proteins are involved or that there exist compensatory mechanisms.

Gla Proteins

Gla proteins contain γ-carboxyglutamic acid (Gla), a calcium-binding amino acid that may facilitate interactions with hydroxyapatite. Bone Gla protein (osteocalcin) is a marker for maturation of osteoblasts, odontoblasts, and cementoblasts and is considered to regulate the extent of mineralization. Matrix Gla protein (MGP) has been identified in periodontal tissues and, based on its suggested role as an inhibitor mineralization, may act to preserve the PDL width. Mice null for MGP exhibit substantial ectopic calcification. However, periodontal development and tooth formation appear to be normal in MGP-null mice; thus additional studies are required to define the role of MGP within periodontal tissues.

Collagens

Type I collagen is the predominant collagen in cementum; in cellular intrinsic fiber cementum, just as in bone, it accommodates mineral deposition. In addition, during early stages of cementogenesis and during development and repair, type III collagen is present in high amounts but is reduced with maturation of this tissue. Type I collagen is also the major collagen within the PDL region, and its main function is to structure the fiber bundles that anchor the tooth to the bone and distribute masticatory forces. Type XII collagen also is abundant within the PDL region, with lower levels noted in cementum. This nonfibrillar collagen interacts with type I collagen and is present in high concentrations in ligamentous tissues; it may assist in maintaining a functional PDL.

Transcription Factors

As we have seen in Chapter 6, Runx-2 (runt-related transcription factor 2), also known as Cbfa 1 (core binding factor alpha 1), and osterix, downstream from Runx-2, have been identified as master switches for differentiation of osteoblasts. Runx-2 now has been found to be expressed in dental follicles cells, PDL cells, and cementoblasts. Based on similarities between cementoblasts (at least in cellular cementum) and osteoblasts, it is likely that both factors may be involved in cementoblast differentiation. The exact factors triggering expression or activation of these key transcription factors currently are being investigated; BMPs already have been identified as factors promoting expression of Runx-2.

Other Factors

Other molecules that are found within the developing and mature periodontal tissues include alkaline phosphatase, several growth factors (e.g., insulin-like growth factor, transforming growth factor β, and platelet-derived growth factor), metalloproteinases, and proteoglycans. The significance of alkaline phosphatase to cementum formation has long been appreciated and is discussed in a previous section. Proteoglycans accumulate at the dentin-cementum junction, and it has been proposed that, together with noncollagenous matrix proteins such as bone sialoprotein and osteopontin, they may mediate initial mineralization and fiber attachment. Mineralized tissues such as bone are turning over continually and require a delicate balance between formative and resorptive cells.

Two key factors that have emerged as critical to this balance are osteoprotegerin and receptor-activated NF-κB ligand (RANKL). Both are produced by osteoblasts and PDL fibroblasts. As discussed in more detail in Chapter 6, RANKL activates osteoclasts by binding to specific osteoclast cell surface receptors (RANK), whereas osteoprotegerin acts as a decoy interfering with the binding of RANKL to RANK. Growth factors and cytokines in the local region of the periodontium have been shown to modulate expression of osteoprotegerin and RANKL and thus may be important for controlling osteoclastic-mediated bone

and root resorption; thus they may be attractive factors in designing therapeutic agents to regulate the behavior of this cell.

Equally important to the process of cell maturation and function are the timed expression of specific cell surface receptors and the ability of certain factors to regulate their expression and, subsequently, the signalling pathways mediated by ligand-receptor interactions.

CEMENTUM VARIETIES

Table 9-2 lists the various types of cementum along with the origin, location, and function of each.

ACELLULAR EXTRINSIC FIBER CEMENTUM (PRIMARY CEMENTUM)

Cementoblasts that produce *acellular extrinsic fiber cementum* differentiate in proximity to the advancing root edge. During root development in human teeth, the first cementoblasts align along the newly formed but not yet mineralized mantle dentin (predentin) surface following disintegration of HERS (Figure 9-7, A and B). The cementoblasts exhibit fibroblastic characteristics, extend cell processes into the unmineralized dentin, and deposit collagen fibrils within it so that the dentin and cementum fibrils intermingle. Mineralization of the mantle dentin starts internally and does not reach the surface until mingling has occurred. Mineralization then spreads across into cementum under the regulatory influence of noncollagenous matrix proteins, thereby establishing the *cementodentinal junction*. In rodents, initial cementum deposition occurs onto the already mineralized dentin surface, preventing the intermingling of fibers (see Figure 9-3, A).

Initial acellular extrinsic fiber cementum consists of a mineralized layer with a short fringe of collagen fibers implanted perpendicular to the root surface (Figure 9-7, D). The cells on the root surface then migrate away from the surface but continue to deposit collagen so that the fine

---

TABLE 9-2   Type, Distribution, and Function of Cementum

TYPE	ORIGIN OF FIBERS	LOCATION	FUNCTION
Acellular (primary)	Extrinsic (some intrinsic fibers initially)	From cervical margin to the apical third	Anchorage
Cellular (secondary)	Intrinsic	Middle to apical third and furcations	Adaptation and repair
Mixed (alternating layers of acellular and cellular)	Intrinsic and extrinsic	Apical portion and furcations	Adaptation
Acellular afibrillar	—	Spurs and patches over enamel and dentin	No known function along the cementoenamel junction

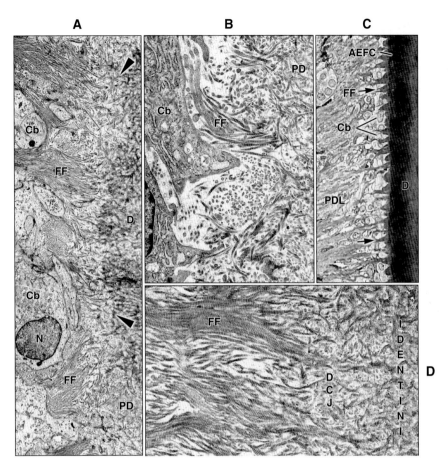

Figure 9-7 Early human acellular extrinsic fiber cementogenesis *(AEFC)*. **A,** Intermingling of collagen fiber bundles with those at the unmineralized dentin (predentin, *PD*) surface. Arrowheads indicate the external dentin mineralization front. **B,** Details of the intermingling. **C,** The final connection between the collagen fiber bundles of acellular (primary) cementum and dentin *(D)* surface are shown. **D,** The fibrous fringe *(FF)* extending from cementum. *Cb,* Cementoblast; *DCJ,* dentinocemental junction; *FF,* fiber fringe; *N,* nucleus; *PDL,* periodontal ligament. *(Courtesy D.D. Bosshardt.)*

fiber bundles lengthen and thicken. These cells also secrete noncollagenous matrix proteins that fill in the spaces between the collagen fibers (Figure 9-8). This activity continues until about 15 to 20 µm of cementum has been formed, at which time the forming PDL fiber bundles become stitched to the fibrous fringe. Thereafter, the cementoblasts will synthesize and secrete only noncollagenous matrix proteins, and the collagen fibrils that embed in the cementum layer will be formed by PDL fibroblasts. Although this cementum variety is called acellular extrinsic fiber cementum, one may question whether its initial part should be classified instead as having intrinsic fibers. As described previously, the collagenous matrix of the first-formed cementum results from cementum-associated cells and is elaborated before the PDL forms; therefore the collagen is of local or intrinsic origin. This cementum variety develops slowly as the tooth is erupting and is considered to be acellular because the cells that form it remain on its surface (Figure 9-7, C).

With the light microscope, acellular extrinsic fiber cementum seems relatively structureless (Figure 9-9, A); however, two sets of striations can be seen with special stains or polarized light. The striations running parallel to the root surface indicate incremental deposition, whereas the short striations at right angles to the root surface indicate the inserted mineralized PDL collagen fiber bundles (Figure 9-10). With the electron microscope, these collagen bundles can be seen clearly to enter cementum, where they become fully mineralized (Figure 9-11). No morphologically distinct layer of cementoid, akin to osteoid or predentin, can be distinguished on the surface of this cementum, which argues for the case that this cementum represents progressive mineralization of the follicle/PDL region by the accumulation of noncollagenous matrix proteins around the fiber bundles. The overall degree of mineralization of this cementum is about 45% to 60%, but soft x-ray examination reveals that the innermost layer is less mineralized and that the outer layers are characterized by

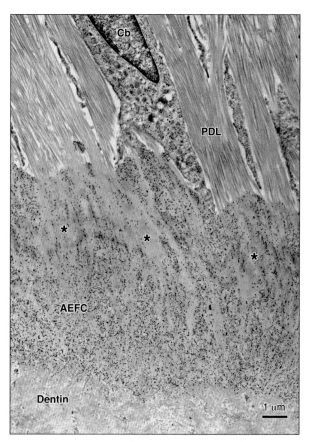

Figure 9-8 Colloidal gold immunocytochemical preparation illustrating the presence and distribution of osteopontin *(black dots)*, a major noncollagenous matrix protein, in rat acellular extrinsic fiber cementum *(AEFC)*. This protein accumulates between the inserted portions of the extrinsic collagen fibers *(asterisks)* and is more concentrated near dentin where collagen fibers are sparse and more loosely arranged. *Cb,* Cementoblast; *PDL,* periodontal ligament.

alternating bands of more and less mineral content that run parallel to the root surface.

CELLULAR INTRINSIC FIBER CEMENTUM (SECONDARY CEMENTUM)

In teeth some teeth (see the following discussion), after at least half the root is formed, a more rapidly formed and less mineralized variety of cementum, *cellular intrinsic fiber cementum*, is deposited on the unmineralized dentin surface near the advancing root edge (see Figure 9-3, *B*). Differentiating cementoblasts extend cell processes into the unmineralized dentin and deposit the collagen fibrils so that fibrils from both layers intermingle. These cells also manufacture various noncollagenous matrix proteins that fill in the spaces between collagen fibrils, regulate mineral deposition, and together with the mineral, impart cohesion to the cementum layer. A layer of

unmineralized matrix, called cementoid, is present at the surface of the mineralized cementum matrix, with a mineralization front between the two layers (Figures 9-11 and 9-13). In contrast to osteoid or predentin, cementoid is not as regular and readily discernible. As cementum deposition progresses, cementoblasts become entrapped in the extracellular matrix they secrete (Figures 9-9, *B*; 9-12; and 9-14). These entrapped cells, with reduced secretory activity, are called *cementocytes*, and, similarly to osteocytes, reside in a *lacuna*. Histologic studies suggest that incorporation of cementoblasts within cementum is more haphazard than that of osteoblasts within bone. Cementocytes have processes that lodge in canaliculi that communicate but do not form a syncytium that extends all the way to the surface, as is the case within bone (see Figure 9-12). Nourishment of the cells is believed to occur essentially by diffusion, and cementocytes in deeper layers may not be vital. With the electron microscope, cementocytes present a variable picture, depending on the distance of their location from the cement surface and their nutritional supply from the PDL. Loss of intracellular organelles and ultimate cell death is progressive in the deeper layers of cellular cementum. Although such features are consistent with loss of cell function, they also may reflect poor tissue preservation in the deeper layers. After a rapid initial phase of matrix formation, the deposition rate slows down and secretion occurs in a more directional manner. This may sometimes lead to the formation of a layer of acellular intrinsic fiber cementum because the cells are not engulfed in their matrix but remain on its surface.

Collagen fibrils are deposited haphazardly during the rapid phase; however, subsequently the bulk of fibrils organize as bundles oriented parallel to the root surface. When the PDL becomes organized, cellular cementum continues to be deposited around the ligament fiber bundles, which become incorporated into the cementum and partially mineralized, thereby creating cellular *mixed* fiber cementum. This constitutes the bulk of secondary cementum, and with the light microscope this tissue is identified easily because of (1) inclusion of cementocytes within lacunae with processes in canaliculi directed toward the tooth surface (see Figure 9-12), (2) its laminated structure, and (3) the presence of cementoid on its surface. Distinguishing between the fine-fibered, densely packed intrinsic fibers running parallel to the root surface and the larger, haphazardly incorporated extrinsic fibers of the PDL running at right angles to the root surface is also easy (see Figure 9-13). The intrinsic fibers are mineralized uniformly, whereas the extrinsic fiber bundles are mineralized variably, with many having a central, unmineralized core.

Cellular (secondary) cementum differs from acellular (primary) cementum in a number of ways. Not only are

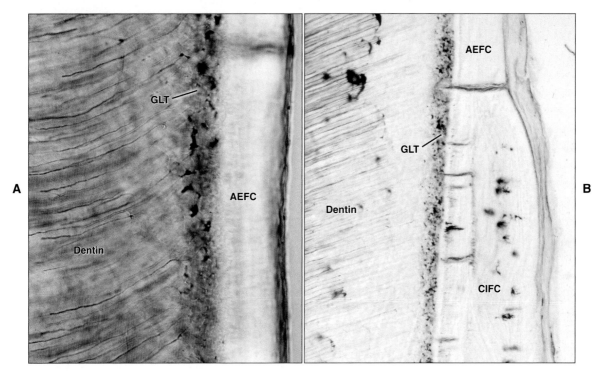

Figure 9-9 Ground sections of human teeth examined by transmitted light illustrating **(A)** acellular extrinsic fiber cementum *(AEFC)* and **(B)** the transition between the former and cellular intrinsic fiber cementum *(CIFC)*. Both appear as a translucent, structureless layer. Cementocytes *(dark, rounded structures)* are present in the cellular intrinsic fiber cementum. *GLT*, Granular layer of Tomes (see Chapter 8).

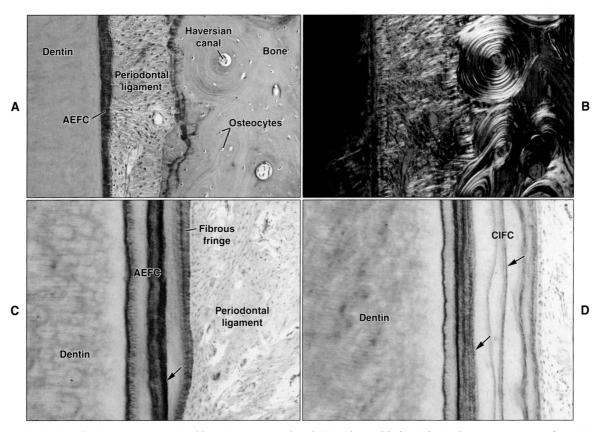

Figure 9-10 Histologic section examined by **(A)** transmitted and **(B)** polarized light. Polarized microscopy reveals striations in the cementum layer. **C** and **D**, Longitudinal *(arrows)* and perpendicular lines are also visible with some histologic stains. The longitudinal layering can appear as thin or thicker lines, essentially denoting the interface between successive layers of cementum. *AEFC*, Acellular extrinsic fiber cementum; *CIFC*, cellular intrinsic fiber cementum. *(**A** and **B** courtesy P. Tambasco de Oliveira.)*

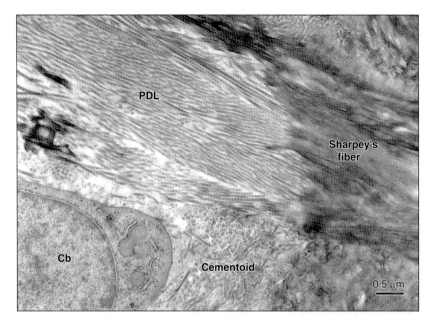

Figure 9-11 Electron micrograph illustrating the insertion of periodontal ligament *(PDL)* fiber bundles into cellular intrinsic fiber cementum. *Cb,* Cementoblast.

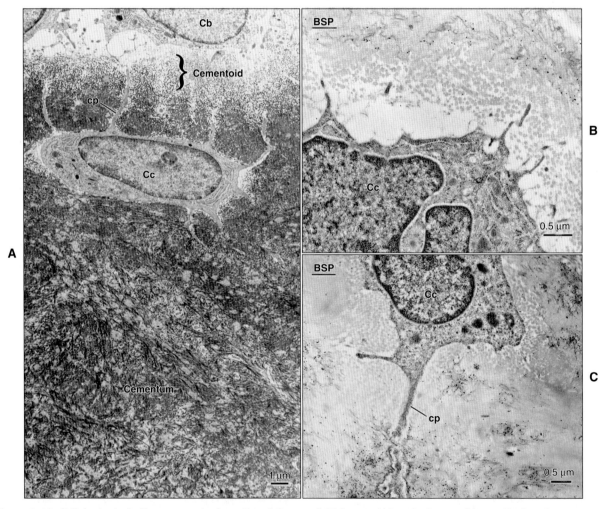

Figure 9-12 Cellular intrinsic fiber cementum from (**A** and **C**) rat and (**B**) human being. **A,** Cementoblasts *(Cb)* line the cementum surface and are apposed against a layer of unmineralized matrix (cementoid). **A** to **C,** Cementocytes *(Cc)* reside within lacunae in cementum and can adopt various shapes. **A,** The cell processes *(cp)* of cementocytes generally are directed toward the surface. **B** and **C,** Immunocytochemical preparations for bone sialoprotein *(BSP)*. This noncollagenous matrix protein (indicated by the presence of *black dots*) accumulates among the mineralized collagen in regions that are generally more electron dense.

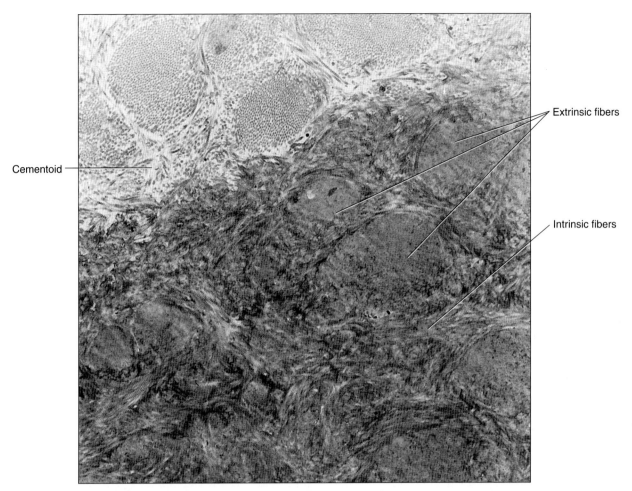

Cementoid

Extrinsic fibers

Intrinsic fibers

Figure 9-13 Electron micrograph of an oblique section through the periodontal ligament–cementum interface. The distinction between extrinsic and intrinsic fibers within cementum is readily apparent, the intrinsic fibers essentially surrounding the embedded portions of the extrinsic fibers, which constitute Sharpey's fibers. *(Courtesy M.A. Listgarten.)*

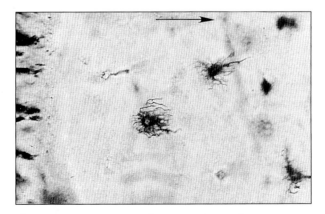

Figure 9-14 Cementocyte lacunae in ground section. Most of the canaliculi point toward the tooth surface *(arrow)*. The indistinct dark patches are other cementocyte lacunae deeper within the ground section (and consequently out of focus).

structural differences obvious in that the cells are incorporated into the matrix, but also the phenotype of the cells producing them may differ. Furthermore, secondary cementum is involved in tooth attachment in a minor and secondary way (this variety of cementum is usually absent from incisor and canine teeth) and is confined to the apical and interradicular regions of the tooth. As one can see, secondary cementum is deposited first as an unmineralized layer, called cementoid, which calcifies gradually at the mineralization front (see Figure 9-13).

ACELLULAR AFIBRILLAR CEMENTUM

The *acellular afibrillar cementum* variety consists of an acellular and afibrillar mineralized matrix with a texture similar to the one found among the collagen fibrils of fibrillar cementum varieties and of bone. This cementum lacks collagen and hence plays no role in tooth attachment. Under the light microscope, acellular afibrillar cementum appears rather uniform, but transmission electron microscopy reveals layers with variable electron density and texture. This cementum is deposited over enamel and dentin in proximity to the cementoenamel junction (Figure 9-15, A).

The cells responsible for the production of acellular afibrillar cementum still have not been identified with precision. For a long time, this cementum variety has been believed to represent a developmental anomaly formed as the result of local disruptions in the reduced dental epithelium that permit follicular cells to come into contact with the enamel surface and differentiate into cementoblasts. This concept has come under questioning because the enamel organ itself has been demonstrated to be able to produce mesenchymal proteins found in bone and cementum. Hence the reduced dental epithelium need not obligatorily retract from the enamel surface to result in deposition of afibrillar cementum.

Researchers also have reported that HERS may produce epithelial products that accumulate on the forming root surface to form a layer, referred to as *intermediate cementum*. To date, however, no study has demonstrated the consistent presence of a distinct matrix layer between dentin and cementum proper. The apparent presence of a layer along the radicular dentin surface in some histologic preparations (see Figure 9-10, C and D) may result from the way dentin and cementum collagen interface and the packing density of noncollagenous matrix proteins among the collagen fibrils.

DISTRIBUTION OF CEMENTUM VARIETIES ALONG THE ROOT

In human beings, acellular afibrillar cementum is limited to the cervical enamel surface and occurs as spurs extending from acellular extrinsic fiber cementum or as isolated patches on the enamel surface close to the cementoenamel junction. Acellular extrinsic fiber cementum, which becomes the principal tissue of attachment, extends from the cervical margin of the tooth and covers two thirds of the root and often more. Indeed, in incisors and canines, this form of cementum is often the only one found, and it extends to the apical foramen.

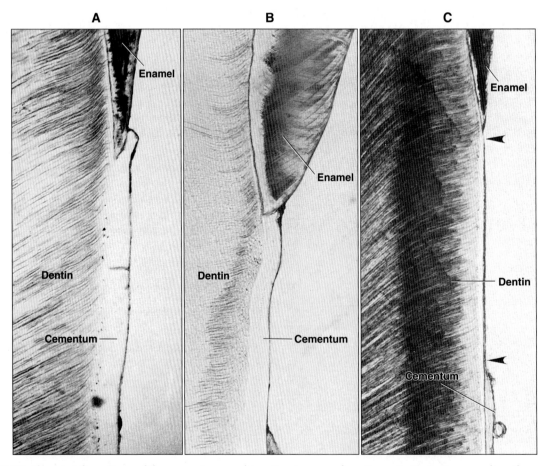

Figure 9-15 Three configurations of the cementoenamel junction in ground sections. **A,** Cementum overlaps the enamel. **B,** A butt joint is visible. **C,** A deficiency of cementum (between the *arrowheads*) leaves root dentin exposed.

At the cervical margin, the cementum is some 50 μm thick and increases in thickness as it progresses apically to some 200 μm. Cellular cementum is confined to the apical third and interradicular regions of premolar and molar teeth. Cellular cementum is often absent from single-rooted teeth, which indicates that its presence is not essential for tooth support. Both fibrillar cementum varieties can overlap. As mentioned before, the type of cementum formed during periodontal wound healing appears to be cellular in origin. Existing data suggest that formation of cementum is important for creating an environment for predictable regeneration of tissues lost as a consequence of periodontal disease.

CEMENTOENAMEL JUNCTION

Classically, in approximately 30% of human teeth the cementum and enamel meet as a butt joint, forming a distinct cementoenamel junction at the cervical margin; 10% have a gap between the cementum and enamel, exposing root dentin; and in about 60% the cementum overlaps the enamel. This information was obtained from the study of ground sections (Figure 9-15), but studies with the scanning electron microscope indicate that the cementoenamel junction may exhibit all of these forms and shows considerable variation when traced circumferentially. The exposure of root dentin at the cervical margin can lead to sensitivity at this site, and some suggestion has been made that such morphology may result in increased risk for idiopathic osteoclast-mediated root resorption and root surface caries.

ATTACHMENT OF CEMENTUM ONTO DENTIN

The attachment mechanism of cementum to dentin is of biologic interest and of clinical relevance because pathologic alterations and clinical interventions may influence the nature of the exposed root surface and hence the quality of the new attachment that forms when repair cementum is deposited. The mechanism by which these hard tissues bind together is essentially the same for acellular extrinsic fiber cementum and cellular intrinsic fiber cementum. Mineralization of the mantle dentin starts internally and does not reach the surface until the collagen fibrils of dentin and cementum have had the time to blend together. Mineralization then spreads through the surface layer of dentin, across the dentin-cementum junction and into cementum, essentially resulting in an amalgamated mass of mineral. Although initiation of dentin mineralization occurs in relation to matrix vesicles, the subsequent spread of mineral deposition is under the regulatory influence of the various noncollagenous matrix proteins. From a biomechanical perspective, this arrangement appears optimal for a strong union between dentin and cementum. In acellular extrinsic fiber cementum of rodent teeth, cementum is deposited onto mineralized dentin, making amalgamation of dentin and cementum impossible and establishing a weakened interface. Indeed, histologic sections of rodent teeth often show a separation between dentin and cementum in the cervical third of the root. Interestingly, repair cementum adheres well to the root surface if a resorptive phase precedes new matrix deposition, implying that odontoclasts not only remove mineral and matrix but also that most likely at the end of the process they precondition the root surface. One possibility is that odontoclasts generate an organic matrix fringe with which the matrix of reparative cementum then can blend, thereby recapitulating the developmental sequence.

ALVEOLAR PROCESS

The *alveolar process* is that bone of the jaws containing the sockets (alveoli) for the teeth (Figure 9-16). The alveolar process consists of an outer (buccal and lingual) *cortical plate*, a *central spongiosa*, and bone lining the alveolus (*alveolar bone*). The cortical plate and alveolar bone meet at the alveolar crest (usually 1.5 to 2 mm below the level of the cementoenamel junction on the tooth it surrounds). Alveolar bone comprises inner and outer components; it is perforated by many foramina, which transmit nerves and vessels; thus it sometimes is referred to as the *cribriform plate*. Radiographically, alveolar bone also is referred to as the *lamina dura* because of an increased radiopacity (Figure 9-17). This increased radiopacity is due to the presence of thick bone without trabeculations that x-rays must penetrate and not to any increased mineral content.

The bone directly lining the socket (inner aspect of alveolar bone) specifically is referred to as *bundle bone*. Embedded within this bone are the extrinsic collagen fiber bundles of the PDL (Figure 9-18), which, as in cellular cementum, are mineralized only at their periphery. Bundle bone thus provides attachment for the PDL fiber bundles that insert into it. Histologically, bundle bone generally is described as containing less intrinsic collagen fibrils than lamellar bone and exhibiting a coarse-fibered texture. Bundle bone is apposed to an outer layer of lamellar bone, but in some cases the alveolar bone can be made up almost completely of bundle bone. This is a simplistic description, however, because the tooth constantly is making minor movements, and therefore the bone of the socket wall constantly must adapt to many forms of stress. Thus practically all histologic forms of bone can be observed lining the alveolus, even in the same field in the same

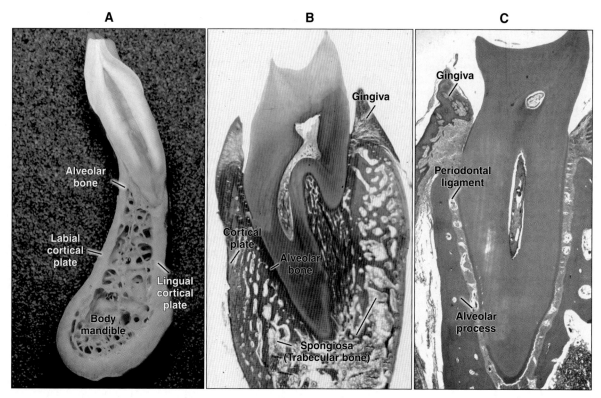

Figure 9-16 A, Trabecular bone *(arrow)* is found between the lingual cortical plate and alveolar bone in the region of the apical third of the root and in the body of the mandible. **B** and **C,** Histologic sections illustrating **(B)** a thick alveolar process with an abundant spongiosa (trabecular bone) between the cortical plates and alveolar bone and **(C)** a thin alveolar process lacking trabecular bone and where the cortical plates and alveolar bone are fused together. *(A courtesy P. Tambasco de Oliveira.)*

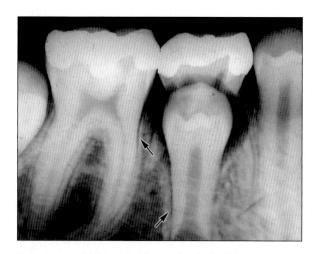

Figure 9-17 Radiograph of an individual whose permanent dentition is still in formation. The second permanent, inferior premolar is erupting between the first permanent premolar and molar. The denser bone *(arrows)* along the roots of the teeth is the lamina dura. The presence of important dental restorations on the deciduous and permanent teeth is notable. *(Courtesy M. Michaud.)*

section (Figure 9-19). This considerable variation reflects the functional plasticity of alveolar bone.

The cortical plate consists of surface layers of lamellar bone supported by compact haversian system bone of variable thickness. The cortical plate is generally thinner in the maxilla and thickest on the buccal aspect of mandibular premolar and molars. The trabecular (or spongy) bone occupying the central part of the alveolar process also consists of bone disposed in lamellae with haversian systems occurring in the large trabeculae. Yellow marrow, rich in adipose cells, generally fills the intertrabecular spaces, although sometimes there also can be some red or hematopoietic marrow. Trabecular bone is absent in the region of the anterior teeth, and in this case, the cortical plate and alveolar bone are fused together. The important part of this complex in terms of tooth support is the bundle bone.

PERIODONTAL LIGAMENT

Understanding the cell populations and their function in healthy, mature periodontal tissues is required for developing predictable regenerative therapies.

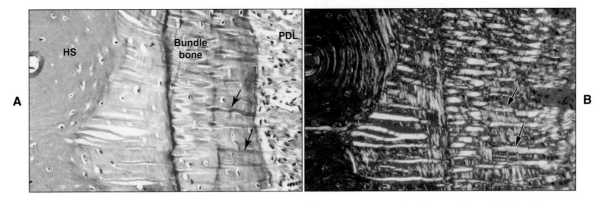

Figure 9-18 Histologic preparations of alveolar bone examined by **(A)** transmitted and **(B)** polarized light microscopy. Periodontal ligament fiber bundles *(arrows)* insert into the bone lining the alveolar socket, giving it the name *bundle bone*. The inserted fibers are referred to as Sharpey's fibers and appear refringent under polarized light. Bundle bone is apposed to trabecular bone with haversian systems *(HS)*. *(Courtesy P. Tambasco De Oliveira.)*

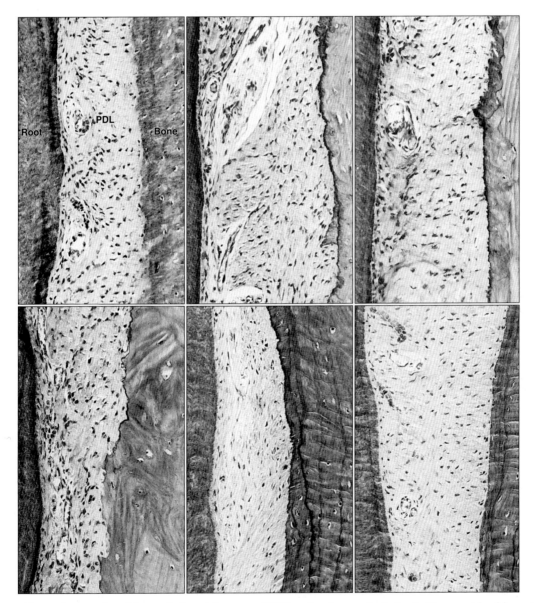

Figure 9-19 Photomicrographs of the periodontal ligament *(PDL)* region from a single tooth. The considerable variation in morphology of the bone lining this alveolus is produced by the resorption and deposition of bone as it responds to functional demands placed on it. The root surface is always on the left and bone on the right.

Investigations to date suggest that the PDL region in health contains a heterogeneous population of mesenchymal cells and that some cells within this population, when triggered appropriately, can differentiate toward an osteoblast or cementoblast phenotype, that is, promote formation of bone and cementum. In addition, perivascular and endosteal fibroblasts, again when appropriately induced, have the capacity to form PDL, cementum, and bone. An important point is that compelling evidence exists indicating that populations of cells within the PDL, during development and during regeneration, secrete factors that can regulate the extent of mineralization. Thus factors secreted by PDL fibroblasts may inhibit mineralization and prevent the fusion of tooth root with surrounding bone, for example, ankylosis. Although much research is still to be done, current knowledge has enabled development of improved strategies for attracting and maintaining cells at a regenerative site.

The PDL is that soft, specialized connective tissue situated between the cementum covering the root of the tooth and the bone forming the socket wall. The PDL ranges in width from 0.15 to 0.38 mm, with its thinnest portion around the middle third of the root (Figures 9-20 and 9-21). The average width is 0.21 mm at 11 to 16 years of age, 0.18 mm at 32 to 52 years, and 0.15 mm

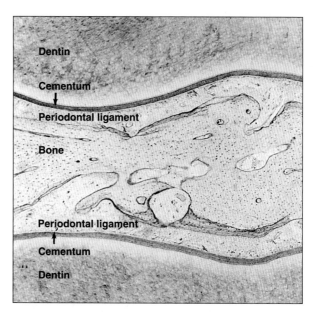

Figure 9-21 Periodontal ligament in a cross section between two teeth.

at 51 to 67 years, showing a progressive decrease with age. The PDL is a connective tissue particularly well adapted to its principal function, supporting the teeth in their sockets and at the same time permitting them to withstand the considerable forces of mastication. The PDL also has the important function, in addition to attaching teeth to bone, of acting as a sensory receptor, which is necessary for the proper positioning of the jaws during normal function.

Apart from recognition that the PDL is formed within the developing dental follicle region, the exact timing of events associated with the development of an organized PDL varies among species, with individual tooth families, and between deciduous and permanent teeth. What follows is a generalized account from several studies undertaken largely on primates. At the commencement of ligament formation the ligament space consists of unorganized connective tissue with short fiber bundles extending into it from the bone and cemental surfaces (Figure 9-22). Next, ligament mesenchymal cells begin to secrete collagen (mostly type I collagen), which assembles as collagen bundles extending from the bone and cementum surfaces to establish continuity across the ligament space and thereby secure an attachment of the tooth to bone. In addition to collagen, several noncollagenous proteins are secreted that appear to play a role in the maintenance of the PDL space. Eruptive tooth movement and the establishment of occlusion then modify this initial attachment. For example, before the tooth erupts, the crest of the alveolar bone is above the cementoenamel junction, and the developing fiber bundles of the PDL are directed obliquely. Because the tooth moves during eruption, the level of the alveolar

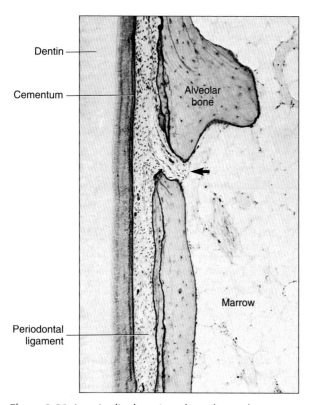

Figure 9-20 Longitudinal section along the tooth root. Note the perforation *(arrow)* in the alveolar bone that transmits neurovascular bundles.

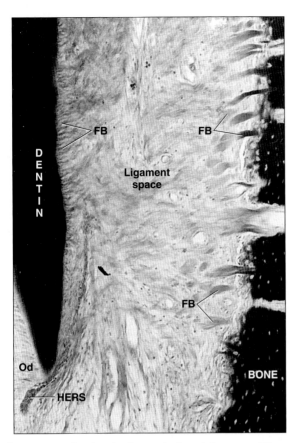

Figure 9-22 The developing periodontal ligament. Fiber bundles *(FB)* extend into the unorganized ligament space from the cement and alveolar bone surfaces. *HERS,* Hertwig's epithelial root sheath; *Od,* odontoblasts.

crest comes to coincide with the cementoenamel junction, and the oblique fiber bundles just below the free gingival fibers become horizontally aligned. During the process of tooth eruption, osteoclast precursors are activated by a variety of factors secreted by cells within the local environment, including NF-κB ligand (RANKL/osteoprotegerin ligand) and macrophage colony-stimulating factor. Functional osteoclasts are critical for the formation of marrow spaces within bone and for tooth eruption. When the tooth finally comes into function, the alveolar crest is positioned nearer the apex. The horizontal fibers, termed the *alveolar crest fibers,* have become oblique once more, with the difference that now the cemental attachment has reversed its relation to the alveolar attachment and is positioned in a coronal direction, as opposed to its previous apical direction (Figure 9-23). Only after the teeth come into function do the fiber bundles of the PDL thicken appreciably.

Similar to all other connective tissues, the PDL consists of cells and an extracellular compartment of collagenous fibers and a noncollagenous extracellular matrix. The cells include osteoblasts and osteoclasts (technically within the ligament but functionally associated with bone), fibroblasts, epithelial cell rests of Malassez, macrophages, undifferentiated mesenchymal cells, and cementoblasts (also technically within the ligament but functionally associated with cementum). The extracellular compartment consists of well-defined collagen fiber bundles (Figure 9-24) embedded in an

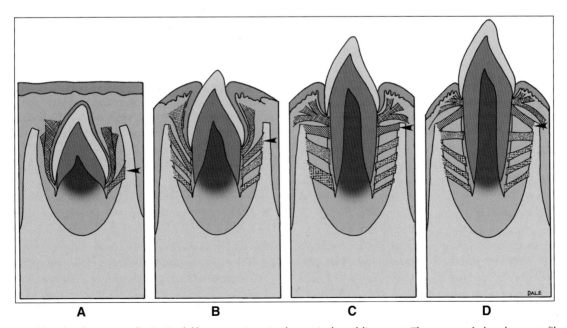

Figure 9-23 The development of principal fiber groupings in the periodontal ligament. The group of alveolar crest fibers *(arrowheads),* first forming in **A,** are initially oblique **(B),** then horizontal **(C),** and then oblique again **(D).**

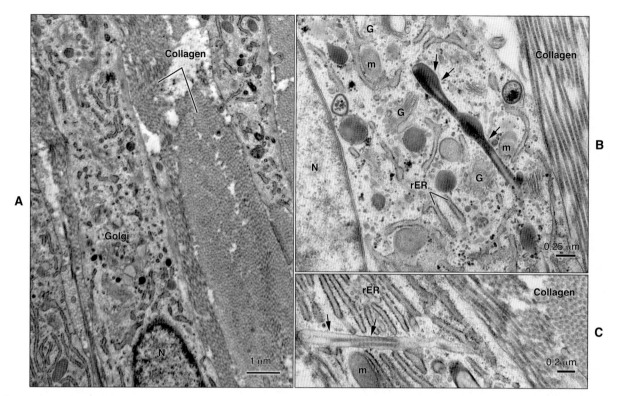

Figure 9-24 Electron micrographs of the periodontal ligament in pig. **A,** Elongated fibroblasts can be seen alternating with distinctive collagen fiber bundles. The clear areas are occupied by ground substance. **B** and **C,** The periodontal ligament undergoes turnover and remodeling during which matrix synthesis and breakdown take place. Some collagen degradation takes place intracellularly following its internalization *(arrows)*. *G,* Golgi complex; *m,* mitochondria; *N,* nucleus; *rER,* rough endoplasmic reticulum.

amorphous background material, known as ground substance, consisting of, among others, glycosaminoglycans, glycoproteins, and glycolipids.

FIBROBLASTS

The principal cells of the PDL are fibroblasts. Although fibroblasts look alike microscopically, heterogeneous cell populations exist between different connective tissues and also within the same connective tissue. In the case of the PDL, its fibroblasts are characterized by an ability to achieve an exceptionally high rate of turnover of proteins within the extracellular compartment, in particular, collagen. PDL fibroblasts are large cells with an extensive cytoplasm containing an abundance of organelles associated with protein synthesis and secretion (i.e., rough endoplasmic reticulum, Golgi complex, and many secretory granules). Ligament fibroblasts also have a well-developed cytoskeleton (see Chapter 4) with a particularly prominent actin network, the presence of which is thought to indicate the functional demands placed on the cells, requiring change in shape and migration.

Ligament fibroblasts also show frequent cell-to-cell contacts of the adherens and the gap junction types. Fibroblasts are aligned along the general direction of the fiber bundles and have extensive processes that wrap around the bundles. The collagen fibrils of the fiber bundles are being remodeled continuously. Visualizing how a concerted and balanced activity of two cell types, the osteoblast and the osteoclast, achieve the remodeling of a bone is straightforward. In the PDL a single cell, the fibroblast, achieves remodeling of collagen; it is capable of simultaneously synthesizing and degrading collagen (see Chapter 4). Because of the exceptionally high rate of turnover of collagen in the ligament, any interference with fibroblast function by disease rapidly produces a loss of the supporting tissue of a tooth. Importantly, in inflammatory situations, such as those associated with periodontal diseases, an increased expression of matrix metalloproteinases occurs that aggressively destroys collagen. Thus attractive therapies for controlling tissue destruction may include host modulators that have the capacity to inhibit matrix metalloproteinases.

TOPICS FOR CONSIDERATION   Fibroblast Contractility

The basic structure and functions of fibroblasts were discussed in Chapter 4, where it was mentioned that fibroblasts exhibit motility, which requires intracelluar contractile proteins, and that fibroblasts in certain tissues have significant contractile properties. These latter cells exhibit features characteristic of smooth muscle cells, such as substantial amounts of intracellular microfilaments and expression of α–smooth muscle actin. Fibroblasts with these features, often called *myofibroblasts*, also make connections with the extracellular matrix through fibronexus. Examples of tissues containing myofibroblasts include the capsules of several organs, such as the spleen and adrenal glands, the perineurium surrounding nerve bundles, the core of the intestinal villus, tendons, and ligaments. Myofibroblasts present in connective tissues undergoing repair and regeneration after wounding are responsible for contraction of the wound. Fibroblasts cultured from regenerating wounds and other tissues are capable of exerting force sufficient to contract their extracellular matrix. Myofibroblasts have been implicated in the contracture of the palmar fascia that leads to Dupuytren's disease. Myofibroblasts also are the predominant cell type in the connective tissue stroma of most carcinomata, where they exhibit a greater rate of proliferation, release of growth factors, and expression of certain extracellular matrix proteins than their counterparts in normal tissues.

Fibroblasts exhibiting myofibroblastic characteristics, specifically abundant actin filaments and fibronexus, are present in the periodontal ligament (PDL). By exerting tension on their extracellular matrix, PDL fibroblasts placed in culture with a slice of root dentin are able to move the piece of dentin. If the growing end of a continuously erupting tooth, such as the rat incisor, is removed, the incisal end of the tooth continues to erupt, apparently as a result of force exerted by the PDL. Based on these and other observations, it has been proposed that the contraction of fibroblasts in the dental follicle and developing PDL is responsible for the process of tooth eruption, essentially "pulling" the tooth into the oral cavity. More recent studies have emphasized the importance of localized bone resorption and formation during the intraosseous phase of tooth eruption. This process appears to be regulated by growth factors and other signaling molecules produced by the dental follicle and stellate reticulum.

Fibroblast contractility probably is of greatest significance during posteruptive tooth movements. These include functional movements during mastication, accommodation for growth of the jaws, and compensation for occlusal and interproximal wear. Fibroblasts are associated intimately with the fibrous components of their matrix and respond to changes in tension and compression in the matrix. Integrins, which bind to extracellular matrix components, serve as mechanotransducers to transmit the stimulus to the cell. In addition to contraction, the response of the cell may encompass the pulling of collagen fibrils back toward the cell, the movement of cell processes or individual receptors on the processes, or a combination of all of these events. The fibroblasts and the collagen align parallel to the direction of the principal strain in the matrix, which probably accounts for the highly ordered arrangement of the PDL fiber bundles.

Mechanical stress also is a significant stimulus for extracellular matrix production by fibroblasts; the repetitive stress to which the PDL is subjected presumably contributes to the high rates of collagen turnover in this tissue. This rapid turnover of matrix components allows the PDL to adapt to the demands of functional tooth movements. Localized changes in tensile and compressive forces during growth, and the mesial drift resulting from interproximal wear, stimulate bone and cementum formation or resorption. In contrast, the absence of these forces, such as when a tooth has no opponent, results in decreased matrix production, increased collagenase (matrix metalloproteinase 1) secretion, and a thinning of the PDL.

Arthur R. Hand, DDS
Department of Pediatric Dentistry
University of Connecticut Health Center
Farmington, Connecticut

EPITHELIAL CELLS

The epithelial cells in the PDL are remnants of HERS, known as the epithelial cell rests of Malassez. The epithelial cells occur close to the cementum as clusters or strands of cells easily recognized in histologic sections because their nuclei generally stain deeply (see Figure 9-6).

UNDIFFERENTIATED MESENCHYMAL CELLS

An important cellular constituent of the PDL is the undifferentiated mesenchymal cell or progenitor cell; these cells have a perivascular location. Although they have been demonstrated to be a source of new cells for the PDL, whether a single progenitor cell gives rise to daughter cells that differentiate into fibroblasts, osteoblasts, and cementoblasts or whether separate progenitors exist for each cell line is not known. The fact that new cells are being produced for the PDL while cells of the ligament are in a steady state means that this production of new cells must be balanced by migration of cells out of the ligament or cell death. Selective deletion of ligament cells occurs by apoptosis (see Chapter 7), and this process provides cell turnover, which in the rat PDL involves approximately 2% of the population at any time.

BONE AND CEMENTUM CELLS

Although technically situated within the PDL, bone and cementum cells are associated properly with the hard tissues they form and are discussed with these tissues.

FIBERS

The predominant collagens of the PDL are types I, III, and XII, with individual fibrils having a smaller average diameter than tendon collagen fibrils. This difference is thought to reflect the short half-life of ligament collagen, meaning that they have less time for fibrillar assembly.

Most collagen fibrils in the PDL are arranged in definite and distinct fiber bundles. Each bundle resembles a spliced rope; individual strands can be remodeled continually, whereas the overall fiber maintains its architecture and function. In this way the fiber bundles are able to adapt to the continual stresses placed on them. These bundles are arranged in groups that can be seen easily in an appropriately stained light microscope section (Figures 9-25 and 9-26). Those bundles running between the tooth and bone represent the *principal fiber bundles* of the PDL. These bundles are as follows:

1. The *alveolar crest group*, attached to the cementum just below the cementoenamel junction and running downward and outward to insert into the rim of the alveolus
2. The *horizontal group*, just apical to the alveolar crest group and running at right angles to the long axis of the tooth from cementum to bone just below the alveolar crest
3. The *oblique group*, by far the most numerous in the PDL and running from the cementum in an oblique direction to insert into bone coronally
4. The *apical group*, radiating from the cementum around the apex of the root to the bone, forming the base of the socket
5. The *interradicular group*, found only between the roots of multirooted teeth and running from the cementum into the bone, forming the crest of the interradicular septum (see Figure 9-25)

At each end, all the principal collagen fiber bundles of the PDL are embedded in cementum or bone (see Figures 9-7, 9-10, 9-11, 9-18, and 9-22). The embedded portion is referred to as *Sharpey's fiber*. Sharpey's fibers in primary acellular cementum are mineralized fully; those in cellular cementum and bone generally are mineralized only partially at their periphery. Occasionally, Sharpey's fibers pass uninterruptedly through the bone of the alveolar process to continue as principal fibers of an adjacent PDL, or they may mingle buccally and lingually with the fibers of the periosteum that cover the outer cortical plates of the alveolar process. Sharpey's fibers pass through the alveolar process only when the process consists entirely of compact bone and contains no haversian systems, which is not common.

Although not strictly part of the PDL, other groups of collagen fibers are associated with maintaining the functional integrity of the periodontium. These groups are found in the lamina propria of the gingiva and collectively form the *gingival ligament* (see Figures 9-25 and 9-26). Five groups of fiber bundles compose this ligament:

1. *Dentogingival group.* These are the most numerous fibers, extending from cervical cementum to lamina propria of the free and attached gingivae.
2. *Alveologingival group.* These fibers radiate from the bone of the alveolar crest and extend into the lamina propria of the free and attached gingivae.
3. *Circular group.* This small group of fibers forms a band around the neck of the tooth, interlacing with other groups of fibers in the free gingiva and helping to bind the free gingiva to the tooth (see Figure 9-25).
4. *Dentoperiosteal group.* Running apically from the cementum over the periosteum of the outer cortical plates of the alveolar process, these fibers insert into the alveolar process or the vestibular muscle and floor of the mouth.
5. *Transseptal fiber system.* These fibers run interdentally from the cementum just apical to the base of the junctional epithelium of one tooth over the alveolar crest and insert into a comparable region of the cementum of the adjacent tooth. Together these fibers constitute the transseptal fiber system, collectively forming an *interdental ligament* connecting all the teeth of the arch (Figure 9-27). The supracrestal fibers, particularly the transseptal fiber system, have been implicated as a major cause of postretention relapse of orthodontically positioned teeth. The inability of the transseptal fiber system to undergo physiologic rearrangement has led to this conclusion. Although the rate of turnover is not as rapid as in the PDL, studies have shown that the transseptal fiber system is capable of turnover and remodeling under normal physiologic conditions, as well as during therapeutic tooth movement. A sufficiently prolonged

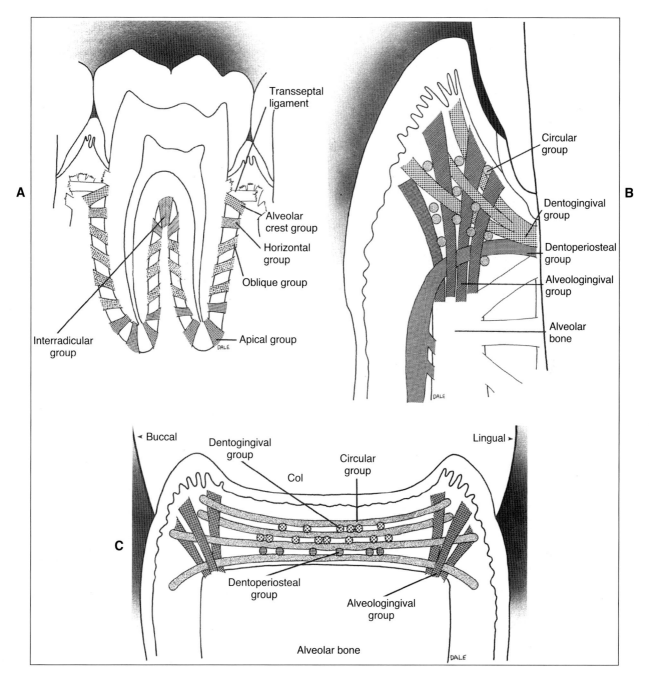

Figure 9-25 The arrangement of the principal fiber groups within the periodontium. **A,** Principal fiber groups. **B,** Fiber groups of the gingival ligament. **C,** Gingival ligament fibers as seen interproximally related to the gingival col.

retention period following orthodontic tooth movement then would seem reasonable to allow reorganization of the transseptal fiber system to ensure the clinical stability of tooth position.

ELASTIC FIBERS

The three types of elastic fibers are *elastin, oxytalan,* and *elaunin*. Only oxytalan fibers are present within the

PDL; however, elaunin fibers also may be found within fibers of the gingival ligament.

Oxytalan fibers (Figure 9-28) are bundles of microfibrils the distribution of which in the PDL is extensive when the ligament is examined in sheets rather than in section. The fibers run more or less vertically from the cementum surface of the root apically, forming a three-dimensional branching meshwork that surrounds the root and terminates in the apical complex

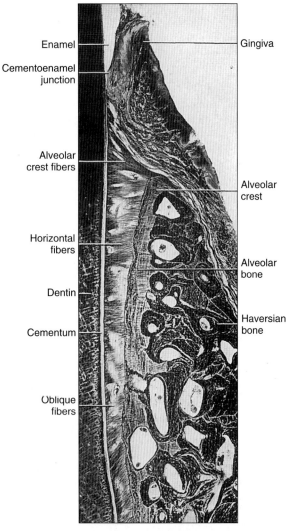

Enamel

Cementoenamel junction

Alveolar crest fibers

Horizontal fibers

Dentin

Cementum

Oblique fibers

Gingiva

Alveolar crest

Alveolar bone

Haversian bone

Figure 9-26 Silver-stained section of some of the fiber groups of the gingival and periodontal ligaments.

of arteries, veins, and lymphatic vessels. The fibers also are associated with neural and vascular elements. Oxytalan fibers are numerous and dense in the cervical region of the ligament, where they run parallel to the gingival group of collagen fibers. Although their function has not been determined fully, they are thought to regulate vascular flow in relation to tooth function. Because they are elastic, they can expand in response to tensional variations, with such variations then registered on the walls of the vascular structures.

GROUND SUBSTANCE

Ground substance is an amorphous background material that binds tissue and fluids, the latter serving for the diffusion of gases and metabolic substances. Ground substance is a major constituent of the PDL, but few studies have been undertaken to determine its exact composition. What information exists indicates similarity to most other connective tissues in terms of its components, with some variation in ratios, so that in the ligament dermatan sulfate is the principal glycosaminoglycan. The PDL ground substance has been estimated to be 70% water and is thought to have a significant effect on the ability of the tooth to withstand stress loads. An increase in tissue fluids occurs within the amorphous matrix of the ground substance in areas of injury and inflammation.

When the periodontium is exposed to increased function, the width of the PDL can increase by as much as 50%, and the principal fiber bundles also increase greatly in thickness. The bony trabeculae supporting the alveoli also increase in number and in thickness, and the alveolar bone itself becomes thicker. Conversely, a reduction in function leads to changes that are the

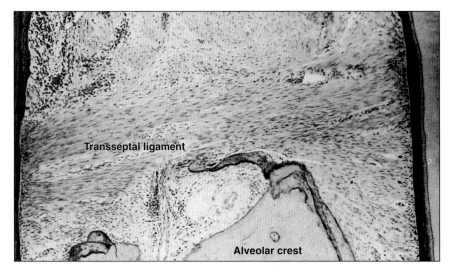

Transseptal ligament

Alveolar crest

Figure 9-27 Transseptal ligament. This fiber grouping is identified in sagittal sections running interdentally between adjacent teeth over the alveolar crest.

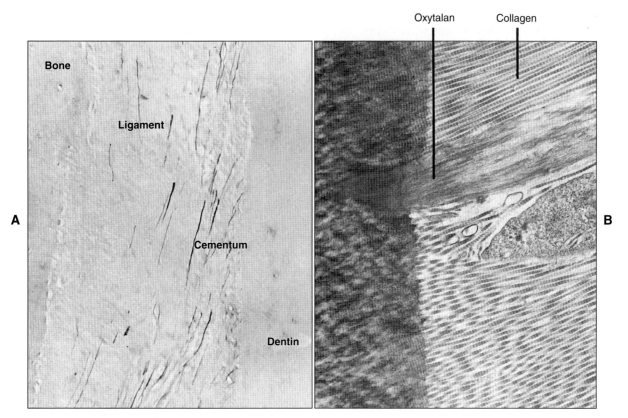

Figure 9-28 Oxytalan fibers seen through **(A)** the light microscope and **(B)** the electron microscope. These fibers run in an oblique direction, often from the cementum to blood vessels.

opposite of those described for excess function. The ligament narrows, the fiber bundles decrease in number and thickness, and the trabeculae become fewer. This reduction in width of the PDL is caused mostly by the deposition of additional cementum (Figure 9-29).

BLOOD SUPPLY

For a connective tissue, the PDL is exceptionally well vascularized, which reflects the high rate of turnover of its cellular and extracellular constituents. The main blood supply of connective tissue is from the superior and inferior alveolar arteries. These arteries pursue an intraosteal course and give off alveolar branches that ascend within the bone as interalveolar arteries. Numerous branches arise from the interalveolar vessels to run horizontally, penetrate the alveolar bone, and enter the PDL space. Because they enter the ligament, they are called *perforating* arteries, and they are more abundant in the PDL of posterior teeth than in that of anterior teeth and are in greater numbers in mandibular than in maxillary teeth. In single-rooted teeth, these arteries are found most frequently in the gingival third of the ligament, followed by the apical third.

This pattern of distribution has clinical importance. In healing of extraction wounds, new tissue invades from the perforations, and the formation of a blood clot occupying the socket is more rapid in its gingival and apical areas. Once within the ligament, these arteries occupy areas (or bays) of loose connective tissue called *interstitial areas* between the principal fiber bundles. Vessels course in an apical-occlusal direction with numerous transverse connections (Figure 9-30). Fenestrated capillaries occur.

Many arteriovenous anastomoses occur within the PDL, and venous drainage is achieved by axially directed vessels that drain into a system of retia (or networks) in the apical portion of the ligament consisting of large-diameter venules (see Figure 9-30). Lymphatic vessels tend to follow the venous drainage.

NERVE SUPPLY

The use of radioautographic and immunocytochemical labeling of neural proteins has greatly improved knowledge about the innervation of the PDL over what previously was based on the results of somewhat unpredictable silver staining techniques. Although species differences have been reported, a general pattern of ligament innervation seems to be present (Figure 9-31). First, the general anatomic configuration is applicable to all teeth, with nerve fibers running from the apical region toward the gingival margin and being

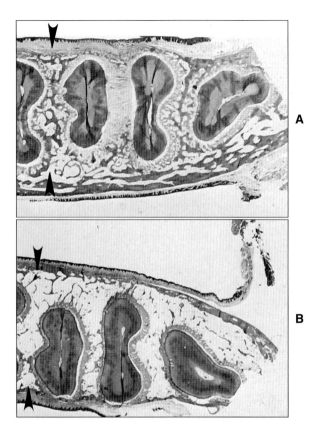

joined by fibers entering laterally through the foramina of the socket wall (see Figure 9-20). These latter fibers divide into two branches, one extending apically and the other gingivally. Second, regional variation occurs in the termination of neural elements, with the apical region of the ligament containing more nerve endings than elsewhere (except for the upper incisors, where not only is the innervation generally denser than in molars but also further dense distributions of neural elements exist in the coronal half of the labial PDL as well as apically, suggesting that the spatial arrangement of receptors is a factor in determining the response characteristics of the ligament). Third, the manner in which these nerve fibers terminate is being clarified. Four types of neural terminations now have been described (Figure 9-32). The first (and most frequent) are free nerve endings that ramify in a treelike configuration. These nerve endings are located at regular intervals along the length of the root, suggesting that each termination controls its own territory, and extend to the cementoblast layer. These nerve endings originate largely from unmyelinated fibers but carry with them a Schwann cell envelope with processes that project into the surrounding connective tissue (Figure 9-33). Such endings are thought to be nociceptors and mechanoreceptors. The second type of nerve terminal is found around the root apex and resembles Ruffini's corpuscles. These nerves appear to be dendritic and end in terminal expansions among the PDL fiber bundles. By electron microscopy, such receptors can be seen to have subdivided further into simple and compound forms, the former consisting

Figure 9-29 Photomicrographs of the effect of nonfunction on the supporting apparatus of the tooth. **A,** Normal appearance of tissues supporting the teeth. **B,** Effect of nonfunction for 6 months. The loss of bone in the area marked by the arrowheads is notable. A narrowing of the ligament also can be distinguished. *(Courtesy D.C. Picton.)*

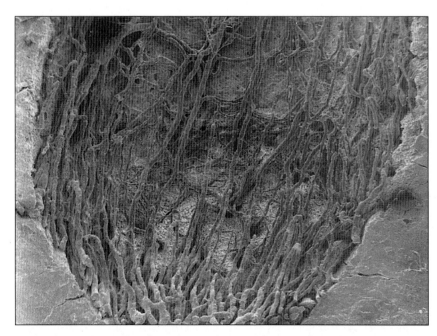

Figure 9-30 Corrosion cast demonstrating the extensive vasculature of the periodontal ligament. Many transverse connections and the thickened venous network at the apex are visible. *(From Selliseth NJ, Selvig KA: J Periodontol 65:1079, 1994.)*

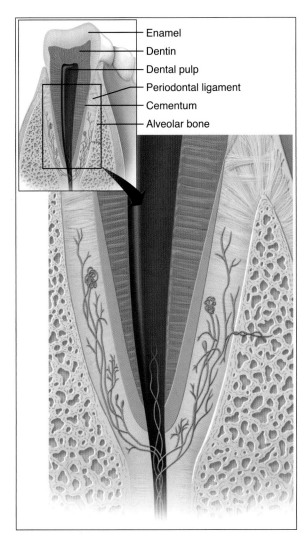

- Enamel
- Dentin
- Dental pulp
- Periodontal ligament
- Cementum
- Alveolar bone

Figure 9-31 Nerve terminals in a human periodontal ligament. *(From Maeda T, Kannari K, Sato O et al:* Arch Histol Cytol *53:259, 1990.)*

of a single neurite and the latter of several terminations following branching. Both receptors have ensheathing Schwann cells that are especially close to collagen fiber bundles (Figure 9-34), which provide morphologic evidence of their known physiologic function as mechanoreceptors. An incomplete fibrous capsule sometimes is found associated with the compound receptors. The third type of nerve terminal is a coiled form found in the midregion of the PDL, the function and ultrastructure of which have not been determined yet. The fourth type (with the lowest frequency) is found associated with the root apex and consists of spindlelike endings surrounded by a fibrous capsule.

The autonomic supply of the PDL has not been worked out fully yet, and the few descriptions available concern sympathetic supply. No evidence indicates the existence of a parasympathetic supply. The many free nerve terminals observed in close association with blood vessels are thought to be sympathetic and to affect regional blood flow.

ADAPTATION TO FUNCTIONAL DEMAND

The structural components of the periodontium have been presented. (The gingiva facing teeth are described in Chapter 12.) Together these components form a functional system that provides an attachment for the tooth to the bone of the jaw while permitting the teeth to withstand the considerable forces of mastication.

A remarkable capacity of the PDL is that it maintains its width more or less over time. The balance between formation and maintenance of mineralized tissues, bone, and cementum versus soft connective tissues of the PDL requires finely regulated control over cells in the local area. Several situations in which this balance is disrupted result in a variety of abnormal pathologic conditions; for example, (1) lack of tooth eruption because of ankylosis of teeth with surrounding bone, often associated with an osteoclast defect, and (2) lack of cementum formation resulting in exfoliation of teeth, as observed in hypophosphatasia.

Compelling evidence exists indicating that populations of cells within the PDL, during development and during regeneration, secrete molecules that can regulate the extent of mineralization and prevent the fusion of tooth root with surrounding bone, for example, ankylosis. Among these molecules, balance between the activities of bone sialoprotein and osteoprotegerin, and the inhibitory activity of MGP. At the cell level, it has been reported that Msx2 prevents the osteogenic differentiation of PDL fibroblasts by repressing Runx2 transcriptional activity. Indeed, Msx2 may play a central role in preventing ligaments and tendons, in general, from mineralizing. At this point, the issue of how the PDL stays uncalcified while it is trapped between two calcified tissues remains unresolved and will require more attention.

The PDL also has the capacity to adapt to functional changes. When the functional demand increases, the width of the PDL can increase by as much as 50%, and the fiber bundles also increase greatly in thickness. Conversely, a reduction in function leads to narrowing of the ligament and a decrease in number and thickness of the fiber bundles. These functional modifications of the PDL also implicate corresponding adaptive changes in the bordering cementum and alveolar bone.

Another major function of the periodontium is sensory, although the nature of this function of the PDL still is being debated. When teeth move in their sockets, undoubtedly they distort receptors in the PDL and trigger

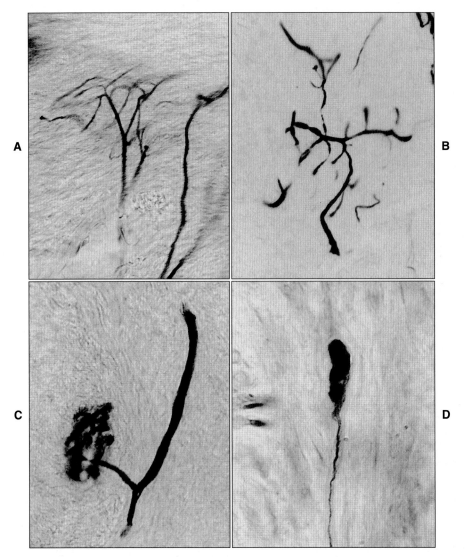

Figure 9-32 The four types of nerve endings found in a human periodontal ligament. **A,** Free endings with treelike ramifications. **B,** Ruffini's ending. **C,** Coiled ending. **D,** Encapsulated spindle-type ending. *(From Maeda T, Kannari K, Sato O et al:* Arch Histol Cytol *53:259, 1990.)*

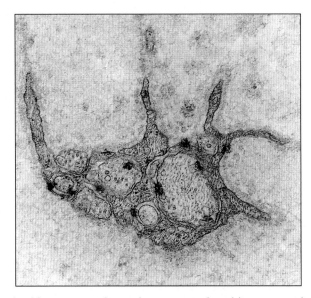

Figure 9-33 Electron micrograph of free nerve ending in human periodontal ligament with an associated Schwann cell sending fingerlike projections into the connective tissue. *(From Lambrichts I, Creemers J, van Steenberghe D:* J Periodontal Res *27:191, 1992.)*

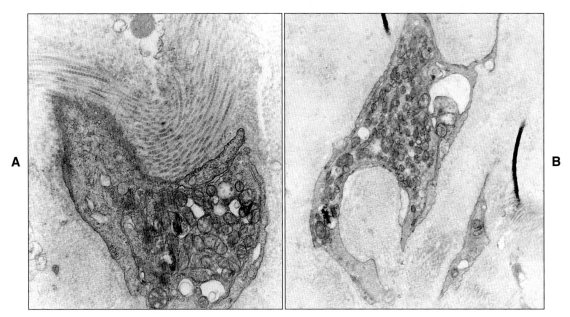

Figure 9-34 Electron micrographs illustrating the close relationship of Ruffini-like endings with collagen fiber bundles. **A,** Insertion of collagen fibrils into the basal lamina of a Schwann cell. **B,** Neurite embracing a bundle of collagen fibrils. *(From Lambrichts I, Creemers J, van Steenberghe D:* J Periodontal Res *27:191, 1992.)*

a response. Thus the PDL contributes to the sensations of touch and pressure on the teeth; in addition, the spatial distribution of receptors is significant. What is equally certain, however, is that the ligament receptors are not the only organs from which sensations arise. For example, when teeth are tapped, vibrations are passed through the bone and detected in the middle ear. Debate also exists about the exact physiologic function of these receptors. Stimulation of the teeth causes a reflex jaw opening, and likewise, stimulation of periodontal mechanoreceptors initiates this response. Whether such a reflex is required for the normal masticatory process or is a protective mechanism to prevent forces applied to the teeth from reaching potentially damaging levels is not known.

RECOMMENDED READING

Bartold PM, Narayanan AS: Molecular and cell biology of healthy and diseased periodontal tissues, *Periodontology 2000* 40:29, 2006.

Beertsen W, McCulloch CA, Sodek J: The periodontal ligament: a unique, multifunctional connective tissue, *Periodontology 2000* 13:20, 1997.

Bosshardt DD: Are cementoblasts a subpopulation of osteoblasts or a unique phenotype? *J Dent Res* 84:390, 2005.

Diekwisch TG, Thomas GH: The developmental biology of cementum, *Int J Dev Biol* 45(5-6):695, 2001.

McCulloch CA, Bordin S: Role of fibroblast sub-populations in periodontal physiology and pathology, *J Periodontal Res* 26:144, 1991.

Saffar JL, Lasfargues JJ, Cherruah M: Alveolar bone and the alveolar process: the socket that is never stable, *Periodontology 2000* 13:76, 1997.

Ten Cate AR: The development of the periodontium: a largely ectomesenchymally derived unit, *Periodontology 2000* 13:9, 1997.

Wesselink PR, Beertsen W: The prevalence and distribution of rests of Malassez in the mouse molar and their possible role in repair and maintenance of the periodontal ligament, *Arch Oral Biol* 38:399, 1993.

Physiologic Tooth Movement: Eruption and Shedding

The jaws of an infant can accommodate only a few small teeth. Because teeth, once formed, cannot increase in size, the larger jaws of the adult require not only more but also bigger teeth. This accommodation is accomplished in human beings with two dentitions. The first is the deciduous or primary dentition, and the second is the permanent or secondary dentition (Figures 10-1 and 10-2).

The early development of teeth has been described already, and the point has been made that the teeth develop within the tissues of the jaw (Figure 10-3). For teeth to become functional, considerable movement is required to bring them into the occlusal plane. The movements teeth make are complex and may be described in general terms as follows:

Preeruptive tooth movement. Made by the deciduous and permanent tooth germs within tissues of the jaw before they begin to erupt
Eruptive tooth movement. Made by a tooth to move from its position within the bone of the jaw to its functional position in occlusion (This phase sometimes is subdivided into intraosseous and extraosseous components.)
Posteruptive tooth movement. Maintaining the position of the erupted tooth in occlusion while the jaws continue to grow and compensate for occlusal and proximal tooth wear

Superimposed on these movements is a progression from primary to permanent dentition, involving the shedding (or exfoliation) of the deciduous dentition. Although this categorization of tooth movement is convenient for descriptive purposes, what is being described is a complex series of events occurring in a continuous process to move the tooth in three-dimensional space.

PREERUPTIVE TOOTH MOVEMENT

When the deciduous tooth germs first differentiate, they are extremely small, and a good deal of space is available for them in the developing jaw. Because they grow

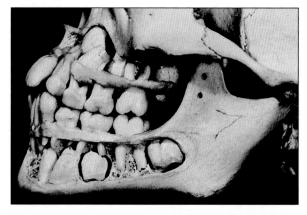

Figure 10-1 Dried skull of a 7-year-old child. The outer cortical plate has been cut away to show the mixed dentition.

268

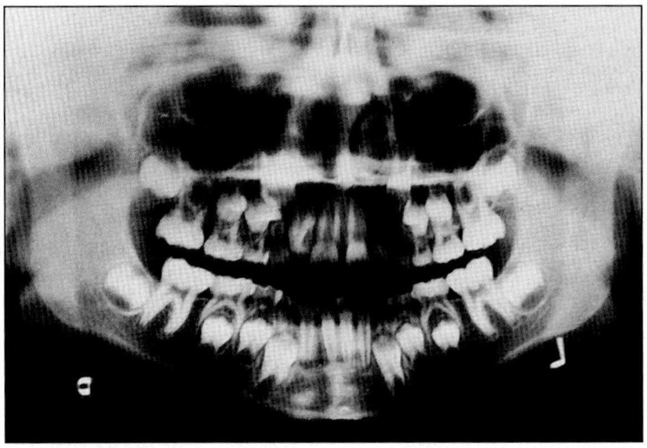

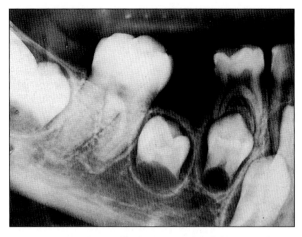

Figure 10-2 Radiograph of the mixed dentition of a 7-year-old child. *(Courtesy D.W. Stoneman.)*

Figure 10-4 Radiograph of a 7-year-old child's jaw. The permanent first premolar is erupting between the divergent roots of the deciduous first molar. The deciduous second molar has been lost early, which could lead to a tipping of the permanent first molar and prevent eruption of the permanent second premolar. *(Courtesy D.W. Stoneman.)*

rapidly, however, they become crowded. A lengthening of the jaws, which permits the deciduous second molar tooth germs to move backward and the anterior germs to move forward gradually, alleviates this crowding. At the same time the tooth germs are moving bodily outward and upward (or downward, as the case may be) with the increasing length and width and height of the jaws.

The origin of the successional permanent teeth was described in Chapter 5. Those tooth germs develop on the lingual aspect of their deciduous predecessors, in the same bony crypt. From this position they shift considerably as the jaws develop. For example, the incisors and canines eventually occupy a position, in their own bony crypts, on the lingual side of the roots of their deciduous predecessors, and the premolar tooth germs, also in their own crypts, finally are positioned between the divergent roots of the deciduous molars (Figures 10-4 and 10-5).

The permanent molar tooth germs, which have no predecessors, develop from the backward extension of the dental lamina. At first, little room is available in the jaws to accommodate these tooth germs. In the upper jaw the molar tooth germs develop first with their

occlusal surfaces facing distally and swing into position only when the maxilla has grown sufficiently to provide room for such movement (Figure 10-6). In the mandible the permanent molars develop with their axes showing a mesial inclination, which becomes vertical only when sufficient jaw growth has occurred.

These preeruptive movements of deciduous and permanent tooth germs are thought of best as the means by which the teeth are placed in a position within the jaw for eruptive movement. Analysis has shown that these preeruptive movements of teeth are a combination of two factors: total bodily movement of the tooth germ and growth in which

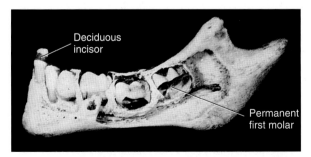

Deciduous incisor

Permanent first molar

Figure 10-3 Dried mandible of a 6-month-old child. The teeth occupy most of the body of the mandible. The first deciduous incisor has erupted. The amount of crown formation in the permanent first molar is notable.

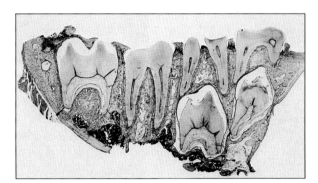

Figure 10-5 Histologic section through the lower jaw of a monkey at approximately the same dental age as a 7-year-old child. The first premolar has started to erupt, causing resorption of the roots of the deciduous first molar. The second premolar is situated between the roots of the second deciduous molar. The permanent first molar is functioning, and the permanent second molar is erupting; one cusp tip has pierced the oral mucosa.

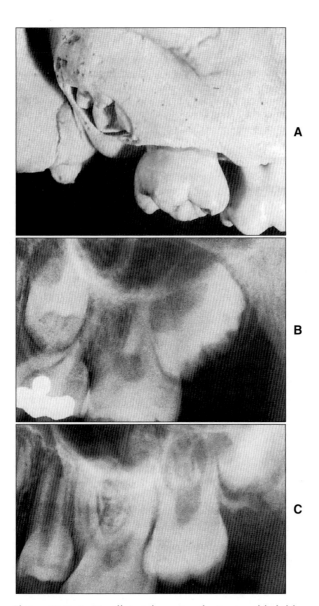

Figure 10-6 A, Maxillary tuberosity of a 4-year-old child. The first molar faces backward. **B** and **C,** Radiographs of the maxilla showing the developing second and third molars with their occlusal surfaces facing backward. (**A** *from Bhaskar SN, editor:* Orban's oral histology and embryology, *ed 11, St Louis, 1991, Mosby;* **B** *and* **C** *courtesy D.W. Stoneman.)*

deposition occurs on the distal wall as a *filling-in* process. During eccentric growth, only bony resorption occurs, thus altering the shape of the crypt to accommodate the altering shape of the tooth germ. Little is known about the mechanisms that determine preeruptive tooth movements. Whether remodeling of bone to position the bony crypt is important as a mechanism or merely represents an adaptive response is debatable (and is discussed further when eruptive movement is considered), but the idea that skeletal development determines tooth position has other parallels: Marrow spaces develop in bones of the appendicular skeleton, and bones grow in length and width by balanced resorption and deposition to determine final shape (bone modeling).

ERUPTIVE TOOTH MOVEMENT

The mechanisms of eruption for deciduous and permanent teeth are similar, resulting in the axial or occlusal movement of the tooth from its developmental position within the jaw to its final functional position in the occlusal plane. The actual eruption of the tooth, when it breaks through the gum, is only one phase of eruption.

HISTOLOGIC FEATURES

Histologically, many changes occur in association with and for the accommodation of tooth eruption. The periodontal ligament (PDL) develops only after root formation has been initiated; once established, the PDL must be remodeled to accommodate continued eruptive tooth movement. The remodeling of PDL fiber bundles is achieved by the fibroblasts, which simultaneously synthesize and degrade the collagen fibrils as required across the entire extent of the ligament (see Chapter 4 and Topics for Consideration, p. 75). One may recall also that the fibroblast has a cytoskeleton, which enables it to contract. This contractility is a property of all fibroblasts but is especially well developed in PDL fibroblasts, which have been demonstrated to exert stronger contractile forces than, for example, gingival or skin fibroblasts. Ligament fibroblasts exhibit numerous (20 to 30 per cell) contacts with one another of the adherens type and exhibit a close relationship to PDL collagen fiber bundles.

The architecture of the tissues in advance of erupting successional teeth differs from that found in advance of deciduous teeth. The fibrocellular follicle surrounding a successional tooth retains its connection with the lamina propria of the oral mucous membrane by means of a strand of fibrous tissue containing remnants of the dental lamina, known as the *gubernacular cord*. In a dried skull, holes can be identified in the jaws on the lingual aspects of the deciduous teeth. These holes, which once contained the gubernacular cords, are termed *gubernacular*

one part of the tooth germ remains fixed while the rest continues to grow, leading to a change in the center of the tooth germ. This growth explains, for example, how the deciduous incisors maintain their position relative to the oral mucosa as the jaws increase in height.

Preeruptive movements occur in an intraosseous location and are reflected in the patterns of bony remodeling within the crypt wall. For example, during bodily movement in a mesial direction, bone resorption occurs on the mesial surface of the crypt wall, and bone

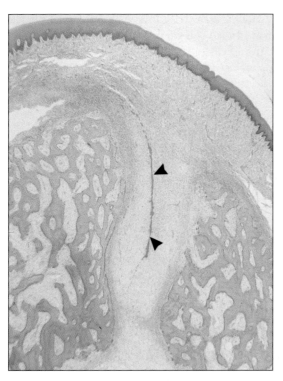

Figure 10-7 Gubernacular canal and its contents in histologic section. The canal is filled with connective tissue that connects the dental follicle to the oral epithelium. Strands of epithelial cells *(arrowheads),* remnants of the dental lamina, are often present.

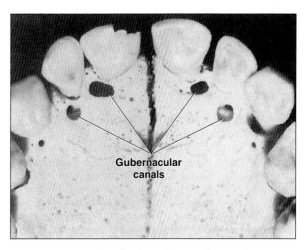

Figure 10-8 Dried skull. The gubernacular canals are located behind the upper deciduous incisors. *(From Bhaskar SN, editor:* Orban's oral histology and embryology, *ed 11, St Louis, 1991, Mosby.)*

canals (Figures 10-7 and 10-8). As the successional tooth erupts, its gubernacular canal is widened rapidly by local osteoclastic activity, delineating the eruptive pathway for the tooth. The rate of eruption depends on the phase of movement. During the intraosseous phase, the rate averages 1 to 10 μm per day; it increases to about 75 μm per day once the tooth escapes from its bony cell. This rate persists until the tooth reaches the occlusal plane, indicating that soft connective tissue provides little resistance to tooth movement.

When the erupting tooth appears in the oral cavity, it is subjected to environmental factors that help determine its final position in the dental arch. Muscle forces from the tongue, cheeks, and lips play on the tooth, as do the forces of contact of the erupting tooth with other erupted teeth. A sustained muscular force of only 4 to 5 g is sufficient to move a tooth. The childhood habit of thumb-sucking is an obvious example of environmental determination of tooth position.

MECHANISMS OF ERUPTIVE TOOTH MOVEMENT

More is known about the possible mechanisms of eruptive tooth movement than about preeruptive tooth movement.

Even so, eruptive mechanisms are not understood fully yet, and most reviews on this subject have concluded that eruption is a multifactorial process in which cause and effect are difficult to separate. Numerous theories for tooth eruption have been proposed; among these, root elongation, alveolar bone remodeling, and to some extent, formation of the PDL provide the most plausible explanation for tooth eruption in human beings. An excellent critical review on the factors involved in tooth eruption has been written by Marks and Schroeder (see Recommended Reading).

Root Formation

At first glance, root formation appears to be an obvious cause of tooth eruption because it undoubtedly causes an overall increase in the length of the tooth that must be accommodated by the growth of the root into the bone of the jaw, by an increase in jaw height, or by the occlusal movement of the crown. Although the last movement is what occurs, it does not follow that root growth is responsible. Indeed, clinical observation, experimental studies, and histologic analysis argue strongly against such a conclusion. For example, if a continuously erupting tooth (e.g., the rodent incisor or guinea pig molar) is prevented from erupting by being pinned to bone, root growth continues and is accommodated by resorption of some bone at the base of the socket and by a buckling of the newly formed root. This experiment yields two conclusions: that root growth produces a force and that this force is sufficient to produce bone resorption. The latter observation is an important aspect of bone biology because it indicates that pressure applied to bone normally results in the removal of bone by osteoclasts. Thus although root growth can produce a force, it cannot be translated into eruptive tooth movement unless some structure exists at the base of the tooth capable of withstanding this force; because no such structure exists, some other mechanism must move the tooth to accommodate root growth. The situation is substantiated further by the facts that rootless teeth erupt, that some teeth erupt a greater distance than the total length of their roots, and that teeth still will erupt after the completion of root formation or when the tissues forming the root (the apical papilla, Hertwig's epithelial root sheath, and periapical tissue) are removed surgically.

In conclusion, root formation is accommodated during tooth eruption and is a consequence, not a cause, of the eruption process. Root formation per se is not required for tooth eruption, although root formation, under certain circumstances, may accelerate tooth eruption. Depending on the rate at which the root elongates, the basal bone will resorb or form to maintain a proper relationship between the root and bone.

Bone Remodeling

Bone remodeling of the jaws has been linked to tooth eruption in that, as in the preeruptive phase, the inherent growth pattern of the mandible or maxilla supposedly moves teeth by the selective deposition and resorption of bone in the immediate neighborhood of the tooth. The strongest evidence in support of bone remodeling as a cause of tooth movement comes from a series of experiments in dogs. When the developing premolar is removed without disturbing the dental follicle, or if eruption is prevented by wiring the tooth germ down to the lower border of the mandible, an eruptive pathway still forms within the bone overlying the enucleated tooth as osteoclasts widen the gubernacular canal. If the dental follicle is removed, however, no eruptive pathway forms. Furthermore, if a metal or s ilicone replica replaces the tooth germ, and so long as the dental follicle is retained, the replica will erupt, with the formation of an eruptive pathway. These observations should be analyzed carefully. First, they clearly demonstrate that some programmed bony remodeling can and does occur (i.e., an eruptive pathway forms in bone without a developing and growing tooth). Second, they show that the dental follicle is involved. The conclusion cannot be drawn that the demonstration of an eruptive pathway forming within bone means that bony remodeling is responsible for tooth movement unless coincident bone deposition also can be demonstrated at the base of the crypt and prevention of such bone deposition can be shown to interfere with tooth eruption. Careful studies using tetracyclines as markers of bone deposition have shown that the predominant activity in

the fundus of an alveolus in a number of species (including human beings) is bone resorption. In human beings, for instance, the base of the crypt of the permanent first and third molars continually resorbs as these teeth erupt, although in the second premolar and molar, some bone deposition on the crypt floor occurs. In the case of the demonstrated eruption of an inert replica, one might think that only bony remodeling could bring this about, but as discussed next, evidence indicates that follicular tissue is responsible for this movement. Therefore the notion that bone deposition on the crypt floor causes axial tooth movement is not proved.

Dental Follicle

Investigations indicate a pattern of cellular activity involving the reduced dental epithelium and the follicle associated with tooth eruption, which facilitates connective tissue degradation and bone resorption as the tooth erupts. In osteopetrotic animals, which lack colony-stimulating factor 1, a factor that stimulates differentiation of osteoclasts, eruption is prevented because no mechanism for bone removal exists. Local administration of this factor permits the differentiation of osteoclasts, and eruption occurs. The reduced enamel epithelium also secretes proteases, which assist in the breakdown of connective tissue to produce a path of least resistance.

It is believed that there is signaling between the reduced enamel epithelium and dental follicle. This signaling could explain the remarkable consistency of eruption times, for the enamel epithelium likely is programmed as part of its functional life cycle. It has been suggested that the stellate reticulum releases factors and by so doing provides a "biologic clock" that regulates the timing of tooth eruption. One should remember, however, that when tooth eruption takes place, the stellate reticulum is reduced greatly and the four cell layers of the enamel organ amalgamate to form the reduced enamel epithelium. Signaling also helps to explain why radicular follicle, which is not associated with reduced enamel epithelium, does not undergo degeneration but instead forms the PDL.

Periodontal Ligament

Formation and renewal of the PDL has been considered a factor in tooth eruption because of the traction power that fibroblasts have and because of experimental results using the continuously erupting rat incisor. The situation is different in teeth with a limited growth period in which the presence of a PDL does not always correlate with resorption. Cases occur in which a PDL is present and the tooth does not erupt, and cases occur in which rootless teeth erupt.

Molecular Determinants of Tooth Eruption

As mentioned previously, tooth eruption is a tightly regulated process involving the tooth organ (dental follicle, enamel organ) and surrounding alveolar tissues. Tooth movement results from a balance between tissue destruction (bone, connective tissue, and epithelium) and tissue formation (bone, PDL, and root). During bone remodeling, osteoclasts are recruited; these derive from circulating monocytes that are attracted chemically at the site where bone resorption takes place. The follicle produces colony-stimulating factor 1, a growth factor that promotes the differentiation of monocytes into macrophages and osteoclasts. Furthermore, interleukin-1α, a promoter of bone resorption, is synthesized by the enamel organ in response to epidermal growth factor and induces follicular cells to produce colony-stimulating factor 1. Monocyte chemotactic protein-1 also may be involved in attracting monocytes along the path of tooth eruption.

As discussed in Chapters 6 and 9, osteoclastogenesis is regulated through signaling via the receptor-activated NF-κB/receptor-activated NF-κB ligand/osteoprotegerin pathway. Osteoprotegerin inhibits osteoclast formation, and its expression is down-regulated in the apical portion of the dental follicle. Finally, differentiation of osteoblasts at the base of the alveolar crypt is accentuated. One may recall that the transcription factor Runx-2 is involved in osteoblast differentiation and function and, as expected, is expressed at high level in the basal portion of the dental follicle. Transforming growth factor β down-regulates expression of Runx-2 in the apical portion of the dental follicle, favoring bone removal along the surface where the tooth erupts. Epidermal growth factor, which increases the level of expression of transforming growth factor β, has been shown to accelerate incisor eruption in rodents.

Table 10-1 lists the various molecules that have been proposed to take part in the paracrine signaling cascade of eruption. Understanding their role may one day offer the possibility to correct eruption effects and achieve molecular orthodontic movements. Along this line, it has been shown using local gene transfer that receptor-activated NF-κB ligand accelerates and osteoprotegerin diminishes orthodontic tooth movement in rats.

POSTERUPTIVE TOOTH MOVEMENT

Posteruptive movements are those made by the tooth after it has reached its functional position in the occlusal plane. They may be divided into three categories: (1) movements to accommodate the growing jaws, (2) those to compensate for continued occlusal wear, and (3) those to accommodate interproximal wear.

TABLE 10-1   Putative Molecules Implicated in the Tooth Eruption Signaling Cascade

MOLECULE	ABBREVIATION
Bone morphogenetic protein-2	BMP-2
Epidermal growth factor	EGF
Epidermal growth factor receptor	EGF-R
Colony-stimulating factor 1	CSF-1
Colony-stimulating factor 1 receptor	CSF-1R
Interleukin 1α	IL-1α
Interleukin 1 receptor	IL-1R
c-Fos	
Nuclear factor κB	NF κB
Monocyte chemotactic protein 1	MCP-1
Transforming growth factor α	TGF-α
Transforming growth factor β₁	TGF-β₁
Parathyroid hormone–related protein	PTHrP
Osteoprotegerin	OPG
Receptor activator of nuclear factor κB ligand	RANKL
Runt-related transcription factor-2	Runx-2

Adapted from Wise GE, Frazier-Bowers S, D'Souza RN: *Crit Rev Oral Biol Med* 13:323, 2002.

ACCOMMODATION FOR GROWTH

Posteruptive movements that accommodate the growth of the jaws are completed toward the end of the second decade, when jaw growth ceases. They are seen histologically as a readjustment of the position of the tooth socket, achieved by the formation of new bone at the alveolar crest and on the socket floor to keep pace with the increasing height of the jaws. Recent studies have shown that this readjustment occurs between the ages of 14 and 18 years, when active movement of the tooth takes place. The apices of the teeth move 2 to 3 mm away from the inferior dental canal (regarded as a fixed reference point). This movement occurs earlier in girls than in boys and is related to the burst of condylar growth that separates the jaws and teeth, permitting further eruptive movement.

Although such movement is seen as remodeling of the socket, one must not assume it brings about tooth movement. The same arguments that apply to bony remodeling for preeruptive and eruptive tooth movement apply in this case.

COMPENSATION FOR OCCLUSAL WEAR

The axial movement that a tooth makes to compensate for occlusal wear most likely is achieved by the same mechanism as eruptive tooth movement. Notably, these axial posteruptive movements are made when the apices of the permanent lower molars are formed fully and the apices of the second premolar and molar are almost complete, which indicates again that root growth is not the factor responsible for axial eruptive tooth movement and further emphasizes the role of the PDL. Compensation for occlusal wear often is stated to be achieved by continued cementum deposition around the apex of the tooth; however, the deposition of cementum in this location occurs only after the tooth has moved.

ACCOMMODATION FOR INTERPROXIMAL WEAR

Wear also occurs at the contact points between teeth on their proximal surfaces; its extent can be considerable (more than 7 mm in the mandible). This interproximal wear is compensated for by a process known as *mesial* or *approximal* drift. Mesial drift and an understanding of its probable causes are important to the practice of orthodontics because the maintenance of tooth position after treatment depends on the extent of such drift. The forces causing mesial drift are multifactorial and include an anterior component of occlusal force, contraction of the transseptal ligament between teeth, and soft tissue pressure.

Anterior Component of Occlusal Force

When teeth are brought into contact (e.g., in clenching the jaws), an anteriorly directed force is generated. This force can be demonstrated easily by placing a steel strip between the teeth and showing that more force is required to remove it when the jaws are clenched. This anterior force is the result of the mesial inclination of most teeth and the summation of intercuspal planes (producing a forward-directed force). In the case of incisors, which are inclined labially, any anterior component of force would be expected to move them in the same direction. The incisors move mesially, but this can be explained by the billiard ball analogy (Figure 10-9). When cusps are selectively ground, the direction of occlusal force can be enhanced or reversed. Paradoxically, one experiment designed to demonstrate this anterior component of force also showed that other factors are involved. When opposing teeth were removed, thereby eliminating the biting force, the mesial migration of teeth was slowed but not halted, indicating the presence of some other force. The transseptal fibers of the PDL have been implicated.

Contraction of the Transseptal Ligament

The PDL plays an important role in maintaining tooth position. The suggestion has been made that its transseptal fibers (running between adjacent teeth across the alveolar process) draw neighboring teeth together and

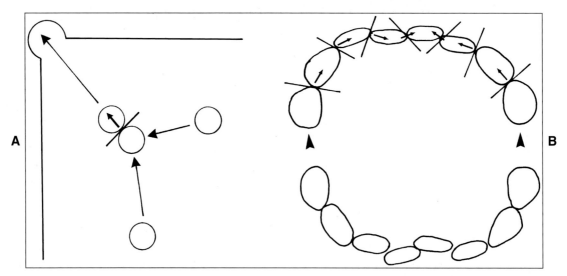

Figure 10-9 Billiard ball analogy. **A,** If the two touching balls are in line with the pocket, no matter how the first ball is struck, the second will enter the pocket because it travels at right angles to the common tangent between the two balls. **B,** In a young dentition the arrowheads indicate the anterior component of force, which drives the first premolars against the canines. Following the example of the billiard balls, the canines and incisors all move in directions at right angles to the common tangents drawn through the contact points *(arrows). (From a discussion by J. Osborn. In Poole DFG, Stack MV, editors:* The eruption and occlusion of teeth, *Colston Papers, No 27, London, 1976, Butterworth Heinemann.)*

maintain them in contact, and some supporting evidence exists. For example, relapse of orthodontically moved teeth is reduced if a gingivectomy removing the transseptal ligament is performed. Also, in experimental demonstration, in bisected teeth the two halves separate from each other, but if the transseptal ligaments are cut previously, this separation does not occur. Furthermore, remodeling by collagen phagocytosis has been demonstrated in the transseptal ligament, with the rate of turnover increasing during orthodontic tooth movement; however, this only shows that the transseptal ligament is capable of adaptation. A simple and elegant experiment indicates that the cause of mesial drift is multifactorial: grinding away proximal contacts provides room for a tooth to move, after which teeth move to reestablish contact. If teeth also are ground out of occlusion and their proximal surfaces are disked, the rate of drift is slowed. Until the contrary has been demonstrated, one must assume that mesial drift is achieved by a contractile mechanism associated with the transseptal ligament fibers and enhanced by occlusal forces.

Soft Tissue Pressures

The pressures generated by the cheeks and tongue may push teeth mesially. When such pressures are eliminated, however, by constructing an acrylic dome over the teeth, mesial drift still occurs, which suggests that soft tissue pressure does not play a major role (if any) in creating mesial drift. Nevertheless, soft tissue pressure does influence tooth position, even if it does not cause tooth movement.

SHEDDING OF TEETH

As the permanent incisors, canines, and premolars develop, increase in size, and begin to erupt, they influence the pattern of resorption of the deciduous teeth and their exfoliation (shedding). For instance, the permanent incisors and canines develop lingually to the deciduous teeth and erupt in an occlusal and vestibular direction. Resorption of deciduous tooth roots occurs on the lingual surface, and these teeth are shed with much of their pulp chamber intact (Figures 10-10 and 10-11).

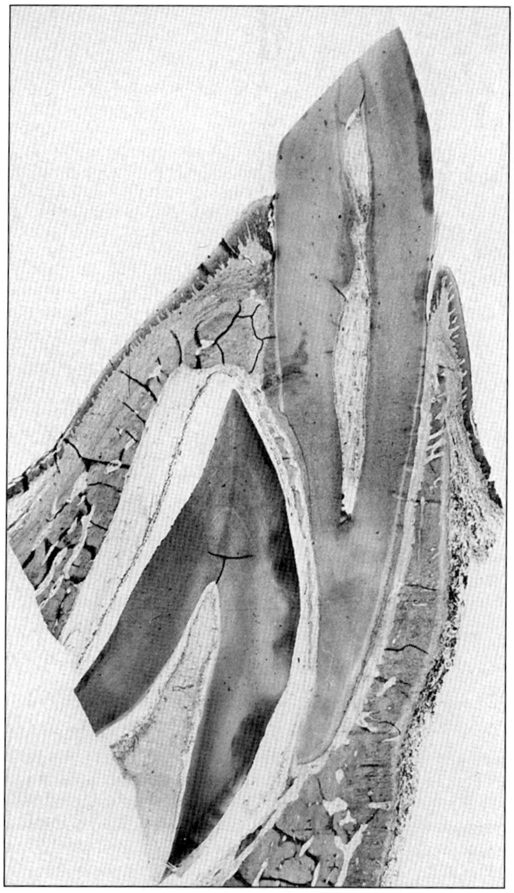

Figure 10-10 Photomicrograph of the relative positions of deciduous and permanent canines. Resorption occurs on the lingual aspect of the deciduous canine, and the tooth often is shed with much of its lingual root intact.

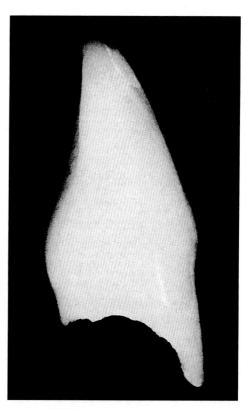

Figure 10-11 Exfoliated deciduous canine. This tooth is shed with a considerable portion of its root remaining on the buccal aspect.

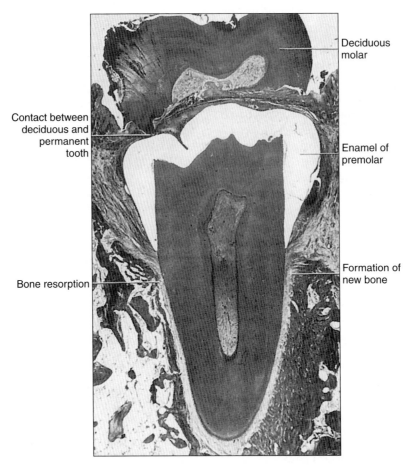

Figure 10-12 Roots of a primary molar completely resorbed. Dentin is in contact with the premolar enamel. *(Courtesy E.A. Grimmer.)*

Permanent premolars develop between the divergent roots of deciduous molars and erupt in an occlusal direction. Hence the resorption of interradicular dentin takes place with some resorption of the pulp chamber, coronal dentin, and sometimes enamel (Figures 10-12 and 10-13).

ODONTOCLAST

The resorption of dental hard tissue is achieved by cells with a histologic nature similar to that of osteoclasts, but because of their involvement in the removal of dental tissue, they are called *odontoclasts* (Figures 10-14 and 10-15). Odontoclasts derive from the monocyte and migrate from blood vessels to the resorption site, where they fuse to form the characteristic multinucleated odontoclast with a clear attachment zone and ruffled border.

Less is known about the resorption of the soft tissues of the tooth (i.e., the pulp and PDL) as it sheds. Although active root resorption is taking place, coronal pulp appears normal, and odontoblasts still line the surface of the predentin. When root resorption is almost complete, these odontoblasts degenerate, and mononuclear cells emerge from the pulpal vessels and migrate to the predentin surface, where they fuse with other mononuclear cells to form odontoclasts actively engaged in the removal of predentin and dentin (Figure 10-16). Just before exfoliation, resorption ceases as the odontoclasts migrate away from the dentin surface, and the remaining pulp cells now deposit a cementlike tissue on it (Figure 10-17). The tooth then sheds, with some pulpal tissue intact. During this process, odontoclasts resorb unmineralized dentin (predentin). Although clast cells generally attach to mineralized surfaces, this is not a unique situation; resorption of osteoid has been observed in situations of physiologic imbalance such as hypocalcemia.

Simple observation of histologic sections shows that the loss of PDL fibers is abrupt (Figure 10-18). Electron microscopic investigation confirms this finding and also shows that cell death in this region occurs without inflammation. Cell death assumes at least two forms. In one instance, fibroblasts exhibit signs of interference with normal cellular processes such as secretion

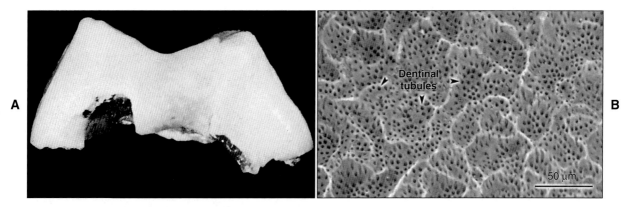

Figure 10-13 **A,** Exfoliated deciduous molar. The roots have been lost completely, and the enamel and coronal dentin have eroded. **B,** Scanning electron microscope view of the eroded dentin surface showing the numerous resorption lacunae created by odontoclasts.

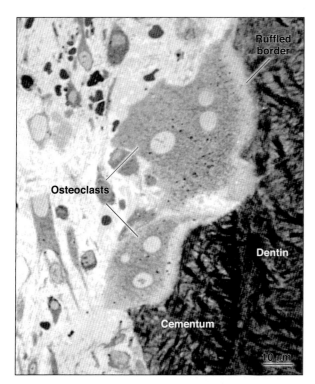

Figure 10-14 Root resorption induced by orthodontic forces in a human premolar. Cementum and dentin have been resorbed by odontoclasts that line the root surface. These large, multinucleated cells with a ruffled border resemble osteoclasts.

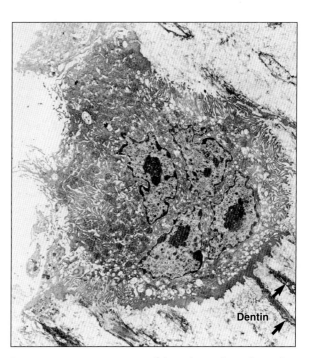

Figure 10-15 Fine structure of the odontoclast. This cell is resorbing dentin, and sends extensions *(arrows)* into the dentinal tubules. The ruffled or brush border can be seen, as can the multinucleated character of the cell. *(From Freulich LS: J Dent Res 50:1047, 1971.)*

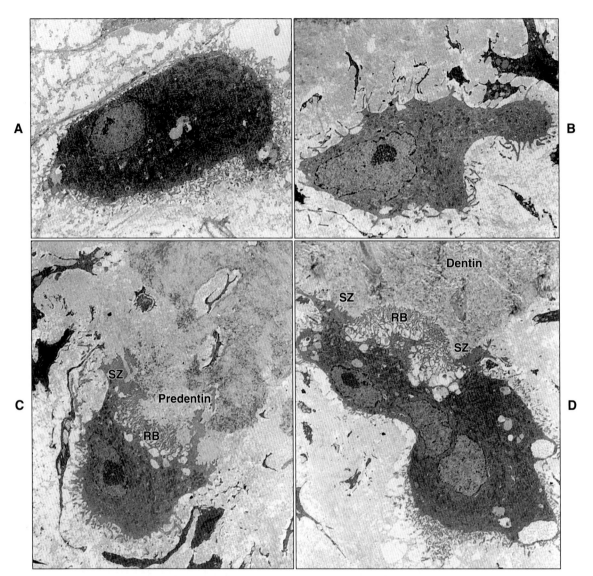

Figure 10-16 Ultrastructure of odontoclasts and their precursors. **A,** Mononuclear precursor cell in the pulp chamber. **B,** Mononuclear precursor cell attached to the predentin surface. **C,** Multinucleate odontoclast resorbing predentin. **D,** Multinucleate odontoclast resorbing dentin. In **C** and **D,** the sealing zones *(SZ)* and the ruffled border *(RB)* are notable. *(From Sahara N, Okafuji N, Toyokia A et al:* Arch Histol Cytol *55:273, 1992.)*

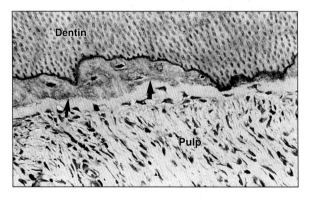

Figure 10-17 Cementlike tissue *(arrows)* deposited on resorbed coronal dentin. *(Courtesy N. Sahara; from Sahara N, Okafuji N, Toyoka A et al:* Acta Anat *147:24, 1993.)*

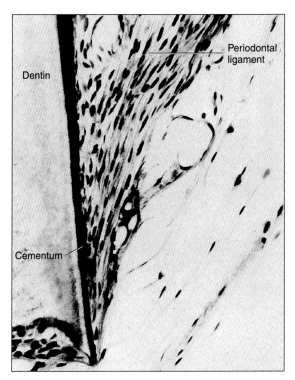

Figure 10-18 Photomicrograph showing the abrupt loss of periodontal ligament in a shedding tooth.

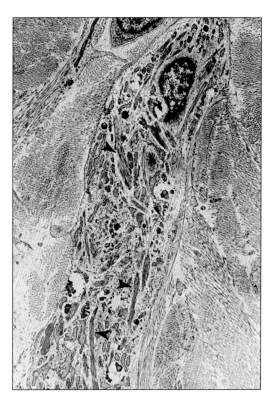

Figure 10-19 Electron micrograph of a periodontal ligament fibroblast in an area preceding the root resorption front. The cytoplasm of the fibroblast is filled with collagen *(arrowheads),* suggesting an interference with the protein synthetic and/or degradative cell physiology.

(Figure 10-19), as well as other cytotoxic alterations that eventually lead to necrosis and cell death. This process is induced in response to local cell insult. In the other, ligament fibroblasts exhibit morphologic features characteristic of apoptotic cell death (Figure 10-20). Apoptosis (see Chapter 7) has been well described and involves *condensation* of the cell with its ultimate phagocytosis by neighboring macrophages or undamaged fibroblasts. The finding of apoptotic cell death in the resorbing PDL suggests that shedding teeth also is a programmed event. Support for this conclusion is obtained from the study of tooth eruption in monozygotic twins, which indicates that shedding is determined mostly (80%) by genetic factors (with the remaining determinants being local).

PRESSURE

Obviously, pressure from the erupting successional tooth plays a role in shedding the deciduous dentition. For instance, if a successional tooth germ is missing congenitally or occupies an aberrant position in the jaw, shedding of the deciduous tooth is delayed. Yet the tooth usually is shed. The suggestion also has been made that increased force applied to a deciduous tooth can initiate its resorption. Growth of the face and jaws and the corresponding enlargement in size and strength of the muscles of mastication probably increase the forces applied

to the deciduous teeth so that the supporting apparatus of the tooth, in particular the PDL, is damaged and tooth resorption is initiated (Figure 10-21).

The superimposition of local pressure and masticatory forces on physiologic tooth resorption is likely to determine the pattern and rate of deciduous tooth shedding. Pressure from an erupting permanent tooth results in some root loss, which in turn means a loss of supporting tissue. As the support of the tooth diminishes, the tooth is less able to withstand the increasing masticatory forces, and thus the process of exfoliation is accelerated.

PATTERN OF SHEDDING

In general, the pattern of exfoliation is symmetrical for the right and left sides of the mouth. Except for second molars, the mandibular primary teeth are shed before their maxillary counterparts. The exfoliation of all four secondary primary molars is practically simultaneous. Exfoliation occurs in girls before it does in boys. The greatest discrepancy between the sexes is observed for the mandibular canines, and the least for the maxillary central incisors. The sequence of shedding in the mandible follows the anterior-to-posterior order of the

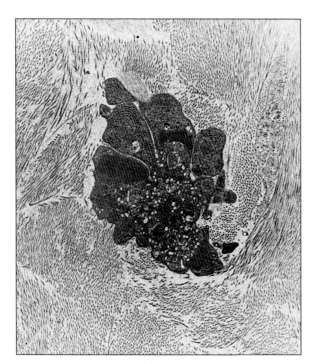

Figure 10-20 A degenerated fibroblast in the periodontal ligament near the root resorption front. This appearance is characteristic of apoptotic (physiologic) cell death.

teeth in that jaw. In the maxilla the first molar exfoliating before the canine disrupts this sequence.

In summary (Figure 10-22), physiologic tooth movement is a complex and multifactorial process. Several related events take place involving bone remodeling and soft tissue removal. Failure of such events to proceed properly delays or prevents eruption. Active tooth eruption begins in a dynamic intraosseous environment that undergoes bone formation and resorption, events that are regulated by the dental follicle and enamel organ. Although the force for eruptive tooth movement might be considered to have been identified, the controlling mechanisms remain to be defined fully. The consistency of eruption dates for the human dentition is remarkable (the so-called 6-year molars as a descriptor for the permanent first molars testifying to this) and surely indicates the involvement of programmed development. The ability of orthodontists to manage clinically and intervene during tooth resorption is limited and includes extraction of primary teeth, surgical removal of bone, and incising of the gingiva. A better understanding of the molecular mediators of eruption, and in particular of the role of products produced by the reduced enamel organ, certainly will increase clinical options. Because the eruption pathway created by osteoclasts determines, at least initially, the direction of tooth eruption and hence its three-dimensional positioning in the forming jaw, one even may ask the question of whether using

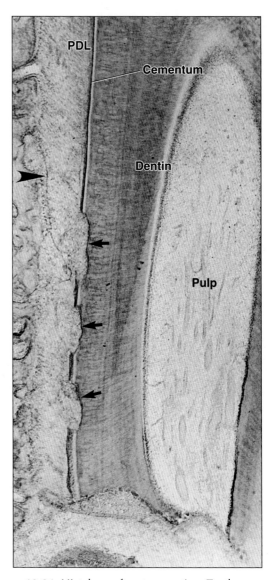

Figure 10-21 Histology of root resorption. Tooth resorption is occurring at the apex of the root, and as a consequence, changes are seen in the periodontal ligament *(PDL)* as this structure becomes less able to cope with the forces applied to it. The downward and oblique orientation of the ligament fibers is progressively lost *(below arrowhead)*, and local pockets of cementum resorption occur *(arrows)*.

some of these mediators to manage the final position and interrelation of teeth could be possible.

ABNORMAL TOOTH MOVEMENT

The steps leading to the development of the final permanent dentition are complex, requiring a balance among tooth formation, jaw growth, and the maintenance of function. Not surprisingly, disturbances in this process often indicate some local or systemic abnormality, and thus the patterns of tooth formation and eruption are of considerable diagnostic significance. The normal pattern is so remarkably consistent that permanent first molars (as just mentioned) often are referred to as *6-year molars* because of their predictable time of eruption.

Earlier than normal tooth eruption is unusual. Sometimes babies are born with a central incisor that is erupted already, but this represents abnormal dental development, and the tooth is extracted to permit suckling. The premature loss of a deciduous tooth occasionally leads to early eruption of its permanent successor. Delayed eruption of teeth is far more common and may be caused by congenital, systemic, or local factors (with local factors predominating). Congenital absence of teeth most commonly occurs with the permanent third molars. Systemic factors involving delays in tooth eruption may be caused by endocrine deficiencies, nutritional deficiencies, and some genetic factors. If teeth have not appeared in an infant during the first year, some underlying cause must be sought. Any systemic lesion delaying eruption of the permanent teeth usually has been identified before the sixth year, when the permanent first molars erupt.

Local factors preventing tooth eruption are many. Examples are early loss of a deciduous tooth, with consequent drifting of the adjacent teeth to block the eruptive pathway (see Figure 10-4), and eruption cysts (derived from the dental lamina). Crowding of teeth in small jaws often provides little room for eruption, with consequent impaction of the teeth (see Figure 10-23). The third molars are particularly prone to impaction because they erupt last, when the least room is available. The upper canine also frequently is impacted because of its late eruption (see Figure 10-24). Although much is known about tooth movement and positioning, at times some clinical conditions cannot be explained. Figure 10-25 illustrates just

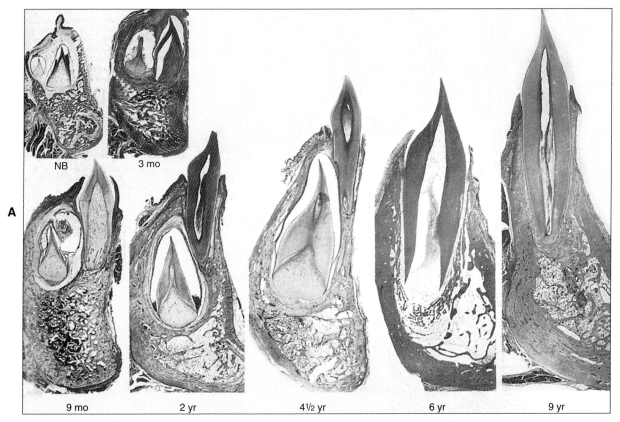

Figure 10-22 Summary of preeruptive and eruptive tooth movement, including the pattern of tooth resorption. **A,** Buccolingual sections through the central incisor region of the mandible at representative stages of development from birth *(NB)* to 9 years of age. At birth the deciduous and permanent tooth germs occupy the same bony crypt. Note how, by eccentric growth and eruption of the deciduous tooth, the permanent tooth germ comes to occupy its own bony crypt apical to the erupted incisor. At 4½ years, resorption of the deciduous incisor has begun. At 6 years the deciduous incisor has been shed and its successor is erupting. The active deposition of new bone at the base of the socket is notable.

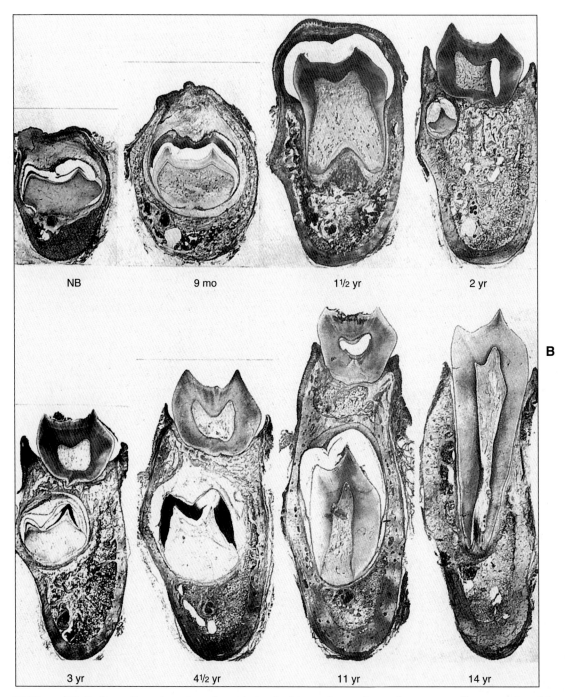

Figure 10-22, cont'd   B, Buccolingual sections through the deciduous first molar and permanent first premolar of the mandible at representative stages of development from birth to 14 years. Note how the permanent tooth germ shifts its position. In the section of a 4½-year-old mandible, the gubernacular canal is clearly visible. Lack of roots in the 2-, 3-, 4½-, and 11-year-old sections results not from resorption but from the section's having been cut in the midline of a tooth with widely diverging roots. *(From Bhaskar SN, editor:* Orban's oral histology and embryology, *ed 11, St Louis, 1991, Mosby.)*

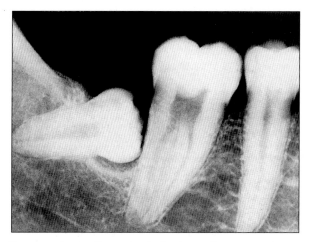

Figure 10-23 Radiograph of a horizontally impacted mandibular third molar. *(Courtesy D.W. Stoneman.)*

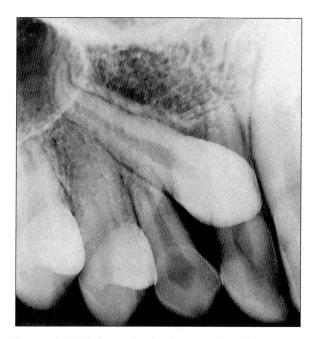

Figure 10-24 Radiograph of an impacted maxillary canine. *(Courtesy D.W. Stoneman.)*

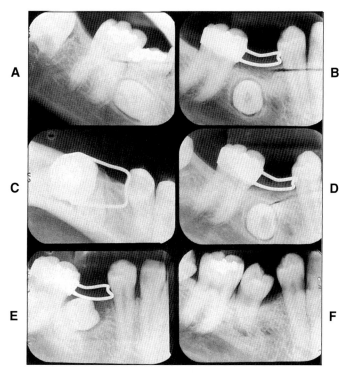

Figure 10-25 Series of radiographs illustrating an instance of unusual tooth movement. **A,** The permanent second premolar is buried beneath the deciduous second molar. **B,** The deciduous molar has been extracted and a space maintainer inserted to prevent tilting and drift of the permanent first molar. **C** is the same as **B** but seen from above. **D,** The premolar has shifted and now occupies a buccolingual position. **E** and **F** show the same tooth erupting and erupted 4 and 5 years later. *(Courtesy F. Pulver.)*

such a case. A tooth has developed in an abnormal location and is lying parallel to the lower border of the mandible. The clinical treatment in this instance was simply to provide room for the tooth to erupt by extraction of the overlying tooth. Then the horizontally inclined tooth righted itself and erupted with no further clinical interference. In this instance the roots of the tooth were formed fully. Explaining how the periodontal tissues knew the direction in which to move the tooth is difficult.

TOPICS FOR CONSIDERATION   Physiologic Tooth Movement: Eruption and Shedding

Clearly, from the material presented in this chapter, tooth eruption is a complex process that involves highly coordinated actions and interactions of cells of the dental (enamel) organ, follicle (osteoclasts), and alveolus (osteoblasts). Despite the advances in understanding the underlying mechanisms of the eruptive process, the precise relationship of molecules involved within signaling pathways remains to be determined. Like the forming skeleton and the developing tooth organ, it is likely that a high level of redundancy is shared by growth factors and cytokines that influence tooth eruption. Transcription factors that are produced in minute amounts within the nucleus are most likely to play specific roles in cell-cell signaling during tooth eruption. To further knowledge on the biologic role(s) and relationship of known key transcription factors, growth factors, cytokines, and the discovery of novel molecules, modern research tools and multipronged approaches that involve mouse and human genetic studies must be used to fullest advantage.

A disturbed eruption process creates a clinical situation that is challenging to diagnose and treat. Disturbances in tooth eruption most commonly are caused by mechanical obstruction from soft tissue overgrowth, supernumerary teeth, crowding, and pathologic lesions. In addition, tooth eruption anomalies also occur in several medical and genetic syndromes. In this group, a condition termed *primary failure of eruption* (PFE) is viewed as one of the most challenging and threatening to treat and diagnose. PFE affects mainly permanent posterior teeth that are normal in appearance but unable to reach the occlusal plane because of a primary defect in the eruption mechanism itself. Teeth affected by PFE are nonankylosed and not impacted by supernumerary teeth or soft tissues. Orthodontic treatments to close accompanying open bites are futile and may result in ankylosis of PFE-affected teeth. Multidisciplinary treatment requiring intervention by oral surgeons, periodontists, and prosthodontists often is warranted.

The genetic and molecular basis of PFE is not known. From a theoretical standpoint, a disruption in function of the dental follicle, periodontal ligament, cementoblasts, osteoblasts, osteoclasts, and osteoblast-osteoclast signaling may contribute to the failure in the primary mechanism. Clearly, the significant advances made in understanding the mechanisms of osteoblast and osteoclast differentiation have opened exciting avenues for new research. For example, mouse models of osteopetrosis have provided definitive evidence of the importance of molecules such as *PU.1*, macrophage colony-stimulating factor, and the transcriptional regulators *c*-fos and NF κB. The role of receptor-activated NF-κB ligand in the stimulation of osteoclastogenesis and osteoprotegerin that directly inhibits the ligand cannot be ignored because the balance between the level of expression of the two genes is responsible for the quantity of bone resorbed during the formation of the eruption pathway. Molecules such as the $\alpha_v\beta_3$ integrin, tumor necrosis factor receptor–associated factor 6, and *c*-Src (a tyrosine kinase) are needed for the osteoclast to "polarize" on bone cells and develop a specialized cytoskeleton that probably permits transport of acidifying substances to the osteocyte. Cathepsin K, carbonic anhydrase II, and hydrogen-adenosinetriphosphatase influence the ability of osteoclasts to resorb bone matrix. Mice deficient in the molecules noted before (osteoprotegerin is an exception; osteoprotegerin deficiency causes osteoporosis, whereas its overexpression leads to osteopetrosis) develop an osteopetrotic phenotype and have defects in early to late stages of osteoclast formation and function. Mice genetically engineered to lack these genes have defects in osteoclast differentiation or function that result in osteopetrosis and failure of tooth eruption. Therefore, these animal models provide useful tools to unravel the complex mechanisms of tooth eruption. The identification of more individuals and families affected by human PFE will open new avenues of research using modern genetic approaches. The search for the candidate gene(s) that are associated with PFE will require the use of the candidate gene approach, in which individual gene sequences can be assessed for disease-causing mutations or genome-wide scans and linkage analysis in which groups of individuals can be pooled. Such research is important and will provide interesting insights into the genetic control of tooth eruption. This information can lead to the development of effective therapies that will provide better control of the eruptive process, thus improving the overall health of dentition.

Rena N. D'Souza, DDS, MS, PhD
*Department of Orthodontics, Dental Branch
University of Texas Health Science Center
Houston, Texas*

ORTHODONTIC TOOTH MOVEMENT

The supporting tissues of the tooth (i.e., the PDL and alveolar bone) have a remarkable plasticity that permits physiologic tooth movement and accommodates to the constant minor movements that the tooth makes during mastication. This plasticity of the supporting tissues of the tooth permits orthodontic tooth movement.

Theoretically, bringing about tooth movement without any tissue damage by using a light force, equivalent to the physiologic forces determining tooth position, to capitalize on the plasticity of the supporting tissues should be possible. The changes that happen under these circumstances are easy to describe: Differentiation of osteoclasts occurs, and they resorb bone of the socket wall on the pressure side. At the same time, remodeling of collagen fibers in the PDL occurs to accommodate the new tooth position. On the tension side, remodeling of collagen fiber bundles also takes place but in association with bone deposition on the socket wall. No changes occur in tooth

structure (e.g., in the cementum). Whether current orthodontic techniques duplicate this ideal situation is doubtful; most involve some degree of tissue damage that varies because the forces applied to move the tooth are not distributed equally throughout the PDL.

Analyzing the tissue reactions in terms of a graph illustrating the typical pattern of orthodontic tooth movement is worthwhile (Figure 10-26). An applied force results in immediate movement of the tooth, which in turn leads to areas of tension and compression within the PDL and to changes within the bone and ligament. Unlike physiologic tooth movement, in which bone resorption of the alveolar wall occurs on its PDL aspect, orthodontic tooth movement also causes some internal or undermining resorption, in which alveolar bone is remodeled from its endosteal face (Figure 10-27).

This difference in resorption is caused by changes within the PDL resulting from compression. The ligament undergoes *hyalinization*, a term from light microscopy

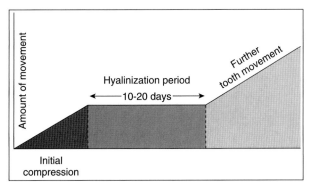

Figure 10-26 Orthodontic tooth movement over time.

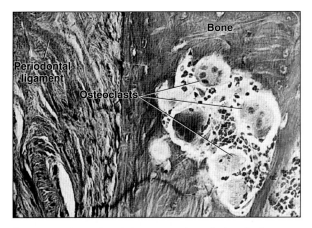

Figure 10-27 Undermining resorption of alveolar bone 7 days after the beginning of tooth movement with a light tipping force. *(From Buck DL, Church DH: Am J Orthod 62:507, 1972.)*

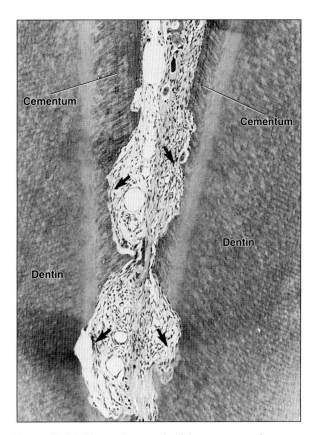

Figure 10-28 Photomicrograph of the response of supporting tissues when the roots of teeth come into contact. The two teeth are tipping into contact as a consequence of malocclusion, but the same picture can be created by excessive orthodontic force. The interdental septum has been lost almost completely, and the root surfaces now are resorbing. Repair of these resorption bays *(arrows)* is possible if the drifting ceases.

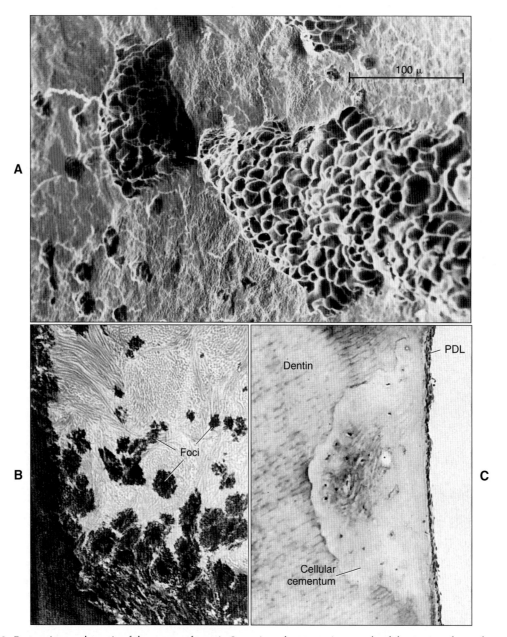

Figure 10-29 Resorption and repair of the root surface. **A,** Scanning electron micrograph of the root surface of a tooth used as an anchor for rapid maxillary expansion showing resorption lacunae on the root surface. **B,** Transmission electron micrograph of a region of cementum repair illustrating the presence of mineralization foci in the collagenous tissue. **C,** A light microscope picture of completed root surface repair. *PDL,* Periodontal ligament. *(A from Barber AF, Sims MR: Am J Orthod 79:630, 1981; B from Furseth R: Arch Oral Biol 13:417, 1968; C from Langford SR, Sims MR: Am J Orthod 81:108, 1982.)*

describing the loss of cells from an area of ligament because of trauma. Obviously, if no cells are present, no bony remodeling can occur. Although hyalinization is present, tooth movement ceases. Only when new cells repopulate the hyalinized portion of the ligament and the bone is removed by osteoclasts does tooth movement begin again. This movement coincides with the active remodeling of ligament collagen by the newly arrived fibroblasts and the deposition of new bone. Obviously, heavier forces cause larger areas of hyalinization, a longer period of repair, and slower tooth movement.

Chapter 9 makes the point that orthodontic tooth movement is possible because of the greater resistance of cementum than bone to resorption. If both tissues were resorbed with equal facility, root loss would follow orthodontic movement; however, even when radiographs show no visible changes in the root surface, that most teeth moved orthodontically undergo some minor degree of root resorption is now appreciated (Figure 10-28), and resorption is followed by repair. This resorption is seen as small lacunae created by odontoclasts that are repaired rapidly by the formation of new cementum (Figure 10-29).

Because cementum is more resistant than bone to resorption, clinically demonstrable resorption usually occurs only after application of heavy force and the movement of teeth for more than 30 days.

In addition to changes within the periodontium, tooth movement demands remodeling of the adjacent gingival tissues (of which little is known) and some adaptation of pulpal tissue. Too rapid a movement can lead to damage of the vessels supplying the pulp, resulting in eventual pulp necrosis, especially when the tooth is tilted too far. An interrupted force of some magnitude

has little effect on the pulp, which is why removable appliances cause little or no pulp damage. With a fixed appliance providing a continuous force, some pulp damage usually occurs; because young pulp usually is involved and the forces are moderate, however, repair follows.

The development of a functional dentition, from its inception through the deciduous to the permanent dentition, has been described fully. Many of the key events in the process, for both dentitions, are summarized in Figures 10-30 and 10-31.

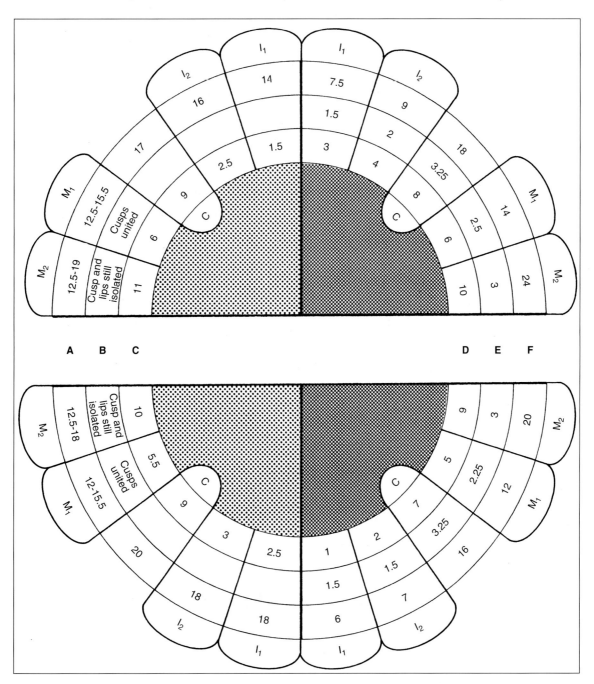

Figure 10-30 Chronology of the human primary dentition. **A,** Mineralization begins (weeks in utero). **B,** Amount of enamel matrix found at birth. **C,** Enamel complete (months). **D,** Eruption sequence. **E,** Root completed (years). **F,** Emergence into the oral cavity (months). *C,* Canine; *I,* incisor; *M,* molar.

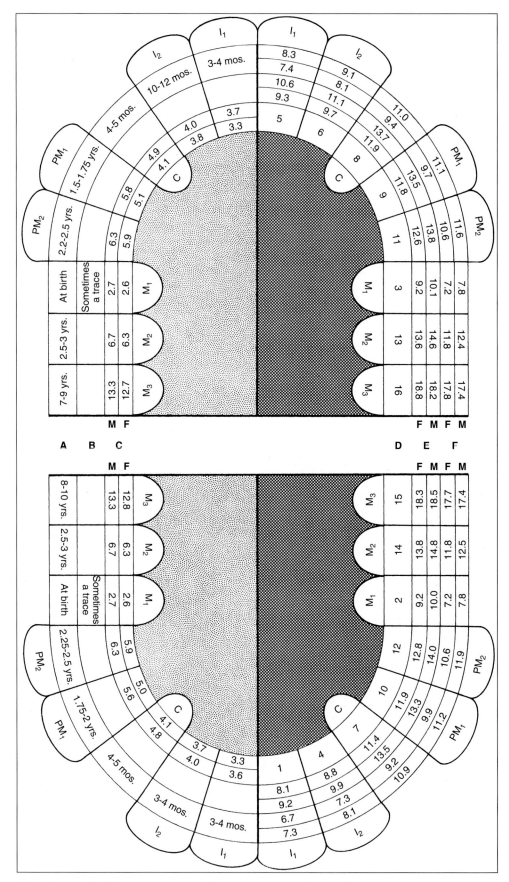

Figure 10-31 Chronology of the human permanent dentition. **A,** Mineralization begins. **B,** Amount of enamel matrix at birth. **C,** Enamel completed (years). **D,** Eruption sequence. **E,** Root completed (years). **F,** Emergence into the oral cavity (years). *F,* Female; *M,* male; *C,* canine; *I,* incisor; *M,* molar; *P,* premolar.

RECOMMENDED READING

Cahill DR: Histological changes in the bony crypt and gubernacular canal of erupting permanent premolars during deciduous premolar exfoliation in beagles, *J Dent Res* 53:786, 1974.

Kardos TB: The mechanism of tooth eruption, *Br Dent J* 181:91, 1996.

Marks SC Jr, Gorski JP, Wise GE: The mechanisms and mediators of tooth eruption: models for developmental biologists, *Int J Dev Biol* 39:223, 1995.

Marks SC Jr, Schroeder HE: Tooth eruption: theories and facts, *Anat Rec* 245:374, 1996.

Ten Cate AR, Deporter DA, Freeman E: The role of fibroblasts in the remodelling of periodontal ligament during physiologic tooth movement, *Am J Orthod* 69:155, 1976.

Wise GE, Frazier-Bowers S, D'Souza RN: Cellular, molecular and genetic determinants of tooth eruption, *Crit Rev Oral Biol Med* 13:323, 2002.

Salivary Glands

Arthur R. Hand

CHAPTER OUTLINE

The oral cavity is kept moist by a film of fluid called *saliva* that coats the teeth and the mucosa. Saliva is a complex fluid, produced by the salivary glands, the most important function of which is to maintain the well-being of the mouth. Individuals with a deficiency of salivary secretion experience difficulty eating, speaking, and swallowing and become prone to mucosal infections and rampant caries.

In human beings, three pairs of *major salivary glands*—the *parotid*, submandibular, and *sublingual*—are located outside the oral cavity, with extended duct systems through which the gland secretions reach the mouth. Numerous smaller *minor salivary glands* are located in various parts of the oral cavity—the *labial*, lingual, palatal, buccal, glossopalatine, and *retromolar glands*—typically located in the submucosal layer (Figure 11-1), with short ducts opening directly onto the mucosal surface.

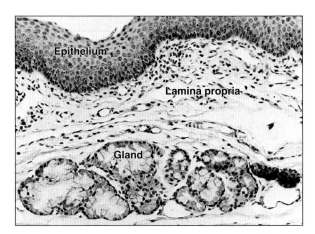

Figure 11-1 Minor mucous salivary gland, located in the submucosa below the epithelium of the oral cavity. The saliva secreted by minor salivary glands reaches the oral cavity through short ducts that connect the glands to the surface epithelium.

TABLE 11-1   Composition of Saliva

PARAMETER	CHARACTERISTICS
Volume	600-1000 mL/day
Electrolytes	Na^+, K^+, Cl^-, HCO_3^-, Ca^{2+}, Mg^{2+}, HPO_4^{2-}, SCN^-, and F^-
Secretory proteins/peptides	Amylase, proline-rich proteins, mucins, histatin, cystatin, peroxidase, lysozyme, lactoferrin, defensins, and cathelicidin-LL37
Immunoglobulins	Secretory immunoglobulin A; immunoglobulins G and M
Small organic	Glucose, amino acids, urea, uric acid, and lipids molecules
Other components	Epidermal growth factor, insulin, cyclic adenosine monophosphate—binding proteins, and serum albumin

FLOW RATE (ml/min)	WHOLE	PAROTID	SUBMANDIBULAR
Resting	0.2-0.4	0.04	0.1
Stimulated	2.0-5.0	1.0-2.0	0.8
pH	6.7-7.4	6.0-7.8	

The composition of saliva is summarized in Table 11-1. The saliva produced by each major salivary gland, however, differs in amount and composition. The parotid glands secrete a watery saliva rich in enzymes such as *amylase*, proteins such as the *proline-rich proteins*, and other glycoproteins. Submandibular saliva, in addition to the components already listed, contains highly glycosylated substances called *mucins*. The sublingual gland produces a viscous saliva rich in mucins. Oral fluid, which is referred to as *mixed*, or *whole*, *saliva*, includes the secretions of the major glands, the minor glands, desquamated oral epithelial cells, microorganisms and their products, food debris, and serum components and inflammatory cells that gain access through the gingival crevice. Moreover, whole saliva is not the simple sum of all of these components, because many of the proteins are removed as they adhere to the surfaces of the teeth and oral mucosa, bind to microorganisms, or are degraded.

FUNCTIONS OF SALIVA

Saliva has many functions (Table 11-2), the most important being protection of the oral cavity.

PROTECTION

Saliva protects the oral cavity in many ways. The fluid nature of saliva provides a washing action that flushes away nonadherent bacteria and other debris. In particular,

TABLE 11-2   Functions of Saliva

FUNCTION	EFFECT	ACTIVE CONSTITUENTS
Protection	Clearance	Water
	Lubrication	Mucins, glycoproteins
	Thermal/chemical insulation	Mucins
	Pellicle formation	Proteins, glycoproteins, mucins
	Tannin binding	Basic proline-rich proteins, histatins
Buffering	pH maintenance	Bicarbonate, phosphate, basic proteins, urea, ammonia
	Neutralization of acids	
Tooth integrity	Enamel maturation, repair	Calcium, phosphate, fluoride, statherin, acidic proline-rich proteins
Antimicrobial activity	Physical barrier	Mucins
	Immune defense	Secretory immunoglobulin A
	Nonimmune defense	Peroxidase, lysozyme, lactoferrin, histatin, mucins, agglutinins, secretory leukocyte protease inhibitor, defensins, and cathelicidin LL-37
Tissue repair	Wound healing, epithelial regeneration	Growth factors, trefoil proteins
Digestion	Bolus formation	Water, mucins
	Starch, triglyceride digestion	Amylase, lipase
Taste	Solution of molecules	Water and lipocalins
	Maintenance of taste buds	Epidermal growth factor and carbonic anhydrase VI

the clearance of sugars from the mouth limits their availability to acidogenic plaque microorganisms. The mucins and other glycoproteins provide lubrication, preventing the oral tissues from adhering to one another and allowing them to slide easily over one another. The mucins also form a barrier against noxious stimuli, microbial toxins, and minor trauma.

BUFFERING

The bicarbonate and, to some extent, phosphate, ions in saliva provide a buffering action that helps to protect the teeth from demineralization caused by bacterial acids produced during sugar metabolism. Some basic salivary proteins also may contribute to the buffering action of saliva. Additionally, the metabolism of salivary proteins and peptides by bacteria produces urea and ammonia, which help to increase the pH.

PELLICLE FORMATION

Many of the salivary proteins bind to the surfaces of the teeth and oral mucosa, forming a thin film, the salivary *pellicle*. Several proteins bind calcium and help to protect the tooth surface. Others have binding sites for oral bacteria, providing the initial attachment for organisms that form *plaque*.

MAINTENANCE OF TOOTH INTEGRITY

Saliva is supersaturated with calcium and phosphate ions. The solubility of these ions is maintained by several calcium-binding proteins, especially the acidic proline-rich proteins and *statherin*. At the tooth surface the high concentration of calcium and phosphate results in a posteruptive maturation of the enamel, increasing surface hardness and resistance to demineralization. Remineralization of initial caries lesions also can occur; this is enhanced by the presence of fluoride ions in saliva.

ANTIMICROBIAL ACTION

Saliva has a major ecologic influence on the microorganisms that colonize oral tissues. In addition to the barrier effect provided by mucins, saliva contains a spectrum of proteins with antimicrobial activity such as the *lysozyme*, lactoferrin, *peroxidase*, and *secretory leukocyte protease inhibitor*. A number of small peptides that function by inserting into membranes and disrupting cellular or mitochondrial functions are present in saliva. These include α-defensins and β-defensins, cathelicidin-LL37, and the histatins. In addition to antibacterial and antifungal activities, several of these proteins and

peptides also exhibit antiviral activity. The major salivary immunoglobulin, *secretory immunoglobulin A* (IgA), causes agglutination of specific microorganisms, preventing their adherence to oral tissues and forming clumps that are swallowed. Mucins, as well as specific *agglutinins*, also aggregate microorganisms.

TISSUE REPAIR

A variety of growth factors and other biologically active peptides and proteins are present in small quantities in saliva. Under experimental conditions, many of these substances promote tissue growth and differentiation, wound healing, and other beneficial effects. However, the role of most of these substances in protection of the oral cavity is presently unknown.

DIGESTION

Saliva also contributes to the digestion of food. The solubilization of food substances and the actions of enzymes such as amylase and *lipase* begin the digestive process. The moistening and lubricative properties of saliva also allow the formation and swallowing of a food bolus.

TASTE

Saliva functions in taste by solubilizing food substances so that they can be sensed by taste receptors located in taste buds. Saliva produced by minor glands in the vicinity of the circumvallate papillae contains proteins that are believed to bind taste substances and present them to the taste receptors. Additionally, saliva contains proteins that have a trophic effect on taste receptors.

ANATOMY

The parotid gland is the largest salivary gland. The superficial portion of the parotid gland is located subcutaneously, in front of the external ear, and its deeper portion lies behind the ramus of the mandible. The parotid gland has a mass between 14 and 28 g and is associated intimately with peripheral branches of the facial nerve (cranial nerve VII; Figure 11-2, A). The duct (*Stensen's duct*) of the parotid gland runs forward across the masseter muscle, turns inward at the anterior border of the masseter, and opens into the oral cavity at a papilla opposite the maxillary second molar. A small amount of parotid tissue occasionally forms an accessory gland associated with Stensen's duct, just anterior to the superficial portion. The parotid gland receives its blood supply from branches of the external carotid artery as they pass through the gland. The parasympathetic

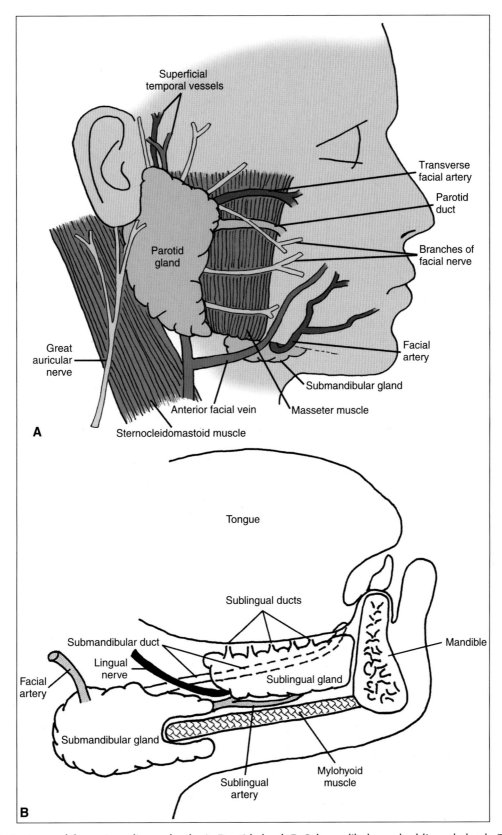

Figure 11-2 Anatomy of the major salivary glands. **A,** Parotid gland. **B,** Submandibular and sublingual glands. The major glands are bilaterally paired and have long ducts that convey their saliva to the oral cavity. *(Modified from Hollinshead WH: Anatomy for surgeons, vol 1,* The head and neck, *New York, 1958, Hoeber.)*

nerve supply to the parotid gland is mainly from the glossopharyngeal nerve (cranial nerve IX). The preganglionic fibers synapse in the otic ganglion; the postganglionic fibers reach the gland through the auriculotemporal nerve. The sympathetic innervation of all of the salivary glands is provided by postganglionic fibers from the superior cervical ganglion, traveling with the blood supply.

The submandibular gland is situated in the posterior part of the floor of the mouth, adjacent to the medial aspect of the mandible and wrapping around the posterior border of the mylohyoid muscle (Figure 11-2, *B*). The gland has a mass between 10 and 15g. The excretory duct (*Wharton's duct*) of the submandibular gland runs forward above the mylohyoid muscle and opens into the mouth beneath the tongue at the sublingual caruncle, lateral to the lingual frenum. The submandibular gland receives its blood supply from the facial and lingual arteries. The parasympathetic nerve supply is derived mainly from the facial nerve (cranial nerve VII), reaching the gland through the lingual nerve and submandibular ganglion.

The sublingual gland is the smallest of the paired major salivary glands; its mass is approximately 2 g. The gland is located in the anterior part of the floor of the mouth between the mucosa and the mylohyoid muscle (see Figure 11-2, *B*). The secretions of the sublingual gland enter the oral cavity through a series of small ducts (*ducts of Rivinus*) opening along the sublingual fold and often through a larger duct (*Bartholin's duct*) that opens with the submandibular duct at the sublingual caruncle. The sublingual gland receives its blood supply from the sublingual and submental arteries. The facial nerve (cranial nerve VII) provides the parasympathetic innervation of the sublingual gland, also via the lingual nerve and submandibular ganglion.

The minor salivary glands, estimated to number between 600 and 1000, exist as small, discrete aggregates of secretory tissue present in the submucosa throughout most of the oral cavity. The only places they are not found are the gingiva and the anterior part of the hard palate. They are predominantly mucous glands, except for the lingual serous glands (*Ebner's glands*) that are located in the tongue and open into the troughs surrounding the circumvallate papillae on the dorsum of the tongue and at the foliate papillae on the sides of the tongue.

DEVELOPMENT

Individual salivary glands arise as a proliferation of oral epithelial cells, forming a focal thickening that grows into the underlying ectomesenchyme. Continued growth results in the formation of a small bud connected

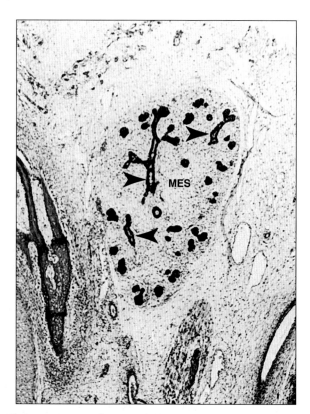

Figure 11-3 Developing salivary gland. Proliferation of the epithelium into the underlying mesenchyme results in long epithelial cords (*arrowheads*) that undergo repeated dichotomous branching. The mesenchyme (*MES*) has condensed around the developing glandular epithelium.

to the surface by a trailing cord of epithelial cells, with mesenchymal cells condensing around the bud (Figure 11-3). Clefts develop in the bud, forming two or more new buds; continuation of this process, called *branching morphogenesis*, produces successive generations of buds and a hierarchic ramification of the gland.

Studies of analogous processes in experimental animals and studies of salivary gland development in vitro have revealed that the process of branching morphogenesis requires interactions between the epithelium and mesenchyme. Several factors that control the location of the branch points and the overall structure of the gland have been identified. Signaling molecules, including members of the fibroblast growth factor protein family, sonic hedgehog, transforming growth factor β, and their receptors, play a major role in the development of branches. The differential contraction of actin filaments at the basal and apical ends of the epithelial cells is thought to provide the physical mechanism underlying cleft formation, and the deposition of extracellular matrix components within the clefts apparently serves to stabilize them. Finally, the specific mesenchyme associated with the salivary glands has

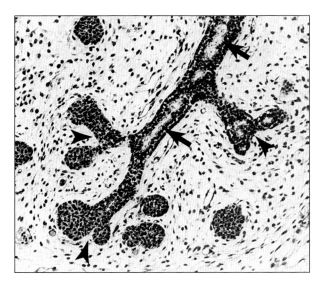

Figure 11-4 Developing salivary gland. Lumen formation *(arrows)* has begun in the ducts. Branching of the distal ends of the epithelial cords is evident *(arrowheads)*.

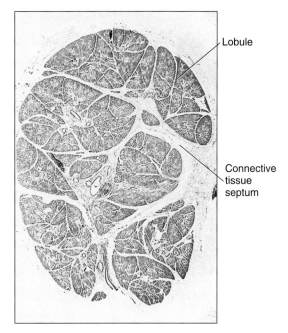

Lobule

Connective tissue septum

Figure 11-5 Salivary gland showing its lobular organization.

been shown to provide the optimum environment for gland development.

The development of a lumen within the branched epithelium generally occurs first in the distal end of the main cord and in branch cords, then in the proximal end of the main cord, and finally in the central portion of the main cord (Figure 11-4). The lumina form within the ducts before they develop within the terminal buds. Some studies have suggested that lumen formation may involve apoptosis of centrally located cells in the cell cords, but further research is required to establish definitively a role for cell death in this process.

Following development of the lumen in the terminal buds, the epithelium consists of two layers of cells. The cells of the inner layer eventually differentiate into the secretory cells of the mature gland, mucous or serous, depending on the specific gland. Some cells of the outer layer form the contractile myoepithelial cells that are present around the secretory end pieces and intercalated ducts. As the epithelial parenchymal components increase in size and number, the associated mesenchyme (connective tissue) is diminished, although a thin layer of connective tissue remains, surrounding each secretory end piece and duct of the adult gland. Thicker partitions of connective tissue (septa), continuous with the capsule and within which run the nerves and blood vessels supplying the gland, invest the excretory ducts and divide the gland into lobes and lobules (Figure 11-5).

The parotid glands begin to develop at 4 to 6 weeks of embryonic life, the submandibular glands at 6 weeks, and the sublingual and minor salivary glands at 8 to 12 weeks. The cells of the secretory end pieces and ducts attain maturity during the last 2 months of gestation.

The glands continue to grow postnatally—with the volume proportion of acinar tissue increasing and the volume proportions of ducts, connective tissue, and vascular elements decreasing—up to 2 years of age.

STRUCTURE

As described in the previous section, a salivary gland consists of a series of branched *ducts*, terminating in spherical or tubular *secretory end pieces* or *acini* (Figure 11-6). An analogy can be made to a bunch of grapes, with the stems representing the ducts and the grapes corresponding to the secretory end pieces. The main *excretory duct*, which empties into the oral cavity, divides into progressively smaller interlobar and interlobular excretory ducts that enter the lobes and lobules of the gland. The predominant intralobular ductal component is the *striated duct*, which plays a major role in modification of the primary saliva produced by the secretory end pieces. Connecting the striated ducts to the secretory end pieces are *intercalated ducts*, which branch once or twice before joining individual end pieces. The lumen of the end piece is continuous with that of the intercalated duct. In some glands, small extensions of the lumen, *intercellular canaliculi*, are found between adjacent secretory cells (Figure 11-7). These intercellular canaliculi may extend almost to the base of the secretory cells and serve to increase the size of the secretory (luminal) surface of the cells.

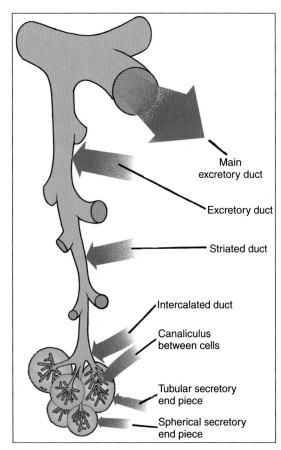

Figure 11-6 Ductal system of a salivary gland. The main excretory duct opens into the oral cavity. Excretory ducts are located in the interlobular connective tissue, and striated ducts are the main intralobular ductal component. Intercalated ducts vary in length and connect the secretory end pieces with the striated ducts. Intercellular canaliculi are extensions of the lumen of the end piece between adjacent secretory cells that serve to increase the luminal surface area available for secretion.

SECRETORY CELLS

The two main types of secretory cells present in salivary glands are *serous cells* and *mucous cells*. Serous and mucous cells differ in structure, as seen in classic histologic and electron microscopic analyses, and in the types of macromolecular components that they produce and secrete. In general, serous cells produce proteins and glycoproteins, many of which have well-defined enzymatic, antimicrobial, calcium-binding, or other activities. These proteins typically are modified by the addition of sugar residues (glycosylation) and thus correctly are called glycoproteins. Typically, serous glycoproteins have N-linked (bound to the β-amide of asparagine) oligosaccharide side chains. The main products of mucous cells are mucins, which have a

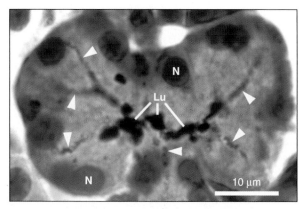

Figure 11-7 Lumen and intercellular canaliculi in a serous end piece. The lumen *(Lu)* and intercellular canaliculi were filled with India ink. Arrowheads indicate intercellular canaliculi extending between adjacent cells. *N,* Nuclei of serous cells. *(From Hand AR. In Provenza DV, Seibel W, editors,* Oral histology: inheritance and development, *ed 2, Philadelphia, 1986, Lea and Febiger.)*

protein core (apomucin) that is organized into specific domains and is highly substituted with sugar residues. Mucins therefore also are glycoproteins, but they differ from most serous cell glycoproteins in the structure of the protein core, the nature (predominantly O-linked; i.e., to the hydroxyl groups of serine or threonine) and extent of glycosylation, and their function. Mucins function mainly to lubricate and form a barrier on surfaces and to bind and aggregate microorganisms. Mucous cells secrete few, if any, other macromolecular components.

In recent years the distinction between serous cells and mucous cells has become somewhat blurred. Serous cells of some salivary glands now are known to produce certain type of mucins, and some mucous cells are thought to produce certain nonglycosylated proteins. Additionally, advances in tissue preservation procedures have demonstrated that the structure of mucous and serous cells is actually similar and that the typical morphology of swollen, fused, and empty-appearing mucous granules is likely a result of artifactual changes occurring during chemical fixation.

Serous Cells

Secretory end pieces that are composed of serous cells are typically spherical and consist of 8 to 12 cells surrounding a central lumen (Figure 11-8). The cells are pyramidal, with a broad base adjacent to the connective tissue stroma and a narrow apex forming part of the lumen of the end piece. The lumen usually has finger-like extensions located between adjacent cells called intercellular canaliculi that increase the size of the luminal surface of the cells. The spherical nuclei are located basally, and occasionally, binucleated cells

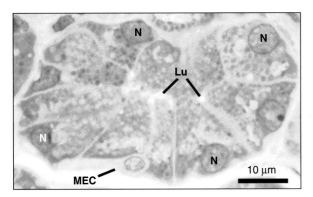

Figure 11-8 Light micrograph of a serous end piece of the human submandibular gland, stained with toluidine blue. The apical cytoplasm of the serous cells contains secretory granules of variable density. *Lu,* Lumen; *MEC,* myoepithelial cell; *N,* nucleus.

are seen. Numerous *secretory granules,* in which the macromolecular components of saliva are stored, are present in the apical cytoplasm (Figures 11-9 and 11-10). The granules may have a variable appearance, ranging from homogeneously electron-dense to a combination of electron-dense and electron-lucent regions arranged in intricate patterns. The basal cytoplasm contains numerous cisternae of rough endoplasmic reticulum, which converge on a large Golgi complex located just apical or lateral to the nucleus (Figure 11-11). Forming secretory granules of variable size and density are present at the *trans* face of the Golgi complex. These granules increase in density as their content condenses, eventually forming the mature secretory granules. Serous cells also contain all of the typical organelles found in other cells, including cytoskeletal components, mitochondria, lysosomes, and peroxisomes.

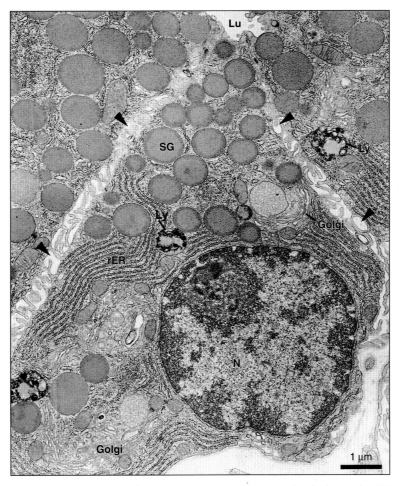

Figure 11-9 Transmission electron micrograph of serous cell of the rat parotid gland. The nuclei *(N)* and rough endoplasmic reticulum *(rER)* are located basally, and numerous electron-dense secretory granules *(SG)* are present in the apical cytoplasm. Portions of the Golgi complex *(Golgi)* are located apical and lateral to the nucleus. *Arrowheads,* Intercellular spaces; *Lu,* lumen; *Ly,* lysosomes. *(From Hand AR:* Am J Anat *135:71, 1972.)*

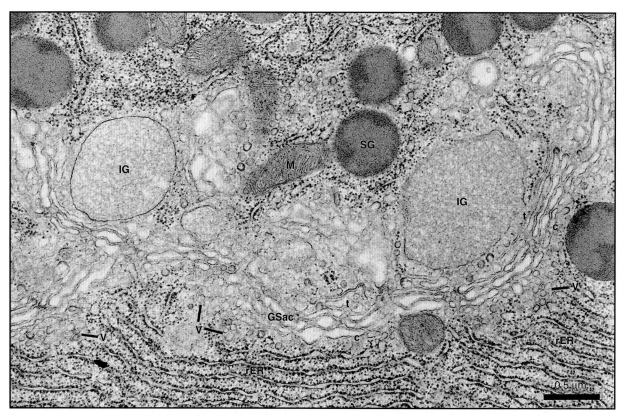

Figure 11-10 Transmission electron micrograph of the Golgi complex of serous cell of the rat parotid gland. The Golgi complex consists of several interconnected stacks of membranous saccules *(GSac)*. Small vesicles *(V)* are located between the rough endoplasmic reticulum *(rER)* and the *cis* face *(c)* of the Golgi complex, and immature granules *(IG)* of variable size and density are present at the *trans* face *(t)*. M, Mitochondrion; SG, mature secretory granules. *(From Hand AR. In Bhaskar SN, editor,* Orban's oral histology and embryology, *ed 11, St Louis, 1991, Mosby.)*

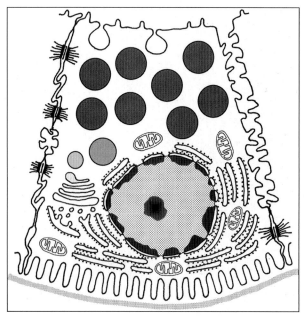

Figure 11-11 Serous cell. Intercellular canaliculi are seen in longitudinal *(right)* and cross section *(left)*.

The plasma membranes of serous cells exhibit several specializations. The luminal surface, including the intercellular canaliculi, is studded with a few short microvilli. The lateral surfaces have occasional folds that interdigitate with similar processes from the adjacent cells. The basal surface is thrown into regular folds, approximately 0.5 μm deep, that extend laterally beyond the borders of the cell to interdigitate with folds of the adjacent cells. The folding of the cell membranes greatly increases the surface area of the cell. Serous cells, as well as mucous cells, also are joined to one another by a variety of intercellular junctions (see Chapter 4). A tight junction (*zonula occludens*), an adhering junction (*zonula adherens*), and a *desmosome (macula adherens)* form a junctional complex that separates the luminal surface from the basolateral surfaces of the cell. The tight junctions help to maintain these cell surface domains and regulate the passage of material from the lumen to the intercellular spaces and vice versa. The tight junctions exhibit a selective permeability, allowing the passage of certain ions and water. Their permeability can be altered by specific neurotransmitters to allow the passage of larger molecules (up to several thousand daltons in size). The adhering junctions, and desmosomes that also are found elsewhere along the lateral cell surfaces, serve to hold adjacent cells together. The secretory cells also are attached to the basal lamina and the underlying connective tissue by hemidesmosomes. Through interactions with cytoplasmic proteins and cytoskeletal elements, these cell-cell and cell-matrix junctions also function in signaling events that provide information to the cells about their immediate environment. Gap (communicating) junctions linking the cytoplasm of adjacent cells also are found along the lateral cell surfaces. These junctions allow the passage of small molecules between cells, such as ions, metabolites, and cyclic adenosine monophosphate (cAMP). They probably serve to coordinate the activity of all of the cells within an end piece, creating a functional unit.

Mucous Cells

Secretory end pieces that are composed of mucous cells typically have a tubular configuration; when cut in cross section, these tubules appear as round profiles with mucous cells surrounding a central lumen of larger size than that of serous end pieces (Figure 11-12). Mucous end pieces in the major salivary glands and some minor salivary glands have serous cells associated with them in the form of a *demilune* or crescent covering the mucous cells at the end of the tubule (Figure 11-13). These serous

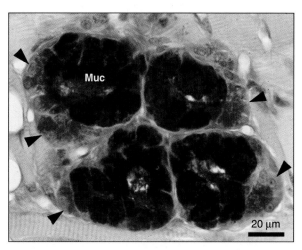

Figure 11-13 Mucous end pieces with serous demilunes *(arrowheads)* in a minor salivary gland stained with periodic acid-Schiff, alcian blue, and hematoxylin. The mucous secretory product *(Muc, dark purple)* stains strongly with periodic acid-Schiff and alcian blue, whereas the glycoproteins of the serous demilune cells stain only with periodic acid-Schiff *(magenta). (From Hand AR. In Provenza DV, Seibel W, editors:* Oral histology: inheritance and development, *ed 2, Philadelphia, 1986, Lea and Febiger.)*

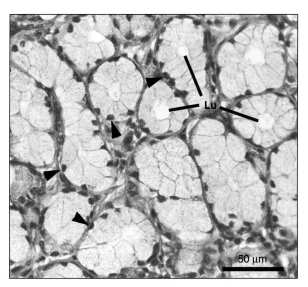

Figure 11-12 Mucous cells in tubular secretory end pieces, stained with hematoxylin and eosin. Poorly stained mucous secretory granules fill the cytoplasm, and the nuclei *(arrowheads)* are flattened and compressed against the basal surfaces of the cells. The lumina *(Lu)* are large compared with those of serous acini.

demilune cells are in all respects similar to the serous end piece cells present in the same gland. Their secretions reach the lumen of the end piece through intercellular canaliculi extending between the mucous cells at the end of the tubule.

The most prominent feature of mucous cells is the accumulation in the apical cytoplasm of large amounts of secretory product (mucus), which compresses the nucleus and endoplasmic reticulum against the basal cell membrane. The secretory material appears unstained in routine histologic preparations, giving an empty appearance to the supranuclear cytoplasm. However, when special stains that reveal sugar residues or acidic groups, such as the periodic acid-Schiff stain or alcian blue, are used, the secretory material is strongly stained (see Figure 11-13). In the electron microscope the mucous secretory granules appear swollen, their membranes are disrupted, and they often are fused with one another. Their content appears electron-lucent but may include some finely filamentous or flocculent material (Figure 11-14). As noted previously, the typical appearance of mucous granules probably is caused by artifacts induced during chemical fixation; when tissue samples are rapidly (a few milliseconds) frozen and subsequently prepared for electron microscopy, the mucous secretory granules are small, dense, have intact membranes, and do not fuse with one another.

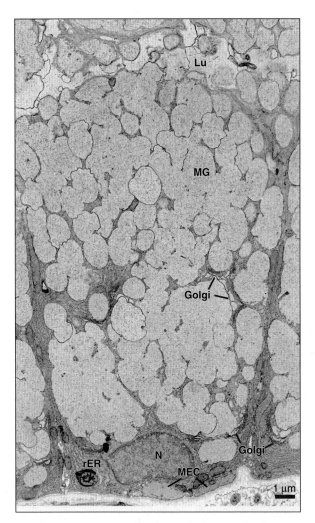

Figure 11-14 Transmission electron micrograph of mucous cell of the mouse sublingual gland. The nucleus *(N)* and rough endoplasmic reticulum *(rER)* are located basally. The supranuclear cytoplasm is filled with pale mucous secretory granules *(MG)* that have a fine fibrillar content. Many granules have disrupted membranes and are fused with adjacent granules. The Golgi complex *(Golgi)* is large, and portions of it are located basally and centrally in the cell. Two myoepithelial cell processes *(MEC)* are present at the basal surface of the mucous cell. *Lu,* Lumen.

Mucous cells have a large Golgi complex, located mainly basal to the mass of secretory granules. Small granules form at the *trans* face of the Golgi complex, increase in size, and join the rest of the granules stored in the apical cytoplasm. The endoplasmic reticulum and most of the other organelles are limited mainly to the basal cytoplasm of the cell (Figure 11-15; see also Figure 11-14). Like serous cells, mucous cells are joined by a variety of intercellular junctions. Unlike serous cells, however, mucous cells lack intercellular canaliculi, except for those covered by demilune cells.

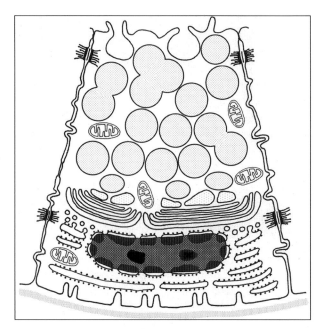

Figure 11-15 Mucous cell.

FORMATION AND SECRETION OF SALIVA

The formation of saliva occurs in two stages. In the first stage, cells of the secretory end pieces and intercalated ducts produce *primary saliva*, which is an isotonic fluid containing most of the organic components and all of the water that is secreted by the salivary glands. In the second stage, the primary saliva is modified as it passes through the striated and excretory ducts, mainly by reabsorption and secretion of electrolytes. The final saliva that reaches the oral cavity is hypotonic.

Macromolecular Components

Like other cells that are specialized for the synthesis and regulated secretion of proteins and glycoproteins, the cells of the secretory end pieces have abundant rough endoplasmic reticula and a large Golgi complex, and they store their products in membrane-bound granules in the apical cytoplasm. Secretory proteins are synthesized by ribosomes attached to the cisternae of the endoplasmic reticulum and translocated to the lumen of the endoplasmic reticulum. The proteins associate with other molecules (chaperones) that ensure proper folding of the protein, and posttranslational modifications such as disulfide bond formation and N- and O-linked glycosylation are initiated. The proteins are transferred by small vesicles to the Golgi complex, where they undergo further modification, followed by condensation and packaging into secretory granules (Figure 11-16).

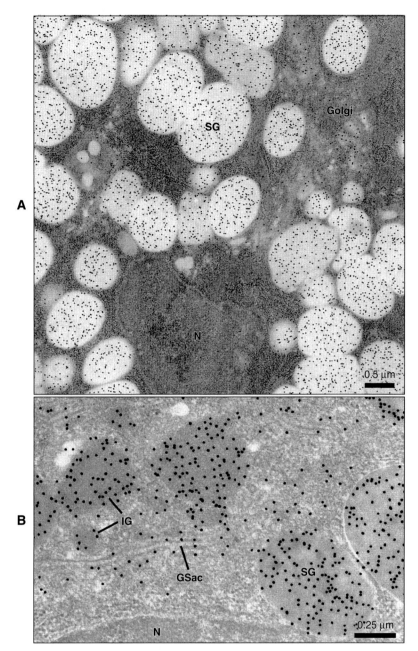

Figure 11-16 Immunogold labeling of secretory proteins in salivary gland cells. **A,** Parotid secretory protein in a serous cell of the rat parotid gland. The section was incubated with an antibody to parotid secretory protein and then with gold particles coupled to staphylococcal protein-A to localize the bound antibody. Gold particles are present over the secretory granules *(SG)* and the Golgi complex *(Golgi)*, indicating the presence of parotid secretory protein in these organelles. **B,** Protein SMGB in a serous demilune cell of the rat sublingual gland. The section was incubated with an antibody to the secretory protein, protein SMGB, and then was treated as in **A.** Gold particles are present over the Golgi saccules *(GSac)* and immature *(IG)* and mature secretory granules *(SG)*. *N,* Nucleus.

The secretory granules are stored in the apical cytoplasm until the cell receives an appropriate secretory stimulus. The granule membranes fuse with the cell membrane at the apical (luminal) surface, and the contents are released into the lumen by the process of *exocytosis* (Figure 11-17). In salivary glands the sympathetic neurotransmitter norepinephrine usually is an effective stimulus of exocytosis. Norepinephrine binds to β-adrenergic receptors on the cell surface. Receptor activation, through guanosine triphosphate-binding proteins, stimulates adenylyl cyclase to produce cAMP. Increased cAMP levels activate protein kinase A,

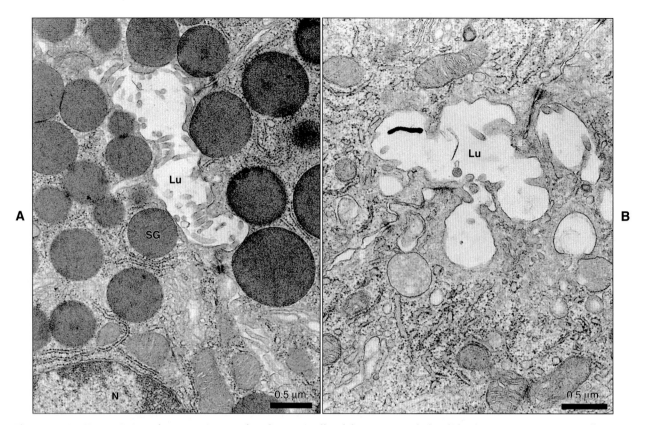

Figure 11-17 Transmission electron micrographs of serous cells of the rat parotid gland demonstrating exocytosis of secretory granules. **A,** The apical cytoplasm of resting (unstimulated) cells is filled with secretory granules *(SG)*. **B,** After administration of isoproterenol, a β-adrenergic drug, the cells are devoid of secretory granules and the lumen *(Lu)* is enlarged because of the fusion of granule membranes during exocytosis. *N,* Nucleus. *(From Hand AR. In Provenza DV, Seibel W, editors:* Oral histology: inheritance and development, *ed 2, Philadelphia, 1986, Lea and Febiger.)*

which phosphorylates other proteins in a cascade that eventually leads to granule exocytosis (Figure 11-18). The fusion of the granule membrane with the cell membrane is mediated by the formation of a protein complex involving proteins of the granule membrane, proteins of the cell membrane, and proteins in the cytoplasm. Following release of the granule content, the granule membrane is internalized by the cell as small vesicles, which may be recycled or degraded.

Fluid and Electrolytes

Secretion of water by the cells of the secretory end pieces is regulated principally by the parasympathetic innervation. Binding of acetylcholine to muscarinic cholinergic receptors activates phospholipase C, resulting in the formation of inositol trisphosphate and the subsequent release of Ca^{2+} from intracellular stores. The increased Ca^{2+} concentration opens Cl^- channels in the apical cell membrane and K^+ channels in the basolateral membrane. The apical Cl^- efflux draws extracellular Na^+ into the lumen, probably through the tight junctions, to balance the electrochemical gradient. The osmotic gradient resulting from the increased luminal Na^+ and Cl^- concentration results in the movement of water into the lumen, probably through the cells via water channels (*aquaporins*) in the apical membrane and possibly through the tight junctions (see Figure 11-18). A $Na^+/K^+/2Cl^-$ cotransporter and the Na^+/K^+-adenosine triphosphatase in the basolateral membrane serve to maintain the intracellular ionic and osmotic balance during active secretion. Thus fluid secretion by the salivary glands is driven by the active transport of electrolytes.

Other receptors also are able to stimulate fluid secretion. Norepinephrine, acting via α-adrenergic receptors, and substance P activate the Ca^{2+}-phospholipid pathway just described. The cells also can secrete fluid using other electrolyte transport mechanisms. The apical Cl^- channel is believed also to transport HCO_3^- into the lumen. At high flow rates, salivary HCO_3^- concentrations increase significantly. A basolateral

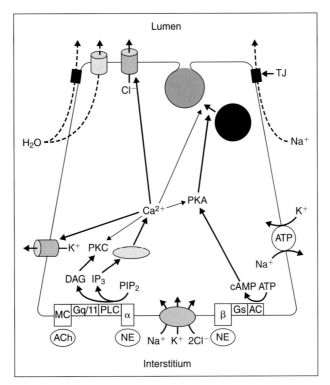

Figure 11-18 Mechanisms of salivary secretion. Protein secretion occurs by exocytosis, that is, the fusion of secretory granules with the luminal membrane to release their contents into the lumen. The binding of the sympathetic transmitter norepinephrine *(NE)* to β-adrenergic *(β)* receptors on the basolateral membrane activates a heterotrimeric G-protein *(Gs)*, which in turn activates adenylyl cyclase *(AC)*, catalyzing the formation of cyclic adenosine monophosphate *(cAMP)* from adenosine triphosphate *(ATP)*. Cyclic adenosine monophosphate activates protein kinase A *(PKA)*, which phosphorylates other proteins in a cascade leading to exocytosis. Fluid and electrolyte secretion is stimulated mainly by the binding of the parasympathetic transmitter, acetylcholine *(ACh)* to muscarinic cholinergic *(MC)* receptors and also by norepinephrine binding to α-adrenergic receptors *(α)*. These receptors activate a heterotrimeric G-protein *(Gq/11)*, causing activation of phospholipase C *(PLC)*, which converts phosphatidylinositol bisphosphate *(PIP$_2$)* to inositol trisphosphate *(IP$_3$)* and diacylglycerol *(DAG)*. Inositol trisphosphate causes the release of Ca^{2+} from intracellular stores, probably the endoplasmic reticulum. The increased Ca^{2+} concentration opens Cl^- channels in the luminal membrane and K^+ channels in the basolateral membrane and activates the basolateral $Na^+/K^+/2Cl^-$ cotransporter. The increased luminal Cl^- is balanced by the movement of extracellular Na^+ across the tight junctions *(TJ)*, and the resulting osmotic gradient pulls water into the lumen through the cell via the water channel aquaporin 5 and through the tight junction. The basolateral $Na^+/K^+/2Cl^-$ cotransporter and the Na^+/K^+-adenosine triphosphatase serve to maintain the intracellular electrolyte and osmotic balances. Calcium also stimulates exocytosis, but to a lesser extent than cyclic adenosine monophosphate, and it modulates the activity of protein kinase A and protein kinase C *(PKC)*. Protein kinase C, in turn, modulates exocytosis and intracellular Ca^{2+} concentrations.

Na^+/H^+ exchanger serves to restore the intracellular pH following the acidification that occurs as a result of HCO_3^- secretion.

Other Mechanisms Modulating Saliva Secretion

The secretion of proteins and fluid and electrolytes by secretory end piece cells may be affected by other signaling molecules. Norepinephrine, acting via α-adrenergic receptors, and substance P, which binds to specific cell-surface receptors, activate the phospholipid-Ca^{2+} pathway described before for muscarinic cholinergic

stimulation, resulting in fluid and electrolyte secretion. Small amounts of protein are secreted in response to certain gastrointestinal hormones (e.g., gastrin and cholecystokinin) and other peptides released from autonomic nerve terminals, such as vasoactive intestinal polypeptide and neuropeptide Y. Substance P, vasoactive intestinal polypeptide, neuropeptide Y, and calcitonin gene-related peptide also exert effects on the glandular vasculature to regulate blood flow. Nitric oxide, produced by parasympathetic nerves, vascular endothelial cells, and glandular secretory cells, stimulates the production of cyclic guanosine monophosphate and the release of Ca^{2+} from intracellular storage sites in secretory cells. These mechanisms most likely act in concert with the β-adrenergic and muscarinic cholinergic signaling pathways to augment or modulate saliva secretion.

Extracellular adenosine triphosphate, which activates the P2X and P2Y purinergic receptors on secretory and duct cells, elevates intracellular Ca^{2+} levels. P2X receptors are nonselective cation channels that allow extracellular Ca^{2+} to enter the cell. P2Y receptors cause release of Ca^{2+} from intracellular storage sites via stimulation of phospholipase C and inositol trisphosphate formation. Purinergic receptors may serve to modulate saliva secretion induced by other signaling pathways, however, only in vitro studies of receptor function have been carried out, and the in vivo source of extracellular adenosine triphosphate is unknown. Thus the physiologic significance of purinergic receptor activation in salivary glands remains elusive.

MYOEPITHELIAL CELLS

Myoepithelial cells are contractile cells associated with the secretory end pieces and intercalated ducts of the salivary glands (Figure 11-19). These cells are located between the basal lamina and the secretory or duct cells and are joined to the cells by desmosomes.

Myoepithelial cells have many similarities to smooth muscle cells but are derived from epithelium. Myoepithelial cells present around the secretory end pieces have a stellate shape; numerous branching processes extend from the cell body to surround and embrace the end piece (Figure 11-20). The processes are filled with filaments of actin and soluble myosin (Figures 11-21 and 11-22). The cell membrane has numerous caveolae, which presumably function in initiating contraction. Most of the other cellular organelles are located in the perinuclear cytoplasm. Myoepithelial cells associated with the intercalated ducts have a more fusiform shape with fewer processes and tend to be oriented lengthwise along the duct.

Contraction of the myoepithelial cells is thought to provide support for the end pieces during active secretion of saliva. The cells also may help to expel the primary saliva from the end piece into the duct system. Contraction of the myoepithelial cells of the intercalated ducts may shorten and widen the ducts, helping to maintain their patency. Recent studies suggest that myoepithelial cells have additional functions that may be more important than their ability to contract. They provide signals to the acinar secretory cells that are necessary for maintaining cell polarity and the structural organization of the secretory end piece.

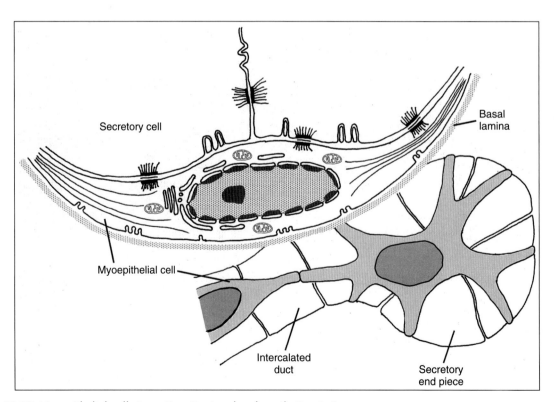

Figure 11-19 Myoepithelial cells in section *(top)* and surface *(bottom)* views.

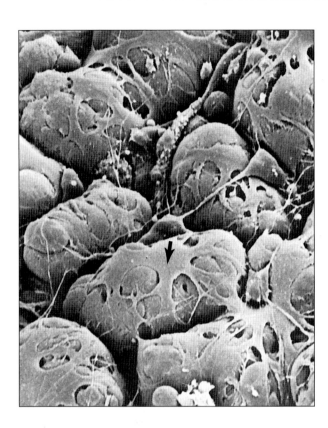

Figure 11-20 Scanning electron micrograph of myoepithelial cells. The basal lamina has been digested away, revealing the basal surfaces of the acinar cells covered by myoepithelial cells *(arrow)* and their branching processes. *(From Nagato T, Yoshida H, Yoshida A et al: Cell Tissue Res 209:1, 1980.)*

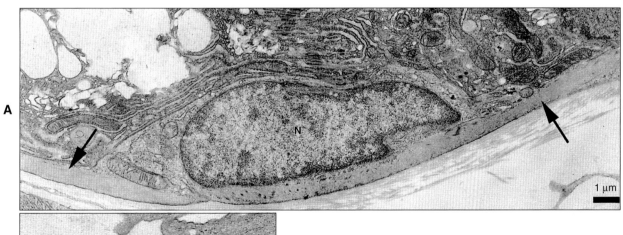

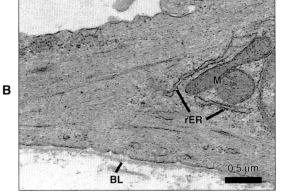

Figure 11-21 A, Transmission electron micrograph of myoepithelial cell at the base of mucous secretory cell of the rat sublingual gland. Processes of the cell *(arrows)* extend from both sides of the cell body. *N,* Nucleus. **B,** The myoepithelial cell processes are filled with actin filaments. A few mitochondria *(M)* and short cisternae of rough endoplasmic reticulum *(rER)* are located in the perinuclear cytoplasm. The myoepithelial cell is located on the epithelial side of the basal lamina *(BL).* *(A from Hand AR. In Bhaskar SN, editor: Orban's oral histology and embryology, ed 11, St Louis, 1991, Mosby.)*

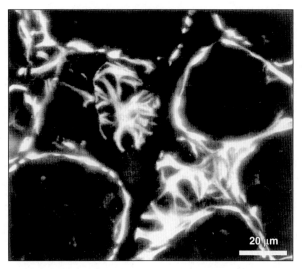

Figure 11-22 Immunofluorescence of myosin in myoepithelial cells of the rat sublingual gland. The section was treated with an antibody to smooth muscle myosin, followed by a fluorescent-labeled secondary antibody. Tangential sections of acini reveal the branching nature of the myoepithelial cells. Myoepithelial cell processes cut in cross and longitudinal section surround adjacent acini. *(Courtesy D. Drenckhahn, Würzburg, Germany. From Hand AR. In Bhaskar SN, editor: Orban's oral histology and embryology, ed 11, St Louis, 1991, Mosby.)*

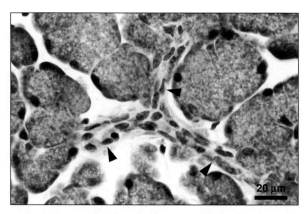

Figure 11-23 Light micrograph of branching intercalated duct *(arrowheads)* joining several serous end pieces in the human submandibular gland. The duct cells are low cuboidal and their cytoplasm stains lightly with eosin. The surrounding serous end piece cells stain with hematoxylin.

The evidence also suggests that myoepithelial cells produce a number of proteins that have tumor suppressor activity, such as proteinase inhibitors (e.g., tissue inhibitor of metalloproteinases) and antiangiogenesis factors, and that these cells may provide a barrier against invasive epithelial neoplasms.

DUCTS

The ductal system of salivary glands is a varied network of tubules that progressively increase in diameter, beginning at the secretory end pieces and extending to the oral cavity (see Figure 11-6). The three classes of ducts are intercalated, striated, and excretory, each with differing structure and function. The ductal system is more than just a simple conduit for the passage of saliva; it actively participates in the production and modification of saliva.

Intercalated Ducts

The primary saliva produced by the secretory end pieces passes first through the intercalated ducts (Figure 11-23). The first cells of the intercalated duct are directly adjacent to the secretory cells of the end piece, and the lumen of the end piece is continuous with the lumen of the intercalated duct. The intercalated ducts

are lined by a simple cuboidal epithelium, and myoepithelial cell bodies and their processes typically are located along the basal surface of the duct. The overall diameter of the intercalated ducts is smaller than that of the end pieces, and their lumina are larger than those of the end pieces. Several ducts draining individual end pieces join to form larger intercalated ducts, and these may join again before emptying into the striated ducts. The length of the intercalated ducts in the different major and minor salivary glands varies.

The intercalated duct cells have centrally placed nuclei and a small amount of cytoplasm containing some rough endoplasmic reticulum and a small Golgi complex (Figures 11-24 and 11-25). A few small secretory granules may be found in the apical cytoplasm, especially in cells located near the end pieces. The apical cell surface has a few short microvilli projecting into the lumen; the lateral surfaces are joined by apical junctional complexes and scattered desmosomes and gap junctions and have folded processes that interdigitate with similar processes of adjacent cells. Because of their small size and lack of distinctive features, intercalated ducts often are difficult to identify in routine histologic sections.

The intercalated ducts contribute macromolecular components, which are stored in their secretory granules, to the saliva. These components include lysozyme and lactoferrin; other currently unknown components probably also are secreted by these cells. A portion of the fluid component of the primary saliva likely is added in the intercalated duct region. Undifferentiated cells, thought to represent salivary gland stem cells, are believed to be present in the intercalated ducts. These cells may proliferate and undergo differentiation to

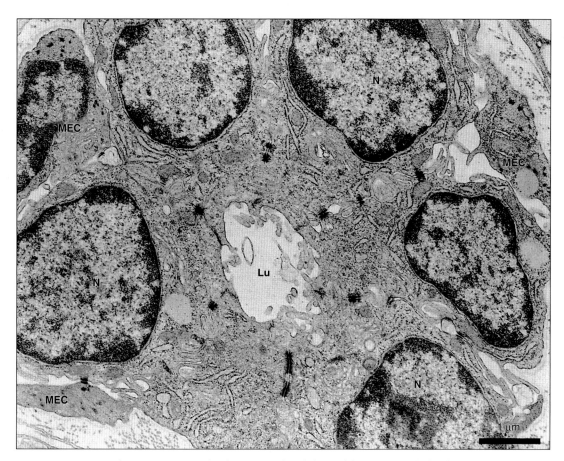

Figure 11-24 Transmission electron micrograph of an intercalated duct of the rat parotid gland. The cuboidal cells have a few endoplasmic reticulum cisternae and a small Golgi complex and are joined by junctional complexes and numerous desmosomes. Myoepithelial cell processes *(MEC)* are present at the basal side of the duct cells. *Lu*, Lumen; *N*, nucleus. *(From Hand AR. In Bhaskar SN, editor:* Orban's oral histology and embryology, *ed 11, St Louis, 1991, Mosby.)*

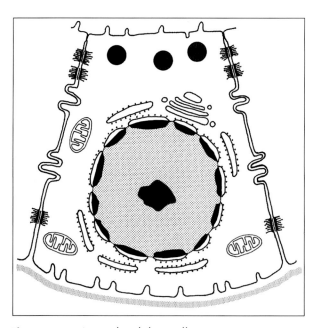

Figure 11-25 Intercalated duct cell.

replace damaged or dying cells in the end pieces and striated ducts.

Striated Ducts

The striated ducts, which receive the primary saliva from the intercalated ducts, constitute the largest portion of the duct system. These ducts are the main ductal component located within the lobules of the gland, that is, intralobular (Figure 11-26). Striated duct cells are columnar, with a centrally placed nucleus and pale, acidophilic cytoplasm (Figure 11-27). In well-preserved tissue, faint radially oriented lines or striations may be observed in the basal cytoplasm of the ducts. The overall diameter of the duct is greater than that of the secretory end pieces, and the lumen is larger than those of the secretory end pieces and intercalated ducts. A basal lamina encloses the striated duct, and a capillary plexus is present in the surrounding connective tissue.

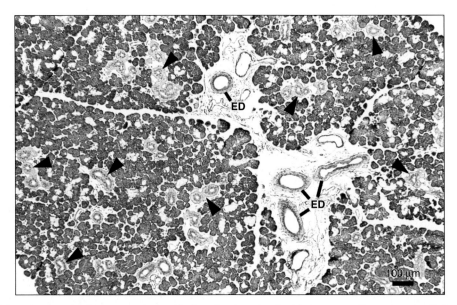

Figure 11-26 Light micrograph of human submandibular gland, stained with hematoxylin and eosin. Striated ducts *(arrowheads)* stain lightly with eosin and are readily identifiable at low power. The serous acini stain with hematoxylin. Larger excretory ducts *(ED)* are present in the interlobular connective tissue.

As described in the following discussion, an important function of striated duct cells is modification of the primary saliva by reabsorption and secretion of electrolytes. The structure of the duct cells reflects this function. The basal striations of the duct cells, when observed by electron microscopy, result from the presence of numerous elongated mitochondria in narrow

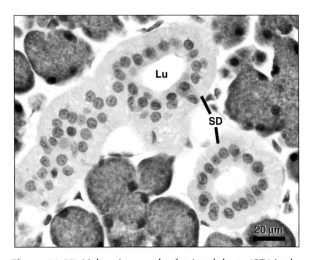

Figure 11-27 Light micrograph of striated ducts *(SD)* in the human submandibular gland. The ducts have large lumina *(Lu)* and are lined by a pale-staining, simple columnar epithelial cells, with centrally placed nuclei and faint basal striations. The duct cell cytoplasm stains lightly with eosin.

cytoplasmic partitions, separated by highly infolded and interdigitated basolateral cell membranes (Figure 11-28). The apical cytoplasm may contain small secretory granules and electron-lucent vesicles. The granules contain kallikrein and perhaps other secretory proteins; the presence of vesicles suggests that the cells may participate in endocytosis of substances from the lumen. The duct cells also contain numerous lysosomes and peroxisomes, and deposits of glycogen frequently are present in the perinuclear cytoplasm. Adjacent cells are joined by well-developed tight junctions and junctional complexes but lack gap junctions. The structure of the striated duct cells is summarized in Figure 11-29.

Excretory Ducts

The excretory ducts are located in the connective tissue septa between the lobules of the gland, that is, in an extralobular or interlobular location. These ducts are larger in diameter than striated ducts and typically have a pseudostratified epithelium with columnar cells extending from the basal lamina to the ductal lumen and small basal cells that sit on the basal lamina but do not reach the lumen (Figure 11-30, A). As the smaller ducts join to form larger excretory ducts, the number of basal cells increases, and scattered mucous (goblet) cells may be present (Figure 11-30, B). The epithelium of the main excretory duct may become stratified near the oral opening.

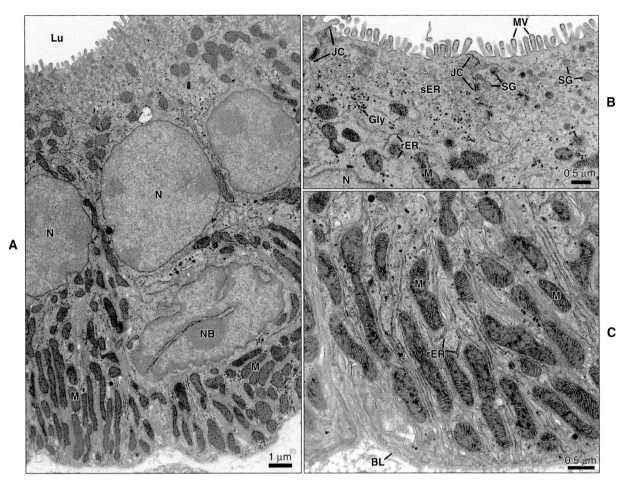

Figure 11-28 Transmission electron micrographs of striated duct cells of the mouse parotid gland. **A,** The columnar duct cells have centrally placed nuclei *(N)*, abundant mitochondria *(M)* between infolded basal membranes, and short microvilli on their apical surface. The basally located nucleus *(NB)* may belong to a dendritic (antigen-presenting) cell. *Lu,* Lumen. **B,** The apical cytoplasm contains irregular cisternae of smooth *(sER)* and rough *(rER)* endoplasmic reticulum, mitochondria near the nucleus, and scattered dense glycogen particles *(Gly)*. Some cells have an accumulation of small secretory granules *(SG)* near the apical membrane. Adjacent cells are held together by junctional complexes *(JC)*. *MV,* Microvilli. **C,** The basal region consists of partitions of cytoplasm containing mitochondria, a few endoplasmic reticulum cisternae, and glycogen particles, separated from other cytoplasmic partitions by extensively infolded cell membranes. The narrow cytoplasmic processes extend laterally beyond the cell boundaries to interdigitate with similar processes from the adjacent cells. *BL,* Basal lamina. *(A from Park K, Evans RL, Watson GE et al:* J Biol Chem *276:27042, 2001.)*

In the smaller excretory ducts the structure of the columnar cells is similar to that of the striated duct cells. As the ducts increase in size, the number of mitochondria and the extent of infolding of the basolateral membranes decrease. The basal cells have numerous bundles of intermediate filaments (tonofilaments) and are attached to the basal lamina by prominent hemidesmosomes. In some instances, basal cells may contain abundant actin filaments and have elongated processes similar to myoepithelial cells. Studies in experimental animals suggest that the columnar cells and the basal cells have a high rate of proliferation.

Small numbers of other types of cells are present in the excretory ducts and to some extent in the striated ducts. *Tuft (caveolated* or *brush) cells,* with long stiff microvilli and apical vesicles, are thought to be receptor cells of some type. Nerve endings occasionally are found adjacent to the basal portions of these cells. Other cells with pale cytoplasm and dense nuclear chromatin may be found toward the base of the duct epithelium. Some of these cells appear to be lymphocytes and macrophages. In other cases the cells have long branching processes that extend between the epithelial cells. These cells presumably are *dendritic cells,* or

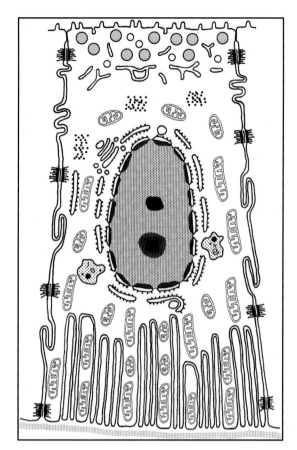

Figure 11-29 Striated duct cell.

antigen-presenting cells, that are involved in immune surveillance and the processing and presentation of foreign antigens to T lymphocytes.

DUCTAL MODIFICATION OF SALIVA

In addition to conveying saliva from the secretory end pieces to the oral cavity, an important function of the striated and excretory ducts is modification of the primary saliva produced by the end pieces and intercalated ducts. This modification occurs principally through reabsorption and secretion of electrolytes. The luminal and basolateral membranes have abundant transporters (Figure 11-31) that function to produce a net reabsorption of Na^+ and Cl^-, resulting in the formation of hypotonic final saliva. The ducts also secrete K^+ and HCO_3^-, but little if any secretion or reabsorption of water occurs in the striated and excretory ducts. The final electrolyte composition of saliva varies, depending on the salivary flow rate. At high flow rates, saliva is in contact with the ductal epithelium for a shorter time, and Na^+ and Cl^- concentrations rise and the K^+ concentration decreases. At low flow rates the electrolyte concentrations change in the opposite direction. The HCO_3^- concentration, however, increases with increasing flow rates, reflecting the increased secretion of HCO_3^- by the acinar cells to drive fluid secretion.

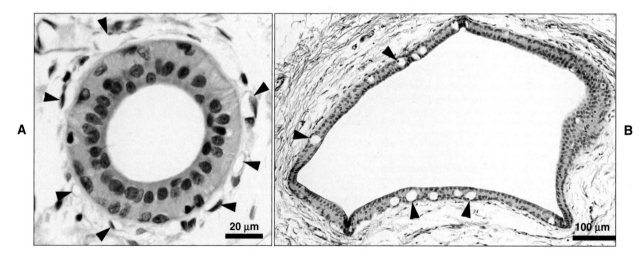

Figure 11-30 Light micrographs of excretory ducts of the human submandibular gland, stained with hematoxylin and eosin. **A,** A small excretory duct in the interlobular connective tissue. The duct epithelium is pseudostratified, with tall columnar cells and a few basal cells. Numerous capillaries and venules *(arrowheads)* are present around the duct. **B,** A large excretory duct is surrounded by dense connective tissue. The pseudostratified epithelium contains several mucous goblet cells *(arrowheads)*.

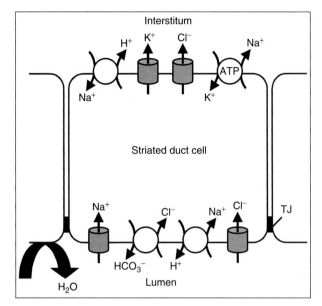

Figure 11-31 Mechanisms of ductal modification of saliva. Striated duct cells reabsorb Na^+ and Cl^- mainly via channels in the luminal membrane; Na^+/H^+ and Cl^-/HCO_3^- exchangers provide additional mechanisms for uptake of these ions. Na^+ exits at the basolateral surface via the Na^+/K^+-adenosinetriphosphatase, and Cl^- exits via a channel. K^+ channels at the basolateral surface maintain electroneutrality, and the Na^+/H^+ exchanger compensates for intracellular acidification. The tight junctions *(TJ)* are relatively "tight," and the duct cells are impermeable to water. *(Modified from Melvin JE: Crit Rev Oral Biol Med 10:199, 1999.)*

Electrolyte reabsorption and secretion by the striated and excretory ducts is regulated by the autonomic nervous system and by mineralocorticoids produced by the adrenal cortex. The sympathetic innervation has a more important role in regulating electrolyte transport in the ducts than in the acini because of a larger number of cAMP-regulated Cl^- channels (the *cystic fibrosis transmembrane conductance regulator*) in the luminal cell membrane.

CONNECTIVE TISSUE

The connective tissue of the salivary glands includes a surrounding capsule, variably developed, that demarcates the gland from adjacent structures. Septa that extend inward from the capsule divide the gland into lobes and lobules and carry the blood vessels and nerves that supply the parenchymal components and the excretory ducts that convey saliva to the oral cavity (see Figures 11-5 and 11-26). As in other locations, the cells of the connective tissue include fibroblasts, macrophages, dendritic cells, mast cells, plasma cells, adipose cells, and occasionally, granulocytes

and lymphocytes. Collagen and elastic fibers along with the glycoproteins and proteoglycans of the ground substance constitute the extracellular matrix of the connective tissue.

Within the lobules of the gland, finer partitions of connective tissue extend between adjacent secretory end pieces and ducts. These partitions carry the arterioles, capillaries, and venules of the microcirculation and the finer branches of the autonomic nerves that innervate the secretory and ductal cells. The same cellular and extracellular connective tissue components are present in these locations.

Plasma cells located adjacent to the secretory end pieces and intralobular ducts produce immunoglobulins that are secreted into the saliva by *transcytosis*. The main immunoglobulin present in saliva is secretory IgA, which is synthesized as a dimer complexed with an additional protein called *J chain*. The salivary gland epithelial cells have receptors for dimeric IgA on their basolateral membranes. The epithelial cells take up the receptor-bound IgA by endocytosis, and the vesicles containing the IgA move from the basolateral cytoplasm to the apical cytoplasm. The bound IgA, along with a portion of the receptor called *secretory component*, is released at the luminal surface of the cell. Small amounts of IgG and IgM also are secreted into the saliva.

NERVE SUPPLY

The salivary glands are innervated by postganglionic nerve fibers of the sympathetic and parasympathetic divisions of the autonomic nervous system. Depending on the gland, preganglionic parasympathetic fibers originate in the superior or inferior salivatory nuclei in the brainstem and travel via the seventh (facial) and ninth (glossopharyngeal) cranial nerves to the submandibular and otic ganglia, where they synapse with postganglionic neurons that send their axons to the glands through the lingual and auriculotemporal nerves. Preganglionic sympathetic nerves originate in the thoracic spinal cord, synapse with postganglionic neurons in the superior cervical ganglion, and reach the glands traveling with the arterial blood supply. During development, the ability of sympathetic axons to reach their targets, and the survival of the postganglionic neurons, critically depend on neurotrophic factors synthesized by the cells of the developing glands.

Within the gland lobules, branches of the nerves follow the blood vessels, eventually forming a plexus of unmyelinated fibers adjacent to arterioles, ducts, and secretory end pieces (Figure 11-32). The axons of each nerve bundle are invested by cytoplasmic processes of Schwann cells. Two different morphologic relationships between the nerves and the epithelial cells exist. In some cases, an axon leaves the nerve bundle, loses its

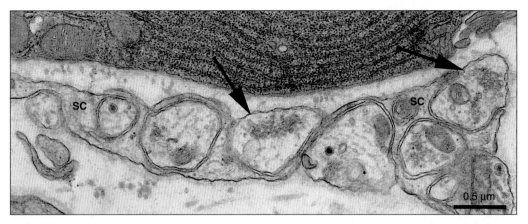

Figure 11-32 Transmission electron micrograph of an autonomic nerve bundle in the rat submandibular gland. Unmyelinated axons are enclosed by Schwann cell *(SC)* cytoplasm. Innervation of the secretory cells occurs where axonal varicosities containing transmitter vesicles lack the Schwann cell covering *(arrows)*. *(From Hand AR. In Provenza DV, Seibel W, editors:* Oral histology: inheritance and development, *ed 2, Philadelphia, 1986, Lea and Febiger.)*

Schwann cell investment, penetrates the epithelial basal lamina, and forms an expanded swelling, or varicosity, in close contact (10 to 20 nm) with the basolateral membrane of the epithelial cell. In the most common relationship the axon forms a varicosity but remains associated with the nerve bundle, and the Schwann cell covering is absent over the varicosity. In this type of innervation the axonal varicosity is separated from the epithelial cells by 100 to 200 nm and the basal laminae surrounding the nerve bundle and the epithelial cell. The type of nerve-epithelial cell relationship, termed *intraparenchymal* and *extraparenchymal*, respectively, varies among the glands and among the different cells within a single gland. For example, intraparenchymal innervation occurs in the human submandibular gland and in the minor glands of the lip, whereas only extraparenchymal innervation occurs in the human parotid gland. Despite the different morphologic relationships, no functional differences between the two patterns of innervation are apparent.

Several varicosities may be present along the length of an axon, and a single nerve may innervate more than one epithelial cell. The axonal varicosities contain small neurotransmitter vesicles; occasional larger, dense-cored vesicles; and mitochondria. These varicosities are believed to be the site of innervation of the gland cells and thus the site of neurotransmitter release. However, no specializations of the axonal or epithelial cell membranes occur at these sites as occur at synapses in the central nervous system. The main parasympathetic neurotransmitter is acetylcholine; the main sympathetic neurotransmitter is norepinephrine. Release of these transmitters and their interaction with cell-surface receptors initiate the response of the cells, that is, fluid and electrolyte secretion, exocytosis, modulation of ductal transport processes, or contraction of myoepithelial cells or arteriolar smooth muscle cells.

BLOOD SUPPLY

Rapid and sustained secretion of saliva, which is 99% water, necessitates an extensive blood supply to the salivary glands. One or more arteries enter the gland and give rise to smaller arteries and arterioles that tend to follow the path of the excretory ducts. The arterioles break up into capillaries that are distributed around the secretory end pieces and striated ducts. In some species the capillaries supplying the secretory end pieces and ducts arise from separate arterioles (i.e., a parallel arrangement), whereas in other species a venous portal system connects the capillary network around the end pieces with that around the ducts. An extensive capillary plexus, also arising from separate arterioles, exists around the excretory ducts. The endothelium of the capillaries and postcapillary venules is fenestrated.

The venous return, except as noted previously, generally follows the arterial supply. However, arteriovenous anastomoses occur in some glands. As blood flow increases during secretion (as much as fifteenfold during maximum secretion), more blood is diverted through these anastomoses, resulting in increased venous and capillary pressures. The resulting increase in fluid filtration across the capillary endothelium provides the fluid necessary to maintain secretion.

SUMMARY OF SALIVARY GLAND STRUCTURE

Salivary glands consist of secretory end pieces that are composed of serous cells or mucous cells, or mucous

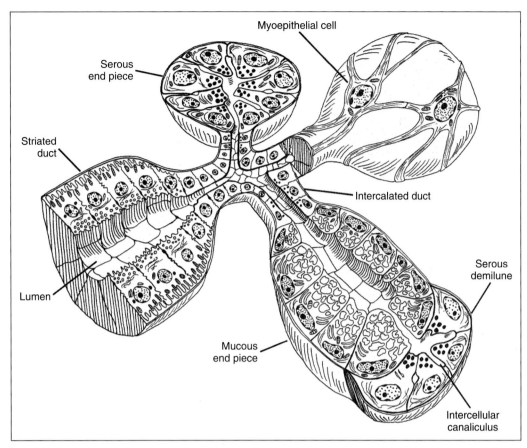

Figure 11-33 Architecture of salivary gland ducts and secretory end pieces and the main features of the parenchymal cells. *(From Hand AR. In Bhaskar SN, editor:* Orban's oral histology and embryology, *ed 11, St Louis, 1991, Mosby.)*

end pieces capped by serous demilunes, and a system of ducts (intercalated, striated, and excretory) that modify the saliva produced by the end pieces and convey it to the oral cavity (Figure 11-33). Contractile myoepithelial cells are distributed around the end pieces and intercalated ducts. The gland is supported by connective tissue, which carries the nerve, vascular, and lymphatic supplies to the parenchymal components and is the location of cells of the innate and adaptive immune systems.

HISTOLOGY OF THE MAJOR SALIVARY GLANDS

PAROTID GLAND

In the parotid gland the spherical secretory end pieces are all serous (Figure 11-34). The pyramidally shaped acinar cells have a spherical, basally situated nucleus and surround a small, central lumen. The basal cytoplasm stains with basophilic dyes, and the secretory granules in the apical cytoplasm usually stain with acidophilic dyes.

Fat cell spaces often are seen in sections of the parotid gland.

Intercalated ducts are numerous and long in the parotid gland. The ducts are lined with cuboidal epithelial cells and have lumina that are larger than those of the acini. Nuclei of myoepithelial cells sometimes may be present at the basal surface of the ducts. The striated ducts are numerous and appear as slightly acidophilic, round, or elongated tubules of larger diameter than the end pieces. The ducts consist of a simple columnar epithelium, with round, centrally placed nuclei. Faint striations, representing the infolded basal cell membranes and mitochondria, may be visible below the nucleus. The lumina are large relative to the overall size of the ducts.

SUBMANDIBULAR GLAND

The submandibular gland contains serous end pieces and mucous tubules capped with serous demilunes (Figure 11-35); thus it is a mixed gland. Although the proportions of serous and mucous secretory end pieces may vary from lobule to lobule and among individual

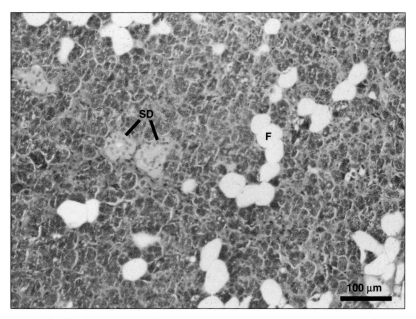

Figure 11-34 Light micrograph of human parotid gland, stained with hematoxylin and eosin. The secretory end pieces are all serous. *F,* Fat cells; *SD,* striated ducts.

glands, serous cells significantly outnumber the mucous cells. The serous end pieces are similar in structure to those found in the parotid gland, with abundant secretory granules, a spherical nucleus, and basophilic cytoplasm. The mucous secretory cells are filled with pale-staining secretory material, and little cytoplasm is usually visible. The nucleus is compressed against the basal cell membrane and contains densely stained chromatin. The lumina of the mucous tubules are larger than those of serous end pieces. Serous demilune cells are similar in structure to the serous end piece cells but discharge their secretions into small intercellular canaliculi that extend between the mucous cells to reach the tubule lumen. The intercalated and striated ducts are less numerous than those in the parotid gland, but otherwise they are structurally similar.

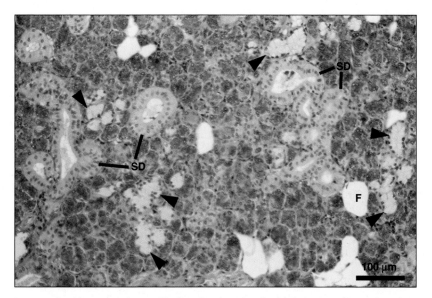

Figure 11-35 Light micrograph of human submandibular gland, stained with hematoxylin and eosin. Serous secretory end pieces predominate, but a few mucous tubules *(arrowheads)* are present. Several lightly stained striated ducts *(SD)* are present. *F,* Fat cells.

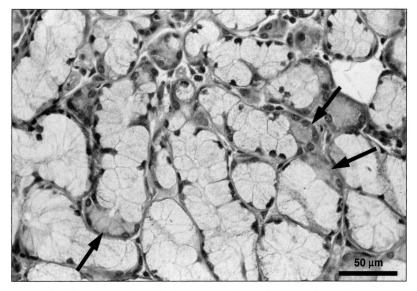

Figure 11-36 Light micrograph of human sublingual gland, stained with hematoxylin and eosin. Mucous tubules are abundant; many have serous demilunes *(arrows)*.

SUBLINGUAL GLAND

The sublingual gland also is a mixed gland, but mucous secretory cells predominate (Figure 11-36). The mucous tubules and serous demilunes resemble those of the submandibular gland. Although serous end pieces may be present, they are rare, and most structures appearing as serous end pieces probably represent sections through demilunes that do not include the mucous tubule. The intercalated ducts are short and difficult to recognize. Intralobular ducts are fewer in number than in the parotid or submandibular glands, and some ducts may lack the infolded basolateral membranes characteristic of striated ducts.

HISTOLOGY OF THE MINOR SALIVARY GLANDS

Minor salivary glands are found throughout the oral cavity, except in the anterior part of the hard palate and the gingiva. These glands consist of aggregates of secretory end pieces and ducts, organized into small lobule-like structures located in the submucosa or between muscle fibers of the tongue (Figure 11-37; see also Figure 11-1). The ducts draining individual glandular aggregates usually open directly onto the mucosal surface. The secretory end pieces of most minor glands are mucous or have a small serous component arranged

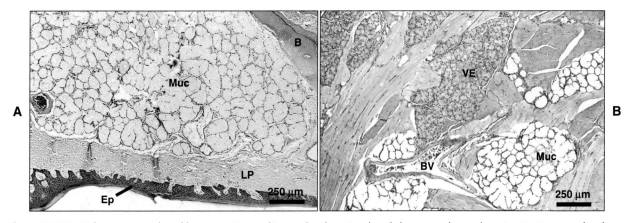

Figure 11-37 Light micrographs of human minor salivary glands stained with hematoxylin and eosin. **A,** Mucous gland *(Muc)* in the lateral portion of the hard palate. *B,* Bone; *Ep,* epithelium; *LP,* lamina propria. **B,** Lingual serous (Ebner's) glands *(VE)* and mucous glands *(Muc)* located between muscle fibers in the posterior part of the tongue. *BV,* Blood vessel.

as occasional demilunes. Intercalated ducts often are poorly developed, and the larger ducts may lack the typical infolded basolateral membranes of the striated ducts of the major glands. In contrast to the usual situation in the minor glands, the lingual serous glands (of Ebner) in the tongue below the circumvallate papillae are pure serous glands. Their secretions are released in regions with significant numbers of taste buds, specifically, the troughs surrounding the vallate papillae, and the clefts between the rudimentary foliate papillae on the sides of the tongue. They secrete digestive enzymes and proteins thought to play a role in the taste process. The fluid component of their secretions is presumed to cleanse the trough and prepare the taste receptors for a new stimulus.

Minor gland saliva typically is rich in mucins, various antibacterial proteins, and secretory immunoglobulins. The minor glands exhibit a continuous slow secretory activity, and thus have an important role in protecting and moistening the oral mucosa, especially at night when the major salivary glands are mostly inactive.

CLINICAL CONSIDERATIONS

AGE CHANGES

With age, a generalized loss of salivary gland parenchymal tissue occurs. A gradual reduction of up to 30% to 60% in the proportional acinar volume of the major salivary glands has been observed. The lost salivary cells often are replaced by adipose tissue. An increase in fibrous connective tissue and vascular elements also occurs. Changes of the duct system, including an increase in nonstriated intralobular ducts, dilatation of extralobular ducts, and degenerative and metaplastic changes, have been reported. Although decreased production of saliva often is observed in older persons, whether this is related directly to the reduction in parenchymal tissue is not clear. Some studies of healthy older individuals, in which the use of medications were controlled carefully, revealed little or no loss of salivary function, suggesting a large functional reserve capacity. Other studies suggest that although resting (unstimulated) salivary secretion is in the normal range, the volume of saliva produced during stimulated secretion is less than normal.

DISEASES

Salivary glands may be influenced by a number of diseases, local and systemic. Several viruses—such as cytomegalovirus, Epstein-Barr virus, and human herpes viruses 6 and 7—infect and replicate within salivary gland cells and are shed into saliva. Viral infections such as mumps and bacterial infections of individual glands may cause inflammation resulting in a painful swelling. Blockage of a duct may cause a transient swelling associated with eating, as blood flow increases and saliva backs up in the gland. Ductal obstruction may result from the formation of *sialoliths* (stones), most common in the submandibular duct, or a mucous plug or the severing of the duct of a minor salivary gland by trauma. The salivary glands also may be affected by a variety of benign and malignant tumors.

The salivary glands may be affected in various endocrine, autoimmune, infectious, and genetic diseases. Diabetes may have significant effects on salivary glands and the secretion of saliva. Parotid gland swelling may occur, and salivary flow is reduced. Increased levels of glucose in saliva may influence plaque metabolism. Studies of experimental diabetes demonstrate changes in the expression of certain secretory proteins. Autoimmune diseases such as *Sjögren's syndrome*, rheumatoid arthritis, or graft-versus-host disease occurring after tissue or organ transplantation may cause destruction of salivary tissue and reduced flow of saliva. Patients with adrenal diseases may have altered salivary electrolyte composition. Salivary function also is affected in individuals with acquired immune deficiency syndrome. Salivary flow rates are decreased, and lower levels of secretory immunoglobulins are present in saliva. Parotid gland enlargement may occur because of lymphadenopathy and lymphoepithelial cysts. Pathologic changes in salivary glands also are observed in individuals with cystic fibrosis. Salivary Na^+ and Cl^- concentrations are increased, and mucus-secreting glands may develop mucous plugs.

DRY MOUTH (XEROSTOMIA)

Dry mouth, or *xerostomia*, is a frequent clinical complaint. A loss of salivary function or a reduction in the volume of secreted saliva may lead to the sensation of oral dryness. Oral dryness occurs most commonly as a side effect of medications taken by the patient for other problems. Many drugs cause central or peripheral inhibition of salivary secretion. Destruction of salivary gland tissue is another common cause of xerostomia. Loss of gland function occurs after radiation therapy for head and neck cancer, because the salivary glands often are included in the radiation field, and salivary gland cells are highly sensitive to the deleterious effects of radiation. Chemotherapy for cancer or associated with bone marrow transplantation also may cause reduced salivary function. Autoimmune diseases, in particular Sjögren's syndrome, may cause progressive loss of salivary function from the invasion of lymphocytes into the gland and the destruction of epithelial cells.

The decreased volume of saliva in the mouth leads to drying of the oral tissues and loss of the protective effects of salivary buffers, proteins, and mucins. The oral tissues are more susceptible to infections, and speech, eating, and swallowing become difficult and painful. The teeth are highly susceptible to caries, especially near the gingival margin. Temporary relief is achieved by frequent sipping of water or artificial saliva. Patients who have some functional salivary tissue may benefit from pharmacologic therapy with oral parasympathomimetic drugs, such as pilocarpine, to increase salivary flow. In the future, satisfactory treatment of patients with xerostomia may include genetic modification of salivary gland cells to increase fluid and protein secretion.

TOPICS FOR CONSIDERATION Xerostomia

Xerostomia, literally *dry mouth*, is caused by decreased secretion of saliva. The decreased volume of saliva and the reduced levels of protective salivary proteins in the mouth lead to drying of the oral tissues, making them more susceptible to infection and diseases such as dental caries and causing movements of the lips and tongue, swallowing, and deglutition to become painful and difficult. The most common causes of decreased saliva secretion are the side effects of medications taken for other conditions. Decreased saliva secretion may occur as a result of immune-mediated hypofunction or destruction of salivary gland tissue. This may occur in certain disease states, such as the autoimmune disease Sjögren's syndrome. Sjögren's syndrome most frequently is diagnosed in middle-aged females and has a population prevalence of about 0.5%. Destruction of salivary gland tissue occurs in patients being treated for head and neck cancer with radiation therapy that includes the region of the salivary glands. Each year, approximately 30,000 new cases of head and neck cancer are treated with radiation therapy in the United States. Decreased saliva secretion also may occur in elderly persons because of a normal loss of salivary gland parenchymal tissue. Because of the growth of this population group, xerostomia is becoming more common.

Treatment of xerostomia depends on the cause of the condition. Patients taking medications that cause dry mouth may find relief by switching to another drug with fewer side effects. If the xerostomia is the result of gland dysfunction or destruction, currently available treatment options are mainly palliative. Some temporary relief is afforded by using artificial saliva solutions that are instilled into the mouth to coat the epithelial surfaces or simply by frequent sipping of water. In cases in which there is functional gland tissue remaining, some relief may be achieved by treatment with drugs that stimulate salivary secretion, such as the parasympathomimetic agents pilocarpine or cevimeline. The challenge to obtaining a satisfactory treatment of this condition is to reduce or eliminate the pathologic processes and/or restore sufficient function of the salivary glands. Recent clinical trials have shown some success with systemically administered immunomodulatory agents in an attempt to reduce or alter the destructive processes occurring in the glands. However, other studies have produced contradictory results, and undesirable side effects may occur with many of these agents. One possible treatment that could have a longer-lasting effect would be to transfect the cells of salivary glands with the genes necessary for production of saliva. An approach currently under investigation involves infecting the salivary glands through the duct opening with a suitable modified virus that contains the missing gene. Incorporation of the gene into the cells would restore the defective function. In animal experiments, in which the gene for a water channel protein (aquaporin) was inserted into the cells remaining after destruction of the salivary glands by radiation, an increase in fluid secretion occurred. A clinical trial to test this approach in human beings recently has been approved. In other experiments using animal models for Sjögren's syndrome, the genes for certain immunomodulatory cytokines or blocking agents have been inserted in order to achieve locally effective concentrations with minimal side effects. Although these gene therapy experiments are promising, certain barriers to their clinical adoption must be overcome. For example, many viral vectors induce only transient expression of the gene, which would necessitate repeated transfections for a lasting effect. Another problem is the development of methods to overcome the normal immune response to the virus and possibly to the expressed protein. Finally, the safety of the modified viruses must be completely assured.

Anders Bennick
Department of Biochemistry
University of Toronto
Toronto, Ontario, Canada

Arthur R. Hand
Department of Craniofacial Sciences
University of Connecticut Health Center
Farmington, Connecticut

RECOMMENDED READING

Cutler LS: Functional differentiation of salivary glands. In Forte J, editor: *Handbook of physiology: salivary, pancreatic, gastric and hepatobiliary secretion*, vol 3, New York, 1989, American Physiological Society.

Dobrosielski-Vergona K, editor: *Biology of the salivary glands*, Boca Raton, Fla, 1993, CRC Press.

Dodds MW, Johnson DA, Yeh CK: Health benefits of saliva: a review, *J Dent* 33:223-233, 2005.

Hand AR: The secretory process of salivary glands and pancreas. In Riva A, Motta PM, editors: *Ultrastructure of the extraparietal glands of the digestive tract*, Boston, 1990, Kluwer Academic.

Kaufman E, Lamster IB: The diagnostic applications of saliva: a review, *Crit Rev Oral Biol Med* 13:197-212, 2002.

Melvin JE, Yule D, Shuttleworth T, Begenisich T: Regulation of fluid and electrolyte secretion in salivary gland acinar cells, *Annu Rev Physiol* 67:445-469, 2005.

Patel VN, Rebustini IT, Hoffman MP: Salivary gland branching morphogenesis. *Differentiation* 74:349-364, 2006.

Tandler B, guest editor: Microstructure of the salivary glands, Part I, *Microsc Res Tech* 26:1-19, 1993.

Oral Mucosa

DEFINITION OF THE ORAL MUCOSA

The term *mucous membrane* is used to describe the moist lining of the gastrointestinal tract, nasal passages, and other body cavities that communicate with the exterior. In the oral cavity this lining is called the *oral mucous membrane*, or *oral mucosa*. At the lips the oral mucosa is continuous with the skin, a dry covering layer the structure of which resembles that of the oral lining in some respects; at the pharynx the oral mucosa is continuous with the moist mucosa lining the rest of the gut. Thus the oral mucosa is located anatomically between skin and gastrointestinal mucosa and shows some of the properties of each.

The skin, oral mucosa, and intestinal lining consist of two separate tissue components: a covering epithelium and an underlying connective tissue. Because these tissues together perform a common function, the oral mucosa (like the skin and the intestinal lining) should be considered an organ. Understanding the complex structure of a tissue or organ often is easier when its function is known. This point is particularly true of the oral mucosa, the structure of which reflects a variety of functional adaptations. The major adaptations are a result of evolutionary changes in the species that have taken place over a long time. Although small and usually reversible changes in structure of oral mucosa may be seen in response to function during the lifetime of an individual, these changes are not heritable.

FUNCTIONS OF THE ORAL MUCOSA

The oral mucosa serves several functions. The major one is protection of the deeper tissues of the oral cavity; others include acting as a sensory organ and serving as the site of glandular activity and secretion.

PROTECTION

As a surface lining, the oral mucosa separates and protects deeper tissues and organs in the oral region from the environment of the oral cavity. The normal activities of seizing food and biting and chewing it expose the oral soft tissues to mechanical forces (compression, stretching, and shearing) and surface abrasions (from hard particles in the diet). The oral mucosa shows a number of adaptations of the epithelium and the connective tissue to withstand these insults. Furthermore, a resident population of microorganisms normally resides within the oral cavity that would cause infection if they gained access to the tissues. Many of these organisms also produce substances that have a toxic effect on tissues. The epithelium of the oral mucosa acts as the major barrier to these threats.

SENSATION

The sensory function of the oral mucosa is important because it provides considerable information about events within the oral cavity, whereas the lips and tongue perceive stimuli outside the mouth. In the mouth, receptors respond to temperature, touch, and pain; the tongue also has taste buds, which are not found anywhere else in the body. Certain receptors in the oral mucosa probably respond to the taste of water and signal the satisfaction of thirst. Reflexes such as swallowing, gagging, retching, and salivating also are initiated by receptors in the oral mucosa.

SECRETION

The major secretion associated with the oral mucosa is saliva, produced by the salivary glands, which contributes to the maintenance of a moist surface. The major salivary glands are situated distant from the mucosa, and their secretions pass through the mucosa via long ducts; however, many minor salivary glands are associated with the oral mucosa (the salivary glands are described fully in Chapter 11). Sebaceous glands frequently are present in the oral mucosa, but their secretions are probably insignificant.

THERMAL REGULATION

In some animals (such as the dog) considerable body heat is dissipated through the oral mucosa by panting; for these animals the mucosa plays a major role in the regulation of body temperature. The human oral mucosa, however, plays practically no role in regulating body temperature, and no obvious specializations of the blood vessels exist for controlling heat transfer, such as arteriovenous shunts.

ORGANIZATION OF THE ORAL MUCOSA

The oral cavity consists of two parts: an outer vestibule, bounded by the lips and cheeks, and the oral cavity proper, separated from the vestibule by the alveolus bearing the teeth and gingivae. The hard and soft palates form the superior zone of the oral cavity proper, and the floor of the mouth and base of the tongue form the inferior border. Posteriorly the oral cavity is bounded by the pillars of the fauces and the tonsils. The oral mucosa shows considerable structural variation in different regions of the oral cavity, but three main types of mucosa can be recognized, identified according to their primary function: masticatory mucosa, lining mucosa, and specialized mucosa. Figure 12-1 shows the anatomic location of each type diagrammatically, and the types are described fully later in the chapter. Quantitatively, the larger part of the oral mucosa is represented by lining mucosa, amounting to 60% of the total area, with masticatory mucosa and specialized mucosa occupying smaller areas (25% and 15%, respectively).

CLINICAL FEATURES

Although the oral mucosa is continuous with the skin, it differs considerably in appearance. Generally, the oral mucosa is more deeply colored, most obviously at the lips (where the bright vermilion border contrasts with the skin tone). This coloration represents the combined effect of a number of factors: the concentration and state of dilation of small blood vessels in the underlying connective tissue, the thickness of the epithelium, the degree of keratinization, and the amount of melanin pigment in the epithelium. Color gives an indication as to the clinical condition of the mucosa; inflamed tissues are red, because of dilation of the blood vessels, whereas normal healthy tissues are a paler pink.

Other features that distinguish the oral mucosa from skin are its moist surface and the absence of appendages. Skin contains numerous hair follicles, sebaceous glands, and sweat glands, whereas the glandular component of oral mucosa is represented primarily by the minor

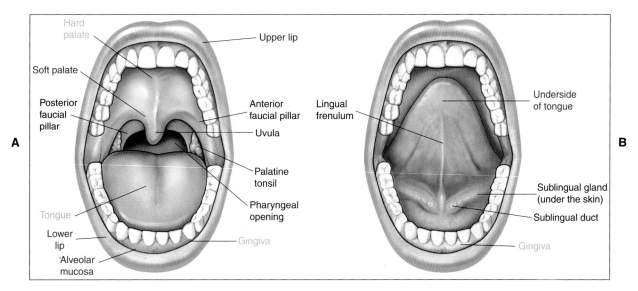

Figure 12-1 **A** and **B,** Anatomic locations occupied by the three main types of mucosa in the oral cavity. *(From Thibodeau G, Patton K:* Anatomy and physiology, *ed 6, St Louis, 2007, Mosby.)*

salivary glands. These glands are concentrated in various regions of the oral cavity, and the openings of their ducts at the mucosal surface are sometimes evident on clinical examination (Figure 12-2, *B*). Sebaceous glands are present in the upper lip and buccal mucosa in about three quarters of adults and have been described occasionally in the alveolar mucosa and dorsum of the tongue (Figure 12-3). Sebaceous glands appear as pale yellow spots and sometimes are called *Fordyce's spots*.

The surface of the oral mucosa tends to be smoother and have fewer folds or wrinkles than the skin, but topographic features are readily apparent on clinical examination. The most obvious are the different papillae on the dorsum of the tongue and the transverse ridges (or rugae) of the hard palate. The healthy gingiva shows a pattern of fine surface stippling, consisting of small indentations of the mucosal surface (Figure 12-2, *A*). In many persons a slight whitish ridge occurs along the buccal mucosa in the occlusal plane of the teeth. This line, sometimes called the *linea alba* (white line), is a keratinized region and may represent the effect of abrasion from rough tooth restorations or cheek biting.

The oral mucosa varies considerably in its firmness and texture. The lining mucosa of the lips and cheeks, for example, is soft and pliable, whereas the gingiva and hard palate are covered by a firm, immobile layer. These differences have important clinical implications for giving local injections of anesthetics or taking biopsies of oral mucosa. Fluid can be introduced easily into loose lining mucosa, but injection into the masticatory

mucosa is difficult and painful. However, lining mucosa gapes when surgically incised and may require suturing, but masticatory mucosa does not. Similarly, the accumulation of fluid with inflammation is obvious and painful in masticatory mucosa, but in lining mucosa the fluid disperses, and inflammation may not be as evident or as painful.

COMPONENT TISSUES AND GLANDS

The two main tissue components of the oral mucosa are a stratified squamous epithelium, called the *oral epithelium*, and an underlying connective tissue layer, called the *lamina propria* (Figure 12-4). In the skin these two tissues are known by slightly different terminology: *epidermis* and *dermis*. The interface between epithelium and connective tissue is usually irregular, and upward projections of connective tissue, called the *connective tissue papillae*, interdigitate with epithelial ridges or pegs, sometimes called the *rete ridges* or *pegs* (see Figure 12-19 later in this chapter). There is a basal lamina at the interface between epithelium and connective tissue that appears as a structureless layer (see Figure 12-19, *A*).

Although the junction between oral epithelium and lamina propria is obvious, that between the oral mucosa and underlying tissue, or submucosa, is less easy to recognize. In the gastrointestinal tract the lining mucosa clearly is separated from underlying tissues by a layer of smooth muscle and elastic fibers, the muscularis mucosae

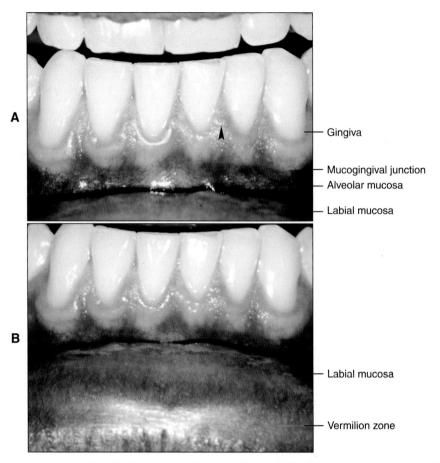

A

Gingiva

Mucogingival junction
Alveolar mucosa
Labial mucosa

B

Labial mucosa

Vermilion zone

Figure 12-2 Healthy oral mucosa. **A,** Attached gingiva and the alveolar and labial mucosae. Gingival stippling is most evident in the interproximal regions *(arrowhead)*. The mucogingival junction between keratinized gingiva and nonkeratinized alveolar mucosa is clearly evident. **B,** Vermilion zone adjoining the labial mucosa. Minor salivary gland ducts open to the surface in this region. *(Courtesy A. Kauzman.)*

(literally, "muscle of the mucosa"; Figure 12-5, *A*) and in functional terms may allow for some isolation of the internal lining from movements of the outer muscular layers of the gut.

The oral mucosa has no muscularis mucosae, and clearly identifying the boundary between it and the underlying tissues is difficult. In many regions (e.g., cheeks, lips, and parts of the hard palate) a layer of loose fatty or glandular connective tissue containing the major blood vessels and nerves that supply the mucosa separates the oral mucosa from underlying bone or muscle. The layer represents the submucosa in the oral cavity (Figure 12-5, *B*), and its composition determines the flexibility of the attachment of oral mucosa to the underlying structures. In regions such as the gingiva and parts of the hard palate, oral mucosa is attached directly to the periosteum of underlying bone, with no intervening submucosa (Figure 12-5, *C*). This arrangement is called a *mucoperiosteum* and provides a firm, inelastic attachment.

The minor salivary glands are situated in the submucosa of the mucosa. Sebaceous glands are less frequent than salivary glands; they lie in the lamina propria and have the same structure as those present in the skin. The sebaceous glands produce a fatty secretion, sebum, the function of which in the oral cavity is unclear, although some claim that the sebum may lubricate the surface of the mucosa so that it slides easily against the teeth. The presence of sebaceous glands in oral mucosa may be an accident of embryologic development by which some of the potential of skin ectoderm is retained in the ectoderm that invaginates to form the lining of the oral cavity.

In several regions of the oral cavity are nodules of lymphoid tissue that consist of crypts formed by invaginations of the epithelium into the lamina propria. Capillaries in the connective tissue carry adhesion molecules such as the endothelial cell leukocyte adhesion molecule, intercellular adhesion molecule, and vascular cell adhesion molecule, which facilitate the

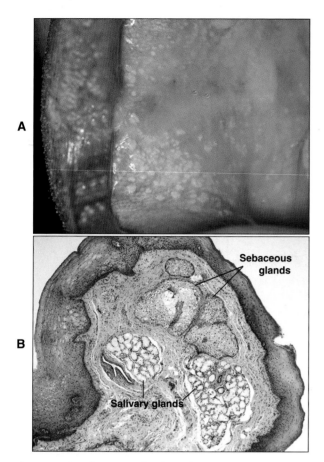

Figure 12-3 Sebaceous glands in the mucosa of the cheek. **A,** Clinically, these appear as clusters of yellowish spots called Fordyce's granules. **B,** Histologic section of a biopsy from this region. Note the presence of minor salivary glands in proximity of the sebaceous glands. *(Courtesy A. Kauzman.)*

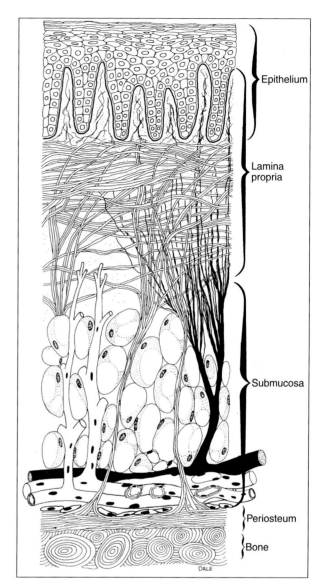

Figure 12-4 Main tissue components of the oral mucosa.

trafficking of leukocytes from the blood. As a result, these areas are infiltrated extensively by lymphocytes and plasma cells. Because of their ability to mount immunologic reactions, such cells play an important role in combating infections of the oral tissues. The largest accumulations of lymphoid tissue are found in the posterior part of the oral cavity, where they form the lingual, palatine, and pharyngeal tonsils, often known collectively as *Waldeyer's ring*. Small lymphoid nodules also may occur sometimes in the mucosa of the soft palate, the ventral surface of the tongue, and the floor of the mouth.

ORAL EPITHELIUM

As the tissue that forms the surface of the oral mucosa, the oral epithelium constitutes the primary barrier between the oral environment and deeper tissues.

The oral epithelium is a stratified squamous epithelium consisting of cells tightly attached to each other and arranged in a number of distinct layers or strata. Like the epidermis and the lining of the gastrointestinal tract, the oral epithelium maintains its structural integrity by a process of continuous cell renewal in which cells produced by mitotic divisions in the deepest layers migrate to the surface to replace those that are shed. The cells of the epithelium thus can be considered to consist of two functional populations: a *progenitor population* (the function of which is to divide and provide new cells) and a *maturing population* (the cells of which continually undergo a process of differentiation or maturation to form a protective surface layer). These two important processes, proliferation and maturation, are next considered in more detail.

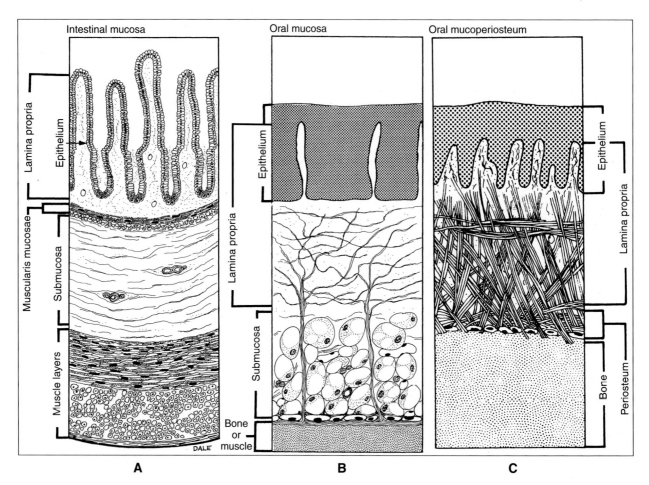

Figure 12-5 Arrangement of tissue components. **A,** Intestinal mucosa. **B,** Oral mucosa. **C,** Oral mucoperiosteum.

EPITHELIAL PROLIFERATION

The progenitor cells are situated in the basal layer in thin epithelia (e.g., the floor of the mouth) and in the lower two to three cell layers in thicker epithelia (cheeks and palate). Dividing cells tend to occur in clusters that are seen more frequently at the bottom of epithelial ridges than at the top. Studies on the epidermis and the oral epithelium indicate that the progenitor compartment is not homogeneous but consists of two functionally distinct subpopulations of cells. A small population of progenitor cells cycles slowly and is considered to represent stem cells, the function of which is to produce basal cells and retain the proliferative potential of the tissue. The larger portion of the progenitor compartment is composed of amplifying cells, the function of which is to increase the number of cells available for subsequent maturation. Despite their functional differences, these proliferative cells cannot be distinguished by appearance. Because it divides infrequently, the epithelial stem cell may be important in protecting the genetic information of the tissue, for DNA is most vulnerable to damage during mitosis.

Regardless of whether the cells are of the stem or amplifying type, cell division is a cyclic activity and commonly is divided into four distinct phases. The only phase that can be distinguished histologically is mitosis, which can be subdivided further into the recognizable stages of prophase, metaphase, anaphase, and telophase. After cell division, each daughter cell recycles in the progenitor population or enters the maturing compartment. Apart from measuring the number of cells in division, estimating the time necessary to replace all the cells in the epithelium is also possible. This is known as *turnover time* of the epithelium and is derived from a knowledge of the time taken for a cell to divide and pass through the entire epithelium.

Different techniques have led to a wide range of estimates of the rate of cell proliferation in the various epithelia, but in general the turnover time is 52 to 75 days in the skin, 4 to 14 days in the gut, 41 to 57 days in the gingiva, and 25 days in the cheek. Regional differences in the patterns of epithelial maturation appear to be associated with different turnover rates; for example, nonkeratinized buccal epithelium turns over faster than keratinized gingival epithelium.

Cancer chemotherapeutic drugs act by blocking mitotic division of rapidly dividing cancer cells, as well as normal host cells. Normal host tissues that have a short turnover time, such as blood cell precursors in bone marrow, intestinal epithelium, and oral epithelium, often are damaged by chemotherapeutic drugs. A significant number of patients taking chemotherapeutic drugs develop oral ulcers (breakdown of the oral squamous epithelium) and thus experience pain and difficulty in eating, drinking, and maintaining oral hygiene.

Mitotic activity also can be affected by factors such as the time of the day, stress, and inflammation. For example, the presence of slight subepithelial inflammatory cell infiltrates stimulates mitosis, whereas severe inflammation causes a reduction in proliferative activity. The mechanism of such action is not known, but the effect may be important in oral epithelium and especially in relation to determining turnover of the epithelium in regions that frequently are inflamed, such as the dentogingival junction.

Scientific views on the mechanisms that control the proliferation and differentiation of oral mucosa, skin, and many other tissues have been clarified by the identification of various *cytokines* that may influence epithelial proliferation. Examples include epidermal growth factor, keratinocyte growth factor, interleukin-1, and transforming growth factors α and β.

EPITHELIAL MATURATION

The cells arising by division in the basal or parabasal layers of the epithelium remain in the progenitor cell population or undergo a process of maturation as they move to the surface. In general, maturation in the oral cavity follows two main patterns: keratinization and nonkeratinization (Table 12-1).

Keratinization

The epithelial surface of the masticatory mucosa (e.g., that of the hard palate and gingiva and in some regions of specialized mucosa on the dorsum of the tongue) is inflexible, tough, resistant to abrasion, and tightly bound to the lamina propria. The mucosal surface results from the formation of a surface layer of keratin, and the process of maturation is called *keratinization* or *cornification*. In routine histologic sections a keratinized epithelium shows a number of distinct layers or strata (Figure 12-6, A). The basal layer (frequently given the Latin name *stratum basale*) is a layer of cuboidal or columnar cells adjacent to the basal lamina. Above the basal layer are several rows of larger elliptical or spherical cells known as the *prickle cell layer* or *stratum spinosum*. This term arises from the appearance of the cells prepared for histologic examination; they frequently shrink away from each other, remaining in contact only at points known as intercellular bridges or desmosomes (Figure 12-7). This alignment gives the cells a spiny or pricklelike profile. The Greek word for prickle, *akanthe*, is used frequently in pathologic descriptions of an increased thickness (acanthosis) or a separation of cells caused by loss of the intercellular bridges (acantholysis) in this layer.

The basal and prickle cell layers together constitute from half to two thirds of the thickness of the epithelium. The next layer consists of larger flattened cells

TABLE 12-1 Major Features of Maturation in Keratinized and Nonkeratinized Epithelium

| Keratinized Epithelium | | Nonkeratinized Epithelium | |
FEATURES	CELL LAYER	FEATURES	CELL LAYER
Cuboidal or columnar cells containing bundles of tonofibrils and other cell organelles; site of most cell divisions	Basal	Cuboidal or columnar cells containing separate tonofilaments and other cell organelles; site of most cell divisions	Basal
Larger ovoid cells containing conspicuous tonofibril bundles; membrane-coating granules appear in upper part of this layer	Prickle cell	Larger ovoid cells containing dispersed tonofilaments; membrane-coating granules appear in upper part of layer; filaments become numerous	Prickle cell
Flattened cells containing conspicuous keratohyaline granules associated with tonofibrils; membrane-coating granules fuse with cell membrane in upper part; internal membrane thickening also occurs	Granular	Slightly flattened cells containing many dispersed tonofilaments and glycogen	Intermediate
Extremely flattened and dehydrated cells in which all organelles have been lost; cells filled only with packed fibrillar material; when pyknotic nuclei are retained, parakeratinization occurs	Keratinized	Slightly flattened cells with dispersed filaments and glycogen; fewer organelles are present, but nuclei persist	Superficial

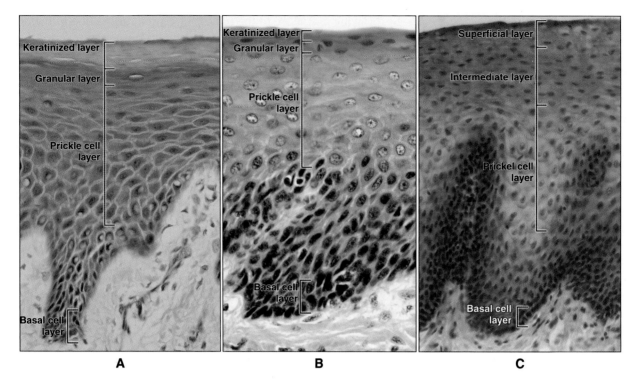

Figure 12-6 Histologic sections of the main types of maturation in human oral epithelium (at the same magnification). **A,** Orthokeratinization in gingiva. The narrow granular layer contains cells with a dark-staining granulation. **B,** Parakeratinization in gingiva. The keratin squames retain their pyknotic nuclei, and the granular layer contains only a few scattered granules. **C,** Nonkeratinization in buccal epithelium. No clear division of strata exists, and nuclei are apparent in the surface layer. The differences in thickness and epithelial ridge pattern, as well as in the patterns of maturation, are apparent.

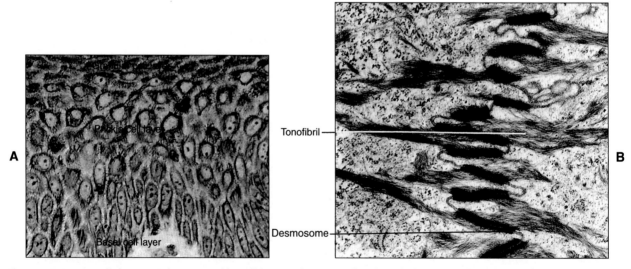

Figure 12-7 Intercellular junctions. **A,** Prickle cell layer in keratinized oral epithelium with the intercellular bridges (prickles) between adjacent cells. Part of the basal and granular layers are also evident. **B,** Electron micrograph of similar tissue after processing for ultrastructural examination. No shrinkage has occurred, so the intercellular bridges are not apparent. In several of the desmosomes, a clear specialized intercellular zone can be seen between the attachment plaques.

containing small granules that stain intensely with acid dyes such as hematoxylin (i.e., they are basophilic). This layer is the *granular* layer, or stratum granulosum, and the granules are called *keratohyalin granules*. In some regions of the masticatory oral epithelium (e.g., the gingiva), these granules are difficult to see clearly under the light microscope. The surface layer is composed of flat (squamous) cells, termed *squames*, that stain bright pink with the histologic dye eosin (i.e., they appear eosinophilic) and do not contain any nuclei. This layer is the keratinized layer or stratum corneum. Other names sometimes used include *cornified layer* and *horny layer*. The pattern of maturation of these cells often is termed *orthokeratinization*.

For masticatory mucosa (e.g., parts of the hard palate and much of the gingiva) to show a variation of keratinization, known as *parakeratinization*, is not unusual. In parakeratinized epithelium (Figure 12-6, *B*), the surface layer stains for keratin, as described previously, but shrunken (or pyknotic) nuclei are retained in many or all of the squames. Keratohyalin granules may be present in the underlying granular layer, though usually fewer than in orthokeratinized areas, so that this layer is difficult to recognize in histologic preparations. Parakeratinization is a normal event in oral epithelium and does not imply disease; this is not true for epidermis, where parakeratinization may be associated with diseases such as psoriasis.

Nonkeratinization

The lining mucosa of the oral cavity, which is present on the lips, buccal mucosa, alveolar mucosa, soft palate, underside of the tongue, and floor of the mouth, has an epithelium that is usually nonkeratinized (Figure 12-6, C).

In many regions the lining mucosa is thicker than keratinized epithelium and shows a different ridge pattern at the connective tissue interface. Epithelium of the cheek, for example, may reach a thickness of more than 500 μm and has broader epithelial ridges than keratinized epithelium.

The basal and prickle cell layers of nonkeratinized oral epithelium generally resemble those described for keratinized epithelium, although the cells of nonkeratinized epithelium are slightly larger and the intercellular bridges or prickles are less conspicuous. For this reason, some persons prefer to avoid the term *prickle cell layer* for nonkeratinized epithelium. No sudden changes in the appearance of cells above the prickle cell layer occur in nonkeratinized epithelium, and the outer half of the tissue is divided rather arbitrarily into two zones: intermediate (*stratum intermedium*) and superficial (*stratum superficiale*). Some refer to the latter as the *stratum distendum*, reflecting its mechanical flexibility. A granular layer is not present, and the cells of the superficial layer contain nuclei that are often plump. This layer does not stain intensely with eosin, as does the surface of keratinized or parakeratinized epithelium.

From the histologic appearance of oral epithelium it is apparent that the tissue shows a well-ordered pattern of maturation and successive layers that contain cells of increasing age (i.e., progressive stages of maturation). Furthermore, the pattern of maturation differs in different regions of the oral mucosa so that two main types can be recognized: keratinization and nonkeratinization. The next section describes the fine structure of the epithelial cell and the main events that take place at the cellular level during maturation of these two types of epithelium (Table 12-2; see also Table 12-1).

	LEVEL IN EPITHELIUM	SPECIFIC STAINING REACTIONS	ULTRASTRUCTURAL FEATURES	FUNCTION
TABLE 12-2 Characteristics of Nonkeratinocytes in Oral Epithelium				
CELL TYPE				
Melanocyte	Basal	Dopa oxidase–tyrosinase; silver stains	Dendritic; no desmosomes or tonofilaments; premelanosomes and melanosomes present	Synthesis of melanin pigment granules (melanosomes) and transfer to surrounding keratinocytes
Langerhans cell	Predominantly suprabasal	CD1a; cell surface antigen markers	Dendritic; no desmosomes or tonofilaments; characteristic Langerhans granule	Antigen trapping and processing
Merkel cell	Basal	Probably periodic acid–Schiff positive	Nondendritic; sparse desmosomes tonofilaments; characteristic electron-dense vesicles and associated nerve axon	Tactile sensory cell
Lymphocyte	Variable	Cell surface antigen markers (CD3— T cells; CD20— B cells)	Large circular nucleus; scant cytoplasm with few organelles; no desmosomes or tonofilaments	Associated with the inflammatory response in oral mucosa

ULTRASTRUCTURE OF THE EPITHELIAL CELL

Cells of the basal layer are the least differentiated oral epithelial cells. They contain not only organelles (nuclei, mitochondria, ribosomes, endoplasmic reticula, and Golgi complexes) commonly present in the cells of other tissues but also certain characteristic structures that identify them as epithelial cells and distinguish them from other cell types. These structures are the filamentous strands called *tonofilaments* and the intercellular bridges or desmosomes. Tonofilaments are fibrous proteins that belong to a class of intracellular filaments called intermediate filaments and form an important structural component within the cell. They often aggregate to form bundles called *tonofibrils* that can be identified with the higher magnifications of the light microscope (Figure 12-7). Chemically the filaments represent a class of intracellular proteins known as *cytokeratins*, which are characteristic constituents of epithelial tissues. Keratins are classified according to their size (i.e., molecular weight) and charge, and the types of keratin present vary between different epithelia and even between the different cell layers of a single stratified epithelium. One name often given to an epithelial cell because of its content of keratin filaments is *keratinocyte*. This serves to distinguish these epithelial cells from the nonkeratinocytes that are described later.

Keratins represent a large family of proteins of differing molecular weights; those with the lowest molecular weight (40 kDa) are found in glandular and simple epithelia; those of intermediate molecular weight, in stratified epithelia; and those with the highest molecular weight (approximately 67 kDa), in keratinized stratified epithelium. A catalog of keratins has been drawn up to represent the different types. Thus all stratified oral epithelia possess keratins 5 and 14, but differences emerge between keratinized oral epithelium (which contains keratins 1, 6, 10, and 16) and nonkeratinized epithelium (which contains keratins 4, 13, and 19).

Stratified epithelia possess a variety of cell surface carbohydrate molecules that show differences between tissues and during differentiation. Much of the research on keratins and cell-surface markers has focused on identifying changes indicative of aberrant maturation to provide early warning of disease processes such as cancer. The research also has enabled distinction of the various types of epithelia making up the dentogingival junction.

An important property of any epithelium is its ability to function as a barrier, which depends to a great extent on the close contact or cohesiveness of the epithelial cells. Cohesion between cells is provided by a viscous intercellular material consisting of protein-carbohydrate complexes produced by the epithelial cells themselves. In addition, modifications of the adjacent membranes of cells occur, the most common of which is the desmosome or *macula adherens* (see Figure 12-7, *B*) into which bundles of intermediate filaments (tonofilaments) insert (see Chapter 4). If the epithelial cells shrink during histologic processing, the desmosomes usually remain intact and so appear as intercellular bridges (see Figure 12-7, *A*). Adhesion between the epithelium and connective tissue is provided by hemidesmosomes, which attach the cell to the basal lamina (see Figure 12-20 later in this chapter). Like desmosomes, hemidesmosomes also possess intracellular attachment plaques with tonofilaments inserted into them. Tonofilaments, (hemi)desmosomes, and basal lamina together represent a mechanical linkage that distributes and dissipates localized forces applied to the epithelial surface over a wide area. In some diseases, such as pemphigus, in which blistering of the epithelium occurs, a splitting of the epithelial layers occurs to form bullous or vesicular lesions within the epithelium. This results from breakdown of certain components of the cellular attachment mechanisms, as a consequence of a genetic defect or as an autoimmune reaction directed against them.

Two other types of connection are seen between cells of the oral epithelium: gap junctions and tight junctions. As shown in Chapter 4, the gap junction is a region where membranes of adjacent cells run closely together, separated by only a small gap. Small interconnections are apparent between the membranes across these gaps. Such junctions may allow electrical or chemical communication between the cells and sometimes are called *communicating junctions* and are seen only occasionally in oral epithelium. Even rarer in oral epithelium is the tight, or *occluding*, junction, where adjacent cell membranes are so tightly apposed as to exclude intercellular space.

CELLULAR EVENTS IN MATURATION

The major changes involved in cell maturation in keratinized and nonkeratinized oral epithelium are presented in Figure 12-8 and Table 12-1. In both types of epithelia the changes in cell size and shape are accompanied by a synthesis of more structural protein in the form of tonofilaments, the appearance of new organelles, and the production of additional intercellular material. A number of changes, however, are not common in both epithelia and serve as distinguishing features. One is in the arrangement of tonofilaments. The cells of both epithelia increase in size as they migrate from the basal to the prickle cell layer, but this increase is greater in nonkeratinized epithelium. A corresponding synthesis of tonofilaments also occurs in

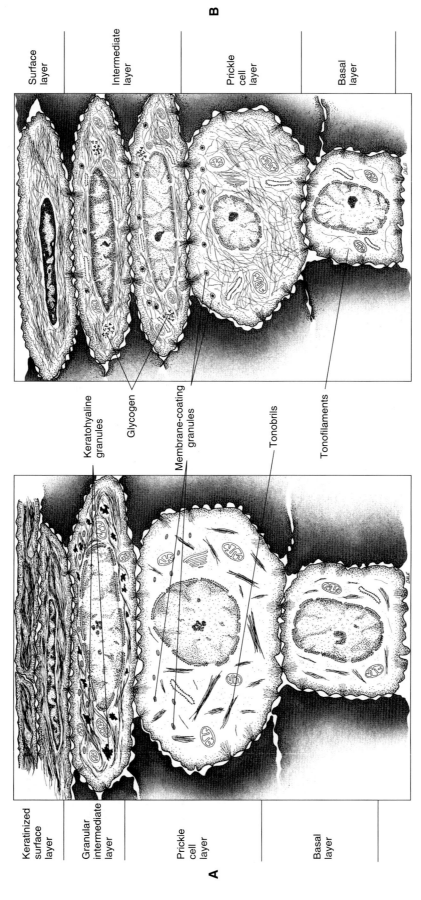

Figure 12-8 Principal structural features of epithelial cells in successive layers. **A,** Orthokeratinized oral epithelium. **B,** Nonkeratinized oral epithelium. *(Adapted from Squier CA, Johnson NW, Hopps RM: Human oral mucosa: development, structure, and function, Oxford, UK, 1976, Blackwell Scientific.)*

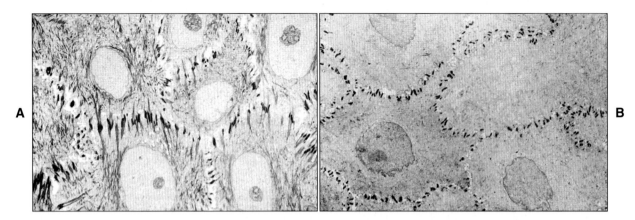

Figure 12-9 Low-magnification electron micrographs of prickle cells from **A** keratinized gingival epithelium and **B** nonkeratinized buccal epithelium. Filaments are assembled into distinct bundles (tonofibrils) in the keratinized tissue but are inconspicuously dispersed in the nonkeratinized epithelium.

both epithelia, but whereas the tonofilaments in keratinized epithelium are aggregated into bundles to form tonofibrils, those in nonkeratinized epithelium remain dispersed and so appear less conspicuous (Figure 12-9). The chemical structure of keratin filaments also is known to differ between layers so that various patterns of maturation can be identified by the keratins that are present.

In the upper part of the prickle cell layer a new organelle appears called the *membrane-coating* or *lamellate* granule. These granules are small, membrane-bound structures about 250 nm in size and containing glycolipid that probably originate from the Golgi complex. In keratinized epithelium the granules are elongated and contain a series of parallel lamellae. In nonkeratinized epithelium, by contrast, the granules appear to be circular with an amorphous core (Figure 12-10). As the cells move toward the surface, these granules become aligned close to the superficial cell membrane.

The next layer, called the granular layer in keratinized epithelium and the *intermediate* layer in nonkeratinized epithelium, contains cells that have a greater volume but are more flattened than those of the prickle cell layer. In the upper part of this layer, in keratinized and nonkeratinized epithelia, the membrane-coating granules appear to fuse with the superficial cell membrane and to discharge their contents into the intercellular space. In keratinized oral epithelium and epidermis the discharge of granule contents is associated with the formation of a lipid-rich permeability barrier that limits the movement of aqueous substances through the intercellular spaces of the keratinized layer. The granules seen in nonkeratinized epithelium probably have a similar function, but the contents have a

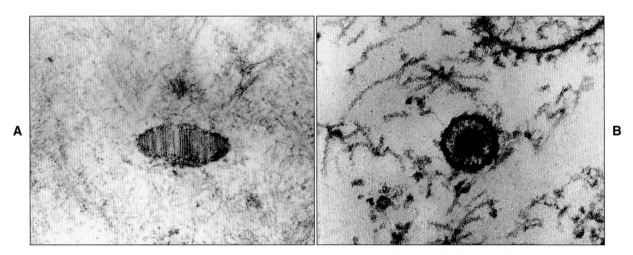

Figure 12-10 Electron micrographs of membrane-coating granules in oral epithelium. **A,** Elongated lamellate type seen in keratinized epithelium. **B,** Circular type with a dense core found in nonkeratinized epithelium.

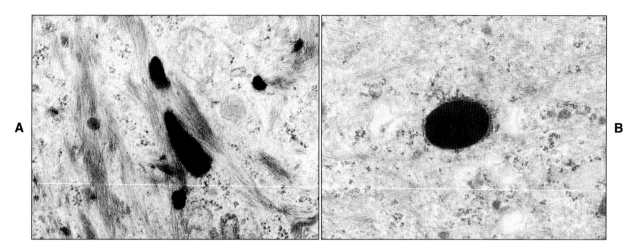

Figure 12-11 Electron micrographs of keratohyaline granules in oral epithelium. **A,** From the granular layer, irregularly shaped granules are associated intimately with tonofilaments. **B,** A granule of the type occasionally seen in nonkeratinized oral epithelium is regular in shape and surrounded by ribosomes but is not associated with tonofilaments.

different lipid composition and do not form as effective a barrier as that in keratinized epithelia.

Cells in the superficial part of the granular layer develop a noticeable thickening on the inner (intracellular) aspect of their membrane that contributes to the considerable resistance of the keratinized layer to chemical solvents. One of the major constituents of this thickening is a protein known as *involucrin*. A similar, but less obvious, thickening often is seen in the surface cells of nonkeratinized epithelia. Despite their name, membrane-coating granules have nothing to do with this thickening. The remaining events during epithelial maturation are greatly different in keratinized and nonkeratinized epithelia and so are described separately.

Keratinized Epithelium

The most characteristic feature of the granular layer of keratinized epithelium is the keratohyalin granules, which appear as basophilic granules under the light microscope and as electron-dense structures in the electron microscope (Figure 12-11). The granules are irregular in shape, usually between 0.5 and 1 nm in size, and probably are synthesized by the ribosomes that can be seen surrounding them. Keratohyalin granules also are associated intimately with tonofibrils, and they are thought to facilitate the aggregation and formation of cross-links between the cytokeratin filaments of the keratinized layer. For this reason the protein making up the bulk of these granules has been named *filaggrin*, although a sulfur-rich component also occurs called *loricrin*. As the cells of the granular layer reach the junction with the keratinized layer, a sudden change in

their appearance occurs (Figure 12-12, *A*). All the organelles, including the nuclei and keratohyalin granules, disappear. The cells dehydrate, and the cells of the keratinized layer become packed with filaments cross-linked by disulfide bonds, which facilitates their dense packing.

The cells of the keratinized layer become dehydrated and flattened and assume the form of hexagonal disks called *squames* (Figure 12-12, *C*). Squames are lost (by the process of *desquamation*) and are replaced by cells from the underlying layers. This process may occur rapidly so that an individual surface squame is shed in a matter of hours rather than days. The mechanism of desquamation is not well understood but probably represents a programmed enzymatic breakdown of lipids and proteins. Rapid clearance of the surface layer is probably important in limiting the colonization and invasion of epithelial surfaces by pathogenic microorganisms, including the common oral fungus *Candida*.

The keratinized layer in the oral cavity may be composed of up to 20 layers of squames and is thicker than that in most regions of the skin except the soles and palms. The tightly packed cytokeratins within an insoluble and tough envelope make this layer resistant to mechanical and chemical damage.

In parakeratinization (see Figure 12-6, *B*), incomplete removal of organelles from the cells of the granular layer occurs so that the nuclei remain as shrunken pyknotic structures, and remnants of other organelles also may be present in the keratinized layer.

When gingival epithelium is prepared for histologic examination with stains such as Mallory's triple stain, a variant of keratinized or parakeratinized epithelium

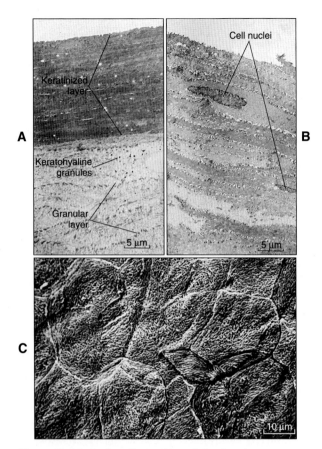

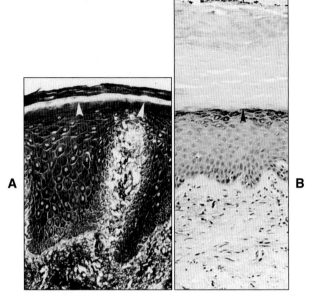

Figure 12-13 Variations in keratinization. **A,** Histologic section of gingiva stained by a modified Mallory method to demonstrate incomplete orthokeratinization. Although normal keratin has formed and appears as a light band *(arrowheads)* beneath the surface of the epithelium, the outermost layers have become hydrated, and their staining pattern reverts to that of the deeper epithelial layers. **B,** Histologic section through the mucosa of hard palate that has developed epithelial hyperkeratosis *(between arrowheads)* as a result of irritation by tobacco smoke. Compare this with the normal palatal epithelium in Figure 12-29.

Figure 12-12 Surface layer of keratinized and nonkeratinized oral epithelium. **A** and **B** are transmission electron micrographs. **A,** The granular and keratinized layers in gingival epithelium. Small keratohyaline granules are visible in the granular layer; the cells (squames) of the keratinized layer are flattened and appear uniformly dense. **B,** The corresponding region of nonkeratinized buccal epithelium. The cells undergo only slight changes as they move to the surface. All the cells appear flattened, and organelles (including cell nuclei) can be seen even in the superficial layers. **C,** Scanning electron micrograph of the surface cells (squames) of keratinized oral epithelium. The squames are flat disks with a polygonal outline, and their surface shows a reticulate pattern of fine ridges. *(**C** courtesy J. Howlett.)*

Nonkeratinized Epithelium

In nonkeratinized oral epithelium the events taking place in the upper cell layers are far less dramatic than those in keratinized epithelium (see Figure 12-12, *A* and *B*). A slight increase in cell size occurs in the intermediate cell layer, as well as an accumulation of glycogen in cells of the surface layer. On rare occasions, keratohyalin granules can be seen at this level, but they differ from the granules in keratinized epithelium and appear as regular spherical structures surrounded by ribosomes but not associated with tonofilaments (see Figure 12-11, *B*). Although they contain no filaggrin, loricrin probably is present and may contribute to the internal thickening of the cell membrane already described. Keratohyalin granules often remain, even in the surface cells, where they may be evident in surface cytologic preparations.

In the superficial layer a few other changes occur. The cells appear slightly more flattened than in the preceding layers and contain dispersed tonofilaments and nuclei, the number of other cell organelles having

sometimes is seen. The outermost squames of the keratinized (or parakeratinized) layer do not look like the rest of the keratin but show a staining similar to that of deeper nucleated cells (Figure 12-13, *A*). Such an appearance is called *incomplete keratinization,* or incomplete parakeratinization, and research suggests that the cells showing this pattern have become rehydrated by taking up fluid from the oral cavity. None of these variants of keratinization, however, seems to have any pathologic significance in oral tissues.

diminished (see Figure 12-12, *B*). The surface layer of nonkeratinized epithelium thus consists of cells filled with loosely arranged filaments that are not dehydrated. They thus can form a surface that is flexible and tolerant of compression and distention.

Although the distribution of keratinized and nonkeratinized epithelium in different anatomic locations is determined during embryologic development, often some variation of this basic pattern occurs in adults (e.g., when the normally nonkeratinized buccal mucosa develops a thin keratin layer, the linea alba, along the occlusal line). Similarly, the normal keratin layer of the palate may become thick in smokers as a result of the irritant effects of tobacco smoke, but such hyperkeratotic epithelium in other ways appears normal (Figure 12-13, *B*). In general, *hyperkeratosis* of oral epithelium that normally is keratinized represents a physiologic response of the epithelium to chronic irritation, similar to that occurring in callous formation on the palms and soles. Hyperkeratosis of nonkeratinized oral epithelium may be physiologic but also can be associated with abnormal cellular changes that eventually lead to cancer of the squamous epithelium. Such hyperkeratotic lesions should be sampled by biopsy so that a diagnosis can be made. The presence of inflammation in regions such as the gingiva can reduce the degree of keratinization so that it appears parakeratinized or even nonkeratinized. This change from one pattern of maturation to another, or the emphasis or depression of an existing trait, is usually reversible when the stimulus is removed.

PERMEABILITY AND ABSORPTION

One function of the oral epithelium is forming an impermeable barrier; unlike the intestinal lining, the oral epithelium does not have an absorptive capacity. Differences in permeability exist between regions, however, depending on the thickness of the epithelial barrier to be traversed and the pattern of maturation. One of the thinnest epithelial regions, the floor of the mouth, may be more permeable than other areas, which is perhaps the reason why certain drugs (e.g., nitroglycerin administered to relieve the pain of angina pectoris) are absorbed successfully when held under the tongue. Nevertheless, the oral mucosa clearly is able to limit the penetration of toxins and antigens produced by microorganisms present in the oral cavity, except in the specialized region of the dentogingival junction.

The permeability barrier is believed to consist of lipids derived from the membrane-coating granules that become aligned in a precise pattern once they have entered the intercellular spaces of the upper cell layer.

NONKERATINOCYTES IN THE ORAL EPITHELIUM

Many histologic sections of oral epithelium contain cells that differ in appearance from other epithelial cells in having a clear halo around their nuclei (Figure 12-14). Such cells have been termed *clear cells,* and what is obvious from ultrastructural and immunochemical studies is that they represent a variety of cell types, including pigment-producing cells (melanocytes), *Langerhans cells, Merkel cells,* and inflammatory cells (e.g., lymphocytes), that together make up as much as 10% of the cell population in the oral epithelium. All of these cells, except Merkel cells, lack desmosomal attachments to adjacent cells so that during histologic processing the cytoplasm shrinks around the nucleus to produce the clear halo. None of these cells contains the large numbers of tonofilaments and desmosomes seen in epithelial keratinocytes, and none participates in the process of maturation seen in oral epithelia; therefore, they often are called collectively *nonkeratinocytes.* Table 12-2 summarizes their structure and function.

MELANOCYTES AND ORAL PIGMENTATION

The color of the oral mucosa is the net result of a number of factors, one of which is pigmentation. Two types of pigmentation occur: endogenous, arising in the tissues from normal physiologic processes, and exogenous, caused by foreign material introduced into the body locally or systemically. The endogenous pigments most commonly contributing to the color of the oral mucosa are *melanin* and *hemoglobin.* Melanin is produced by

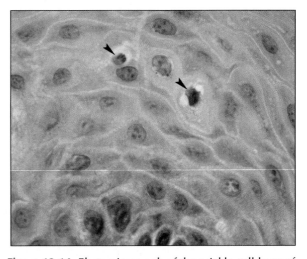

Figure 12-14 Photomicrograph of the prickle cell layer of gingival epithelium. The clear cells *(arrowheads)* have dark nuclei surrounded by a light halo.

specialized pigment cells, called melanocytes, situated in the basal layer of the oral epithelium and the epidermis. Melanocytes arise embryologically from the neural crest ectoderm (see Chapter 2) and enter the epithelium at about 11 weeks of gestation. In the epithelium they divide and maintain themselves as a self-reproducing population. Melanocytes lack desmosomes and tonofilaments but possess long dendritic (branching) processes that extend between the keratinocytes, often passing through several layers of cells. Melanin is synthesized within the melanocytes as small structures called *melanosomes* (Figure 12-15), which are inoculated (or injected) into the cytoplasm of adjacent keratinocytes by the dendritic processes of melanocytes. Groups of melanosomes often can be identified under the light microscope in sections of heavily pigmented tissue stained with hematoxylin and eosin. These groups are referred to as melanin granules. In lightly pigmented tissues the presence of melanin can be demonstrated only by specific histologic and histochemical stains.

Lightly and darkly pigmented individuals have the same number of melanocytes in any given region of skin or oral mucosa; color differences result from the relative activity of the melanocytes in producing melanin and from the rate at which melanosomes are broken down in the keratinocytes. In persons with heavy melanin pigmentation, cells containing melanin may be seen in the connective tissue. These cells are probably macrophages that have taken up melanosomes produced by melanocytes in the epithelium and sometimes are termed *melanophages*. The regions of the oral mucosa where melanin pigmentation is seen most commonly clinically are the gingiva (Figure 12-16), buccal mucosa, hard palate, and tongue. Despite considerable individual variation, a direct relationship tends to be seen between the degrees of pigmentation in the skin and in the oral mucosa. Light-skinned persons rarely show any oral melanin pigmentation.

Melanocytes are involved in the development of several pigmented lesions in the oral mucosa. *Oral melanotic macule* appears clinically similar to a freckle and microscopically shows increased production of melanin pigment without proliferation of melanocytes. The condition is harmless. A *nevus* (mole) is a benign proliferation of melanocytes and in the oral cavity is not easy to distinguish clinically from melanoma. A mole should be removed completely. *Melanoma* is a malignant tumor of melanocytes. In the oral cavity, melanoma is rare but usually fatal. Treatment is surgical removal.

One of the most common *exogenous* pigments is amalgam accidentally forced into the gingiva during placement of a restoration. This circumstance gives rise to patches of bluish gray discoloration known as amalgam tattoo. Certain metals (e.g., lead and bismuth), when present systemically, can give rise to pigmentation of the gingival margin (sometimes called *Burton's line*) and may be indicative of systemic poisoning.

LANGERHANS CELLS

Another dendritic cell sometimes seen above the basal layers of epidermis and oral epithelium is Langerhans cell.

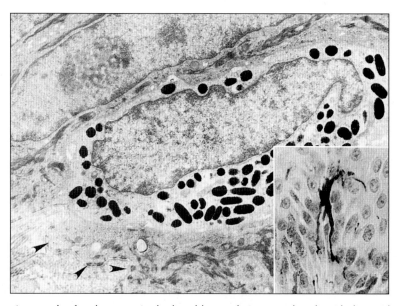

Figure 12-15 Electron micrograph of melanocyte in the basal layer of pigmented oral epithelium. The dense melanosomes are abundant. Arrowheads indicate the basal lamina. *Inset,* Photomicrograph of histologic section showing a dendritic melanocyte. The cell appears dark because it has been stained histochemically to reveal the presence of melanin.

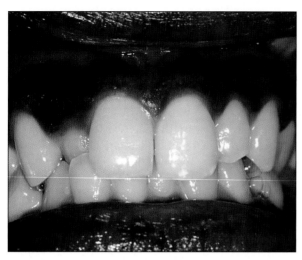

Figure 12-16 Melanin pigmentation of the attached gingiva in a dark-skinned person. *(Courtesy A. Kauzman.)*

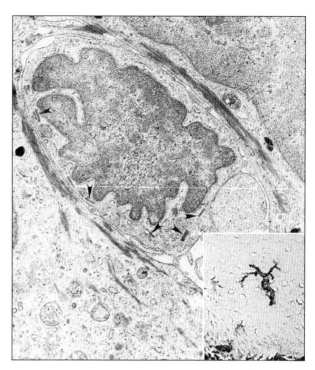

Figure 12-17 Electron micrograph of Langerhans cell from the oral epithelium. The cell has a convoluted nucleus and lacks tonofilaments and desmosome attachments to adjacent cells but contains a number of characteristic rodlike granules *(arrowheads)*. The dark granules in the neighboring cells are melanin pigment. *Inset,* Dendritic Langerhans cell in a light microscope preparation. Revealed by adenosinetriphosphatase staining, the cell is visible in its characteristic suprabasal location. *(Inset preparation courtesy I.C. Mackenzie.)*

This cell lacks desmosomal attachments to surrounding cells and therefore appears as a clear cell in histologic sections. The Langerhans cell is characterized ultrastructurally by a small rod- or flask-shaped granule, sometimes called the *Birbeck granule* (after the person who first described it under the electron microscope; Figure 12-17). The Langerhans cell usually is demonstrated by specific immunochemical reactions that stain cell surface antigens.

Langerhans cells appear in the epithelium at the same time as, or just before, the melanocytes, and they may be capable of limited division within the epithelium. Unlike melanocytes, they move in and out of the epithelium, and their source is the bone marrow. Evidence suggests that Langerhans cells have an immunologic function, recognizing and processing antigenic material that enters the epithelium from the external environment and presenting it to T lymphocytes. Langerhans cells probably can migrate from epithelium to regional lymph nodes.

MERKEL CELLS

The Merkel cell is situated in the basal layer of the oral epithelium and epidermis. Unlike the melanocyte and Langerhans cell, the Merkel cell is not dendritic and does possess keratin tonofilaments and occasional desmosomes linking it to adjacent cells. As a result, the Merkel cell does not always resemble the other clear cells in histologic sections. The characteristic feature of Merkel cells is the small membrane-bound vesicles in the cytoplasm, sometimes situated adjacent to a nerve fiber associated with the cell (Figure 12-18). These granules may liberate a transmitter substance across the synapselike junction between the Merkel cell

and the nerve fiber and thus trigger an impulse. This arrangement is in accord with neurophysiologic evidence suggesting that Merkel cells are sensory and respond to touch. These cells may arise from division of an epithelial cell (keratinocyte).

INFLAMMATORY CELLS

When sections of epithelium taken from clinically normal areas of mucosa are examined microscopically, a number of inflammatory cells often can be seen in the nucleated cell layers. These cells are transient and do not reproduce themselves in the epithelium as the other nonkeratinocytes do. The cell most frequently seen is the lymphocyte, although the presence of polymorphonuclear leukocytes and mast cells is not uncommon. Lymphocytes often are associated with Langerhans cells, which are able to activate T lymphocytes. A few inflammatory cells are commonplace in the oral epithelium and can be regarded as a normal component of the nonkeratinocyte population.

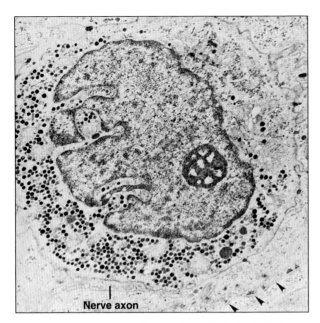

Figure 12-18 Electron micrograph of Merkel cell in the basal layer of oral epithelium. The cytoplasm of this cell is filled with small, dense vesicles situated close to an adjacent unmyelinated nerve axon. Arrowheads point to the site of the basal lamina. *(Courtesy S.Y. Chen.)*

Clearly, the association between nonkeratinocytes and keratinocytes in skin and oral mucosa represents a subtle and finely balanced interrelationship in which cytokines are the controlling factors. Thus keratinocytes produce cytokines that modulate the function of Langerhans cells. In turn, the Langerhans cells produce cytokines such as interleukin-1, which can activate T lymphocytes so that they are capable of responding to antigenic challenge. Interleukin-1 also increases the number of receptors to melanocyte-stimulating hormone in melanocytes and so can affect pigmentation. The influence of keratinocytes extends to the adjacent connective tissue, where cytokines produced in the epithelium can influence fibroblast growth and the formation of fibrils and matrix proteins.

JUNCTION OF THE EPITHELIUM AND LAMINA PROPRIA

The region where connective tissue of the lamina propria meets the overlying oral epithelium is an undulating interface at which papillae of the connective tissue interdigitate with the epithelial ridges. The interface consists of connective tissue ridges, conical papillae, or both projecting into the epithelium (Figure 12-19).

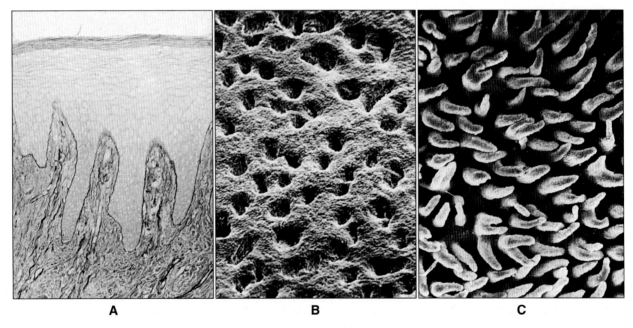

A   **B**   **C**

Figure 12-19 Junction between epithelium and connective tissue. **A,** Photomicrograph of section through gingival epithelium, stained by the periodic acid–Schiff method, demonstrating the basal lamina and extensive interdigitations between epithelium and connective tissue. Staining of the intercellular substance also occurred, particularly around the keratinized epithelial squames. **B** and **C,** Scanning electron micrographs of the interface between epithelium and connective tissue in the palate. **B** shows the underside of oral epithelium and the circular orifices into which the cone-shaped papillae of connective tissue fit that are illustrated in **C.** *(B and C from Klein-Szanto AJP, Schroeder HE: J Anat 123:93, 1977.)*

This arrangement makes the surface area of the interface larger than a simple flat junction and may provide better attachment, enabling forces applied at the surface of the epithelium to be dispersed over a greater area of connective tissue. In this respect, masticatory mucosa interestingly has the greatest number of papillae per unit area of mucosa; in lining mucosa the papillae are fewer and shorter. The junction also represents a major interface for metabolic exchange between the epithelium and connective tissue, for the epithelium has no blood vessels.

Basal laminae cannot be visualized directly by light microscopy using conventional stains such as hematoxylin-eosin. In histologic sections of oral mucosa stained by the periodic acid–Schiff reaction, the basal lamina appears as a bright, structureless band at the interface between the epithelium and subjacent connective tissue (see Figure 12-19, A). The basal lamina runs parallel to the basal cell membrane of the epithelial cells and at the ultrastructural level consists of three zones: the *lamina lucida*, *lamina densa*, and *lamina fibroreticularis* (also called sublamina densa). The lamina densa appears as a homogeneous, finely fibrillar planar assembly of extracellular matrix molecules separated from the adjacent cell by the lamina lucida that appears as a clear zone (see Figure 12-20, C). The lamina lucida is slightly thinner (~40 nm) than the lamina densa (~50 nm) and is not seen with all tissue preservation methods. Some believe it is an artifact of tissue preparation. The lamina densa consists essentially of a network of polymers formed by type IV collagen and laminins. Additional proteins such as heparan sulfate proteoglycan (perlecan), nidogen and fibulin reinforce the double polymer scaffold (see Figure 12-20, C). The lamina lucida essentially contains those proteins that attach the cell to the basal lamina, that is, the interacting portions of hemidesmosome-associated membrane proteins (collagen XVII, integrins) and laminin-5. *Anchoring fibrils*, consisting of collagen type VII, insert into the lamina densa and form a flexible attachment between the basal lamina and subjacent connective tissue. All the basal lamina, except the components of the lamina fibroreticularis, now is believed to be synthesized by the epithelium. Seen under the light microscope the basal lamina is a much thicker structure than the combined lamina lucida and lamina densa seen under the electron microscope. Most probably the special histological stains used to reveal the basal lamina also react with part of the adjacent subepithelial connective tissue.

Several genetic defects and autoimmune diseases cause defects in the basal lamina. When the mucosa blisters, as in the lesions of pemphigoid, separation of the epithelium from connective tissue occurs at the level of the lamina lucida. This separation is thought to result from an individual producing antibodies that attack a specific component (the bullous pemphigoid antigen, collagen XVII) of the basal lamina. Mutations in the laminin-5 or integrin genes also can cause blistering.

LAMINA PROPRIA

The connective tissue supporting the oral epithelium is termed *lamina propria* and for descriptive purposes can be divided into two layers: the superficial papillary layer (associated with the epithelial ridges) and the deeper reticular layer (which lies between the papillary layer and the underlying structures). The term *reticular* in this case means netlike and refers to the arrangement of the collagen fibers.

The difference between these two layers is defined poorly but reflects the relative concentration and arrangement of the collagen fibers (Figure 12-21, A). In the papillary layer, collagen fibers are thin and loosely arranged, and many capillary loops are present. By contrast, the reticular layer has collagen fibers arranged in thick bundles that tend to lie parallel to the surface plane.

The lamina propria consists of cells, blood vessels, neural elements, and fibers embedded in an amorphous ground substance (Figure 12-21, B and C). Like the overlying oral epithelium, the lamina propria shows regional variation in the proportions of its constituent elements, particularly in the concentration and organization of fibers.

CELLS

The lamina propria contains several different cells: fibroblasts, macrophages, mast cells, and inflammatory cells. Table 12-3 lists the major cells of the lamina propria.

Fibroblasts

The principal cell in the lamina propria of oral mucosa is the fibroblast, which is responsible for the elaboration and turnover of fiber and ground substance. The fibroblast thus plays a key role in maintaining tissue connective integrity and was described in Chapter 4. Under the light microscope, fibroblasts are cigar-shaped (fusiform) or star-shaped (stellate) with long processes that tend to lie parallel to bundles of collagen fibers and are not easily visible with the light microscope (Figure 12-22). Ultrastructurally, active fibroblasts exhibit numerous mitochondria, an extensive rough endoplasmic reticulum, a prominent Golgi complex, and numerous membrane-bound vesicles. Fibroblasts have a low rate of proliferation in adult oral mucosa except during wound healing, when their numbers increase because of

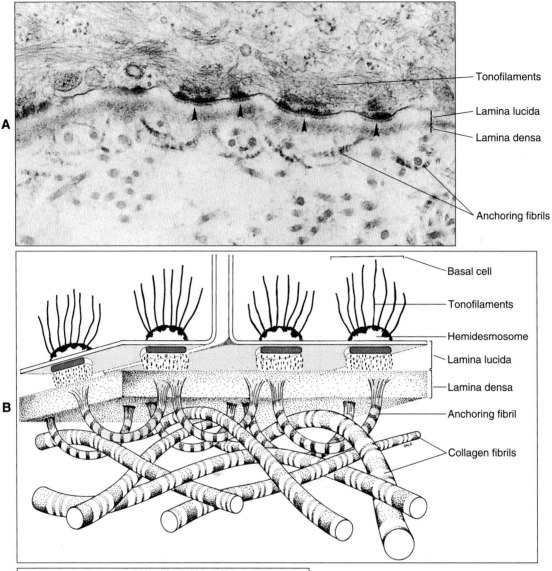

A — Tonofilaments, Lamina lucida, Lamina densa, Anchoring fibrils

B — Basal cell, Tonofilaments, Hemidesmosome, Lamina lucida, Lamina densa, Anchoring fibril, Collagen fibrils

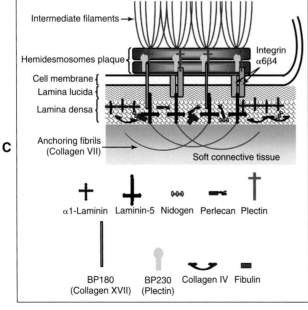

C — Intermediate filaments, Hemidesmosomes plaque, Integrin α6β4, Cell membrane, Lamina lucida, Lamina densa, Anchoring fibrils (Collagen VII), Soft connective tissue

α1-Laminin Laminin-5 Nidogen Perlecan Plectin

BP180 (Collagen XVII) BP230 (Plectin) Collagen IV Fibulin

Figure 12-20 Ultrastructure of basal lamina. **A,** High-magnification electron micrograph of the complex in oral mucosa. Hemidesmosomes *(arrowheads)* at the plasma membrane of epithelial basal cells receive bundles of intermediate filaments (tonofilaments). Adjacent to the membrane are the lamina lucida and lamina densa. Several striated anchoring fibrils loop into the lamina densa, and some contain within their loops cross sections of collagen fibrils. **B,** Schematic representation of the junction between epithelium and connective tissue. **C,** Presents the location of principal molecular constituents of the junction. (**C** *adapted by R. Wazen from McMillan JR, Akiyama M, Shimizu H:* J Dermatol Sci *31:169, 2003; and Schneider H, Mühle C, Pacho F:* Eur J Cell Biol *Sep 23, 2006 [electronic pub].)*

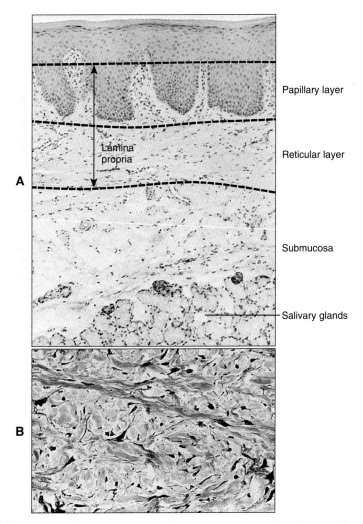

Figure 12-21 **A,** Photomicrograph of palatal mucosa showing the approximate boundaries of the papillary and reticular layers. The group of minor salivary glands in the submucosa is apparent. **B,** Photomicrograph of the lamina propria (reticular layer) of oral mucosa demonstrating cells and cell processes, most of which are fibroblasts.

TABLE 12-3	Cell Types in the Lamina Propria of Oral Mucosa		

CELL TYPE	MORPHOLOGIC CHARACTERISTICS	FUNCTION	DISTRIBUTION
Fibroblast	Stellate or elongated with abundant rough endoplasmic reticulum	Secretion of fibers and ground substance	Throughout lamina propria
Histiocyte	Spindle-shaped or stellate; often dark-staining nucleus; many lysosomal vesicles	Resident precursor of functional macrophage	Throughout lamina propria
Macrophage	Round with pale-staining nucleus; contains lysosomes and phagocytic vesicles	Phagocytosis, including antigen processing	Areas of chronic inflammation
Mast cell	Round or oval with basophilic granules staining metachromatically	Secretion of certain inflammatory mediators and vasoactive agents (histamine, heparin, and serotonin)	Throughout lamina propria; often subepithelial
Polymorphonuclear leukocyte (neutrophil)	Round with characteristic lobed nucleus; contains lysosomes and specific granules	Phagocytosis and cell killing	Areas of acute inflammation within lamina propria; may be present in epithelium
Lymphocyte	Round with dark-staining nucleus and scant cytoplasm with some mitochondria	Some lymphocytes participate in humoral or cell-mediated immune response	Areas of acute and chronic inflammation
Plasma cell	Cartwheel nucleus; intensely basophilic cytoplasm with abundant rough endoplasmic reticula	Synthesis of immunoglobulins	Areas of chronic inflammation, often perivascularly
Endothelial cell	Normally associated with a basal lamina; contains numerous pinocytotic vesicles	Lining of blood and lymphatic channels	Lining vascular channels throughout lamina propria

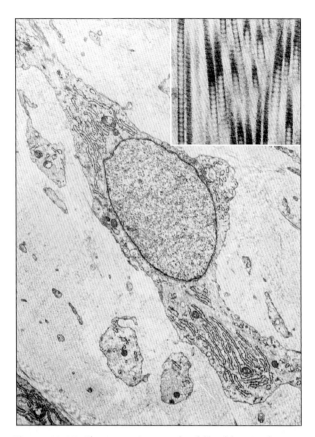

Figure 12-22 Electron micrograph of fibroblast in the lamina propria. *Inset,* Collagen type I fibrils. The typical cross-banding pattern is apparent.

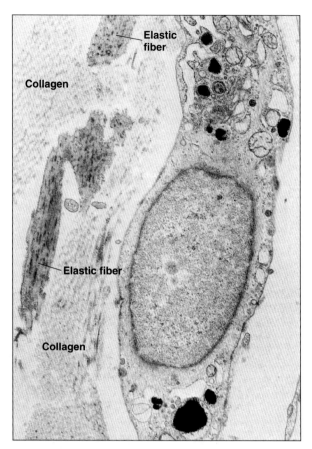

Figure 12-23 Electron micrograph of part of a macrophage in the lamina propria. The cell has a number of phagosomes filled with extremely dense material. Adjacent to the cell are elastic fibers composed of dark filaments embedded in a less dense matrix; they appear distinctly different from the adjacent collagen.

fibroblast division in the adjacent uninjured tissues. Fibroblasts can become contractile and participate in wound contraction, in which case their actin content increases. In certain disease states (e.g., the gingival overgrowth sometimes seen with phenytoin, calcium channel blockers such as nifedipine, and cyclosporine A, an immunosuppressant drug used in organ transplants), fibroblasts may be activated and secrete more ground substance than normal.

Macrophages

Under the light microscope the fixed macrophage (*histiocyte*) is also a stellate or fusiform cell; unless the macrophage is actively phagocytosing extracellular debris, it may be distinguished from a fibroblast only with difficulty. Ultrastructurally, macrophages have smaller and denser nuclei and less granular endoplasmic reticula than fibroblasts, and their cytoplasm contains membrane-bound vesicles that can be identified as lysosomes (Figure 12-23).

The macrophage has a number of functions, the principal one being to ingest damaged tissue or foreign material in phagocytic vacuoles that fuse, intracytoplasmically, with lysosomes and initiate breakdown of these materials. The processing of ingested material by the macrophage may be important in increasing its antigenicity before it is presented to cells of the lymphoid series for subsequent immunologic response. Another important function is the stimulation of fibroblast proliferation necessary for repair.

In the lamina propria of the oral mucosa two special types of macrophages can be identified specifically: the *melanophage* and the *siderophage*. The melanophage, which is common in pigmented oral mucosa, is a cell that has ingested melanin granules extruded from melanocytes within the epithelium. The siderophage is a cell that contains hemosiderin derived from red blood cells that have been extravasated into the tissues as a result of mechanical injury. This material can persist within the siderophage for some time, and the resultant brownish color appears clinically as a bruise.

Mast Cells

The mast cell is a large spherical or elliptical mononuclear cell (Figure 12-24). The nucleus of the mast cell is small relative to the size of the cell and in histologic preparations frequently is obscured by the large number of intensely staining granules that occupy its cytoplasm. These granules stain with certain basic dyes such as methylene blue because of the presence of heparin within the granules. In human beings the principal contents of the granules are histamine and heparin.

Because these cells frequently are found in association with small blood vessels, the suggestion has been made that they play a role in maintaining normal tissue stability and vascular homeostasis. Although histamine is known to be important in initiating the vascular phase of an inflammatory process, the way it is released from the mast cells is understood poorly.

Inflammatory Cells

Histologically, the lymphocyte and plasma cell may be observed in small numbers scattered throughout the lamina propria, but apart from specialized regions such as the lingual tonsil, other inflammatory cells are found in significant numbers only in connective tissue, following an injury (e.g., a surgical incision) or as part of a disease process. When inflammatory cells are present in significant numbers, they influence the behavior of the overlying epithelium by releasing cytokines.

As in other parts of the body, the type of inflammatory cell depends on the nature and duration of the injury. In acute conditions, polymorphonuclear leukocytes are the dominant cell type, whereas more chronic conditions (e.g., periodontal disease) are associated with lymphocytes, plasma cells, monocytes, and macrophages. All these inflammatory cells show the same morphologic features as their circulating counterparts.

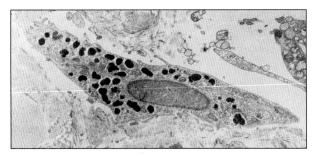

Figure 12-24 Electron micrograph of mast cell from the lamina propria. The dense granules in the cytoplasm, characteristic of this cell type in human beings, are apparent.

FIBERS AND GROUND SUBSTANCE

The intercellular matrix of the lamina propria consists of two major types of fibers, collagen and elastin, together with fibronectin embedded in a ground substance composed of glycosaminoglycans and serum-derived proteins, all of which are highly hydrated.

Collagen

Collagen in the lamina propria is primarily type I and type III, with types IV and VII occurring as part of the basal lamina. Type V may be present in inflamed tissue (a full account of the biology of collagen is given in Chapter 4).

Elastic Fibers

Elastic fibers consist of two protein components that are distinctly different in amino acid composition and morphology. The principal protein of the mature fiber is elastin, which is responsible for the elastic properties of the fiber. The second component is a glycoprotein with a microfibrillar morphology. Initially, elastic fibers consist entirely of aggregates of microfibrils, each 10 to 20 nm in diameter. As they mature, however, elastin is laid down within the microfibril matrix as a granular material until it becomes the predominant component, accounting for more than 90% of the fiber (see Figure 12-23).

When stained using specific methods, some elastic fibers can be seen in most regions of the oral mucosa, but they are more abundant in the flexible lining mucosa, where they function to restore tissue form after stretching. Unlike collagen fibers, elastic fibers branch and anastomose and run singly rather than in bundles.

Ground Substance

Although the ground substance of the lamina propria appears by light and electron microscopy to be amorphous at the molecular level, it consists of heterogeneous protein-carbohydrate complexes permeated by tissue fluid. Chemically these complexes can be subdivided into two distinct groups: proteoglycans and glycoproteins.

The proteoglycans consist of a polypeptide core to which glycosaminoglycans (consisting of hexose and hexuronic acid residues) are attached. In the oral mucosa the proteoglycans are represented by hyaluronan, heparan sulfate, versican, decorin, biglycan, and syndecan. Proteoglycans in the matrix are different from those associated with the cell surface, and interaction between them and with cell surface molecules (e.g., integrins) is probably important in modulating the behavior and function of the cell. The glycoproteins, by contrast, have a branched polypeptide chain to which only a few simple hexoses are attached.

BLOOD SUPPLY

The blood supply of the oral mucosa (Table 12-4) is rich and is derived from arteries that run parallel to the surface in the submucosa or, when the mucosa is tightly bound to underlying periosteum and a submucosa is absent, in the deep part of the reticular layer. These vessels give off progressively smaller branches that anastomose with adjacent vessels in the reticular layer before forming an extensive capillary network in the papillary layer immediately subjacent to the basal epithelial cells. From this network, capillary loops pass into the connective tissue papillae and come to lie close to the basal layer of the epithelium (Figure 12-25).

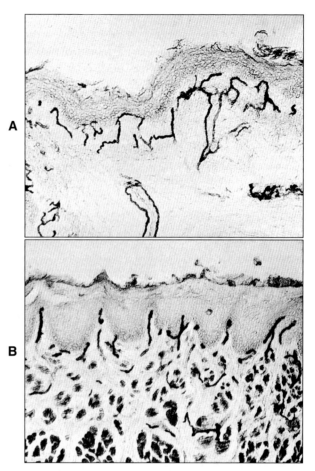

Figure 12-25 Micrographs showing the relationships between capillaries in the lamina propria and overlying epithelium. Mucosal epithelium is from the floor of the mouth **A,** and the cheek **B.** The sections were prepared to demonstrate histochemically the distribution of alkaline phosphatase. In **B** some staining of the muscle also occurred. *(Courtesy G. Zoot.)*

TABLE 12-4 Arterial Blood Supply to the Oral Mucosa

ORAL REGION	SUBTERMINAL BRANCHES
Upper lip	Superior labial artery (anastomoses with buccal artery)
Upper gingiva	
Anterior	Anterior superior alveolar artery
Lingual	Major palatine artery
Buccal	Buccal artery
Posterior	Posterior superior alveolar artery
Hard palate	Major palatine artery
	Nasopalatine artery
	Sphenopalatine artery
Soft palate	Minor palatine artery
Cheek	Buccal artery
	Some terminal branches of facial artery
	Posterior alveolar artery
	Infraorbital artery
Lower lip	Inferior labial artery (anastomoses with buccal artery)
	Mental artery
	Branch of inferior alveolar artery
Lower gingiva	
Anterior buccal	Mental artery
Anterior lingual	Incisive artery and sublingual artery
Posterior lingual	Inferior alveolar artery and sublingual artery
Posterior buccal	Inferior alveolar artery and buccal artery
Floor of mouth	Sublingual artery
	Branch of lingual artery
Tongue (dorsal and ventral surfaces)	
Anterior two thirds	Deep lingual artery
Posterior third	Dorsal lingual artery, to base of tongue, about posterior third

From Stablein MJ, Meyer J. In Meyer J, Squier CA, Gerson SJ, editors: The structure and function of oral mucosa, New York, 1984, Pergamon Press.

The arrangement in oral mucosa is much more profuse than in skin, where capillary loops are found only in association with hair follicles (which may explain the deeper color of oral mucosa).

Regional modifications occur in this basic pattern. For example, in the cheek a single capillary loop passes into each papilla, but in the tongue each filiform papilla receives a variable number of capillaries; in the larger fungiform and circumvallate papillae, arterioles reach into them before giving off capillary loops. In tissues such as the cheek, where the connective tissues may undergo extensive deformation, the arterioles follow a tortuous path and show more extensive branching.

Blood flow through the oral mucosa is greatest in the gingiva, but in all regions of the oral mucosa, blood flow is greater than in the skin at normal temperatures. To what extent inflammation of the gingiva (gingivitis), which is almost inevitably present, may be responsible for this greater flow is uncertain. Postcapillary venules beneath oral sulcular and gingival epithelia express adhesive molecules such as endothelial cell leukocyte adhesion molecule and intercellular adhesion molecule that facilitate leukocyte trafficking even in health. Unlike the skin, which plays a role in temperature regulation, human oral mucosa lacks arteriovenous shunts but does have rich anastomoses of arterioles and capillaries, which undoubtedly contribute to its ability to heal more rapidly than skin after injury.

NERVE SUPPLY

Because the mouth is the gateway to the alimentary and respiratory tracts, the oral mucous membrane is innervated densely so that it can monitor all substances entering. A rich innervation also serves to initiate and maintain a variety of voluntary and reflexive activities involved in mastication, salivation, swallowing, gagging, and speaking. The nerve supply to the oral mucous membrane is therefore overwhelmingly sensory (Table 12-5).

TABLE 12-5   Principal Sensory Nerve Fibers Supplying the Oral Mucosa

ORAL REGION	INNERVATION
Upper lip and vestibule	Twigs from infraorbital branch of maxillary nerve
Upper gingivae	Anterior, posterior, and (when present) middle superior alveolar branches of maxillary nerve
Hard palate	Greater, lesser, and sphenopalatine branches of maxillary nerve
Soft palate	Lesser palatine branch of maxillary nerve; tonsillar branch of glossopharyngeal nerve; and nerve of pterygoid canal (taste; originating from facial nerve)
Cheek	Twigs from infraorbital branch of maxillary nerve; superior alveolar branch of maxillary nerve; buccal branch of mandibular nerve; and possibly some terminal branches of facial nerve
Lower lip and vestibule	Mental branch of inferior alveolar nerve and buccal branch of mandibular nerve
Lower gingivae: buccal, lingual	Inferior alveolar branch of mandibular nerve; buccal branch of mandibular nerve; and sublingual branch of lingual nerve
Anterior two thirds of by tongue	Lingual branch of mandibular nerve (taste) provided fibers carried in lingual nerve but originating in facial nerve and passing by way of chorda tympani to lingual nerve
Posterior third of tongue, facial, and tonsillar	Glossopharyngeal nerve (taste and general sensation)

From Holland GR. In Meyer J, Squier CA, Gerson SJ, editors: The structure and function of oral mucosa, *New York, 1984, Pergamon Press.*

The efferent supply is autonomic, supplies the blood vessels and minor salivary glands, and also may modulate the activity of some sensory receptors. The nerves arise mainly from the second and third divisions of the trigeminal nerve; but afferent fibers of the facial (VII), glossopharyngeal (IX), and vagus (X) nerves also are involved. The sensory nerves lose their myelin sheaths and form a network in the reticular layer of the lamina propria that terminates in a subepithelial plexus.

The sensory nerves terminate in free and organized nerve endings. Free nerve endings are found in the lamina propria and within the epithelium, where they frequently are associated with Merkel cells. Apart from the nerves associated with Merkel cells, intraepithelial nerve endings have a sensory function. Such nerves are not surrounded by Schwann cells as in connective tissue but run between the keratinocytes (which may ensheathe the nerves and so form a mesaxon). These nerves terminate as simple endings in the middle (or upper) layers of the epithelium (Figure 12-26).

Within the lamina propria, organized nerve endings usually are found in the papillary region. They consist of groups of coiled fibers surrounded by a connective tissue capsule. These specialized endings have been grouped according to their morphology as *Meissner's* or *Ruffini's corpuscles*, *Krause's bulbs*, and the mucocutaneous end-organs. The density of sensory receptors is greater in the anterior part of the mouth than in the posterior region, with the greatest density where the connective tissue papillae are most prominent.

The primary sensations perceived in the oral cavity are warmth, cold, touch, pain, and taste. Although specialized nerve endings are differentially sensitive to particular modalities (e.g., Krause's bulbs appear to be most sensitive to cold stimuli and Meissner's corpuscles to touch), no evidence indicates that any one receptor is responsible for detecting only one type of stimulus. Possibly, however, each modality is served by specific fibers associated with each termination.

Sensory nerve networks are more developed in the oral mucosa lining the anterior than in the posterior regions of the mouth, and this pattern is paralleled by the greater sensitivity of this region to a number of modalities. For example, touch sensation is most acute in the anterior part of the tongue and hard palate. By comparison, the sensitivity of the fingertips falls between those of the tongue and the palate. Touch receptors in the soft palate and oropharynx are important in the initiation of swallowing, gagging, and retching. Similarly, temperature reception is more acute in the vermilion border of the lip, at the tip of the tongue, and on the anterior hard palate than in more posterior regions of the oral cavity. The detection of pain is understood poorly. The sensation of pain appears to be initiated by noxious stimuli causing tissue damage and

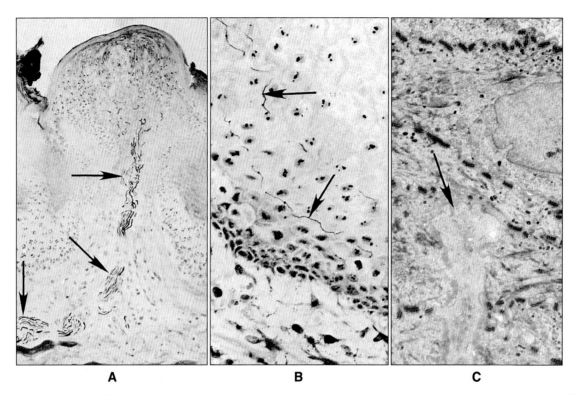

Figure 12-26 Nerves in the oral mucosa. **A,** A nerve bundle *(arrows)* running into the epithelium of a fungiform papilla on the dorsum of the tongue. **B,** The appearance of intraepithelial nerves *(arrows)* running between cells of the buccal epithelium. **C,** An electron micrograph of free nerve ending *(arrow)* between the upper prickle cells in human gingiva. *(A and B courtesy of the late John Linder.)*

thereby activating polypeptides in the interstitial fluid, which in turn act on free nerve endings of slow-conducting unmyelinated and thin myelinated nerves.

A specialized receptor that occurs only in the oral cavity and pharynx is the taste bud. Although some taste buds lie within the epithelium of the soft palate and pharynx, most are found in the fungiform, foliate, and circumvallate papillae of the tongue (Figures 12-27 and 12-28).

Histologically, the taste bud is a barrel-shaped structure composed of 30 to 80 spindle-shaped cells (see Figure 12-28, C). At their bases the cells are separated from underlying connective tissue by the basal lamina, whereas their apical ends terminate just below the epithelial surface in a taste pit that communicates with the surface through a small opening, the taste pore.

The cells of the taste bud have been divided into three types: light (type I), dark (type II), and intermediate (type III). Type I cells are the most common, representing about half of all cells in the taste bud. Type II cells are morphologically similar but contain numerous vesicles and are adjacent to the intraepithelial nerves. They are replaced continually, and their existence depends on a functional gustatory nerve. The apical ends of these cells are joined tightly together by junctional complexes, somewhat like those in intestinal mucosa, so that the initial events stimulating sensation of taste appear to involve the amorphous material within the taste pits and the microvilli of constituent cells that project into those pits.

Taste stimuli probably are generated by the adsorption of molecules onto membrane receptors on the surface of the taste bud cells, which activates a signaling cascade mediated by membrane-associated proteins such as transducin and gustducin. The change in membrane polarization that follows stimulates release of transmitter substances, which in turn stimulate unmyelinated afferent fibers of the glossopharyngeal nerve (IX) that surround the lower half of the taste cells. Taste bud cells, with Merkel cells, are the only truly specialized sensory cells in the oral mucosa.

Although the sensitivity of taste buds to sweet, salty, sour, and bitter substances shows regional variation (sweet at the tip, salty and sour on the lateral aspects, and bitter and sour in the posterior region of the tongue), no distinct structural differences have been observed among taste buds in these regions. The identification of different substances likely depends on binding different membrane receptors.

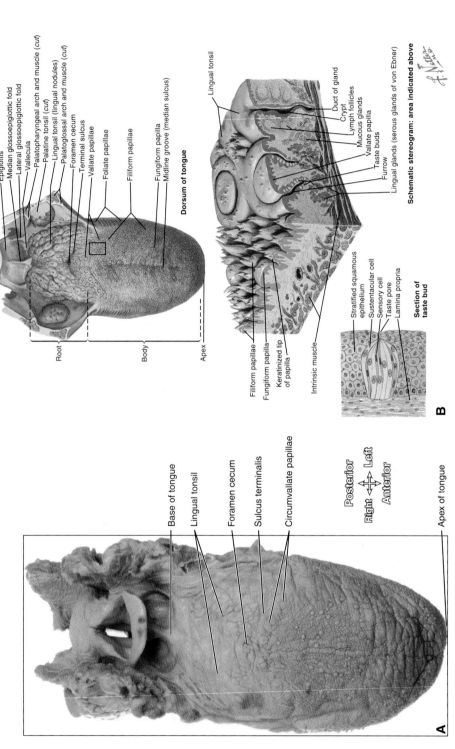

Figure 12-27 A, Macroscopic view of the tongue, showing the distribution and types of lingual papillae on its dorsal surface. **B,** Schematic representation of the papillae. (*A from Norton NS: Netter's head and neck anatomy for dentistry, Philadelphia, 2007, Saunders; B from Logan BM, Reynold PA, Hutching RT: McMinn's color atlas of head and neck anatomy, ed 3, London, 2004, Mosby Ltd.*)

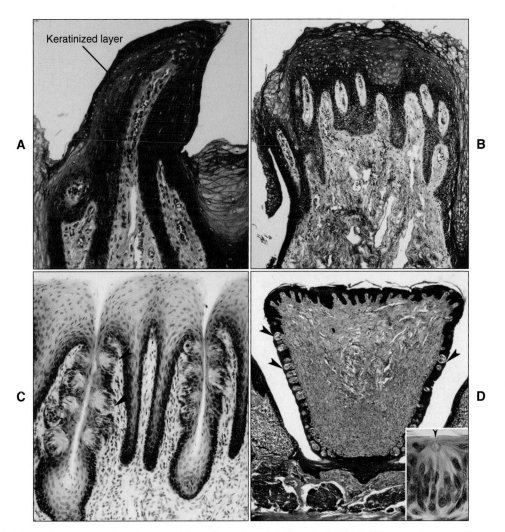

Figure 12-28 Histologic sections of three types of lingual papillae. **A,** Filiform papilla and **B,** a fungiform papilla from the anterior part of the tongue. The epithelium of the filiform papillae is keratinized; that of the fungiform papilla is keratinized thinly or nonkeratinized. **C,** Section through foliate papillae. The nonkeratinized epithelium covering the papilla contains numerous taste buds *(arrowheads)* situated laterally. **D,** Histologic section through a circumvallate papilla from the dorsum of the tongue. A deep groove runs around the papilla, and the glands of Ebner empty into it. The arrowheads indicate the numerous taste buds on the lateral walls of the papilla. *Inset,* Enlarged view of a taste bud with its barrel-like appearance and apical pore *(arrowhead).*

A special type of receptor the function of which is to detect the taste of water has been postulated by physiologists. This function seems localized to the region of the circumvallate papillae of the tongue, but the morphologic structures responsible for it have not been described.

STRUCTURAL VARIATIONS

By now it should be apparent that the human oral mucosa shows considerable variation in structure, not only in the composition of the lamina propria, form of the interface between epithelium and connective tissue, and type of surface epithelium but also in the nature of the submucosa and how the mucosa is attached to underlying structures. Fortunately, the organization of component tissues shows similar patterns in many regions. The oral mucosa can be divided into three main types: masticatory, lining, and specialized. The areas occupied by each type are illustrated in Figure 12-1. In the following sections, each type of mucosa is described. A summary of the structures within the various anatomic regions occupied by each appears in Table 12-6. Finally, a brief account is given of several junctions between different types of mucosa that are of morphologic interest and clinical importance.

MASTICATORY MUCOSA

Masticatory mucosa covers those areas of the oral cavity such as the hard palate (Figure 12-29) and gingiva

TABLE 12-6 Structure of the Mucosa in Different Regions of the Oral Cavity

REGION	COVERING EPITHELIUM	LAMINA PROPRIA	SUBMUCOSA
Lining Mucosa			
Soft palate	Thin (150 μm), nonkeratinized stratified squamous epithelium; taste buds present	Thick with numerous short papillae; elastic fibers forming an elastic lamina; highly vascular with well-developed capillary network	Diffuse tissue containing numerous minor salivary glands
Ventral surface of tongue	Thin, nonkeratinized, stratified squamous epithelium	Thin with numerous short papillae and some elastic fibers; a few minor salivary glands; capillary network in subpapillary layer; reticular layer relatively avascular	Thin and irregular; may contain fat and small vessels; where absent, mucosa is bound to connective tissue surrounding tongue musculature
Floor of mouth	Very thin (100 μm), nonkeratinized, stratified squamous epithelium	Short papillae; some elastic fibers; extensive vascular supply with short anastomosing capillary loops	Loose fibrous connective tissue containing fat and minor salivary glands
Alveolar mucosa	Thin, nonkeratinized, stratified squamous epithelium	Short papillae, connective tissue containing many elastic fibers; capillary loops close to the surface supplied by vessels running superficially to the periosteum	Loose connective tissue, containing thick elastic fibers attaching it to periosteum of alveolar process; minor salivary glands
Labial and buccal mucosa	Very thick (500 μm), nonkeratinized, stratified squamous epithelium	Long, slender papillae; dense fibrous connective tissue containing collagen and some elastic fibers; rich vascular supply giving off anastomosing capillary loops into papillae	Mucosa firmly attached to underlying muscle by collagen and elastin; dense collagenous connective tissue with fat, minor salivary glands, sometimes sebaceous glands
Lips: vermilion zone	Thin, orthokeratinized, stratified squamous epithelium	Numerous narrow papillae; capillary loops close to surface in papillary layer	Mucosa firmly attached to underlying muscle; some sebaceous glands in vermilion border, minor salivary gland and fat in intermediate zone
Lips: intermediate zone	Thin, parakeratinized, stratified squamous epithelium	Long, irregular papillae; elastic and collagen fibers in connective tissue	—
Masticatory Mucosa			
Gingiva	Thick (250 μm), orthokeratinized or parakeratinized, stratified squamous epithelium often showing stippled surface	Long, narrow papillae; dense collagenous connective tissue; not highly vascular but has long capillary loops with numerous anastomoses	No distinct layer; mucosa firmly attached by collagen fibers to cementum and periosteum of alveolar process (mucoperiosteum)
Hard palate	Thick, orthokeratinized (often parakeratinized in parts), stratified squamous epithelium thrown into transverse palatine ridges (rugae)	Long papillae; thick, dense collagenous tissue, especially under rugae; moderate vascular supply with short capillary loops	Dense collagenous connective tissue attaching mucosa to periosteum (mucoperiosteum); fat and minor salivary glands are packed into connective tissue in regions where mucosa overlies lateral palatine neurovascular bundles
Specialized Mucosa			
Dorsal surface of tongue	Thick, keratinized and nonkeratinized, stratified squamous epithelium forming three types of lingual papillae, some bearing taste buds	Long papillae; minor salivary glands in posterior portion; rich innervation especially near taste buds; capillary plexus in papillary layer; large vessels lying deeper	No distinct layer; mucosa is bound to connective tissue surrounding musculature of tongue

(Figure 12-30, A) that are exposed to compressive and shear forces and to abrasion during the mastication of food. The dorsum of the tongue has the same functional role as other masticatory mucosa, but because of its specialized structure, it is considered separately.

The epithelium of masticatory mucosa is moderately thick and frequently is orthokeratinized, although normally parakeratinized areas of the gingiva and occasionally of the palate do occur. Both types of epithelial surface are inextensible and well adapted to withstanding abrasion. The junction between epithelium and underlying lamina propria is convoluted, and the numerous elongated papillae probably provide good mechanical attachment and prevent the epithelium from being stripped off under shear force. The lamina propria is thick, containing a dense network of collagen

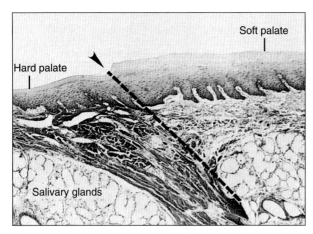

Figure 12-29 Photomicrograph of the junction *(dashed line)* between mucosa covering the hard and the soft palate. The difference in thickness and the ridge pattern between keratinized epithelium of the hard palate and nonkeratinized epithelium of the soft palate is apparent. The section has been stained by the van Gieson's method to demonstrate collagen; the thick dense bundles in the lamina propria of the hard palate appear different from the thinner fibers in the soft palate. Minor salivary glands occur beneath the mucosa.

fibers in the form of large, closely packed bundles. They follow a direct course between anchoring points so that the tissue has little slack and does not yield on impact, enabling the mucosa to resist heavy loading.

Masticatory mucosa covers immobile structures (e.g., the palate and alveolar processes) and is bound firmly to them directly by the attachment of lamina propria to the periosteum of underlying bone—such as in mucoperiosteum—or indirectly by a fibrous submucosa. In the lateral regions of the palate, this fibrous submucosa is interspersed with areas of fat and glandular tissue that cushion the mucosa against mechanical loads and protect the underlying nerves and blood vessels of the palate.

The firmness of masticatory mucosa ensures that it does not gape after surgical incisions and rarely requires suturing. For the same reason, injections of local anesthetic into these areas are difficult and often painful, as is any swelling arising from inflammation.

LINING MUCOSA

The oral mucosa covering the underside of the tongue (Figure 12-31), inside of the lips (Figure 12-32), cheeks, floor of the mouth, and alveolar processes as far as the gingiva (see Figure 12-30) is subject to movement. These regions, together with the soft palate, are classified as lining mucosa.

The epithelium of lining mucosa is thicker than that of masticatory mucosa, sometimes exceeding 500 μm in the cheek, and is nonkeratinized. The surface

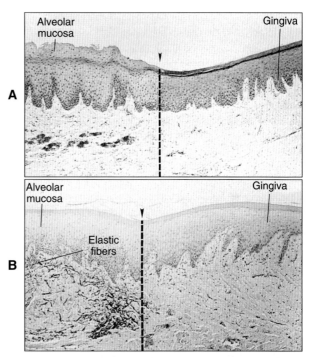

Figure 12-30 Sections through the mucogingival junction *(dashed line)*. In **A** the differences in thickness, ridge pattern, and keratinization between epithelium of the gingiva and alveolar mucosa are seen. The preparation was stained by Papanicolaou's method, which reveals variations in keratinization. The junction in **B** was stained by Hart's method to demonstrate elastic fibers in the connective tissue. Although little change in the epithelium occurs in this specimen, a striking difference appears in the concentration of elastic fibers in the lamina propria between masticatory mucosa of the gingiva and lining mucosa of the alveoli. *(From Squier CA, Johnson NW, Hopps RM: Human oral mucosa: development, structure, and function, Oxford, UK, 1976, Blackwell Scientific.)*

is thus flexible and able to withstand stretching. The interface with connective tissue is smooth, although slender connective tissue papillae often penetrate into the epithelium.

The lamina propria is generally thicker than in masticatory mucosa and contains fewer collagen fibers, which follow a more irregular course between anchoring points. Thus the mucosa can be stretched to a certain extent before these fibers become taut and limit further distention. Associated with the collagen fibers are elastic fibers that tend to control the extensibility of the mucosa. Where lining mucosa covers muscle, the mucosa is attached by a mixture of collagen and elastic fibers. As the mucosa becomes slack during masticatory movements, the elastic fibers retract the mucosa toward the muscle and so prevent it from bulging between the teeth and being bitten.

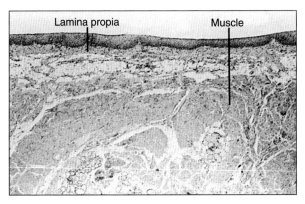

Figure 12-31 Photomicrograph of lining mucosa from the underside of the tongue. The nonkeratinized epithelium is thin, with only a slight ridge pattern, and is bound to the underlying muscle by a narrow lamina propria. Between this lamina and the muscle is a layer of fat, appearing as light areas.

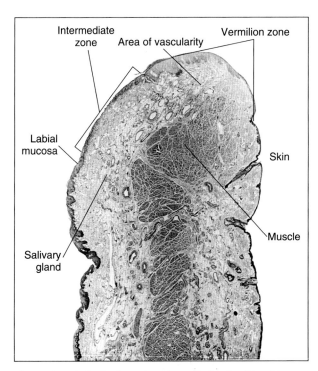

Figure 12-32 Sagittal section through the lip. The skin covering the external aspect has a thin epidermis and contains hair follicles. Continuous with this is the vermilion zone, which has a thin epithelium overlying an area of extensive vascularity. Between the vermilion zone and the labial mucosa of the oral cavity is the intermediate zone. Minor salivary glands occur beneath the labial mucosa, and the extensive muscular tissue represents part of the orbicularis oris.

The alveolar mucosa and mucosa covering the floor of the mouth are attached loosely to the underlying structures by a thick submucosa. Elastic fibers in the lamina propria of these regions tend to restore the mucosa to its resting position after distention. By contrast, mucosa of the underside of the tongue is bound firmly to the underlying muscle. The soft palate is flexible but not highly mobile, and its mucosa is separated from the loose and highly glandular submucosa by a layer of elastic fibers.

The tendency for lining mucosa to be flexible, with a loose and often elastic submucosa, means that surgical incisions frequently require sutures for closure. Injections into such regions are easy because dispersion of fluid occurs readily in the loose connective tissue; however, infections also spread rapidly.

SPECIALIZED MUCOSA

The mucosa of the dorsal surface of the tongue is unlike that anywhere else in the oral cavity because, although covered by what is functionally a masticatory mucosa, it is also a highly extensible lining and in addition has different types of lingual papillae. Some of them possess a mechanical function, whereas others bear taste buds and therefore have a sensory function.

The mucous membrane of the tongue (see Figure 12-27) is composed of two parts, with different embryologic origins (see Chapter 3) and is divided by the V-shaped groove, the sulcus terminalis (terminal groove). The anterior two thirds of the tongue, where the mucosa is derived from the first pharyngeal arch, often is called the *body*, and the posterior third, where the mucosa is derived from the third pharyngeal arch, the *base*. The mucosa covering the base of the tongue contains extensive nodules of lymphoid tissue, the lingual tonsils.

FUNGIFORM PAPILLAE

The anterior portion of the tongue bears the *fungiform* (funguslike) and *filiform* (hairlike) papillae (see Figure 12-28, A). Single fungiform papillae are scattered between the numerous filiform papillae at the tip of the tongue. The fungiform papillae are smooth, round structures that appear red because of their highly vascular connective tissue core, visible through a thin, nonkeratinized covering epithelium. Taste buds normally are present in the epithelium on the superior surface.

FILIFORM PAPILLAE

Filiform papillae cover the entire anterior part of the tongue and consist of cone-shaped structures, each with a core of connective tissue covered by a thick keratinized epithelium (see Figure 12-28, A). Together they form a tough, abrasive surface that is involved in compressing and breaking food when the tongue is apposed to the hard palate. Thus the dorsal mucosa of the tongue functions as a masticatory mucosa. Buildup of keratin results in elongation of the filiform papillae in some patients. The dorsum of the tongue then has a hairy appearance called *hairy tongue*.

The tongue is highly extensible, with changes in its shape accommodated by the regions of nonkeratinized, flexible epithelium between the filiform papillae.

FOLIATE PAPILLAE

Foliate (leaflike) papillae sometimes are present on the lateral margins of the posterior part of the tongue, although they are seen more frequently in mammals other than human beings. These pink papillae consist of 4 to 11 parallel ridges that alternate with deep grooves in the mucosa, and a few taste buds are present in the epithelium of the lateral walls of the ridges (see Figure 12-28, B).

CIRCUMVALLATE PAPILLAE

Adjacent and anterior to the sulcus terminalis are 8 to 12 *circumvallate* (walled) papillae, large structures each surrounded by a deep, circular groove into which open the ducts of minor salivary glands (the glands of Ebner; see Figures 12-27, C, and 12-28, C). These papillae have a connective tissue core that is covered on the superior surface by a keratinized epithelium. The epithelium covering the lateral walls is nonkeratinized and contains taste buds.

JUNCTIONS IN THE ORAL MUCOSA

Within the oral mucosa are three junctions that merit further discussion: the mucocutaneous (between the skin and mucosa), the mucogingival (between the gingiva and alveolar mucosa), and the dentogingival (interface between the gingiva and the tooth). The latter is of considerable anatomic and clinical importance because it represents the first line of defense in periodontal diseases.

MUCOCUTANEOUS JUNCTION

The skin, which contains hair follicles and sebaceous and sweat glands, is continuous with the oral mucosa at the lips (see Figure 12-32). At the mucocutaneous junction is a transitional region where appendages are absent except for a few sebaceous glands (situated mainly at the angles of the mouth). The epithelium of this region is keratinized but thin, with long connective tissue papillae containing capillary loops. This arrangement

brings the blood close to the surface and accounts for the strong red coloration in this region, called the *red* (or *vermilion*) *zone* of the lip. The line separating the vermilion zone from the hair-bearing skin of the lip is called the *vermilion border*. In young persons this border is demarcated sharply, but as a person is exposed to ultraviolet radiation, the border becomes diffuse and poorly defined.

Because the vermilion zone lacks salivary glands and contains only a few sebaceous glands, it tends to dry out, often becoming cracked and sore in cold weather. Between the vermilion zone and the thicker, nonkeratinized labial mucosa is an intermediate zone covered by parakeratinized oral epithelium. In infants this region is thickened and appears more opalescent, which represents an adaptation to suckling called the *suckling pad*.

MUCOGINGIVAL JUNCTION

Although masticatory mucosa meets lining mucosa at several sites, none is more abrupt than the junction between attached gingiva and alveolar mucosa. This junction is identified clinically by a slight indentation called the *mucogingival groove* and by the change from the bright pink of the alveolar mucosa to the paler pink of the gingiva (see Figure 12-2, B).

Histologically, a change occurs at this junction, not only in the type of epithelium but also in the composition of the lamina propria (see Figure 12-30). The epithelium of the attached gingiva is keratinized or parakeratinized, and the lamina propria contains numerous coarse collagen bundles attaching the tissue to periosteum. The stippling seen clinically at the surface of healthy attached gingiva probably reflects the presence of this collagen attachment, the surface of the *free* gingiva being smooth. The structure of mucosa changes at the mucogingival junction, where the alveolar mucosa has a thicker, nonkeratinized epithelium overlying a loose lamina propria with numerous elastic fibers extending into the thick submucosa. These elastic fibers return the alveolar mucosa to its original position after distention by the labial muscles during mastication and speech.

Coronal to the mucogingival junction is another clinically visible depression in the gingiva, the free gingival groove, the level of which corresponds approximately to that of the bottom of the gingival sulcus. This demarcates the free and attached gingivae, although unlike the mucogingival junction, no significant change in the structure of the mucosa occurs at the free gingival groove.

DENTOGINGIVAL JUNCTION

The region where the oral mucosa meets the surface of the tooth is a unique junction of considerable importance because it represents a potential weakness in the otherwise continuous epithelial lining of the oral cavity. The bacteria that are inevitably present on the tooth surface continually produce toxins capable of eliciting inflammation and damage if they enter the mucosal tissues. The junction between the epithelium and the enamel (Figure 12-33) is the principal seal between the oral cavity and the underlying tissues, and understanding the nature of this union is important.

In the average human mouth, in which mild gingival inflammation is invariably present, the *gingival sulcus* (see Figure 12-33, A) has a depth of 0.5 to 3 mm, with an average of 1.8 mm. Any depth greater than 3 mm generally can be considered pathologic; a sulcus this deep is known as a periodontal pocket. When the tooth first becomes functional, the bottom of the sulcus usually is found on the cervical half of the anatomic crown; with age a gradual migration of the sulcus bottom occurs that eventually may pass on to the cementum surface. The sulcus contains fluid that has passed through the junctional epithelium and contains a mixture of desquamated epithelial cells from the junctional and sulcular epithelia and neutrophils that also have passed through the junctional epithelium.

The floor of the sulcus and the epithelium cervical to it, which is applied to the tooth surface is termed *junctional epithelium*. The walls of the sulcus are lined by epithelium derived from and continuous with that of the rest of the oral mucosa. This has been designated *oral sulcular epithelium* and has the same basic structure as nonkeratinized oral epithelium elsewhere in the oral cavity. The orthokeratinized or parakeratinized surface of the free gingiva (or oral epithelium) is continuous with the oral sulcular epithelium at the level of the gingival crest (see Figure 12-33, A).

Junctional epithelium is derived from the reduced enamel (or dental) epithelium of the tooth germ. As the tooth erupts and the crown penetrates the overlying oral epithelium, a fusion occurs between the reduced enamel epithelium and the oral epithelium so that epithelial continuity is never lost. The junctional epithelium is

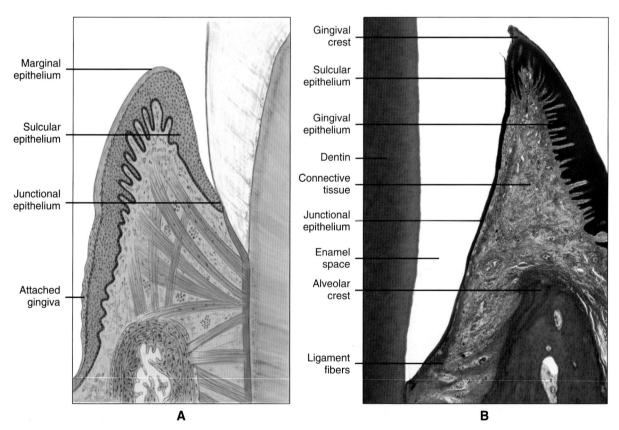

Figure 12-33 The dentogingival junction. **A,** Diagram of the different types of gingival epithelia in the oral cavity; these are the gingival epithelium, sulcular epithelium, and junctional epithelium. Together, the sulcular and junctional epithelium constitute the dentogingival junction. The junctional epithelium attaches to the tooth surface. **B,** Histologic section showing the tissues illustrated in **A.** Decalcification of the specimen has removed the tooth enamel, leaving an enamel space. The sulcular epithelium is short in this preparation because the tooth is not fully erupted. *(**A** from Bath-Balogh M, Fehrenbach MJ: Dental embryology, histology and anatomy, St Louis, 2006, Saunders.)*

basically a stratified squamous nonkeratinizing epithelium the cells of which derive from basal cells situated away from the tooth surface. The basal cells rest on a typical basal lamina that interfaces with the subjacent dermal connective tissue (Figure 12-34, A). This so-called *outer basal lamina* is similar to that which attaches epithelium to connective tissue elsewhere in the oral mucosa. Suprabasal cells have a similar appearance; they are flattened cells oriented parallel to the tooth surface and tapering from three to four layers in thickness apically to 15 to 30 layers coronally. Remarkably, these cells maintain some ability to undergo cell division and turn over rapidly, at least in some species. The most superficial cell layer provides the actual attachment of gingiva to the tooth surface (enamel or sometimes cementum) by means of a structural complex called the *epithelial attachment*. This complex consists of an *inner basal lamina* formed and maintained by the flattened superficial cells that adheres to the tooth surface and to which the cells are attached by hemidesmosomes (Figure 12-34, B). This basal lamina is unique because it binds to calcified surfaces rather than connective tissues. For many years, the only information about its composition was that it is enriched in glycoconjugates. It has now been demonstrated that basal laminae applied to tooth surfaces (also the basal lamina associated with maturation stage ameloblasts; see Chapter 7)

contain laminin-5, whereas components such as γ1 chain-containing laminins and type IV and VII collagens are not present, setting them apart functionally and compositionally. Recently, it has been reported that the inner basal lamina of the junctional epithelium contains amelotin, a novel secreted protein that as shown in Chapter 7 also is expressed by maturation stage ameloblasts.

The junctional epithelium is not simply an area of nonkeratinized oral epithelium but a unique and poorly differentiated tissue. Thus the ultrastructural characteristics of junctional epithelial cells are relatively constant throughout the epithelium and differ considerably from those of other oral epithelial cells. Junctional epithelial cells contain fewer tonofilaments and desmosomal junctions, and the cytokeratins present represent those seen in basal epithelial cells (K5, K14, and K19) and in simple epithelia (K8 and K18). Although the cells of the junctional epithelium divide and migrate to the surface, they show no sign of differentiation to form a keratinized surface epithelium. These features, as well as the frequent presence of infiltrating neutrophil leukocytes and mononuclear cells, may contribute to the permeability of the tissue. This has been studied extensively, and a variety of substances ranging from cells to tissue fluid and small protein molecules have been shown to be capable of traversing the epithelium.

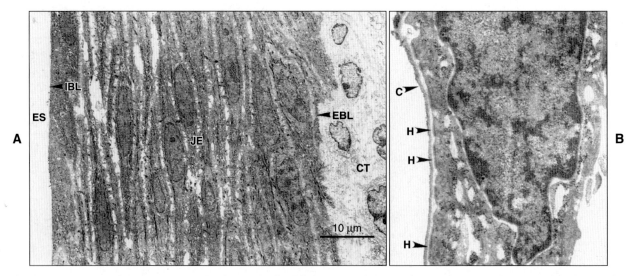

Figure 12-34 A, An electron micrograph of junctional epithelium *(JE)* showing the attachment to the enamel surface at the internal basal lamina *(IBL)* and to the connective tissue *(CT)* by the external basal lamina *(EBL)*. The lack of differentiation of the epithelium and the wide intercellular spaces are notable. *ES,* Enamel space. **B,** An electron micrograph showing the fine structure of the attachment of a junctional epithelial cell to the enamel surface via the internal basal lamina. Hemidesmosomes *(H)* are evident at the surface of the cell, and a lamina lucida and lamina densa are continuous with a dental cuticle *(C)*. *(A from Schroeder HE, Listgarten MA: Fine structure of the developing attachment of human teeth, Basel, Switzerland, 1977, S Karger.)*

As in all epithelia, the deeper cells adjacent to the connective tissue undergo cell division to replenish those lost at the surface. The rate of cell division is high, and those cells produced move to within two or three cell layers of the tooth surface (where the cells are attached to the tooth surface) and then join a main migratory route in a coronal direction, paralleling the tooth surface, to be desquamated into the gingival sulcus.

One of the remarkable properties of the junctional epithelium is that it readily regenerates from the adjacent oral sulcular or oral epithelium if it is damaged or surgically excised. The new junctional epithelium has all the characteristics of the original tissue, including the same types of cytokeratins and an attachment to the tooth that is indistinguishable from the original one. This raises interesting questions as to the nature of the signals responsible for inducing the formation of a junctional epithelium. Contact with a mineralized surface and a connective tissue influence may be implicated.

Connective Tissue Component

Examination of the connective tissue supporting epithelium of the dentogingival junction shows the tissue to be structurally different from connective tissue supporting the oral gingival epithelium in that even in clinically normal gingiva it contains an inflammatory infiltrate thought to be initiated at the time of tooth eruption. Cells of the inflammatory series, particularly polymorphonuclear leukocytes, continually migrate into the junctional epithelium and pass between the epithelial cells to appear in the gingival sulcus and eventually in the oral fluid.

Evidence indicates that the connective tissue supporting junctional epithelium is also functionally different from the connective tissue supporting the rest of the oral epithelium, and such a difference has important connotations for the pathogenesis of periodontal disease and regeneration of the dentogingival junction after periodontal surgery.

Tissue recombination experiments have shown that connective tissue plays a key role in determining epithelial expression. Therefore, subepithelial connective tissues (the lamina propria) provide instructive influences for the normal maturation of a stratified squamous epithelium. Such influences are absent from deep connective tissue, which possesses only "permissive" factors required to maintain the epithelium in a poorly differentiated, or immature, state. Thus epithelium combined with deep connective tissue does not mature but instead persists in a state closely resembling that of junctional epithelium. At the dentogingival junction the gingival and sulcular epithelia, supported by an instructive connective tissue, are believed to be able to mature, whereas junctional epithelium is contact with deep connective tissue remains undifferentiated.

This presumably would allow it to form an epithelial attachment.

That the connective tissue associated with the dentogingival junction is inflamed already has been stated. This inflammation also influences epithelial expression. Thus the oral sulcular epithelium, in distinction to the gingival epithelium, is nonkeratinized, yet both are supported by gingival lamina propria. This difference in epithelial expression may be a direct consequence of the inflammatory process because, if inflammation is reduced by implementation of a strict regimen of oral hygiene combined with antibiotic coverage in experimental animals, the oral sulcular epithelium keratinizes.

The junctional epithelium also is influenced by inflammation. Epithelia maintained experimentally in association with deep connective tissue show little capacity to proliferate but can be induced to do so by the introduction of inflammation into the system. Clinically, in most persons a slow apical migration of the attachment level occurs with age (sometimes referred to as *passive eruption*) that probably is caused by the low-level inflammation in its supporting connective tissue. When inflammation increases, active proliferation and migration of the junctional epithelium occurs, resulting in a periodontal pocket and apical movement of attachment level.

A similar set of biologic events occurs in relation to the proliferation of epithelial cell rests of Malassez and dental cyst formation. Cell rests are supported by the deep connective tissue of the periodontal ligament and proliferate only in the presence of inflammation within that connective tissue.

Col

The previous description of the dentogingival junction applies to all surfaces of the tooth, even though interdentally the gingiva seems to be different. Interdental gingiva appears to have the outline of a *col* (or depression), with buccal and lingual peaks guarding it (Figure 12-35). Col epithelium is identical to junctional epithelium, has the same origin (from enamel epithelium), and is replaced gradually by continuing cell division. No evidence indicates that the structural elements of the col increase vulnerability to periodontal disease. Rather the incidence of gingivitis interdentally is greater than in other areas because the contours between the teeth allow bacteria, food debris, and plaque to accumulate in this location.

Blood Supply

The blood supply to the gingiva is derived from vessels in the periosteum of the alveolar process. Branches from

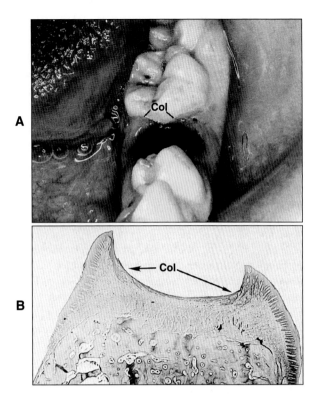

Figure 12-35 Dental col. **A,** Clinical appearance. **B,** Histologic section. The distinction between the keratinized gingival epithelium and the epithelium of the col is evident.

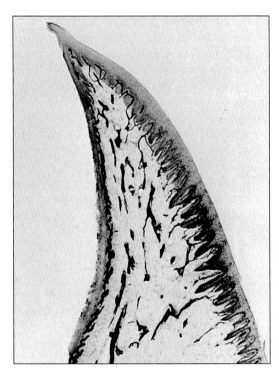

Figure 12-36 Photomicrograph of the blood supply to the dentogingival junction. The differences in shape of vessels related to the gingiva and the dentogingival junction are apparent. *(From Egelberg J:* J Periodontal Res *1:163, 1966.)*

these vessels are perpendicular to the surface and form loops within the connective tissue papillae of the gingiva. Vessels supplying the dentogingival junction are derived from the continuation of interalveolar arteries as they pierce the alveolar crest. These vessels are parallel to the sulcular epithelium and form a rich network just below the basal lamina (Figure 12-36).

For descriptive purposes the blood supply to the periodontium can be divided into three zones: (1) that to the periodontal ligament, (2) that to the gingiva facing the oral cavity, and (3) that to the gingiva facing the tooth. Connections among the three permit collateral circulation.

Nerve Supply

The gingival component of the periodontium is innervated by terminal branches of periodontal nerve fibers and by branches of the infraorbital and palatine, or lingual, mental, and buccal nerves. In the attached gingiva, most nerves terminate within the lamina propria, and only a few endings occur between epithelial cells. In the dentogingival junction of rat molars, a rich innervation of the junctional epithelium has been demonstrated, with free nerve endings between epithelial cells at the connective tissue and the tooth surface of

the epithelium. Vesicular structures and neuropeptides have been demonstrated in these nerve endings.

Why the junctional apparatus should have such an extensive blood and nerve supply is an interesting question. As has been pointed out, when the tooth erupts, inflammation occurs in the connective tissue related to the junction, and this inflammation persists as an almost normal feature of the dentogingival junction. A relationship exists among vascular elements, immunocompetent cells, and secreted neuropeptides, and the described vascular and neural supply may reflect this relationship and function.

DEVELOPMENT OF THE ORAL MUCOSA

The primitive oral cavity develops by fusion of the embryonic stomatodeum with the foregut after rupture of the buccopharyngeal membrane, at about 26 days of gestation, and thus comes to be lined by epithelium derived from ectoderm and endoderm. The precise boundary between these two embryonic tissues is defined poorly, but structures that develop in the branchial arches (e.g., tongue, epiglottis, and pharynx) are covered by epithelium derived from endoderm, whereas the epithelium covering the palate, cheeks, and gingivae is of ectodermal origin (see Chapter 2).

By 5 to 6 weeks of gestation the single layer of cells lining the primitive oral cavity has formed two cell layers, and by 8 weeks a significant thickening occurs in the region of the vestibular dental lamina complex. In the central region of this thickening, cellular degeneration occurs at 10 to 14 weeks, resulting in separation of the cells covering the cheek area and the alveolar mucosa and thus forming the oral vestibule. At about this time (8 to 11 weeks), the palatal shelves elevate and close, so that the future morphology of the adult oral cavity is apparent.

The lingual epithelium shows specialization at about 7 weeks when the circumvallate and foliate papillae first appear, followed by the fungiform papillae. Within these papillae, taste buds soon develop. The filiform papillae that cover most of the anterior two thirds of the tongue become apparent at about 10 weeks. By 10 to 12 weeks the future lining and masticatory mucosa show some stratification of the epithelium and a different morphology.

Those areas destined to become keratinized (e.g., hard palate and alveolar ridge of gingiva) have darkly staining, columnar basal cells that are separated from the underlying connective tissue by a prominent basal lamina. Low connective tissue papillae also are evident. By contrast, the epithelium that will form areas of lining mucosa retains cuboidal basal cells, and the epithelium-connective tissue interface remains flat. Between 13 and 20 weeks of gestation, all the oral epithelia thicken (Figure 12-37), and with the appearance of sparse

keratohyalin granules, a distinction between the prickle cell and granular layer can be made. Differences are evident between the cytokeratins of epithelia of the developing masticatory and lining regions. During this period, melanocytes and Langerhans cells appear in the epithelium. The surface layers of the epithelium show parakeratosis; orthokeratinization of the masticatory mucosa does not occur until after the teeth erupt during the postnatal period.

While these changes are occurring in the oral epithelium, the underlying ectomesenchyme shows progressive changes. Initially the ectomesenchyme consists of widely spaced stellate cells in an amorphous matrix, but by 6 to 8 weeks, extracellular reticular fibers begin to accumulate. As in the epithelium, regional differences can be seen in the ectomesenchyme. The connective tissue of lining mucosa contains fewer cells and fibers than that of the future masticatory mucosa. Between 8 and 12 weeks, capillary buds and collagen fibers can be detected; although the collagen initially shows no particular orientation, as the fibers increase in number, they tend to form bundles. Immediately subjacent to the epithelium these bundles are perpendicular to the basal lamina. Elastic fibers become prominent only in the connective tissue of lining mucosa between 17 and 20 weeks.

AGE CHANGES

Clinically, the oral mucosa of an elderly person often has a smoother and dryer surface than that of a youngster and may be described as atrophic or friable, but these changes likely represent the cumulative effects of systemic disease, drug therapy, or both, rather than an intrinsic biologic aging process of the mucosa.

Histologically, the epithelium appears thinner, and a smoothing of the epithelium-connective tissue interface results from the flattening of epithelial ridges. The dorsum of the tongue may show a reduction in the number of filiform papillae and a smooth or glossy appearance, such changes being exacerbated by any nutritional deficiency of iron or B complex vitamins. The reduced number of filiform papillae may make the fungiform papillae more prominent, and patients erroneously may consider it to be a disease state.

Aging is associated with decreased rates of metabolic activity, but studies on epithelial proliferation and rate of tissue turnover in healthy tissue are inconclusive. Langerhans cells become fewer with age, which may contribute to a decline in cell-mediated immunity. Vascular changes may be prominent, with the development of varicosities. A striking and common feature in elderly persons is nodular varicose veins on the undersurface of the tongue (sometimes called *caviar tongue*;

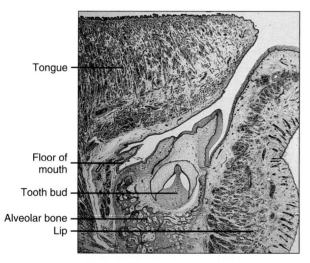

Tongue

Floor of mouth

Tooth bud

Alveolar bone

Lip

Figure 12-37 Sagittal section through the oral cavity of a human embryo showing the tongue, floor of the mouth, alveolar bone ridge with a tooth bud, and lip. Differences in thickness are already apparent between the epithelia of the labial mucosa, alveolar ridge, floor of the mouth, and tongue; however, keratinization has not yet begun.

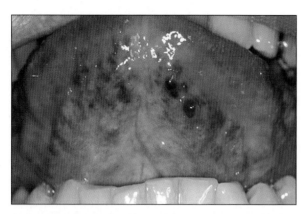

Figure 12-38 Ventral surface of the tongue in an elderly patient showing varicosities. *(Courtesy A. Kauzman.)*

Figure 12-38). Although such changes appear to be unrelated to the cardiovascular status of the patient, they are more frequent in patients with varicose veins of the legs. In the lamina propria a decreased cellularity occurs with an increased amount of collagen, which is reported to become more highly cross-linked. Sebaceous glands (Fordyce's spots) of the lips and cheeks also increase with age, and the minor salivary glands show considerable atrophy with fibrous replacement.

Elderly patients, particularly postmenopausal women, may have symptoms such as dryness of the mouth, burning sensations, and abnormal taste. Whether such symptoms reflect systemic disturbances or local tissue changes is not clear.

TOPICS FOR CONSIDERATION   Oral Epithelium, Premalignant and Malignant Lesions

The oral mucosa can be affected by a number of pathologic conditions. Among these, *squamous cell carcinoma* (SCC), the most common form of oral cancer, carries the worst outcome. Oral cancer accounts for 2% to 4% of malignancies in the West, whereas in the Indian subcontinent and in a number of developing countries it represents one of the most common, if not the most common, form of cancer.

The risk of developing oral SCC increases with age and with *tobacco* use and *alcohol* consumption. In addition, a number of factors, including the human papillomavirus, have been linked to oral carcinogenesis. Oral SCC can also develop in young patients and in non-users of tobacco and alcohol. This has been linked to genetic predisposition.

Prognosis of oral SCC is still very poor, despite the development of new treatment modalities and attempts made at organ preservation. In fact, the 5-year survival rate of oral SCC has remained unchanged—around 50%—over the past few decades. Morbidity and poor quality of life following therapy are important prognostic considerations in oral SCC. The poor outcome associated with this malignancy is primarily due to the advanced stage of disease at diagnosis. This may be caused either by patients not seeking medical advice for unusual, often asymptomatic, oral lesions or by health care workers not thoroughly investigating suspicious mucosal lesions. It is therefore essential for dentists to recognize the early clinical manifestations of oral SCC.

A significant proportion of oral SCCs develop from premalignant lesions, which could present clinically as white, red, or red and white mucosal lesions. *Leukoplakia,* which literally means "white patch," is the most common oral premalignant lesion. The white color is essentially due to epithelial *hyperplasia* and *hyperkeratosis.* The superficial layer in these lesions could be either *orthokeratinized* or *parakeratinized,* or could show a mixture of ortho- and parakeratin.

In some leukoplakias, the epithelium shows both architectural and cellular alterations, known as *epithelial dysplasia.* In these cases, the epithelial cells show an *altered maturation pattern* and cytologic changes such as cellular and nuclear pleomorphism, nuclear hyperchromatism, increased nuclear/cytoplasmic ratio, prominent nucleoli, and increased mitotic activity. Dysplasia could be classified as mild, moderate, or severe, depending on the thickness of the epithelial layers involved. It is important to recognize that in epithelial dysplasia the *basal lamina* is intact and that no dysplastic epithelial cells have breached its continuity. It is recognized that dysplastic epithelial lesions are more likely to progress to oral SCC than nondysplastic lesions. Therefore early diagnosis and treatment of dysplastic lesions is thought to represent an essential step toward reducing the mortality and morbidity associated with oral SCC.

Carcinogenesis is a complex, multistep process in which molecular pathways governing cell physiology are altered. Dysregulation of the cell cycle machinery is an essential event in cancer development where control of *cellular proliferation, differentiation,* and apoptosis (programmed cell death) is lost. Tumors develop following *tumor suppressor gene* inactivation and *proto-oncogene* activation. The order of events may vary, but the end result is an accumulation of genetic alterations that ultimately lead to transformation of a cell from a normal to a profound malignant state.

Similar to many human malignancies, the molecular profile of oral SCC is very complex and appears to dictate the biologic behavior of the disease. In addition, molecular differences exist between oral SCC in smokers and nonsmokers, and between young and old patients affected by the disease, suggesting that different subgroups of oral SCC exist. Furthermore, it is

TOPICS FOR CONSIDERATION   Oral Epithelium, Premalignant and Malignant Lesions—cont'd

important to recognize whether a genetic alteration is an early or late event in tumor development because of the possible clinical implications.

One of the most common genetic alterations in oral SCC is the loss of the 9p21-22 chromosome region, which harbours the *p16/p14^{ARF}* tumor suppressor genes. Deletion of the short arm of chromosome 3 is a common event in oral SCC as well. These molecular alterations are detected in hyperplastic and dysplastic squamous epithelium and hence are thought to represent early genetic events in oral SCC development. Inactivation of the *p53* tumor suppressor gene is commonly identified in oral SCC, and several studies have shown an association between *p53* mutation and tobacco use. The *p53* gene is located on the short arm of chromosome 17 and is one of the most frequently altered genes in human neoplasia. Amplification of the 11q13 region is identified in a number of oral SCC cases. This chromosome location harbors a number of oncogenes, including the *cyclin D1* gene. *Cyclin D1* amplification favors cell proliferation, which can contribute to tumorigenesis. Overexpression of epidermal growth factor receptor (EGFR) and its ligand transforming growth factor alpha (TGF-α) is a frequent event in oral SCC.

Laboratory research is involved in elucidating genetic targets involved in oral SCC development. We hope that soon clinicians will be able to use these sophisticated molecular techniques to *screen* high-risk patients for potential molecular markers of cancer predisposition or to *detect* premalignant lesions that carry a higher risk of malignant transformation. Similarly, these molecular markers can help pathologists to *determine* whether surgical margins are molecularly sound and to *predict* the biologic behavior and response to adjuvant therapy of a given tumor in a specific clinical setting. Most important, this type of research aims at developing targeted *molecular therapies* directed either at blocking tumor cell proliferation, favoring apoptosis, or replacing lost gene functions.

Adel Kauzman, DMD, MSc, FRCD(c)
Specialist in Oral Pathology and Oral Medicine
Associate Professor
Department of Stomatology
Faculty of Dentistry
University of Montreal
Montreal, Quebec, Canada

RECOMMENDED READING

Presland RB, Dale BA: Epithelial structural proteins of the skin and oral cavity: function in health and disease, *Crit Rev Oral Biol Med* 11:383, 2000.

Schroeder HE: *Differentiation of human oral stratified epithelia*, Basel, Switzerland, 1981, S Karger.

Temporomandibular Joint

The articulation of the lower jaw with the cranium and upper facial skeleton involves two separate joints and the teeth when in occlusion. The joints, although anatomically distinct, function in unison, and independent movements are not possible.

The bones involved are the mandible and the temporal bone, and the joint therefore is designated the temporomandibular joint (TMJ). The joint is unique to mammals. In other vertebrates the lower jaw is compound, consisting of several bones including the dentary bone (bearing teeth) and the articular bone (formed from the posterior part of Meckel's cartilage), and articulates with the quadrate bone of the skull (Figure 13-1). As mammals evolved, the compound lower jaw was reduced to a single bone (the mandible) bearing teeth that articulate with the newly developed articulating surface on the temporal bone. Thus in phylogenetic terms the TMJ is a secondary joint. The primary vertebrate jaw joint is still present in human anatomy (as the incudomalleolar articulation), with the bones involved (incus and malleus) now positioned in the middle ear (Figure 13-2).

CLASSIFICATION OF JOINTS

Joints are classified in several ways. Figure 13-3 shows a common and simplistic classification.

FIBROUS JOINTS

In a fibrous joint, two bones are connected by fibrous tissue. Three types are described: The first is the *suture*, a joint that permits little or no movement. The histology of the suture clearly indicates that its function is to permit growth because its articulating surfaces are covered by an osteogenic layer responsible for new bone formation to maintain the suture as the skull bones are separated by the expanding brain. The second type of fibrous joint is the *gomphosis*, the socketed attachment of tooth to bone by the fibrous periodontal ligament. Functional movement is restricted to intrusion and recovery in response to biting forces (long-term movement of teeth in response to environmental pressures or orthodontic treatment represents remodeling of the joint rather than functional movement). The third type of fibrous joint is the *syndesmosis*, examples of which are the joints between the fibula and tibia and between the radius and ulna. The two bony components are some distance apart but are joined by an interosseous ligament that permits limited movement.

CARTILAGINOUS JOINTS

In a *primary cartilaginous joint*, bone and cartilage are in direct apposition. An example is the costochondral junction. In a *secondary cartilaginous joint*, the tissues

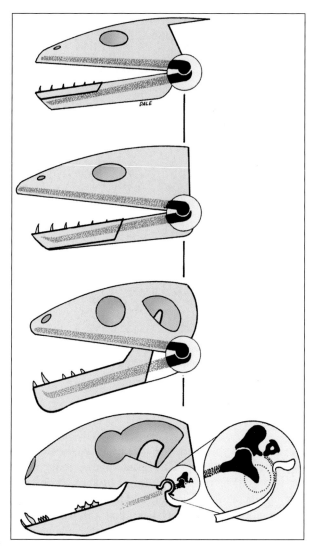

Figure 13-1 Evolution of the mammalian jaw joint. **A,** Amphibian skull. The teeth are confined to the dentary bone. The articulation is between the terminal portion of Meckel's cartilage (the articular) and the palatoquadrate bar. **B,** Reptile skull. The jaw joint is still between the articular and the palatoquadrate, but the dentary bone is of increased size. **C,** The skull of a fossil mammal-like reptile. The dentary bone is enlarged greatly and has a coronoid process. The jaw articulation, however, is still between the articular and palatoquadrate. In mammals **(D),** the dentary bone has formed an articulation with the temporal bone. The original joint now constitutes part of the inner ear. *(Redrawn from DeBrul EL. In Sarnat BG, Laskin DM: The temporomandibular joint, ed 4, Philadelphia, 1992, WB Saunders.)*

SYNOVIAL JOINTS

In a synovial joint, which generally permits significant movement, two bones (each with an articular surface covered by hyaline cartilage) are united and surrounded by a capsule that thereby creates a joint cavity. This cavity is filled with *synovial fluid* formed by a *synovial membrane* that lines the nonarticular surfaces. The cavity in some joints may be divided by an *articular disk.* Various ligaments are associated with synovial joints to strengthen the articulation and check excess movement. Synovial joints are classified further by the number of axes in which the bones involved can move (uniaxial, biaxial, or multiaxial) and by the shapes of the articulating surfaces (planar, ginglymoid [hinged], pivot, condyloid, saddle, and ball-and-socket). Movements of a synovial joint are initiated and effected by muscles working together in a highly coordinated manner. This coordination is achieved in part through the sensory innervation of the joint; according to Hilton's law, the muscles acting on a joint have the same nerve supply as the joint.

TYPE OF JOINT

The temporomandibular articulation is a synovial joint. The anatomy of the TMJ varies considerably among mammals, depending on masticatory requirements, so that a single, all-embracing descriptive classification is not possible. In carnivores, for example, movement is restricted to a simple hinge motion by the presence of well-developed anterior and posterior bony flanges that clasp the mandibular condyle. The badger provides an extreme example of this—the flanges clasp and envelop the condyle to such an extent that it is not possible to dislocate the mandible from the skull. In human beings a different situation exists; the masticatory process demands that the mandible be capable not only of opening and closing movements but also of protrusive, retrusive, and lateral movements and combinations thereof. To achieve them, the condyle undertakes translatory and rotary movements; therefore the human TMJ is described as a *synovial sliding-ginglymoid joint* (Figure 13-4).

DEVELOPMENT OF THE JOINT

Meckel's cartilage (see Chapter 3) provides the skeletal support for development of the lower jaw and extends from the midline backward and dorsally, where it terminates as the malleus (or, in cephalometric terminology, the *articulare*). Meckel's cartilage articulates with the incal cartilage (the quadrate in nonmammals); if any

of the articulation occur in the sequence as bone-cartilage-fibrous tissue-cartilage-bone. An example is the pubic symphysis. Cartilaginous joints and fibrous joints permit little if any movement between the bones involved.

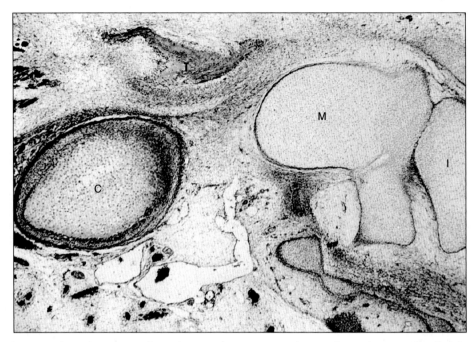

Figure 13-2 Sagittal section through a 67-mm fetus showing the primary and secondary jaw joints. The developing temporal bone *(T)* and condylar blastema *(C)* together form the secondary joint. The malleus *(M)* and incus *(I)* represent the primary joint. *(From Perry HT, Yu Y, Forbes DP: Cranio 3:125, 1985.)*

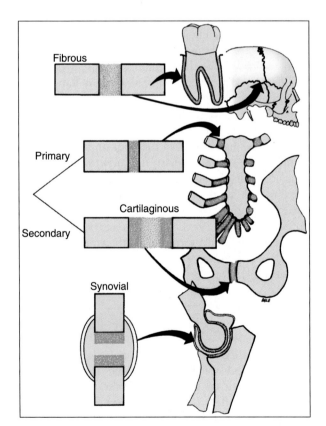

Figure 13-3 Classification of joints.

movement of the early jaw occurs, it occurs between these two cartilages. This primary jaw joint exists for about 4 months until the cartilages ossify and become incorporated in the middle ear. At 3 months of gestation the secondary jaw joint, the TMJ, begins to form. The first evidence of TMJ development is the appearance of two distinct regions of mesenchymal condensation, the temporal and condylar blastemata. The temporal blastema appears before the condylar, and initially both are positioned some distance from each other. The condylar blastema grows rapidly in a dorsolateral direction to close the gap. Ossification begins first in the temporal blastema (Figure 13-5, *A*). While the condylar blastema is still condensed mesenchyme, a cleft appears immediately above it that becomes the inferior joint cavity (Figure 13-5, *B*). The condylar blastema differentiates into cartilage (condylar cartilage), and then a second cleft appears in relation to the temporal ossification that becomes the upper joint cavity (Figure 13-5, *C*). With the appearance of this cleft, the primitive articular disk is formed.

BONES OF THE JOINT

The bones of the temporomandibular articulation are the *glenoid fossa* (on the undersurface of the squamous part of the temporal bone) and the *condyle* (supported by

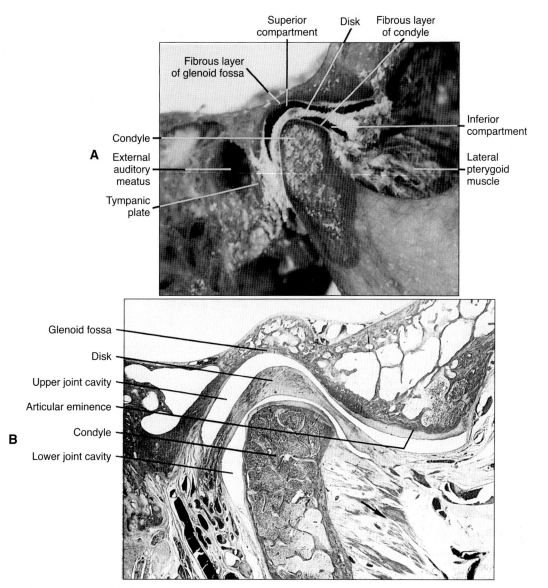

Figure 13-4 The temporomandibular joint. **A,** The macroscopic appearance of the joint is depicted. **B,** Histologic section through the joint. *(A from Liebgott WB:* The anatomical basis of dentistry, *St Louis, 1986, Mosby;* **B** *from Griffin CJ, Hawthorn R, Harris R:* Monogr Oral Sci *4:1, 1975.)*

TOPICS FOR CONSIDERATION Characteristic Origin and Differentiation of Condylar Cartilage

The condylar cartilage performs two distinct biologic functions: (1) as a cartilaginous primordium that provides a provisional supportive template for enlarging tissues and (2) as an articular cartilage with physical properties capable of resisting compressive forces.

Condylar and epiphyseal cartilages are important growth sites in mandible and long bone, respectively. However, the condylar cartilage has a number of characteristic features unlike those of epiphyseal cartilage. For example, condylar cartilage appears later

than the other cartilaginous tissues in development, originates from mandibular periosteum-like cells, displays unique mode of proliferation and differentiation, and responds differentially to humoral factors and mechanical loading (see the table).

It has been suggested that chondrocytes of the condylar cartilage have a close association with the mandible and originate from the mandibular periosteum. The anlage of condylar cartilage on embryonic day 14.0 (E14.0) in mice consists of

Continued

TOPICS FOR CONSIDERATION — Characteristic Origin and Differentiation of Condylar Cartilage—cont'd

Characteristic Features of Condylar Cartilage at Initial Development

	EPIPHYSEAL CARTILAGE	CONDYLAR CARTILAGE
Origin	Mesenchyme	Mandibular periosteum
Type of collagen	Type II (Type X in later stage)	Type I, II, and X
Requirement of *Runx2* gene for initial development	Not essential	Essential

condensed mesenchymal cells, and the first appearance of cartilaginous tissue is on day E14.5 to E15.0. The mesenchymal cells in the condylar anlage exhibit alkaline phosphatase activity and express Runx2 (also called Cbfa1) and Osterix. These typical markers for the preosteoblastic phenotype are found only in mesenchymal cells in the condylar anlage and are not seen at other cartilaginous sites.

Another interesting feature of mesenchymal cells in the condylar anlage is that they have bipotentiality and can differentiate into chondrocytes and osteoblasts. These cells have been called skeletoblasts, and it has been suggested that biomechanical forces are one of the factors determining their differentiation pathway.

Runx2 is a transcription factor essential for osteogenesis. Homozygous *Runx2*-knockout mice completely lack bone tissue, including mandibular bone. The initial appearance of cartilage is not affected in these mutant mice, except for the condylar cartilage. The latter is totally absent, and a condensation of alkaline phosphatase–positive mesenchymal cells is seen only in the corresponding area.[1] This suggests that *Runx2* gene is required for the differentiation toward chondrocytes in condylar cartilage but not in other cartilages. The precise mechanism of condylar chondrocytic differentiation remains to be determined. Whether the *Runx2* gene exerts direct regulation on mesenchymal cells to condylar chondrocytes is unclear. However, it is clear that mandibular bone formation is essential for the appearance and development of condylar cartilage.

The condylar cartilage also has a characteristic expression of extracellular matrix. Chondrocytes in condylar and epiphyseal cartilages express type II collagen. Interestingly, condylar chondrocytes also express type I collagen, which is not seen in epiphyseal cartilage. Moreover, numerous condylar chondrocytes show rapid differentiation to the hypertrophic phenotype and express type X collagen with types I and II soon after their appearance.

A unique mode of proliferation and differentiation of condylar chondrocytes has been reported during the development. Hypertrophic chondrocytes in the epiphyseal cartilage are known to show apoptosis and are not proliferative, although some of them may undergo transdifferentiation into osteoblasts. In contrast, a proportion of the condylar hypertrophic chondrocytes are believed to survive and to be released into the primary spongiosa at the late embryonic stage. PTHrP is known as an autocrine and paracrine factor regulating chondrocytic differentiation and proliferation in long bone cartilage. The receptor for this factor is termed *type 1 PTH/PTHrP receptor* (PTH1R), and the signal transduced from PTH1R promotes proliferation and suppresses chondrocytic hypertrophy. Homozygous *PTHrP*-knockout mice exhibit a dramatic reduction in thickness of the type X collagen negative resting and proliferating zones of the epiphyseal cartilage compared with that of normal mice. The thickness in type X collagen positive hypertrophic zone is not affected, however.[2] Interestingly, in the condylar cartilage the thickness of both type X collagen negative and positive zones is not altered in the mutant mice. Discrepancies between these two cartilages can be explained as follows: Hypertrophic chondrocytes in the condylar cartilage, unlike those in the epiphyseal cartilage, express PTH1R and are regulated by PTHrP. In the normal developmental process, PTHrP promotes proliferation of condylar hypertrophic chondrocytes, and these cells are not in the apoptotic cell cycle (see the figure). In the case of PTHrP deficiency (in homozygous PTHrP-knockout mice), however, these cells hardly proliferate and undergo apoptotic cell death. To be exact, condylar hypertrophic chondrocytes do not maintain this characteristic mode of proliferation and differentiation throughout the life and gradually loose their proliferative activity.

TOPICS FOR CONSIDERATION   Characteristic Origin and Differentiation of Condylar Cartilage—cont'd

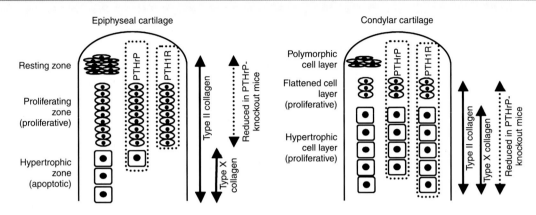

PTHrP; Parathyroid hormone-related protein
PTH1R; Type I PTH/PTHrP receptor

Mode of proliferation and differentiation in chondrocytes of condylar and epiphyseal cartilages.

The fate of nonapoptotic hypertrophic chondrocytes in condylar cartilage is still unclear. Some studies suggest that they can transdifferentiate into osteogenic cells of the mandibular bone, but further studies are needed to clarify their exact fate and characteristic differentiation pathway.

Naoto Suda, DDS, PhD
Lecturer, Maxillofacial Orthognathics
Graduate School
Tokyo Medical and Dental University
Tokyo, Japan

REFERENCES
1. Shibata S, Suda N, Yoda S et al: Runx2-deficient mice lack mandibular condylar cartilage and have deformed Meckel's cartilage, *Anat Embryol* 208:273-280, 2004.
2. Suda N, Shibata S, Yamazaki K et al: Parathyroid hormone-related protein regulates proliferation of condylar hypertrophic chondrocytes, *J Bone Miner Res* 14:1838-1847, 1999.

the condylar process of the mandible). The glenoid fossa is limited posteriorly by the squamotympanic and petrotympanic fissures. The glenoid fossa is limited medially by the spine of the sphenoid and laterally by the root of the zygomatic process of the temporal bone. Anteriorly, the glenoid fossa is bounded by a ridge of bone described as the articular eminence, which also is involved in the articulation (Figure 13-6). The middle part is a thin plate of bone, the upper surface of which forms the middle cranial fossa (housing the temporal lobe of the brain). The condyle is the articulating surface of the mandible. Viewed sagittally, the glenoid fossa is 15 to 20 mm long (from medial to lateral extreme) and 8 to 12 mm thick, superficially resembling a date stone perched atop a column. The articular surface of the condyle is strongly convex in the anteroposterior direction and slightly convex mediolaterally. The medial and lateral ends are termed *poles*. The medial pole extends farther beyond the condylar neck than the lateral pole does and is positioned more posteriorly so that the long axis of the condyle deviates posteriorly and meets a similar axis drawn from the opposite condyle at the anterior border of the foramen magnum. Variations in the shape of the condyle are frequent, and often the condylar surface is divided by a sagittal crest into medial and lateral slopes.

Unlike most synovial joints, the articular surfaces of which are covered with hyaline cartilage, the temporomandibular articulation is covered by a layer of fibrous tissue. This histologic distinction has been used to argue that the TMJ is not a weight-bearing joint, but the reality for this distinction can be found in the developmental history of the joint. The only other synovial joints with articular surfaces covered by fibrous tissue are the acromioclavicular and sternoclavicular, linking the clavicle to the appendicular skeleton. The mandible and the clavicle are bones formed directly from an intramembranous ossification center and are not preformed in cartilage, cartilage that persists in the long bones to cover articular surfaces following the appearance of ossification centers.

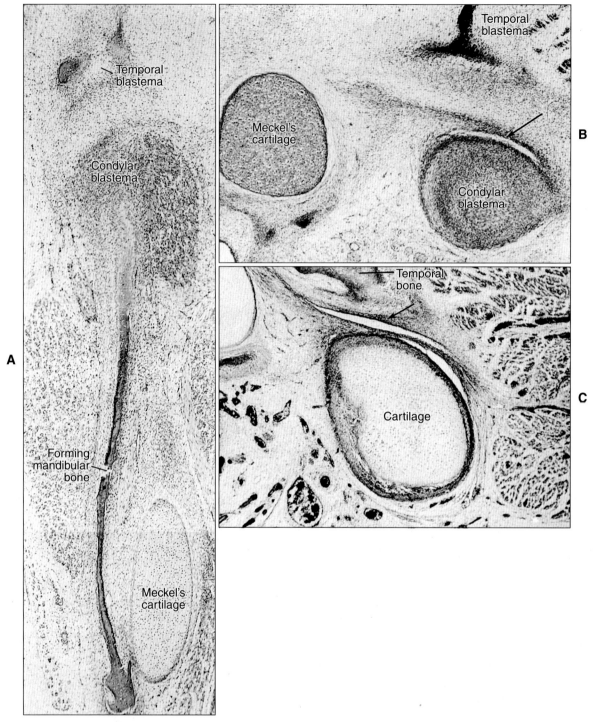

Figure 13-5 Developing temporomandibular articulation. **A,** Coronal section through a 12-week (61-mm crown-rump) fetus. Bone formation has begun in the temporal blastema. The condylar blastema is still undifferentiated. The membranous bone forming the body of the mandible on the lateral aspect of Meckel's cartilage is apparent. **B,** Sagittal section of the temporomandibular joint in a fetus (67-mm crown-rump) showing the developing inferior joint cavity *(arrow)*. Bone formation has begun in the temporal blastema, but the condylar blastema still consists of undifferentiated cells. Meckel's cartilage is to the left of the developing joint. **C,** Sagittal section of the temporomandibular joint of a fetus (70-mm crown-rump) showing the developing superior joint cavity *(arrow)*. Cartilage has formed in the condylar blastema, and the developing temporal bone is indicated. *(A from Chi JG, et al: Sequential atlas of human development, Seoul, 1997, Medical Publishing; B and C from Perry HT, Xu Y, Forbes DP: Cranio 3:125, 1985.)*

The fibrous layer covering the condyle consists of fibroblasts scattered through a dense, largely avascular layer of type I collagen (the *lamina splendens*; Figure 13-7). The fibrous layer sits on a proliferative zone of cells associated with the formation of condylar cartilage. Whether this proliferative zone also contributes to the cellular content and renewal of the fibrous zone is undecided (and indeed unlikely). Studies in rats indicate that cell division occurs within fibroblasts occupying the deeper part of the fibrous layer. Because no convincing demonstration shows that cells from the proliferative layer contribute to the fibrous layer, one must assume that the fibrous articular layer is a self-contained and self-replicating structure.

The glenoid fossa always is covered by a thin fibrous layer that directly overlies the bone, much as periosteum does (Figure 13-8), but this layer becomes appreciably thicker where it covers the slope of the articular eminence (Figure 13-9).

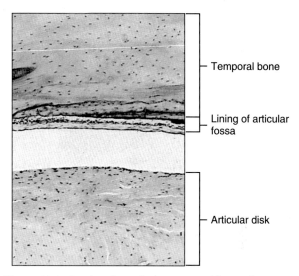

Figure 13-8 Section through the temporal bone showing the thin lining of the articular surface of the glenoid fossa. *(From Blackwood HJJ. In Cohen B, Kramer IRH, editors: Scientific foundations of dentistry, London, 1976, William Heinemann Medical Books.)*

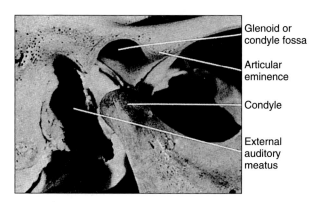

Figure 13-6 Bones involved in the temporomandibular articulation.

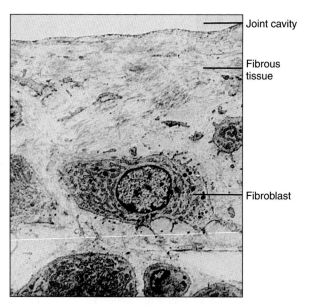

Figure 13-7 Transmission electron micrograph showing the fibrous articular tissue covering the mandibular condyle. *(From Goose DH, Appleton J: Human dentofacial growth, New York, 1982, Pergamon Press.)*

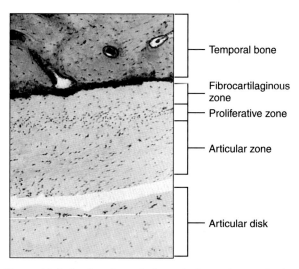

Figure 13-9 Section through the articular eminence in the adult mandibular joint showing the thick articular covering of this area of the joint. *(From Blackwood HJJ. In Cohen B, Kramer IRH, editors: Scientific foundations of dentistry, London, 1976, William Heinemann Medical Books.)*

CARTILAGE ASSOCIATED WITH THE JOINT

Earlier accounts of TMJ histology indicated that the surface coverings of the joint consist of fibrocartilage rather than fibrous tissue. Although with age the fibrous covering layer might contain some cartilage cells, no evidence indicates that this is normal. However, firm evidence indicates that fibrocartilage is associated with the articulation deep to the fibrous layer, in the condyle and on the articular eminence (Figure 13-10). The occurrence of such cartilage has a developmental explanation: a secondary growth cartilage associated with the developing TMJ forms within the blastema the *condylar cartilage* and is in some ways akin to the epiphyseal cartilage of a developing long bone. The condylar cartilage consists essentially of a proliferative layer of replicating cells that function as progenitor cells for the growth cartilage (Figure 13-11). These cells become *chondroblasts* and elaborate an extracellular matrix of proteoglycans and type II collagen to form the extracellular matrix of cartilage, in which they become entrapped as *chondrocytes*. At the same time, an increase in the size of the chondrocytes occurs (hypertrophy). Following the production of this cartilage, endochondral ossification occurs involving mineralization of the cartilage, vascular invasion, loss of chondrocytes, and differentiation of osteoblasts to produce bone on the mineralized cartilaginous framework (Figure 13-12; see also Figure 13-11). The only difference in this process between condylar and epiphyseal cartilages in long bones is the absence of ordered columns of cartilaginous cells (which characterize the epiphyseal growth cartilage and results from chondroblast cell division). The absence of well-defined, elongated columns of chondroblast daughter cells in condylar cartilage has key significance. A typical long bone epiphyseal plate characterized by well-defined columns is committed to an essentially unidirectional mode of growth; that is, the proliferation of cells by mitotic division is such that the whole bone necessarily elongates in a manner determined by the columns of dividing cells. The mandibular condyle, by contrast, has a multidirectional growth capacity, and its cartilage can proliferate in any combination of superior and posterior directions as needed to provide for the best anatomic placement of the mandibular arch. Research also has established that in rat condylar cartilages, cell proliferation and enlargement and extracellular matrix production contribute to the growth of cartilage.

A transient growth cartilage also has been found in association with development of the articular eminence. No eminence exists at birth; its development starts with a slender strip of growth cartilage (involving the same layers as already described for the condyle) situated along the slope of the eminence. Whereas the life span of these cartilages differs—the condylar cartilage existing until the end of the second decade, the eminence cartilage lasting a much shorter time—the subsequent history is the same for both. The proliferative activity of cells in the proliferative layer ceases, but the cells persist (Figure 13-13; see also Figure 13-9). The cartilage immediately below converts to fibrocartilage and in the mandible eventually mineralizes to a degree even

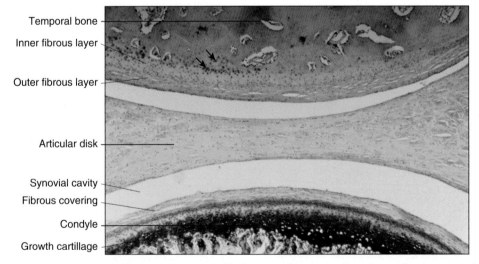

Temporal bone
Inner fibrous layer
Outer fibrous layer
Articular disk
Synovial cavity
Fibrous covering
Condyle
Growth cartilage

Figure 13-10 Histologic section through the temporomandibular joint illustrating the relationship between the temporal bone, the articular disk, and the head of the condyle. Occasionally, chondrocytes are found in the inner fibrous layer of the temporal bone covering (*arrows*).

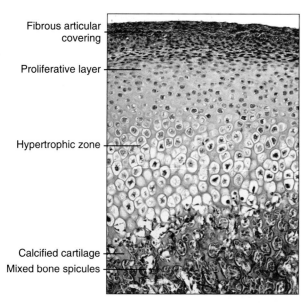

Figure 13-11 Section through the growth cartilage of the condyle illustrating endochondral transformation into bone.

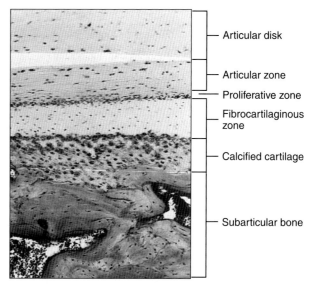

Figure 13-13 Section through the articular covering of the adult mandibular condyle. *(From Blackwood HJJ. In Cohen B, Kramer IRH, editors:* Scientific foundations of dentistry, *London, 1976, William Heinemann Medical Books.)*

greater than that of the mineralized bone (Figure 13-14). Thus fibrocartilage is found in the mandible and on the slope of the articular eminence. Certainly in both instances cells of the proliferative layer can resume their proliferative activity, if the occasion demands. Thus remodeling of the articular surfaces can occur in response to functional changes throughout life and in response to orthodontic treatment. Additions to the

joint surfaces may occur, increasing the vertical dimension of the face. Regressive remodeling creates a loss of the vertical dimension, and peripheral remodeling adds tissue to the margins of the articulation (often an arthritic change). Remodeling also compensates for the changing relationships of the jaws brought about by tooth wear and loss.

In summary, although fibrocartilage is associated with the temporomandibular articulation, it does not form part of the articulation and has no formal functional role to play in the everyday movements occurring between the two bones of the joint.

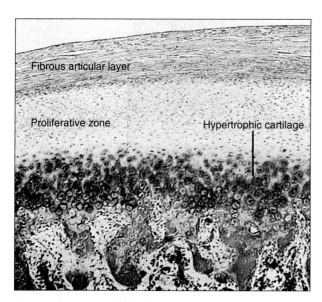

Figure 13-12 Section through the growing condylar cartilage of 13-year-old child. *(From Goose DH, Appleton J:* Human dentofacial growth, *New York, 1982, Pergamon Press.)*

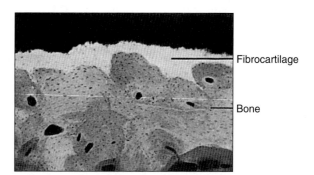

Figure 13-14 Microradiograph showing the subarticular bone and mineralization of the adjacent fibrocartilaginous layer. *(From Blackwood HJ:* J Dent Res *45[suppl 3]:480, 1966.)*

CAPSULE, LIGAMENTS, AND DISK OF THE JOINT

The capsule of a synovial joint is an important structure. The capsule consists of dense collagenous membrane that seals the joint space and provides passive stability, enhanced by increased local thickenings in its walls to form anatomically recognizable ligaments, as well as active stability from proprioceptive nerve endings in the capsule. Furthermore, extensions of the fibrous capsule into the joint cavity in some joints, including the TMJ, form disks that function as articular surfaces and divide the joint into two compartments (Figure 13-15; see also Figures 13-10 and 13-11). The disk consists of coarse collagen fibers with numerous interdispersed fibroblastic cells (see Figure 13-15, A). In some regions the collagen fibers appear wavy, which is believed to relate to their ability to accommodate tensional forces (see Figure 13-15, B). The usual practice of describing the TMJ by treating the disk and capsule separately has led to confusion in describing the capsule as a distinct structure enveloping the joint. Actually, the disk posteriorly and anteriorly divides into two lamellae or sheets, which fuse with the temporal bone and mandible, respectively. The issue is whether these lamellations occur within the capsule or whether they form the wall of the capsule. The former has been the usual interpretation, but the latter has been established as fact.

Recognizing the disk as an extension of the capsule, the capsule of the TMJ can be described as a fibrous, nonelastic membrane surrounding the joint, which is attached above to the squamotympanic fissure posteriorly, the margins of the glenoid fossa laterally, and the articular eminence anteriorly. Inferiorly, the capsule is attached to the neck of the condyle. Above the disk the capsule is fairly lax, whereas below, it is attached tightly to the condyle. The lateral aspect of the capsule is thickened to form a fan-shaped ligament known as the *temporomandibular ligament*, which runs obliquely backward and downward from the lateral aspect of the articular eminence to the posterior aspect of the condylar neck. The ligament consists of two parts: (1) an outer oblique portion arising from the outer surface of the articular eminence and extending backward and downward to insert into the outer surface of the condylar neck and (2) an inner horizontal portion with the same origin but inserting into the lateral pole of the condyle (Figure 13-16). The capsule and its lateral thickening form the ligament of the joint. Joint ligaments restrict and limit the movements a joint can make in that they limit the distance that the bones forming the articulation can be separated from each other without causing tissue damage. The temporomandibular ligament restricts displacement of the mandible in three different planes. First, the ligament functions in a way similar to collateral ligaments of other joints because of the bilateral nature of the articulation. By preventing lateral dislocation of one joint, it prevents medial dislocation of the other. Second, its oblique component limits the amount of inferior displacement, and third, its horizontal component prevents or limits posterior displacement.

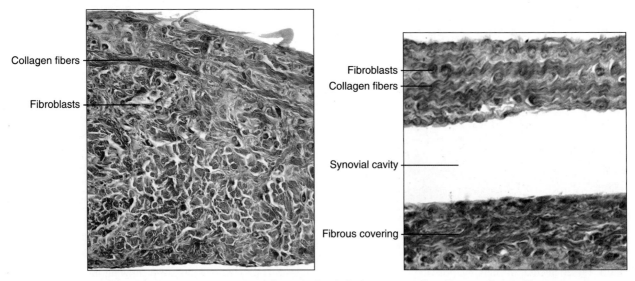

Figure 13-15 A and **B,** Light microscope images of the articular disk showing **(A)** the coarse collagen fiber network constituting it and interposed fibroblastic cells, and **(B)** the wavy appearance of the fibers in some regions that contributes to the biomechanical properties.

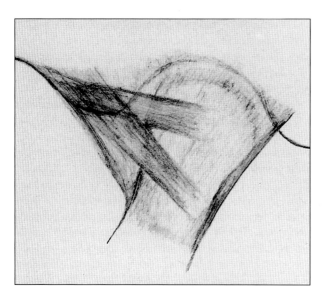

Figure 13-16 The lateral (or temporomandibular) ligament. This diagram emphasizes two functional components of the capsular ligament preventing posterior and inferior displacement. The total ligament also prevents lateral and medial displacement (of the opposite joint).

This anatomic configuration means that, if dislocation occurs, it is forward with the head of the condyle slipping in front of the articular eminence. Two other ligaments are included in conventional descriptions of the joint, although neither has a functional role. The first is the *sphenomandibular ligament,* running from the lingula and shielding the opening of the interior alveolar canal to the spine of the sphenoid. This ligament represents the residual perichondrium of Meckel's cartilage. The second is the *stylomandibular ligament,* running from the styloid process of the temporal bone to the angle of the mandible. This ligament represents the free border of the deep cervical fascia.

An inward circumferential extension of the capsule forms a tough, fibrous disk that divides the joint into upper and lower compartments, provides an articular surface for the head of the condyle, and because the lower half of the capsule is tightly bound to the condyle, moves with the condyle during translation. The disk consists of dense fibrous tissue (see Figure 13-4), and its shape conforms to that of the apposed articular surfaces. Thus the lower surface of the disk is concave and generally matches the convex contour of the condyle. The upper surface of the disk also presents a concave surface because its posterior and anterior components are considerably thickened, delimiting a central thinner component. At rest, this central thinner component of the disk separates the anterior slope of the condyle from the slope of the articular eminence. The thickened posterior portion occupies the gap

between the condyle and the floor of the glenoid fossa, and the anterior portion lies slightly anterior to the condyle. The type I collagen bundles that constitute the disk generally are arranged loosely and are oriented randomly, except in the central region, where they are more tightly bound in organized bundles. Coronal sections of the disk show it to be thicker medially.

The anterior portion of the disk fuses with the anterior wall of capsule. Above the point of fusion, the capsule runs forward to blend with the periosteum of the anterior slope of the articular eminence. Below, the capsule merges with the periosteum of the front of the neck of the condyle. As explained previously, this appearance in section creates the impression that the anterior portion of the disk splits into two lamellae. Posteriorly, the disk also appears to divide into two lamellae, but again these lamellae represent the posterior wall of the capsule. The upper part of the capsule, or lamella, consists of fibrous and elastic tissue (the only part of the capsule where elastic fibers are found) and inserts into the squamotympanic fissure. The lower part of the capsule, consisting of collagen only and nonelastic, blends with the periosteum of the condylar neck.

Between these two lamellae a space is created that is filled with a loose, highly vascular connective tissue. The disk is well supplied with vascular and neural elements at its periphery but is avascular and not innervated in its central region (Figure 13-17). During function, the disk makes only short movements in a passive manner to fit best with the changing relationships of the condylar head and the glenoid fossa and articular eminence. Such adaptation is permitted by the shape of the disk and the slippery environment of the joint cavity, although some influence also is exerted by superior fibers of the lateral pterygoid and the tight relationship created by taut capsular fibers running from the margins of the disk to the condyle.

SYNOVIAL MEMBRANE

The capsule is lined on its inner surface by a *synovial membrane* (Figure 13-18). An exact description of this delicate membrane in the human TMJ is not easy to give; several locations and structures have been described, which probably reflect the difficulty of obtaining adequately fixed specimens of the structure. Generally, the synovial membrane is considered to line the entire capsule, with folds or villi of the membrane protruding into the joint cavity, especially in its fornices and its upper posterior aspect. These folds increase in number with age and are also more prominent in joints affected by a pathologic process. The synovial membrane does not cover the articular surfaces of the joint or the disk, except for its bilaminar posterior region.

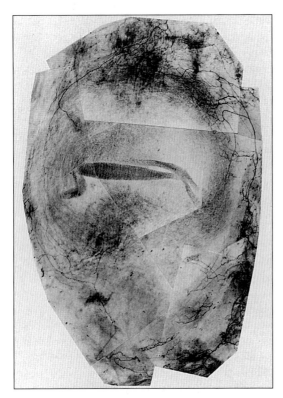

Figure 13-17 Nerve distribution shown in a whole mount preparation of the rat disk. The absence of nerves from the central portion of the disk is notable. *(From Shimizu S, Kido MA, Kiyoshima T et al: Anat Rec 245:568, 1996.)*

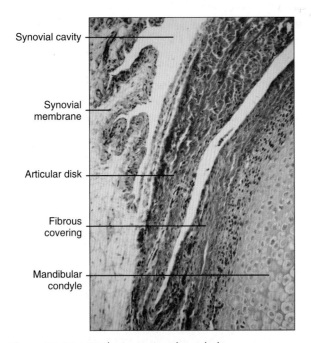

Figure 13-18 Histologic section through the temporomandibular joint showing the synovial membrane, articular disk and articular surface of the condyle. The synovial membrane is a bilayered structure with folds or villi that regulates formation of the synovial fluid that fills the joint cavities and lubricates articular surfaces.

The histology of the synovial membrane is also difficult to describe because different regions of the joint capsule vary. Essentially, any synovial membrane consists of two layers: a cellular intima resting on a vascular subintima (Figure 13-19) and the fibrous tissue of the capsule into which the subintima blends. The subintima is a loose connective tissue containing vascular elements together with scattered fibroblasts, macrophages, mast cells, fat cells, and some elastic fibers, which prevent folding of the membrane. The intima varies in structure, having one to four layers of synovial cells embedded in an amorphous, fiber-free intercellular matrix. Often cellular deficiencies exist so that the subintimal connective tissue directly borders the joint cavity. These cells are not connected by junctional complexes and do not rest on a basal lamina. The joint cavity therefore is not lined by epithelium. The cells forming this discontinuous layer are of two types, a predominant type A (macrophage-like) cell and a type B (fibroblast-like) cell. Type A cells have surface filopodia, many plasma

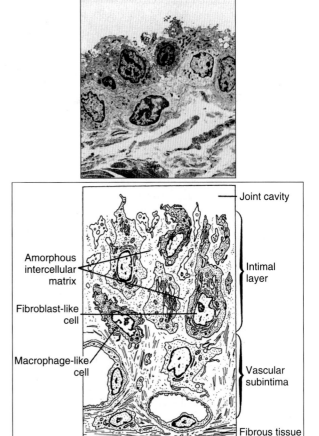

Figure 13-19 Synovial membrane. *Top,* Electron micrograph. *Bottom,* Diagrammatic representation. *(Micrograph courtesy W. Feagens.)*

membrane invaginations, and associated pinocytotic vesicles. The cytoplasm of type A cells contains numerous mitochondria and lysosomal elements and a prominent Golgi complex. Profiles of rough endoplasmic reticulum are few. Type B cells, by contrast, contain many profiles of rough endoplasmic reticula. Type A cells exhibit significant phagocytotic properties, and type B cells synthesize the hyaluronate found in synovial fluid.

The chemical composition of synovial fluid indicates that it is a dialysate of plasma supplemented with proteins and proteoglycans. The synovial membrane is responsible for controlling the passage of plasma components and producing the additional components. Synovial fluid also may contain a small population of varying cell types such as monocytes, lymphocytes, free synovial cells, and occasionally polymorphonuclear leukocytes. Synovial fluid is characterized by well-defined physical properties of viscosity, elasticity, and plasticity. The function of this fluid is to provide (1) a liquid environment for the joint surfaces and (2) lubrication to increase efficiency and reduce erosion. Whether the synovial fluid also provides nutrition for the disk and articular surfaces of the joint is debatable. Synovial fluid also is believed to act as a nutrient fluid for the avascular tissues covering the articular surfaces and for the disk.

MUSCLES THAT CAUSE MOVEMENT

Before the muscles of mastication are described in detail, some general features of muscle architecture and structure should be recalled. Muscles may be described in a number of ways. One is by the arrangement of their fiber bundles, or fasciculi. In strap muscles, all fasciculi run parallel from origin to insertion. In fusiform muscles, essentially the same arrangement exists, except that the parallel-running fiber bundles converge at the site of origin and the site of insertion of the muscle. Finally (in this grouping), the fan-shaped muscle has fasciculi that extend from a broad linear origin to a narrow insertion. Another description schema for muscles involves those that have a central tendon extending into a fleshy belly to which bundles of muscle fibers attach in an oblique direction. If all the muscle fiber bundles attach on one side of such a tendon, the muscle is described as unipennate; if attachment occurs on both sides, bipennate; and if multiple central tendons exist, multipennate.

MUSCLE CONTRACTION

Muscle cells (fibers) that make up the bundles (fasciculi) are long and narrow. A fiber can be several centimeters long and up to 0.1 mm in diameter. In any given muscle, the fibers tend to be of uniform length. The cell membrane of the fiber is called the *sarcolemma*, immediately beneath which the nucleus of the cell is found. Within each cell, the sarcoplasm is packed with myofibrils, arranged in such a way that their close packing creates the pattern of striations seen under the light microscope (standard histology textbooks should be consulted for a detailed account of the molecular basis of muscle contraction). Another feature of the muscle fiber is its sarcoplasmic reticulum, a branching endoplasmic network that surrounds each myofibril. Muscle contraction depends on the availability of calcium ions, which are transferred back and forth from the sarcoplasmic reticulum. Finally, the sarcoplasm contains variable numbers of mitochondria, glycogen, and myoglobin (the last acts as an oxygen-storing pigment).

The distinction between red meat and white meat is a familiar one. This distinction reflects the greater amounts of myoglobin (a pigment similar to hemoglobin) in red meat, which is characterized as muscle and is capable of slow but sustained contraction, as opposed to the more rapidly contracting fast muscle of white meat.

This distinction is mirrored in the histology and histochemistry of the individual muscle fiber, so that the slow-twitch fiber (type I) is generally narrower than the fast-twitch (type II) fiber, has poorly defined myofibrils, contains slow myosin, possesses many mitochondria, and exhibits high oxidative enzyme and low phosphorylase activity. This last trait reflects the fact that slow fibers also have a well-developed aerobic metabolism. As a result, they resist fatigue. By contrast, the type II or fast-twitch fibers have fewer mitochondria, possess an extensive sarcoplasmic reticulum, contain fast myosin, and show a lower oxidative enzyme activity (which is balanced by increased phosphorylase activity). Fast-twitch fibers thus rely more on anaerobic (glycolytic) activity and fatigue more easily.

With this distinction understood, it is important to recognize that most if not all muscles contain a mixture of fast and slow fibers in varying proportions reflecting the function of that muscle (Figure 13-20). Also important is recognition that individual muscle fibers can be transformed (e.g., as a result of training) and that the innervation of the fibril determines its characteristics. In experiments in which nerves to red and white muscle fibers are cut, crossed, and reconnected, the fibers change their morphology and physiology accordingly.

Histochemical analyses of muscle fibers involving the demonstration of activity of the enzyme adenosinetriphosphatase easily show the distinction between type I and type II fibers and also indicate that some fibers fall into an intermediate category. Furthermore, by varying the pH of the substrate during the histochemical

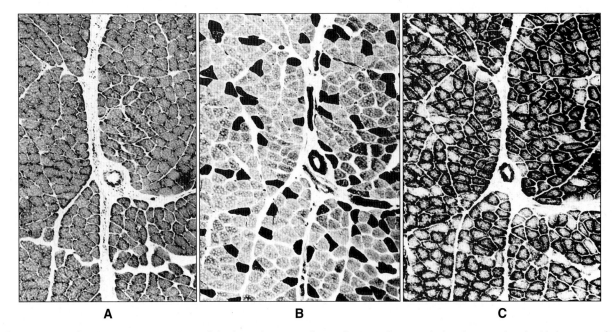

Figure 13-20 Three successive sections of the lateral pterygoid muscle. In **A** the muscle has been stained with hematoxylin and eosin, and all the fibers appear the same. In **B** the muscle has been stained to demonstrate adenosinetriphosphatase activity, and this treatment clearly distinguishes two types of fiber, the slow oxidative (unstained) and the fast glycolytic. The same muscle is stained in **C** to demonstrate reduced nicotinamide adenine dinucleotide. The majority of fibers that stained strongly with adenosinetriphosphatase now are not stained, but some indicate a fast oxidative fiber.

reaction, differentiating subtypes of type II fibers (i.e., types IIA, IIB, and IIC) is possible. Types IIA and IIB contain fast myosin exclusively but can be distinguished based on an inhibition of enzyme activity that occurs at pH 4.6 in the type IIA fiber. The type IIA fiber is more fatigue resistant. Type IIC differs from IIA and IIB in that it contains a mixture of slow and fast myosins, with fast myosin predominating. Intermediate fibers also contain a mixture of fast and slow myosins, but in this case the slow myosins predominate. Although intermediate fibers generally are thought to be those undergoing transformation, evidence from studies of the muscles of mastication indicate that at least some intermediate fibers are part of a stable population of fibers in muscle.

MOTOR UNIT

Voluntary skeletal muscle obviously requires innervation for contraction to take place. A single nerve may innervate a single muscle fiber (fine control) or, by branching, supply as many as 160 fibers. No matter the pattern, the complex is known as a *motor unit* (Figure 13-21), and innervation is achieved through a structure known as the *motor end plate*. At the site of innervation, the nerve loses its myelin sheath, but not the covering of Schwann cells, and forms a terminal dilation that

comes to occupy a corresponding dimple in the muscle cell surface. Between the nerve termination and the sarcolemma is a gap, the synaptic cleft, where the sarcolemmal surface is thrown into a series of junctional folds. A motor unit supplies fibers of a single type.

Two other neuronal structures need to be described in relation to muscle contraction: the muscle spindle and the Golgi tendon organ.

Muscle Spindle

The muscle spindle is an encapsulated proprioceptor that detects changes in length. The spindle consists of a connective tissue sac 5 mm long and 0.2 mm in diameter containing 2 to 12 specially adapted muscle fibers, designated as intrafusal fibers. Intrafusal fibers are narrower than extrafusal fibers and assume two forms. The first is described as a nuclear bag fiber because of the concentration of many nuclei in its centrally expanded portion, and the second, as a nuclear chain fiber because its nuclei are aligned in a single row. The nuclear bag fiber is innervated by a nerve that spirals around the bag, the primary afferent. The nuclear chain fiber is innervated from a primary terminal supplying the central region of the chain and a secondary terminal on either side of the primary (Figure 13-22). The primary terminal is thought to be involved with responses to

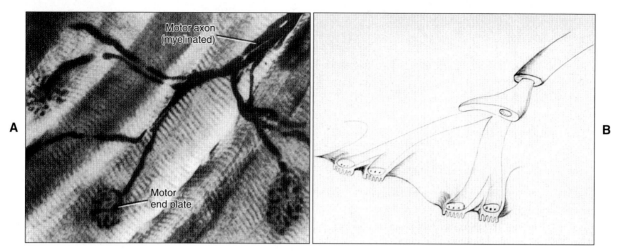

Figure 13-21 A, Motor end plates on skeletal muscle fibers (stained with gold chloride). **B,** Functional relationship between the nerve and muscle fiber. *(From Cormack DH:* Introduction to histology, *Philadelphia, 1984, Williams and Wilkins.)*

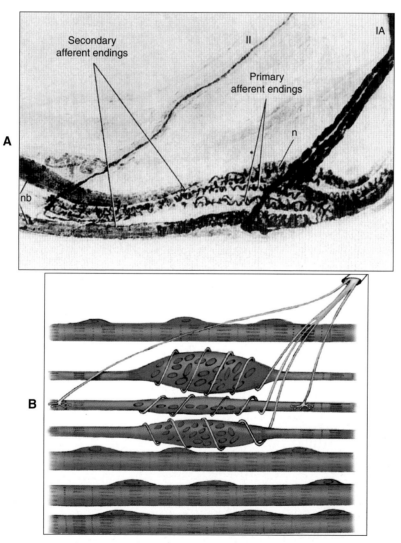

Figure 13-22 A, Photomicrograph of the structure and innervation of a muscle spindle (cat; stained with gold chloride) showing primary annulospiral afferent endings *(right)* and secondary flower spray endings *(left).* **B,** The spindle. (For clarity the capsule has been omitted.) Primary annulospiral fibers envelop the nuclear bag and the nuclear chain intrafusal fibers. The flower spray secondary endings are associated with the nuclear chain fiber. *nb,* nuclear bag; *n,* nuclear chain fibers. *(A from Boyd IA:* Philos Trans R Soc Lond B Biol Sci *245:81, 1962.)*

the degree and rate of stretch, the secondary terminal only with the degree of stretch. Muscle spindle intrafusal fibers retain their efferent supply.

Golgi Tendon Organ

Golgi tendon organs are found at the junctions between muscles and the tendons or aponeuroses on which they pull. Golgi tendon organs are approximately half the size of a muscle spindle and consist of a capsule surrounding a group of collagen fibrils. The afferent nerve breaks up within the capsule, and the terminal fibers ramify between the collagen bundles. The nerves are stimulated by compression between the bundles when the tendon is under compression.

From this abbreviated account of muscle, its heterogeneity can be appreciated as providing the tremendous

adaptation of structure necessary to function, which is especially evident in the muscles of mastication.

MUSCLES OF MASTICATION

Classically, the muscles of mastication are the masseter, the medial (inferior) pterygoid, the lateral (superior) pterygoid, and the temporalis (Figure 13-23). In functional terms, other muscle groups are involved in mastication, such as the postcervical group (which stabilizes the cranial base) and the infrahyoid group (which stabilizes the hyoid bone and permits the mylohyoid muscle and anterior belly of the digastric muscle to influence mandibular position). The anatomic configurations of all these muscles are well described.

The masseter and medial pterygoid muscles together have a slinglike configuration clasping the angle of

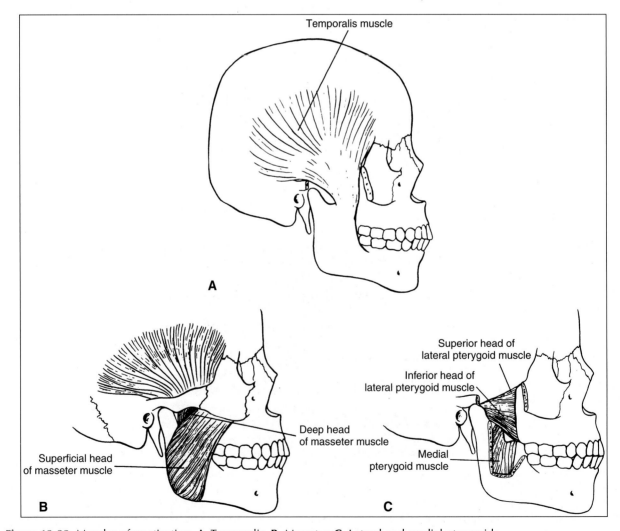

Figure 13-23 Muscles of mastication. **A,** Temporalis. **B,** Masseter. **C,** Lateral and medial pterygoids.

the mandible and are the principal elevators of the jaw. Both muscles are multipennate and quadrate, and each has two heads.

The masseter consists of a superficial portion and a deep portion (or head), which, though originating separately, have a common insertion and blend together at the anterior border of the muscle. The superficial head has a tendinous portion, originating from the zygomatic process of the maxilla, and a fleshy portion, arising from the inferior border of the anterior two thirds of the zygomatic arch. The fibers of the superficial head run inferoposteriorly to insert into the angle and lower border of the mandibular ramus. They cover the fibers of the deep portion of the muscle, which arise from the inner aspect and inferior border of the posterior third of the zygomatic arch and run almost vertically downward to insert into the upper border and lateral aspect of the ramus. Although anatomically this muscle has two components, the components can be distinguished readily and can be seen in functional terms to consist of four components: deep anterior, deep posterior, superficial anterior, and superficial posterior.

The medial pterygoid also has two portions or heads. The bulk of the muscle originates from the medial aspect of the lateral pterygoid plate, with a slip of fibers originating from the maxillary tuberosity. Little functional significance can be attributed to the latter origin.

Analysis of fiber composition of these two powerful elevator muscles confirms regional differences. Both muscles exhibit a preponderance of type I fibers, indicating a muscle that (in conjunction with the multipennate structure) is adapted to resisting fatigue at low force levels. The posterior portions of both muscles, however, are characterized by possessing a high concentration of type IIB fibers. Thus these fibers belong to fast-twitch rapidly contracting motor units and are sensitive to fatigue; they are able to generate large forces intermittently in the molar region of the mandible.

The temporalis is a fan-shaped muscle arising from the side of the skull that inserts into the coronoid process and the anteromedial border of the mandibular ramus. The muscle is covered by a strong sheet of fascia attached (above) to the superior temporal line and (below) to the medial and lateral aspects of the zygomatic arch, the undersurface of which also provides origin for fleshy muscle fibers. The temporalis is bipennate. An inner layer of fibers converges vertically down the lateral wall of the cranium to form a central tendon that inserts into the coronoid process and the anterior edge of the ascending ramus. The outer layer fibers (arising from the temporal fascia) descend in a more medial direction.

Functionally, the temporalis acts as two muscles: its anterior fibers as an elevator and its posterior horizontally disposed fibers as a retractor of the mandible.

The muscle also shows variation in its fiber composition. The bipennate superficial portion has 50% type IIB fibers, indicating a capacity for acceleration coupled with an ability to develop tension. The posterior portion, however, contains a preponderance of type I fibers and many muscle spindles (indicating adaptation to a postural function). Thus in general the masseter and the medial pterygoid are power producers and the temporalis is concerned more with moving and stabilizing the mandible.

Some controversy still exists about the lateral pterygoid concerning not only its anatomy but also its exact functional role. The muscle has two heads, superior and inferior, arising from the roof of the infratemporal fossa and the lateral pterygoid plate, respectively. No debate exists over the insertion of fibers of the lower head; they run posteriorly, inferiorly, and slightly laterally to insert into the pterygoid fovea (on the anterior surface of the condylar neck) and on contraction bring about downward-forward and medial movement of the condyle. The insertion of the fibers of the superior head is what is debatable, and the debate ranges around whether some of the superior fibers insert into the disk. No doubt exists that most of the fibers of this head insert into the pterygoid fovea on the condyle. The upper fibers of the muscle are what show some variation. These (1) may gain insertion into the condyle by merging with the central tendon of the muscle, (2) may insert directly into the pterygoid fovea, or (3) may insert directly into the disk at its most medial aspect. In dissected cadavers, if the upper fibers are pulled manually, the condyle and disk move in unison, suggesting that the muscle directly or indirectly exerts some effect on the disk. Because the bulk of the muscle inserts into the condyle, however, its main activity (obviously) is to move the condyle. Electromyographic studies indicate a reciprocal activation of the two heads of the muscle, with the inferior head involved in opening the jaw and the superior head involved in closure (by seating the condylar head against the posterior slope of the articular eminence). The attachment of the upper fibers to the disk directly or indirectly is thought to stabilize the disk at closure. Again, these functional differences are reflected in fiber composition, with the type I fiber predominating (indicating a capacity for endurance during continuous work at low force levels). Some have argued that the high proportion of type IIC and intermediate fibers in the muscles of mastication indicates such fibers to be permanent residents in masticatory muscle, suggesting special functional characteristics for them.

Finally, the intrafusal fibers of muscle spindles in the masseter not only have a different enzyme profile from that in the extrafusal fibers but also are different from the intrafusal fibers in the limbs and trunk.

This suggests special functional characteristics for this masticatory muscle.

BIOMECHANICS OF THE JOINT

The muscles act on the TMJ to achieve opening and closure of the jaw, protrusion and retrusion, and alternate lateral movements and to provide stability. Because these movements rarely occur in isolation, most involve complex combinations of muscle activity. The role of the muscles in providing stability should not be overlooked, for during mastication the forces applied to the joint not only are great but also are changing constantly; when this is considered with the destabilizing effects of translatory movement, the functional role of muscle becomes more obvious. An example is biting, which demands that the disk be stabilized in a slightly forward position. This stabilization is achieved by the upper fibers of the lateral pterygoid muscle.

Based on the anatomic configuration of the muscles and remembering that most movements of the joint involve rotatory and translatory movement, muscle function now can be grouped as follows (Figure 13-24):

1. The masseter, medial pterygoid, anterior part of the temporalis, and upper head of the lateral pterygoid combine to close the jaw.
2. The inferior head of the lateral pterygoid and the anterior belly of the digastric and the mylohyoid (the latter two not strictly muscles of mastication as defined) are responsible for opening movements.
3. The inferior head of the lateral pterygoid and the elevator group bring about protrusive movement, and the posterior fibers of the temporalis and the elevator group retrude the mandible.
4. Lateral movement is achieved by combined action of the elevator muscles, the posterior part of the temporalis (retrusion on the working side), and the lateral pterygoid (protrusion on the nonworking side).

Because movements at the joint involve rotation and translation, the functional significance of the disk becomes more apparent (Figure 13-25). The disk is not comparable to the meniscus in some other joints but is a unique feature of the temporomandibular articulation in that it enables a complexity of movement to be performed that cannot be done in any other joint. As has been pointed out already, the disk moves passively according to and dictated by its shape and the changing relationships of the bones involved in the temporomandibular articulation. The description is simplistic, however, because the direct and indirect relationships of the superior head of the lateral pterygoid to the disk clearly play a part in its function. At present, the cumulative evidence is that at rest a few slips of the upper head function to maintain the position of the disk, opposing the retractive forces created by elastic fibers in the upper lamella that connect the posterior aspect of the disk to the capsule of the joint. This muscle attachment also may compensate for the weaker attachment of the medial surface of the disk to the condyle than exists laterally, or possibly the lateral attachment is stronger because of the medial muscle attachment.

INNERVATION OF THE JOINT

The innervation of any joint (the TMJ included) involves four types of nerve endings: The first (type I) are *Ruffini's corpuscles*; the second (type II), *Pacini's corpuscles*; the third (type III), *Golgi tendon organs*; and the fourth (type IV), *free nerve endings*. The first three types are encapsulated, with the first two (Ruffini's and Pacini's corpuscles) limited to the capsule of a joint and the third (Golgi tendon organs) confined to the ligaments associated with the joint. Free nerve endings have a wider distribution. Ruffini's corpuscles show a striking resemblance to Golgi tendon organs (already described) so that making a distinction between them other than to point out that Golgi tendon organs are located specifically in tendons or ligaments is difficult to justify. The Pacini's corpuscle has a characteristic microanatomy. The corpuscle is an ovoid encapsulated structure, 1 to 2 mm long and 0.5 to 1 mm in diameter. Within the capsule, concentric layers of modified elongated Schwann cells wrap around a central axon much like the successive layers of an onion, with the inner layers compacted and the outer ones having wider connective tissue spaces between the cells. The corpuscle is adapted to register changes in pressure and vibration.

The TMJ is no different from other joints with respect to its innervation. Free nerve endings are the most abundant, with Ruffin's, Golgi, and Pacini's endings following in descending order. Generally, the anatomic and functional designations for each type of nerve ending, with its reflex role, are listed as in Table 13-1. However, neurophysiologic studies are limited in their ability to attribute single nerve discharges to specific endings. In particular, the role of free nerve endings is confusing because elsewhere in the body such endings are sensitive to thermal, mechanical, and noxious stimuli.

Regardless, a common pattern for innervation of the TMJ can be summarized as follows: Ruffini's endings exist in clusters in the superficial layers of the joint capsule and are thought always to be active in every

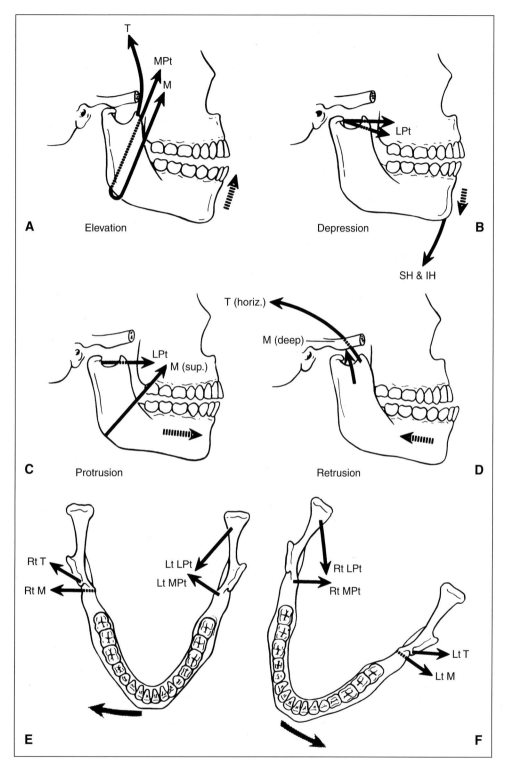

Figure 13-24 Actions of the muscles of mastication. **A,** Elevation. *M,* Masseter; *MPt,* medial pterygoid; *T,* temporalis. **B,** Depression. *IH,* Infrahyoid; *LPt,* lateral pterygoid; *SH,* suprahyoid. **C,** Protrusion. *M (sup.),* Masseter, superficial fibers. **D,** Retrusion. *M (deep),* Masseter, deep fibers; *T (horiz.),* temporalis, horizontal fibers. **E,** Right lateral excursion of the mandible. *Lt MPt,* Left medial pterygoid; *Lt LPt,* left lateral pterygoid; *Rt M,* right masseter; *Rt T,* right temporalis. **F,** Left lateral excursion of the mandible. *Lt M,* Left masseter; *Lt T,* left temporalis; *Rt LPt,* right lateral pterygoid; *Rt MPt,* right medial pterygoid. *(Redrawn from Liebgott B:* The anatomical basis of dentistry, *ed 2, St Louis, 2001, Mosby.)*

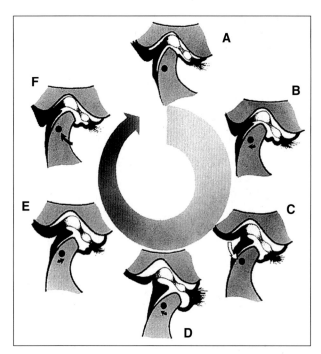

Figure 13-25 Changing position of the mandible during opening and closing. **A** to **D,** During opening. **E** and **F,** During closing. *(Redrawn from Rees LA: Br Dent J 96:126, 1954.)*

position of the joint (even when the joint is immobile) so that they signal static joint position, changes in intraarticular pressure, and the direction, amplitude, and velocity of joint movements. Pacini's corpuscles are rapidly acting mechanoreceptors with a low threshold found mainly in the deeper layers of the capsule that signal joint acceleration and deceleration. Golgi tendon

TABLE 13-1	Anatomic and Functional Designations for Nerve Endings
ANATOMIC DESIGNATION	FUNCTIONAL DESIGNATION
Ruffini's corpuscle	Posture (proprioception)—dynamic and static balance
Pacini's corpuscle	Dynamic mechanoreception—movement accelerator
Golgi tendon organ	Static mechanoreception—protection (ligament)
Free nerve ending	Pain (nociception)—protection (joint)

organs, limited as they are to the ligaments and sparsely distributed in the superficial layers of the lateral ligament, remain completely inactive in immobile joints, becoming active only when the joint is at the extremes of its range of movement. The distribution and significance of free nerve endings in joints usually are considered secondary to the roles of the other specialized receptors, yet they are the most frequently occurring terminal in a joint, are generally thought to be associated with nociception, and are distributed widely. Some debate has occurred as to whether free nerve endings occur in the disk of the TMJ and the synovial membrane. Immunocytochemical studies have shown that nerves do indeed occupy the periphery of the disk (see Figure 13-14) and the synovial membrane, where (it is speculated) they may function to control the activity of macrophagelike cells.

As previously mentioned, Hilton's law states that the trigeminal nerve (cranial nerve V) provides the afferent innervation to a joint, and this is also the case with branches supplying the joint. Branches of the mandibular division of the fifth cranial nerve (i.e., the auriculotemporal, deep temporal, and masseteric) supply the joint.

BLOOD SUPPLY TO THE JOINT

The vascular supply to the TMJ comes from branches of the superficial temporal, deep auricular, anterior tympanic, and ascending pharyngeal arteries, all of which are branches of the external carotid artery (Table 13-1).

RECOMMENDED READING

Edwards JC: The nature and origins of synovium: experimental approaches to the study of synoviocyte differentiation, *J Anat* 184:493, 1994.

Nozawa-Inoue K, Amizuka N, Ikeda N et al: Synovial membrane in the temporomandibular joint—its morphology, function and development, *Arch Histol Cytol* 66:289, 2003.

Schmolke C: The relationship between the temporomandibular joint capsule, articular disc and jaw muscles, *J Anat* 184:335, 1994.

Repair and Regeneration of Oral Tissues

One purpose of studying the formation and structure of dental tissues is to understand how they respond to insult caused by function, trauma, or dental disease and how this response can and should determine subsequent clinical practice. Over the next few decades, the understanding of developmental events and molecular mediators of cellular activity is expected to lead to novel, biologic approaches to treating oral diseases and trauma. Enamel matrix-derived proteins and growth factors, such as bone morphogenetic proteins and platelet-derived growth factor, are good examples of therapeutic molecules. Such progress in understanding will reflect not only on the treatment management plan but also on the education and training of the oral health practitioner.

The response of the body to tissue destroyed by an insult can lead to complete restoration of tissue architecture and function (regeneration) or to restoration of function and of tissue continuity but with distortion of the normal architecture (repair). Although the term regeneration often is used, particularly with respect to the periodontium, true regeneration capacity has been essentially lost from mammals (after birth) but is still found in certain amphibians. Comparative studies between amphibians and mammals eventually may lead to approaches to reactivate the lost regenerative potential and thus the ability to replace tissues and organs

completely and naturally. Predictive clinical outcomes can be achieved only if biologic aspects of wound healing and tissue repair/regeneration are taken into consideration. In time, the dentist, in pace with other fields of medicine, will routinely use tissue engineering approaches and gene therapy to heal and rebuild oral tissues. A recent review on the use of biologic therapies has concluded that "craniofacial tissue engineering is likely to be realized in the foreseeable future, and represents an opportunity that dentistry cannot afford to miss."[1]

WOUND HEALING IN ORAL MUCOSA

To explain the repair process in oral tissues, this chapter first considers wound healing in oral mucosa. Skin and oral mucosa have the primary functions of protecting the underlying tissues and limiting entry of microorganisms and toxins. Interruption in the continuity of these covering and lining tissues compromises these functions. Therefore, an effective system of wound healing is

[1]Mao JJ, Giannobile WV, Helms JA et al: *J Dent Res* 85:966, 2006.

required to restore the structure and function (protection, barrier) of the tissue after damage.

Damage to the oral mucosa may result from direct physical insult, radiation, chemical irritation, or colonization by microorganisms. Afterward, a rapid, well-coordinated response involving the epithelium and the underlying connective tissue occurs. This response involves the complex interaction of extracellular matrix molecules, various resident cells, and infiltrating leukocytes and involves the following four overlapping phases.

INITIAL RESPONSE TO WOUNDING: HEMOSTASIS

Damage to the mucosal surface usually causes vascular damage and hemorrhaging into the tissue defect, which results in the deposition of fibrin, aggregation of platelets, and coagulation to form a clot within minutes of wounding. This clot forms a hemostatic barrier that unites the wound margins and protects the exposed tissues. The clot also provides a provisional scaffold for the subsequent migration of reparative cells. However, because of the moist environment of the oral cavity and salivary flow, the clot does not resemble the hard, dry clots in skin tissue; rather it is a soft coagulum that is easily lost. After several minutes, vasodilation and increased vascular permeability allow plasma proteins to leak into the wound site and stimulate leukocyte migration. At this time, the integrity of the protective barrier has been compromised, and microorganisms, toxins, and antigens likely have entered into the mucosal tissues, stimulating an inflammatory response.

INFLAMMATORY CELL ACTIVATION, MIGRATION, AND FUNCTION

Tissue injury causes an immediate acute inflammatory reaction. Polymorphonuclear leukocytes, mononuclear leukocytes (phagocytic cell macrophages and lymphocytes), and mast cells are the major cells involved in inflammation and wound healing. Inflammatory cells in a wound derive from three sources: cells normally present in tissues, cells extravasated when blood vessels are damaged, and cells carried in intact blood vessels adjacent to the wound that exit by means of a process called *diapedesis*. Platelet-derived cytokines recruit leukocytes to the site of tissue damage by a process known as *chemotaxis*.

Polymorphonuclear leukocytes, mainly neutrophils, are the first inflammatory cells to invade the wound. They appear within a few hours of injury and become activated in response to phagocytic stimuli or by binding of chemotactic mediators, antigen-antibody complexes to specific receptors on the cell membrane, and components of the complement system. These cells reach a maximum concentration at about 24 hours and have a short life span at the wound site before they die. Neutrophils contain various enzymes and reactive oxygen metabolites (oxygen-derived free radicals) that kill engulfed bacteria but that also can destroy damaged and normal tissue when the cells die. Neutrophils function primarily to manage bacterial invasion and hence infection, thus their absence in noninfected wounds does not hinder the repair process.

Macrophages and other mononuclear leukocytes enter the wound after 24 hours and are the predominant cell type in damaged tissue at 5 days (Figure 14-1). Macrophage infiltration into the wound site is mediated by various chemotactic factors that are released by platelets in the fibrin clot, keratinocytes at the wound margins, fibroblasts, and leukocytes. These cells also are activated through receptor-mediated processes that result in cellular and humoral responses and in phagocytosis of damaged tissue components and foreign material. They also release many potent growth factors (transforming growth factor β [TGF-β], platelet-derived growth factor, interleukin-1, and others), cytokines, and chemokines. These soluble mediators are critical for the next phase of wound repair involving cell recruitment and differentiation and the commencement of rebuilding damaged tissues. Macrophages are a major source of cytokines involved in lymphocyte chemotaxis and later constitute the most prominent leukocyte subset in wounds. TGF-β in particular stimulates fibroblasts to proliferate and synthesize extracellular matrix proteins.

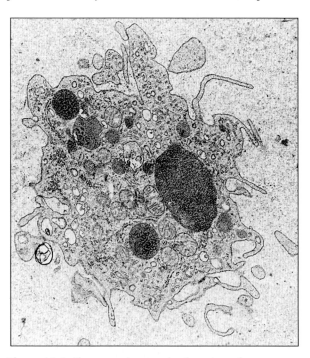

Figure 14-1 Electron micrograph of portion of a macrophage in a defect 24 hours after wounding.

In the absence of macrophages, fewer fibroblasts are stimulated during healing, so that healing is slowed and less repair tissue is produced.

Mast cells represent are an important source of proinflammatory mediators and cytokines that promote inflammation and vascular changes.

Another interesting cytokine is osteopontin, which accumulates in calcified tissues. Osteopontin is expressed widely by a variety of inflammatory cells, including T lymphocytes and macrophages. Osteopontin also is known as *early T lymphocyte activation-1* and is implicated in macrophage recruitment and activation. Locally produced osteopontin and some found in serum and tissue fluids may act as an *opsonin* that facilitates uptake of material, possibly including bacteria, by macrophages. Mutant mice lacking a functional osteopontin gene show an aberrant skin healing response and are more susceptible to infection. Thus by direct action and ability to stimulate fibroblasts, macrophages have a direct effect on the repair process.

REPARATIVE PHASE

Successful repair of the injured tissues requires resolution of the inflammatory reaction. As the acute inflammatory phase subsides, regeneration of the tissue begins, occurring first in the epithelium and then in the connective tissue.

Damage to the epithelium results in mobilization and migration of epithelial cells at the wound margin. The cells lose their close attachment to each other and to the underlying connective tissue within 24 hours of wounding; this is apparent histologically as a widening of the intercellular spaces (Figure 14-2). Twenty-four to 48 hours after wounding, cell division in the basal epithelium increases a short distance behind the wound margin, and those cells immediately adjacent to the margin begin to migrate laterally beneath the clot or coagulum (Figure 14-3). As they migrate, the epithelial cells deposit basal lamina constituents that facilitate movement through the subepithelial connective tissue. Migration and subsequent adhesion of epithelial cells to the basal lamina implicates remodeling of the cytoskeleton and redistribution of integrin membrane receptors, interaction with laminin-5, and ultimately the formation of hemidesmosomes.

Initially, basal cells move, but suprabasal cells slide or *roll* over the basal cells subsequently. Epithelial cells continue to migrate until they reach the cells from the opposing wound margin, when contact inhibition restricts further movement. At this time an increase in cell division leads to stratification and differentiation, reestablishing a normal epithelial tissue.

Initially, the wounded connective tissue consists of fibrin, necrotic tissue, and an acute inflammatory cell infiltrate. Fibroblasts migrate into and proliferate within the healing connective tissue within 24 hours. The fibroblasts involved in wound repair derive from two sources: division of undamaged fibroblasts at the wound periphery (Figure 14-4, A) and undifferentiated connective tissue (mesenchymal) cells (Figure 14-4, B). The resulting daughter cells from both sources migrate into

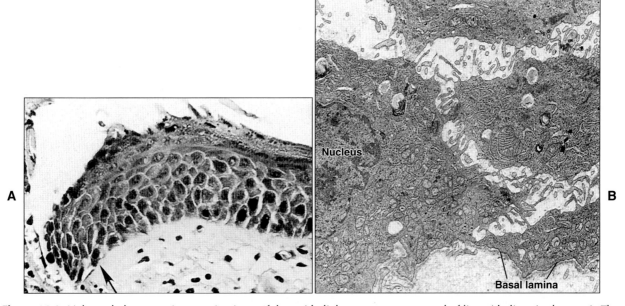

Figure 14-2 Light and electron microscopic views of the epithelial response to a wound of lip epithelium in the rat. **A,** The epithelial cells bordering the wound margin *(arrow)* are beginning to separate from each other before migrating across the defect. **B,** The migrating cells show widened intercellular spaces.

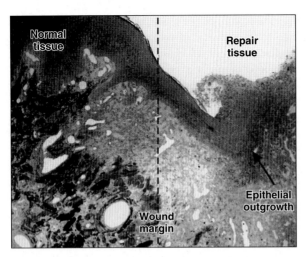

Figure 14-3 Healing of an excisional wound of the palatal epithelium at 3 days after wounding. The epithelium already has migrated almost 1 mm from the original wound margin *(dotted line)*. The tip of the epithelial outgrowth *(arrow)* is migrating under a slough of inflammatory cells and necrotic tissue debris. The underlying connective tissue is highly cellular and contains fibroblasts, endothelial cells, and inflammatory cells.

the wound defect to form the collagen of scar tissue (Figure 14-5). Moreover, endothelial cells proliferate and capillaries develop from preexisting vessels at the wound margin. New blood vessels play an essential role in tissue healing by participating in connective tissue formation, providing nutrients and oxygen, secreting

bioactive substances (endothelial cells), and allowing for inflammatory cell migration to the site of injury. Angiogenesis is a complex event regulated by growth factors acting in synergy. Vascular endothelial growth factor, fibroblast growth factor, and TGF-β are major components in wound angiogenesis. Extracellular matrix molecules, such as fibronectin, laminin, and collagens, are also important in vessel growth by acting as a scaffold for cell migration and reservoir for growth factors.

At 3 days the healing lamina propria is predominantly cellular, consisting of inflammatory cells, developing capillaries, and abundant fibroblasts among fibrin remnants and new collagen fibrils (see Figure 14-3). Between days 5 and 20 after wounding, collagen is deposited rapidly in the wound, with a corresponding increase in tissue tensile strength, although up to 150 days may be required to regain normal tissue strength (Figure 14-6). The relative proportion of cells and fibers approaches that of unwounded tissue by 20 days.

Persistence of the inflammatory response delays wound healing by generating unbalanced proteolytic activity and tissue destruction at the repair site. Infiltrating macrophages and neutrophils produce numerous proteinases, including various matrix metalloproteinases. Resident cells at the wound site, such as keratinocytes, fibroblasts, and endothelial cells, also up-regulate production of proteinases. Bacterial components and degraded tissue perpetuate the problem by sustaining continued influx of inflammatory cells.

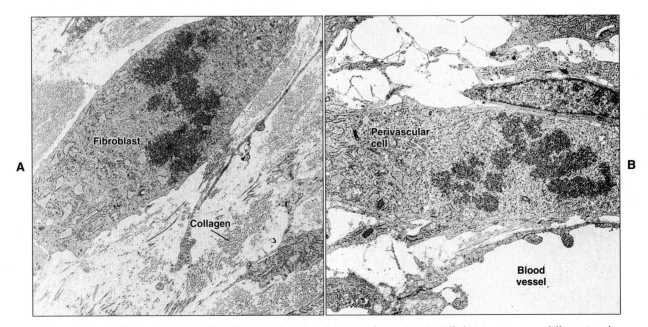

Figure 14-4 **A,** Cell division within a fibroblast peripheral to the wound margin. **B,** Cell division in an undifferentiated perivascular cell.

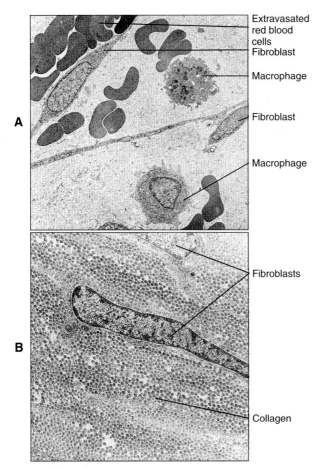

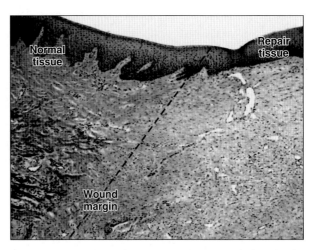

Figure 14-6 Healing of an excisional wound of the palatal epithelium at 20 days after wounding. The epithelium forms a continuous covering over the wound, but the differences between the normal fibrous connective tissue at the wound margin and the healing connective tissue in the wound are obvious *(dotted line)*. The wound connective tissue contains numerous fibroblasts, capillaries, and immature collagen fibers.

Figure 14-5 A, Migration of pioneer fibroblasts into the wound defect. **B,** Electron micrograph of scar tissue showing a dense mass of collagen fibrils (cut in cross section) and two quiescent fibroblasts.

WOUND CONTRACTION AND SCARRING

Scar formation is a physiologic and inevitable outcome of wound repair in mammals, the function of which is to restore tissue integrity quickly. Evidence indicates that scar formation is linked intimately to the inflammatory phase of repair. By controlling infection, the rapid initial inflammatory response allows the wound to heal quickly but ultimately results in the production of a tissue of lesser quality. Interestingly, repair in early fetal life shows no typical inflammatory phase, and healing of the skin, for instance, is scarless.

In skin the first fibroblasts that enter the wound contain abundant actin and myosin and have contractile properties, so that they often are called *contractile fibroblasts* or *myofibroblasts*. These cells have junctions with one another and with connective tissue fibrils. By contracting, myofibroblasts are able to draw the edges of the wound together, thereby reducing the surface area and facilitating healing. Myofibroblasts are

believed to derive from a clonal population within the connective tissue.

Collagen that is laid down may form scar tissue and lead to rigidity and immobilization of the area, with impairment of function. Myofibroblasts and wound contraction have been described in oral mucosa, but scar tissue that is formed usually is remodeled so that most surgery within the mouth can be undertaken without fear of producing disabling scar tissue. The reason for the differences in wound healing between skin and oral mucosa is not understood, but increasing evidence indicates that fibroblasts in oral mucosa are phenotypically different from those of skin and more closely resemble fetal fibroblasts. Such differences can be seen in the synthesis of glycosaminoglycans and in the response to the cytokine TGF-β. Figure 14-7 provides a summary of this simple account of repair.

WOUND HEALING AT THE DENTOGINGIVAL JUNCTION

If *gingivitis* progresses to *periodontitis*, the junctional epithelium migrates apically and is responsible for the formation of the pocket epithelium. This process requires not only cell proliferation but also migration of the cells over the connective tissue substratum that has been modified by the inflammatory process. Recent studies have identified variable expression of *integrins* and other adhesion molecules at the epithelial-connective tissue interface during the inflammatory process and

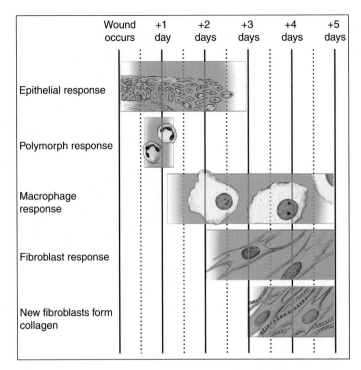

Figure 14-7 Schematic summary of tissue repair. The epithelial response is achieved by proliferation and migration of cells to cover the defect. The connective tissue response involves successively a polymorph response (12 to 24 hours), a macrophage response (2 to 5 days), and a fibroblast response (2 days and on) from undifferentiated perivascular cells and undamaged fibroblasts. The new fibroblasts form collagen that may result in scar tissue in skin but not in oral mucosa.

subsequent migration of the junctional epithelium. When healing occurs, a new structure with the same histologic characteristics as the original junctional epithelium develops from the phenotypically different oral (or gingival) epithelium.

The underlying connective tissue is believed to play a significant role in determining the formation of the junctional epithelium. Connective tissue is destroyed during periodontal disease, and the junctional epithelium therefore extends until it reaches intact connective tissue that provides the signal to stop its migration, forming a long junctional epithelium. Some believe that lack of mechanical stability at the wound site favors formation of a long junctional epithelium and that following periodontal surgery, formation of a fibrin clot against the denuded root surface favors formation of a connective tissue attachment that prevents apical migration of the gingival epithelium.

REPAIR OF ENAMEL

Enamel cannot reform after it is destroyed because the cells that formed it no longer exist, but enamel is capable of some limited repair by physicochemical means. If the carious process is arrested and the enamel surface layer has not broken down, remineralization can occur in the subsurface enamel. This result depends on an added supply of calcium and phosphate ions from the saliva, and if fluoride is present, the remineralized enamel becomes more resistant than normal enamel to further demineralization. One interesting prospect over the next few years is the potential use of matrix proteins that regulate mineralization, or knowledge derived from studying their function, to restore lost enamel naturally.

REPAIR OF THE DENTIN-PULP COMPLEX

Dentin is a vital tissue, and its repair is complex and varied because of several factors that affect the basic reparative process described for the oral mucosa. These factors include the extent and duration of the stimulus, the variability of dentin structure, and the age of the tooth. For example, slowly progressing attrition and cavity preparation invoke differing degrees of response. The former represents a gentle and protracted insult that provides time for a measured response, whereas cavity preparation represents an immediate crisis to the cellular elements of the complex. Considerable variation exists within the tubular compartment of dentin, which may contain a process, may be sclerosed, or may be plugged with collagen, and these variations influence the

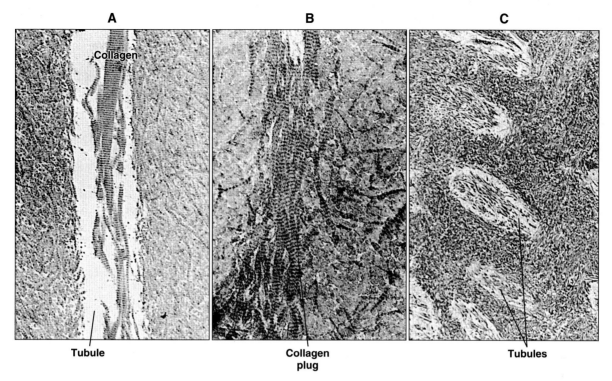

A   **B**   **C**

Collagen

Tubule

Collagen plug

Tubules

Figure 14-8 Occlusion of dentinal tubules with collagen (all sections demineralized). In **A,** collagen fibrils occupy the patent tubule. In **B,** they have occluded the tubule. **C** shows a number of collagen-containing tubules in cross section.

response of dentin. The age of the tooth also must be considered. Formation of dentin continues throughout life, so that the pulp chamber becomes increasingly smaller. At the same time, the cellularity of dentin decreases, its collagen content increases, and the ground substance loses water. The blood supply is diminished, as is the nerve supply, and these events influence the reparative response of the dentin-pulp complex.

Because of this variability, the responses of the complex can be described best in two ways. First, in response to prolonged insult of slow onset, such as attrition or dental caries, a number of different events may cause occlusion of the tubule within the tubular compartment. Increased collagen deposition by the odontoblast process may plug the tubule (Figure 14-8), or mineral may be deposited in the tubule by extension of the peritubular dentin or reprecipitation of mineral salts released by the carious process (Figure 14-9). At the same time, the odontoblast responds by laying down regular tubular reparative or reactionary dentin. All these reactions are aimed at depositing a calcified barrier to protect the dental pulp.

Second, if the insult is severe and rapid in onset (fracture of the tooth or cavity preparation), the issue is whether the odontoblast survives this degree of trauma. If the odontoblast survives, it is capable of depositing further reactionary dentin. If the odontoblast does not survive, the wounded pulp reacts by the classic repair

mechanism involving cellular proliferation and scar tissue formation to form a *bridge* of reparative dentin that seals off the site of exposure. Which population of cells proliferates has not been established with certainty, and two possibilities exist. The cells may come from undifferentiated mesenchymal cells situated perivascularly or from mesenchymal cells forming the subodontoblast layer and that were exposed to all the influences required

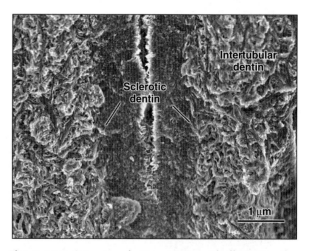

Intertubular dentin

Sclerotic dentin

1 μm

Figure 14-9 Scanning electron micrograph illustrating the almost complete occlusion of a dentinal tubule by peritubular (sclerotic) dentin. A difference in texture is apparent between the sclerotic and intertubular dentin.

for odontoblast differentiation except the final epithelial influence, as described in Chapter 8. A long-standing puzzle has been how these newly differentiated cells, from whatever source, assume odontoblastic characteristics in the absence of epithelially produced mediators required for normal development. Apparently, epithelial peptides necessary for odontoblast differentiation may be trapped in dentin as it forms and are released when dentin is damaged. These newly differentiated cells migrate toward the wounded surface and deposit *scar tissue* in the form of reparative dentin. Importantly, reparative dentin differs from primary and secondary dentin in that it contains less collagen and is enriched in noncollagenous matrix proteins normally found in small amounts. Understanding what triggers this change and the eventual transformation of such matrix into true tubular dentin is essential for predictable approaches for dentin-pulp repair.

Dental pulp is essentially a connective tissue. Whenever dental pulp is injured, the immune system triggers an inflammatory response similar to that which would take place in any other connective tissues in the body. What distinguishes dental pulp is its anatomic location within a calcified chamber formed by circumpulpal and radicular dentin. This position within a rigid, enclosed space has led to the widespread notion that, unlike for other connective tissues, the exudate associated with inflammation could lead to its *self-strangulation* and eventually pulp necrosis. Indeed, this occurs in some circumstances, but clinical experience indicates that pulp inflammation usually resolves without necrosis.

Even in advanced cases of pulp damage, residual vital tissue can be found in root canals.

Next, the responses of enamel and dentin are analyzed in terms of the carious process and the clinical procedures undertaken to restore the structural damage from that process, namely, cavity preparation.

DENTAL CARIES

Under the light microscope one can distinguish three zones in the early carious lesion. At the inner advancing edge is a translucent zone, which is followed by a dark zone. The third zone is the body of the lesion, which occupies the space between the dark zone and the intact enamel surface (Figure 14-10). The inner translucent zone represents the first area of change in enamel observable by light microscopy, and research has well established that removal of mineral occurs in this region. The dark zone represents an area that previously was demineralized but now is undergoing remineralization. Thus the carious process is dynamic, with alternating phases of demineralization and remineralization, rather than a static simple continuing dissolution of material. The body of a lesion is where the bulk of mineral is lost and where over time the most destructive morphologic changes occur.

An important characteristic of the early carious lesion is that demineralization occurs below the surface, so that a mineralized surface layer remains in place for some time. This surface zone remains intact because calcium and phosphate ions reprecipitate in it from

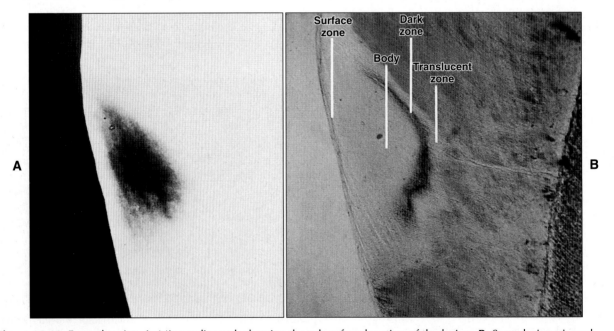

Figure 14-10 Enamel caries. **A,** Microradiograph showing the subsurface location of the lesion. **B,** Same lesion viewed with polarized light. The translucent zone, dark zone, body of the lesion, and surface zone are visible. *(From Silverstone L. In Cohen B, Kramer RH, editors:* The scientific foundation of dentistry, *London, 1976, William Heinemann Medical Books.)*

subsurface dissolution or the saliva. Little ultrastructural change can be identified in the translucent and dark zones: damage to the crystals is observed primarily in the body of the lesion.

In summary, the carious process within enamel consists of a cyclic demineralization of enamel crystals by bacterial acids with periods of remineralization, with demineralization ultimately dominating the process. If the surface of the enamel remains intact and the bacterial infection is removed, remineralization predominates with restoration of enamel integrity.

When the carious process reaches dentin, the response is sequential. Frequently at this stage the surface enamel is still intact and bacterial invasion has not occurred. The lesion, however, has increased the permeability of enamel to acid and various other chemical stimuli, which stimulates a response from the dentin-pulp complex. The nature of the initial response reflects an increased activity of odontoblasts, with a possible retraction of processes and an increase in collagen deposition in the periodontoblastic process space, plus the formation of sclerotic dentin by the mechanisms described in Chapter 8 (Figure 14-11; see also Figure 14-9). This response then can lead to the deposition of reactionary dentin by the vital odontoblasts. Once the enamel cavitates, bacteria eventually reach the dentin surface, and destruction of dentin begins. Superimposed on this process are the death of odontoblasts, a mild inflammatory reaction in the pulp, and the bacterial invasion of dentin. Because bacteria that infect dentin are acidogenic, acid diffuses ahead of them and demineralizes the dentin; consequently, an additional mechanism comes into play,

involving reprecipitation to enhance the zone of sclerotic dentin within dentinal tubules (Figure 14-12). Bacteria are at first confined to the tubules (Figure 14-13, A) but later escape this confinement and destroy the dentin matrix (Figure 14-13, B). At this stage, pulp cells have been recruited and lay down reparative dentin as previously described.

If the carious process within dentin is to be arrested (naturally or by surgical intervention to remove infected dentin), the reparative dentin must provide an effective mineralized barrier. Surgical intervention is achieved, of course, by cavity preparation and the restoration of lost tooth tissue by substitute materials.

CAVITY PREPARATION

Cavity preparation in a tooth involves the removal of enamel and dentin. Enamel covers the dentin-pulp complex, which is a connective tissue with a repair response similar in many ways to that described for skin and oral mucosa (Table 14-1).

The major difference between teeth and mucosa is the absence of any epithelial response because the cells that form enamel (ameloblasts) are lost at the time of tooth eruption. To overcome this deficiency, dentistry has formulated substitute materials that not only must mimic the hardness of enamel but also must serve as effective sealants

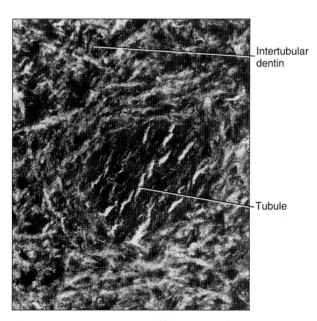

Figure 14-11 Translucent zone in dentinal caries (undemineralized section). The tubule is filled with mineral. *(Courtesy N.W. Johnson.)*

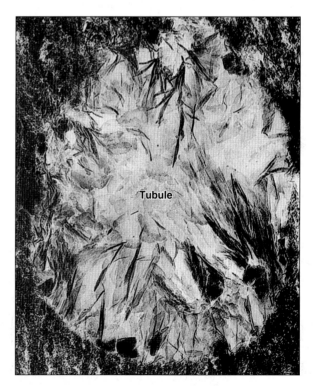

Figure 14-12 Remineralization in dentinal tubule. Crystals are present within the lumen of the tubule. *(Courtesy N.W. Johnson.)*

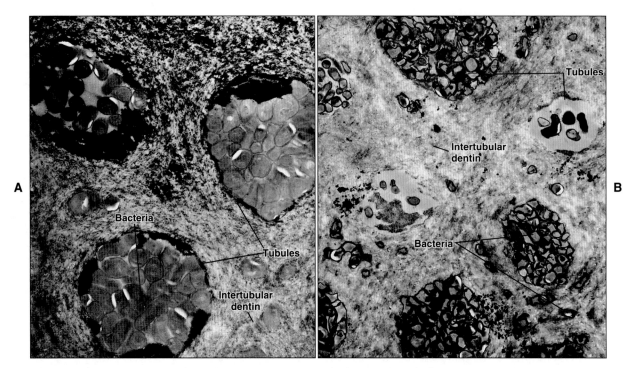

Figure 14-13 Dentinal caries. **A,** Although microorganisms are confined to the tubules, demineralization of the dentin has occurred. **B,** Microorganisms have escaped the boundaries of the dentinal tubules. *(Courtesy N.W. Johnson.)*

against the external environment to protect the underlying dentin-pulp complex. The latter property has been particularly difficult to replicate, and microleakage around restorative materials is a problem that can lead to a continuing low-grade inflammation within the dental pulp that hinders its reparative potential. Although improvement in the properties of restorative materials (e.g., materials that

would expand on polymerization or hardening) one day may resolve the problem of microleakage, controlled bioengineering of mineral from exposed surfaces during cavity preparation remains the goal.

The basic nature of the dentin-pulp response is harnessed and involves occlusion of the dentinal tubules and, if odontoblasts are undamaged, the further deposition of dentin. At this point the extent of the odontoblast processes and their response to severance become an issue. If cavity preparation involves odontoblast death or pulp exposure, recruitment of pulp cells ensues to form a dentinlike layer as already described.

REPAIR FOLLOWING TOOTH EXTRACTION

The wound created by extracting a tooth differs from an incisional skin or mucosal wound in that substantially greater soft tissue loss occurs. Even so, the repair process uses the same basic mechanisms already described. After the tooth has been extracted, the defect is filled immediately by a blood clot (the hemostatic response). Sometimes the clot can be dislodged; when this happens, infection may intervene and lead to what is known as dry socket, a painful infection of the bone lining the socket. The epithelial cells bordering the socket rim begin to proliferate and migrate across the clot so that after about

TABLE 14-1 Comparison of Repair Responses in Skin and Teeth

REPAIR RESPONSE	IN SKIN	IN TEETH
Epithelial response	Proliferation and migration of cells to cover the defect	No epithelial response because ameloblasts are lost at time of tooth eruption
Connective tissue response	Polymorph response Macrophage response Fibroblast response from undifferentiated perivascular cells and undamaged fibroblasts New fibroblasts form collagen	Polymorph response Macrophage response Fibroblast response by division of undamaged pulpal and perivascular cells New fibroblasts form collagen, which mineralizes to form dentin

10 days the socket is epithelialized. Within the clot the inflammatory response takes place, involving first neutrophils and then macrophages. The proliferative and synthesizing phase differs from that in skin because the cells invading the clot are not fibroblasts but cells from the adjacent bone marrow that have osteogenic potential. Once in the clot, these cells begin to form bone. Bone formation begins about 10 days after tooth extraction; by 10 to 12 weeks the extraction site can no longer be distinguished (Figure 14-14).

REPAIR OF THE PERIODONTIUM

Healthy periodontal tissues are required to provide the necessary support to maintain teeth in adequate function. The tissues that compose the periodontium are divided into four principal components; namely, the gingiva, periodontal ligament, alveolar bone, and cementum. Each of these tissues has a distinct anatomic location, biochemical composition, and tissue architecture. These four tissues, however, function as a single unit, with the various extracellular matrix components within each compartment being capable of influencing the cellular and structural functions of adjacent structures. With recent advances in the understanding of the cell and molecular biology of the periodontal connective tissues, new concepts are evolving regarding the likely biologic processes involved in the repair and regeneration of the tissues destroyed by periodontitis.

ALTERATIONS TO THE PERIODONTAL CONNECTIVE TISSUES WITH THE DEVELOPMENT OF PERIODONTAL INFLAMMATION

With the development of inflammatory periodontal diseases, significant qualitative and quantitative changes occur in the molecular composition of the periodontal connective tissues. As dental plaque accumulates adjacent to the gingival margins, an inflammatory response is induced within the gingival connective tissues (Figure 14-15). Within 3 to 4 days, histologic evidence clearly indicates connective issue destruction resulting in up to 70% of the collagen being lost within the foci of inflammation. If left untreated, the inflammatory response continues, and the amount of tissue destruction extends deeper toward the periodontal ligament and alveolar bone. At the same time the inflammatory response is causing tissue destruction, a form of frustrated repair also is initiated, resulting in fibrosis and scarring coexisting at foci of inflammation. In this case,

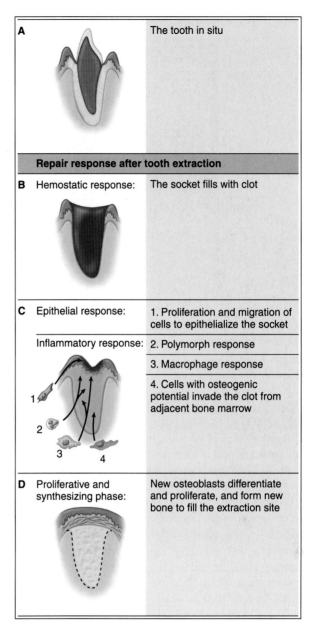

Figure 14-14 Repair response after tooth extraction. **A,** The tooth in situ. **B,** After extraction the socket is filled with clot. **C,** The clot resolves by (*1*) the polymorph response, (*2*) the macrophage response, and (*3*) the fibroblast response. In addition, the bony defect becomes colonized by new osteoblasts (*4*) that form new bone as the collagen scar is remodeled **(D).**

gingivitis may be contained and periodontitis does not follow; the latter occurs only if the host response is unable to contain the gingival inflammation. As the lesion of periodontitis develops, numerous quantitative and qualitative biochemical changes occur to the extracellular matrix components of the gingival, alveolar bone, and periodontal ligament collagen, resulting in further tissue destruction.

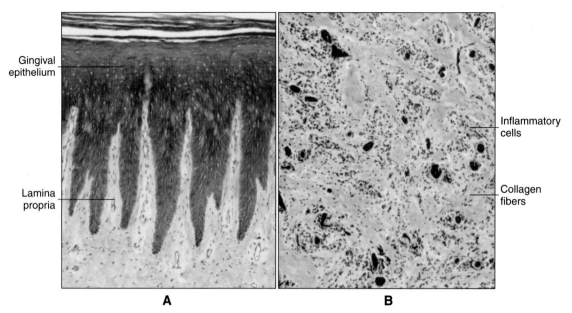

Gingival epithelium

Lamina propria

Inflammatory cells

Collagen fibers

A　　　　　　　　　　　**B**

Figure 14-15 Histologic appearance of normal **(A)** and inflamed **(B)** human gingival tissues following plaque accumulation. **B,** Dense inflammatory cell infiltration occurs together with loss of collagen fibers at these sites. *(Courtesy P.M. Bartold.)*

REPAIR POTENTIAL OF THE PERIODONTIUM

A significant goal of clinical periodontics in recent years has been the regeneration of periodontal tissues to their original form, architecture, and function after they have been affected by periodontitis; however, as noted previously, *perfect* repair actually may not take place. The process of periodontal regeneration is extraordinarily complex and involves significant communication between all of the cellular and matrix components of the periodontium to induce the inherent regenerative or repair capacity of this tissue.

A well-accepted principle is that the effects of gingival inflammation encountered during the development of gingivitis are reversible provided the causative agent(s) can be removed. However, once the destructive phase reaches the alveolar bone and periodontitis ensues, periodontal regeneration no longer becomes a clinically predictable event. A major reason why periodontal regeneration is such a challenge is the need for restoration of not one, but four different tissues; namely, gingiva, periodontal ligament, cementum, and bone.

MECHANISMS OF REPAIR AND REGENERATION OF PERIODONTAL CONNECTIVE TISSUES

Regeneration of the periodontium is unique because of the need for new connective tissue fibers to insert into cementum and bone. Fiber insertion requires the healing components of all the soft and hard connective tissues of the periodontium to be integrated fully. Consequently, the molecular and cellular events associated with periodontal regeneration are extraordinarily complex. For full integration to occur, a coordinated sequence of events must be induced. These events include stimulation of an initial inflammatory response, followed by recruitment of specific cell populations, induction of their proliferation, cellular differentiation, and combined efforts of several cell types including fibroblasts for soft connective tissues, cementoblasts for cementogenesis, osteoblasts for bone formation, and endothelial cells for angiogenesis. These events are controlled largely by a number of soluble mediators.

Repair of the periodontal ligament also may use a previously described important biologic phenomenon: the ability of fibroblasts to remodel collagen. Skin repair involves formation of scar tissue. Repair of the periodontal ligament after, for example, tooth movement involves the same mechanism as that found in skin without scar formation. The reason is that although the repair mechanism is identical to that in skin, this scar tissue almost immediately is remodeled by the ligament fibroblasts to restore normal architecture. The adult periodontal connective tissues contain heterogeneous populations of cells with diverse properties, functions, and potential that gives rise to progeny with specific phenotypes. For example, fibroblasts originate from precursors within gingival and periodontal ligament connective tissues, whereas cementoblasts are believed to originate from cells located perivascularly in the ligament and bone and perhaps reactivated epithelial cell rests of Malassez. For regeneration to occur, the cells responsible for each tissue must be able to participate in these processes at the right location and in the correct temporal sequence. In addition, exclusion of unwanted cells (for example, epithelial cells) from the healing site is important.

One of the methods in current clinical practice in periodontology involves raising a flap of tissue away from the tooth, cleaning the root surface by planing it to remove cementum (thought to have accumulated bacterial toxins), and then repositioning the flap with the intention that new attachment will form against the now cleansed root surface. This procedure, however, also removes the surface layer of dentin, which in normal development is implicated in cementum attachment (one may recall the intermingling of collagen fibrils from mantle predentin and cementum before mineralization takes place). Although short dentin collagen fringes may be present, indirect evidence suggests that reparative cementum is apposed or weakly attached to the cleansed root surface. Early efforts to improve periodontal regeneration focused on *root surface conditioning* to try to create conditions conducive for the selective repopulation of root surfaces by cells responsible for regeneration. Demineralization with citric acid to decontaminate the root surface and expose dentin collagen was advocated. Unfortunately, this procedure often resulted in ankylosis and root resorption as side effects instead of regeneration. An alternative approach of coating root surfaces with molecules such as fibronectin also was considered to be advantageous; however, over time the lack of clinical benefit from this procedure became apparent.

With the recognition that the down-growth of junctional epithelium was a significant negative influence on the induction of periodontal regeneration, a procedure was developed in which a physical barrier is introduced at the time of periodontal surgery by placing a membrane between connective tissue of the periodontal flap and the curetted root surface. The biologic basis for this procedure was in the premise that the membrane not only would prevent apical migration of gingival (epithelial) cells onto the root surface but also would exclude unwanted gingival connective tissue from the healing site and facilitate the repopulation of the wound with periodontal ligament cells. This procedure was termed *guided tissue regeneration*, and although the clinical results varied, it demonstrated for the first time that regeneration/repair of root cementum, alveolar bone, and periodontal ligament and new attachment formation was possible (Figure 14-16).

More recently and in line with improving understanding of the molecular processes associated with tissue repair and regeneration, polypeptide growth factors applied to root surfaces have been used to facilitate new cementum and connective tissue formation. Examples of growth factors studied to date include epidermal growth factor, fibroblast growth factor, insulin-like growth factor, platelet-derived growth factor, and TGF-β. Another promising group of polypeptide growth factors is the bone morphogenetic proteins, which offer good potential for stimulating bone and cementum regeneration. In addition to single growth factor preparations, *mixtures* of growth factors such as those present in platelet-rich plasma preparations also have been advocated as useful aids in promoting periodontal regeneration (Figure 14-17).

At the same time that polypeptide growth factors were being considered for use in periodontal regeneration, another approach was being developed. Through the application of knowledge concerning the embryologic processes involved in root formation, attempts were made to *recreate* these processes in adults. On the premise that enamel-like proteins participate in root formation (discussed in Chapter 9, this still remains to be confirmed), extracts of enamel matrix have been applied to root surfaces at the time of periodontal surgery with the aim of inducing periodontal regeneration through the recreation of the molecular events of cementogenesis. Whether these proteins act as instructional messengers, similar to growth factors, for cells to undergo the processes of regeneration or merely alter the periodontal environment, permitting regeneration to proceed more efficiently, is unclear. Nonetheless, clinical results have been encouraging (Figure 14-18), and these proteins appear capable of helping regeneration of periodontal tissues, albeit not in a completely predictable or consistent manner.

Some evidence suggests that new cementum formation must occur for periodontal repair to take place. Because the connective tissue matrix of cementum sequesters a battery of polypeptides, which mediate cell adhesion and spreading, the extracellular matrix of cementum itself has been proposed to have the potential to regulate the differentiation of precursor cells into cementoblasts and the subsequent formation of cementum matrix and fiber insertion. Thus cementum components may be capable of providing informational signals for the recruitment, proliferation, and differentiation of periodontal cells and may regulate the regeneration of cementum and adjacent periodontal components.

NEW PERSPECTIVES

Although significant advances have been made regarding the understanding of periodontal regeneration, the desired clinical end point of a procedure that results in predictable regeneration of the periodontal tissues damaged by inflammation to their original form and function remains elusive. Future developments in

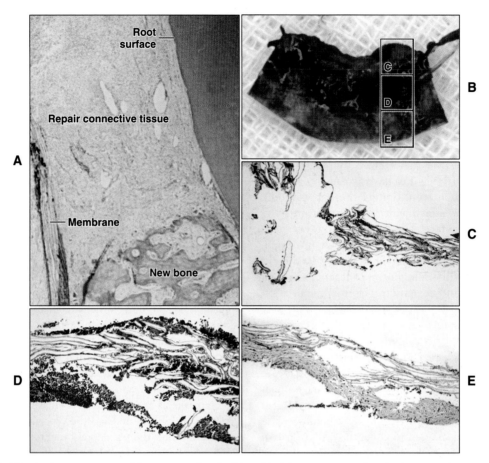

Figure 14-16 Histologic appearance of tissues associated with guided tissue regeneration. In **A,** a membrane can be seen draped over the bone and forming a space underneath to allow new connective tissue formation to occur between the membrane and the débrided root surface. New bone formation is evident. **B** shows the appearance of the membrane at time of removal. **C** to **E** show stained sections of this membrane in the coronal, middle, and apical one third of the membrane, respectively. Excluded epithelial cells in the coronal portion of the membrane are evident. In the middle third a mild inflammatory reaction has occurred, and the apical third shows evidence of healthy new fibrous tissue. *(Courtesy P.M. Bartold.)*

connective tissue biochemistry, cell biology, and molecular biology will continue to have a significant effect on managing the anatomic changes resulting from periodontitis. Tissue engineering, which is the science of developing techniques for the fabrication of new tissues to replace damaged tissues, is an emerging discipline and provides new horizons in the field of periodontal regeneration. The principles of tissue engineering take into account the notion that treatment of periodontal defects with an agent or procedure requires that each functional stage of reconstruction be grounded in a biologically directed process. Tissue engineering for periodontal regeneration undoubtedly will embrace further emerging fields within bioengineering and nanotechnology (the science of bioengineering at the molecular level to produce materials of hitherto unknown, and unthought-of, properties). As a result, biodegradable scaffolds will be developed that incorporate the necessary instructional molecular messengers for the selection of adult stem cells as the basis of periodontal regeneration in the new millennium.

Another promising development is *gene transfer*, which consists of the insertion of a transgene into a host cell to achieve overextended periods of expression of a therapeutic protein to modulate periodontal cell activity and regenerative capacity. Such *gene therapy* overcomes problems associated with delivery of the protein itself. Most gene transfer studies have been conducted using viral vectors such as adenoviruses and adeno-associated viruses. Viral vectors derived from the human immunodeficiency virus (HIV) (Figure 14-19) and nonviral vectors also are being explored for introducing genetic

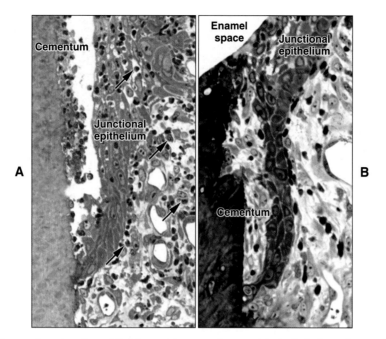

Figure 14-17 Gingival flap and root surface débridement in a porcine model. **A,** At 5 days after surgical treatment the reforming junctional epithelium and underlying connective tissue are heavily infiltrated by numerous inflammatory cells *(arrows);* the epithelium descends along the root and fails to attach to its surface. **B,** When the wound site is treated at the time of surgery with a growth factor cocktail extracted from platelets, the inflammatory infiltrate is much less important, and downgrowth of epithelial cells is limited.

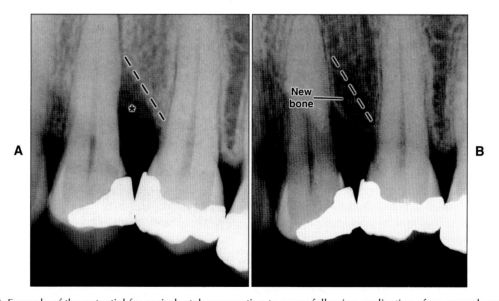

Figure 14-18 Example of the potential for periodontal regeneration to occur following application of an enamel matrix derivative. **A,** Before application, localized bone loss (*) occurs adjacent to the distal surface of the upper left first premolar. **B,** Six months after application of enamel matrix proteins, radiographic evidence shows bone fill on the distal surface of the upper left first premolar. *(Courtesy P.M. Bartold.)*

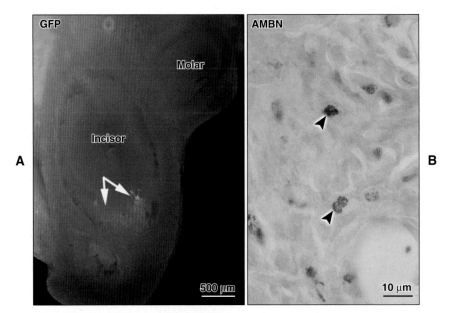

Figure 14-19 Local gene transfer in the rat hemimandible using a lentiviral vector derived from the human immunodeficiency virus (HIV). **A,** Whole-mount preparation showing the localized expression in dental and periodontal tissues of the green fluorescent protein (GFP), a cytoplasmic marker used to monitor gene transfer by the vector. **B,** The gene for ameloblastin (AMBN), a protein produced by ameloblasts during enamel formation, was introduced in osteoblasts. Immunolabeling reveals the presence of this ectopic protein in the Golgi apparatus *(arrowheads)* of these cells.

material into cells. Viral vectors can be delivered at target sites by injection or slow infusion or by being implanted with a scaffold. An alternative approach is to transduce cells in vitro, and expand and implant them at the desired site (ex vivo technique). Virus-mediated gene transfer has been used to study periodontal tissue formation, repair, and pathologic loss. For example, treatment of periodontal defects with an adenovirus encoding for platelet-derived growth factor (PDGF) and bone morphogenic proteins (BMPs) has produced promising results.

Although significant progress has been made in recent years to warrant optimism for the development and clinical application of gene therapy, this approach remains problematic for calcified tissues. So far, vector delivery has been limited to readily accessible anatomic sites (joints and synovial spaces) and in postsurgical, traumatized, or congenital bone defects. Another challenge is the relatively large amounts of vector and its persistence at the site of administration required to infect a sufficient number of cells. Periodontal tissue formation is a complex process in which several factors and molecules interact over time. Therefore, much emphasis is now placed on developing vectors encoding for multiple genes and on generating systems for regulated viral expression to control the inflammatory response or promote tissue formation. Gene therapy also can be coupled with the concepts of tissue engineering described previously and the seeding of cells containing

transgenes coding for specific regenerative instructional messages.

In summary, the oral tissues use a basic mechanism for repair, but local factors benefit and hinder this process. The absence of ameloblasts prevents the repair of enamel (although physicochemical mechanisms permit a limited form of repair). Thus substitutes for an epithelial response, in the form of dental restorative materials, are used in restorative dentistry. Dentin is capable of repair with basic mechanisms, but the scar tissue that forms becomes mineralized. This basic response has been obscured in the past by the occurrence of microleakage and by age changes (which are particularly evident in the pulp). The repair of dental supportive tissues depends on the degree of damage. If the damage is minimal and programmed follicular cells are available, repair involving scar tissue formation occurs, but this scar is rapidly remodeled to restore normal architecture. If damage is more extensive, the outcome depends on the repopulation of the cells in the defect. Finally, although the oral mucosa has many similarities to skin and uses the same principle of repair, wounds of the oral mucosa, especially the gingiva, often heal without the formation of scar tissue. Scar tissue does form but is remodeled quickly to restore normal architecture, just as in the periodontal ligament and using the same mechanism. Therefore, surgery within the mouth can be undertaken without fear of producing disabling scar tissue.

TOPICS FOR CONSIDERATION   Future Prospects for Gene Therapy in Periodontology

The promise of being able to modify genetic material to treat injury or disease has long been a hope for scientists, clinicians, and patients. The possibilities of replacing deficient or missing genes offer much in treating congenital and acquired genetic defects. The use of DNA delivery systems may serve as an alternative method of targeting proteins to tissue defects, including periodontal wounds, to engineer or replace defective tissues. Current approaches for protein administration of tissue healing factors to chronic periodontal lesions are difficult to control. The periodontal wound microenvironment represents a harsh setting loaded with a variety of proteases that rapidly destroy topically applied polypeptides such as growth factors. Furthermore, the bioavailability of proteins may be limited because of the difficulty in targeting proteins to the desired site of action along the tooth root surface and base of the periodontal defect.

Gene therapy has demonstrated significant potential in the treatment of a variety of oral and craniofacial disorders, including the periodontium. Research is active in areas ranging from tooth tissue engineering to gene therapy of periodontia and alveolar bone[1-3] to salivary gland repair.[4] At the basic level, work in stem cell biology as it relates to cell transplantation of genetically modified cells for the repair of oral, craniofacial, and periodontal defects has shown good promise.[5] Materials science and biomedical engineering fields have been critical at the basic developmental level for dental tissue engineering for gene delivery.

A major challenge that has not been emphasized is the modulation of the exuberant host response to microbial contamination that plagues the periodontal wound microenvironment. For improvements in the outcomes in periodontal regenerative medicine using gene delivery strategies, scientists will need to examine dual delivery of host modifiers or antiinfective agents to optimize the results of gene therapy. The future is exciting, and gene therapy represents an important potential tool to treat periodontal diseases.

William V. Giannobile
Michigan Center for Oral Health Research
Department of Periodontics and Oral Medicine
School of Dentistry
University of Michigan
Ann Arbor, Michigan

REFERENCES
1. Dunn CA, Jin Q, Taba M Jr et al: BMP gene delivery for alveolar bone engineering at dental implant defects, *Mol Ther* 11:294-299, 2005.
2. Jin Q, Anusaksathien O, Webb SA et al: Engineering of tooth-supporting structures by delivery of PDGF gene therapy vectors, *Mol Ther* 9:519-526, 2004.
3. Jin QM, Anusaksathien O, Webb SA et al: Gene therapy of bone morphogenetic protein for periodontal tissue engineering, *J Periodontol* 74:202-213, 2003.
4. Voutetakis A, Kok MR, Zheng C et al: Reengineered salivary glands are stable endogenous bioreactors for systemic gene therapeutics, *Proc Natl Acad Sci U S A* 101:3053-3058, 2004.
5. Mao JJ, Giannobile WV, Helms JA et al: Craniofacial tissue engineering by stem cells, *J Dent Res* 85:966-979, 2006.

RECOMMENDED READING

Eming SA, Krieg T, Davidson JM: Inflammation in wound repair: molecular and cellular mechanisms, *J Invest Dermatol* 127:514, 2007.

Kirkwood KL, Cirelli JA, Rogers JE, Giannobile WV: Novel host response therapeutic approaches to treat periodontal diseases, *Periodontol 2000* 43:294-315, 2007.

Mao JJ, Giannobile WV, Helms JA et al: Craniofacial tissue engineering by stem cells, *J Dent Res* 85:966, 2006.

Index

Page numbers followed by f indicate figures; t, tables; b, boxes.

Enhance your understanding and prepare for the National Board Dental Exam!

Expand your knowledge of oral histology and apply what you've learned with fun and engaging exercises on the enclosed companion CD.

■ **A full-color image collection** gives you instant access to high-quality visual references from the text to help you better understand difficult concepts.

■ **Over 400 multiple-choice questions** provide topic-specific self-assessment opportunities that prepare you for Part I of the board exam.

■ **More than 100 labeling exercises** challenge your knowledge and provide valuable exam practice.

COMPANION CD

Ten Cate's
Oral Histology
Development, Structure, and Function
SEVENTH EDITION

MOSBY
ELSEVIER

Antonio Nanci

WIN/MAC

9996025276

Copyright © 2008 by Mosby, Inc.,
an affiliate of Elsevier Inc.
All rights reserved.
Produced in the USA.

Get the most out of your study time!
Start using your CD now!

MOSBY
ELSEVIER